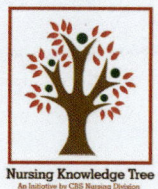
Nursing Knowledge Tree
An Initiative by CBS Nursing Division

Textbook of
NURSING MANAGEMENT
and LEADERSHIP

As per the Revised INC Syllabus (2021-22) for BSc Nursing

Johny Kutty Joseph MSc (N), RN

Assistant Professor
Shri Mata Vaishno Devi College of Nursing
Katra, Jammu and Kashmir

Babitha K Devu MSc (N), RN

Assistant Professor
Shri Mata Vaishno Devi College of Nursing
Katra, Jammu and Kashmir

Foreword

Judie Arulappan

Shailla Cannie
(NFNA - 2020 Awardee)

CBSPD
Dedicated to Education

CBS Publishers & Distributors Pvt Ltd

• New Delhi • Bengaluru • Chennai • Kochi • Kolkata • Lucknow • Mumbai
• Hyderabad • Jharkhand • Nagpur • Patna • Pune • Uttarakhand

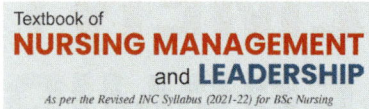

Textbook of
NURSING MANAGEMENT
and **LEADERSHIP**
As per the Revised INC Syllabus (2021-22) for BSc Nursing

ISBN: 978-93-90619-40-5

Reprint: 2025

First Edition: 2022

Published by **Satish Kumar Jain** and produced by **Varun Jain** for

CBS Publishers and Distributors Pvt Ltd

4819/XI Prahlad Street, 24 Ansari Road, Daryaganj, New Delhi 110 002, India.
Ph: +91-11-23289259, 23266861, 23266867   Website: www.cbspd.com
Fax: 011-23243014
e-mail: delhi@cbspd.com; cbspubs@airtelmail.in.

Corporate Office: 204 FIE, Industrial Area, Patparganj, Delhi 110 092
Ph: +91-11-4934 4934   Fax: 4934 4935
e-mail: feedback@cbspd.com; bhupesharora@cbspd.com

Branches

- **Bengaluru:** Seema House 2975, 17th Cross, K.R. Road, Banasankari 2nd Stage, Bengaluru-560 070, Karnataka
  Ph: +91-80-26771678/79   Fax: +91-80-26771680   e-mail: bangalore@cbspd.com

- **Chennai:** 7, Subbaraya Street, Shenoy Nagar, Chennai-600 030, Tamil Nadu
  Ph: +91-44-26680620, 26681266   Fax: +91-44-42032115   e-mail: chennai@cbspd.com

- **Kochi:** 68/1534, 35, 36-Power House Road, Opp. KSEB, Cochin-682018, Kochi, Kerala
  Ph: +91-484-4059061-65   Fax: +91-484-4059065   e-mail: kochi@cbspd.com

- **Kolkata:** Hind Ceramics Compound, 1st Floor, 147, Nilganj Road, Belghoria, Kolkata-700056, West Bengal
  Ph: +91-033-2563-3055/56   e-mail: kolkata@cbspd.com

- **Lucknow:** Basement, Khushnuma Complex, 7-Meerabai Marg (Behind Jawahar Bhawan), Lucknow-226001, Uttar Pradesh
  Ph: +0522-4000032   e-mail: tiwari.lucknow@cbspd.com

- **Mumbai:** PWD Shed, Gala No. 25/26, Ramchandra Bhatt Marg, Next to J.J. Hospital Gate No. 2, Opp. Union Bank of India, Noor Baug, Mumbai-400009, Maharashtra
  Ph: +91-22-66661880/89   Fax: +91-22-24902342   e-mail: mumbai@cbspd.com

Representatives

Hyderabad	+91-9885175004	**Jharkhand**	+91-9811541605	**Nagpur**	+91-9421945513
Patna	+91-9334159340	**Pune**	+91-9623451994	**Uttarakhand**	+91-9716462459

Printed at: SDR Printers Trans Delhi Signature City Ghaziabad (U.P.)

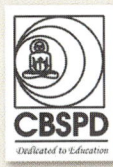

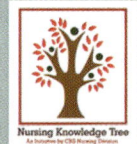

Extends its Tribute to

Florence Nightingale

"

For glorifying the role of women as nurses,
For holding the title of "The Lady with the Lamp,"
For working tirelessly for humanity—
Florence Nightingale will always be
remembered for her
selfless and memorable services to the
human race.

"

Florence Nightingale
(May 1820 – August 1910)

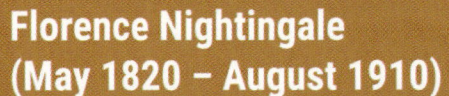

Foreword

This book, written by Johny Kutty Joseph and Babitha K Devu with a fascinating title *Textbook of Nursing Management and Leadership*, is about fundamental management principles for the nursing students. The management principles are made simple and the book is easy to read because it is written in simple English. The Units include Health Care and Development of Nursing Services in India; Management Basics Applied to Nursing and Management Process; Planning Nursing Services; Organizing; Staffing (Human Resource Management); Directing and Leading; Leadership; Controlling; Organizational Behavior and Human Relations; Financial Management; Nursing Informatics/Information Management: Review; Personal Management Review; Establishment of Nursing Educational Institutions; Planning and Organizing of Nursing Educational Institutions; Faculty and Student Selection in Nursing Educational Institutions, Directing and Controlling Educational Institution; Professional Considerations and Professional Advancement. This book suits the current needs of nursing students and is prepared to meet the educational needs of both BSN and MSN students.

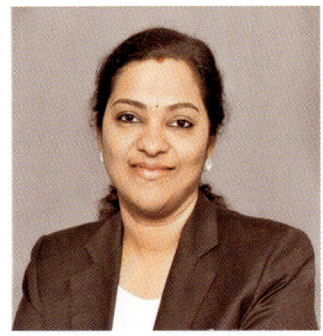

Johny Kutty Joseph and Babitha K Devu are known to me as BSN students since 2005. They both are very studious and intelligent and committed academic professionals with 11 years of experience in various academic roles. They are currently working in Shri Mata Vaishno Devi College of Nursing, Jammu and Kashmir (UT). They are industrious and innovative with a proven history of strong student rapport; dedicated and skilled in classroom management with focus on research-oriented teaching/learning. They are passionate about fostering academic development and success for every student; well-versed in academic advisement and driving student's learning objectives. Besides the authors are creative and reliable academic success coaches with expertise in motivating students to reach their academic potential.

I wish both of them good luck in all their professional endeavors.

Judie Arulappan
MSc (N), PhD, DNSc
Assistant Professor/HOD, Department of Maternal and Child Health
College of Nursing, Sultan Qaboos University, Muscat, Sultanate of Oman

Foreword

I am writing this Foreword with great pride and bliss to appreciate Johny Kutty Joseph and Babitha K Devu, my colleagues, over their innovative approach to the conception of this title. Currently working in Shri Mata Vaishno Devi College of Nursing, Jammu and Kashmir, they have a proven track record of academic and professional excellence with a rich experience over 10 years under various capacities.

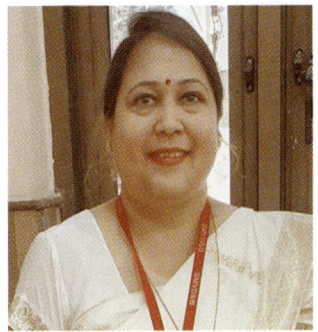

The concepts of management and administration are spread across all sectors of every discipline. The health care system in India is too complex and in a developing stage. Every nurse has to be highly skilled and knowledgeable in order to manage and lead health care providers and their services. The revised syllabus of BSc Nursing (2021) is designed with comprehensive approach to develop these abilities among graduate nurses. This book, authored by Johny Kutty Joseph and Babitha K Devu, has been prepared and organized as per the latest syllabus of Indian Nursing Council, 2021 keeping in view the essential learning outcomes desired.

The book is based on the latest concepts, and adequate emphasis has been given to clarify the concepts through simple and well-structured content. The title covers **18 units** covering the core concepts, such as Health Care System of India, Basic Concepts of Management and Administration, Concepts Related to Organizational Management (both education and service), Nursing Informatics, Personnel Management, and Concepts of Professional Development. This book efficiently covers the learning needs of undergraduate as well as postgraduate students of Nursing Sciences.

To each of you, the readers, who are expanding your knowledge and skills to be more effective nurse leaders *Textbook of Nursing Management and Leadership,* will be a rich resource and primer within nursing education.

My best wishes and prayers for all their future endeavors!

Shailla Cannie

MSc (N), PhD (NFNA - 2020 Awardee)
Dean, Faculty of Nursing, Shri Mata Vaishno Devi University
Principal, Shri Mata Vaishno Devi College of Nursing
Kakryal, Katra, Jammu and Kashmir (India)

Preface

The technological advancements, knowledge explosion, and increasing health care demands pose a challenge to nurse's competence, skills, knowledge and commitment. As health care workers, nurses are an integral part of health care delivery system, and are constantly in contact with people under various roles. To deal with this dynamism and responsibility, nurses require to have knowledge and skills of management. It is quite evident that understanding the skills of leadership which are required to get work done by individuals, is extremely necessary for nurses in their professional lives. In addition, proactive leaders who have a mission and inspire their colleagues to collaborate for mutual goals, help the organization succeed and even prosper through rapid change.

This book offers theoretical and realistic insights that will enable the trained nurses to fulfill the needs of ever-changing health care programs operated within a diverse adaptive framework. The book is designed to teach nursing students the process of management and leadership with a view to supply practicing nurses the needed information on nursing administration as management skills are as important for the nurse administrators as clinical skills and knowledge.

Nursing has a major role to play, so each and every nurse needs to be a leader and speaker for patients in order to provide safe and quality nursing care. It also provides input to multiple types of healthcare providers on changes in the healthcare system. In view of these needs, this book includes many teaching-learning features. This book comprises 18 Units which have been specially designed for the graduate and postgraduate students of nursing science to become expert nurse leaders, managers and administrators. All the units have been thoroughly reviewed, updated and streamlined, and synthesized information have been incorporated along with learning objectives and review questions. Every attempt has been made to maintain simplicity and lucidity of language and style so that readers could enjoy reading this book to a great extent.

Johny Kutty Joseph
Babitha K Devu

Acknowledgments

We are thankful to the Lord Almighty for His grace and abundant blessings as He has been our guiding force behind all our endeavors. A work like this, certainly requires lots of time and efforts. Our family members deserve much credit to this account and we express our sincere thanks to them for their inspiration, love and encouragement. We sincerely thank our daughters Ms Amiya Johny & Ms Zarah Johny for their compromises which enabled us to spend time on this work.

We are also thankful to the Chairman and Members of the Governing Body, Shri Mata Vaishno Devi College of Nursing, for their encouragement and support. We are indebted to Dr Shailla Cannie, Dean & Principal, Shri Mata Vaishno Devi College of Nursing, Judie Arulappan, Assistant Professor/HOD, Department of Maternal and Child Health, College of Nursing, Sultan Qaboos University, Muscat, Sultanate of Oman and our colleagues for their motivation, support and necessary help toward completion of this book. Our special thanks are due to all our teachers, senior professionals in nursing, our friends, well-wishers and students for their consistent persuasion and constructive judgment.

We would like to thank **Mr Satish Kumar Jain** (Chairman) and **Mr Varun Jain** (Managing Director), M/s CBS Publishers and Distributors Pvt Ltd for providing us the platform in bringing out the book. We have no words to describe the role, efforts, inputs and initiatives undertaken by **Mr Bhupesh Aarora** [Sr. Vice President – Publishing and Marketing (Health Sciences Division)] for helping and motivating us.

We sincerely thank the entire CBS team for bringing out the book with utmost care and attractive presentation. We would like to thank Ms Nitasha Arora (Assistant General Manager Publishing – Medical and Nursing), Ms Daljeet Kaur (Assistant Publishing Manager) and Dr Anju Dhir (Sr. Product Manager and Medical Development Editor) for their publishing support. We would also extend our thanks to Mr Shivendu Bhushan Pandey (Sr. Manager and Team Lead), Ms Surbhi Gupta (Sr. English Editor), Mr Ashutosh Pathak (Sr. Proofreader cum Team Coordinator) and all the production team members for devoting laborious hours in designing and typesetting the book.

Reviewers

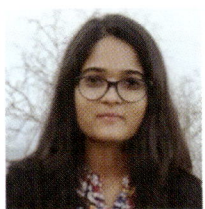

Deeksha Patel
MSc Nursing (Oncology)
Nursing Officer
All India Institute of Medical Sciences
(AIIMS)
Bhopal (MP)

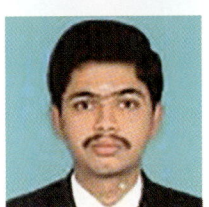

K Shesha Kumar
MSc (Pediatric Nursing)
Community Health Officer
Health and Wellness Centre
Chittoor, Andhra Pradesh

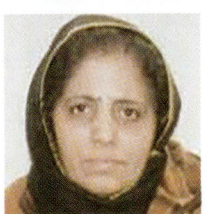

Mehmooda Regu MSc (N), PhD
Principal
Alamdar Memorial College of Nursing
and Medical Technology
Islamic University of Science &
Technology
Awantipora, Pulwama, J&K

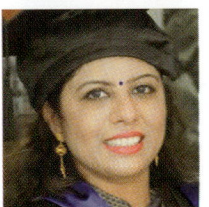

Monika Kankarwal
PhD (Critical Care Nursing)
Nursing Officer
All India Institute of Medical Sciences
(AIIMS)
New Delhi

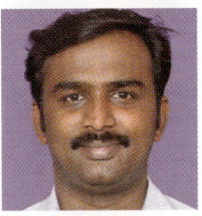

Poovaragavan V RN
Vice-Principal
Vignesh Nursing College
Kizhanaikarai
Tiruvannamalai, Tamil Nadu

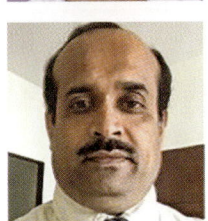

Rajesh Konnur PhD, RN
Professor
Kurji Holy Family College of Nursing
Kurji Holy Family Hospital (KHFH)
Patna, Bihar
Dean
Eudoxia Research Centre, India

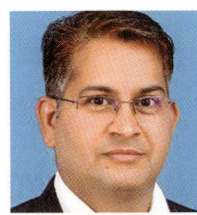

Rajesh Kumar PhD (N), RN
Associate Professor
All India Institute of Medical Sciences
(AIIMS)
Rishikesh, Uttarakhand

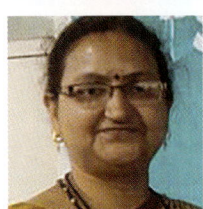

Sangita Singh MSc (N)
Assistant Professor
Indira Gandhi Institute of Medical
Sciences
Patna, Bihar

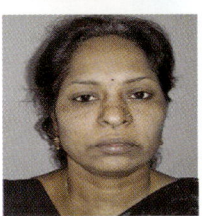

Shanthi Ida RN, RM, MSc (N), PhD (N)
Professor and HOD (OBG)
SNSR, Sharda University
Greater Noida, Uttar Pradesh

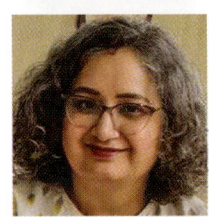

Smriti Arora MSc (N), PhD
Professor and PhD Coordinator
ACON, AUH
Amity College of Nursing
Manesar, Gurugram, Haryana

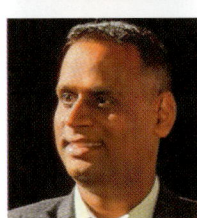

Sushil Kumar Maheshwari
MSc (N), PhD
Associate Professor
Baba Farid University of Health
Sciences
Faridkot, Punjab

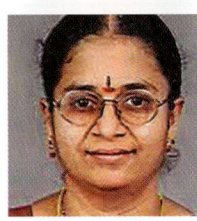

Tamil Selvi A MSc (N), PhD
Principal
Amity College of Nursing
Amity University
Manesar, Gurugram, Haryana

Publisher's Desk

Dear Reader,

Nursing Education has a rich history, often characterized by traditional teaching techniques that have evolved over time. Primarily, teaching took place within classroom settings. Lectures, textbooks, and clinical rotations were the core teaching tools; and students majorly relied on textbooks by local or foreign publishers for quality education. However, today, technology has completely transformed the field of nursing education, making it an integral part of the curriculum. It has evolved to include a range of technological tools that enhance the learning experience and better prepare students for clinical practice.

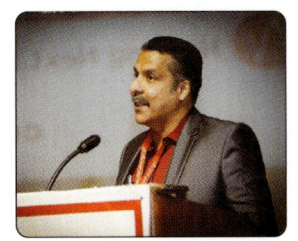

As publishers, we've been contributing to the field of Medical Science, Nursing and Allied Sciences and earned the trust of many. By supporting **Indian authors**, coupled with **nursing webinars and conferences**, we have paved an easier path for aspiring nurses, empowering them to excel in national and state level exams. With this, we're not only enhancing the quality of patient care but also enabling future nurses to adapt to new challenges and innovations in the rapidly evolving world of healthcare. Following the ideology of **Bringing learning to people instead of people going for learning**, so far, we've been doing our part by:

- Developing quality content by qualified and well-versed authors
- Building a strong community of faculty and students
- Introducing a smart approach with Digital/Hybrid Books, and
- Offering simulation Nursing Procedures, etc.

Innovative teaching methodologies, such as modern-age Phygital Books, have sparked the interest of the Next-Gen students in pursuing advanced education. The enhancement of educational standards through **Omnipresent Knowledge Sharing Platforms** has further facilitated learning, bridging the gap between doctors and nurses.

At Nursing Next Live, a sister concern of CBS Publishers & Distributors, we have long recognized the immense potential within the nursing field. Our journey in innovating nursing education has allowed us to make substantial and meaningful contributions. With the vision of strengthening learning at every stage, we have introduced several plans that cater to the specific needs of the students, including but not limited to **Plan UG** for undergraduates, **Plan MSc** for postgraduate aspirants, **Plan FDP** for upskilling faculties, **SDL** for integrated learning and **Plan NP** for bridging the gap between theoretical & practical learning. Additionally, we have successfully completed seven series of our **Target High** Book in a very short period, setting a milestone in the education industry. We have been able to achieve all this just with the sole vision of laying the foundation of diversified knowledge for all. With the rise of a new generation of educated, tech-savvy individuals, we anticipate even more remarkable advancements in the coming years.

We take immense pride in our achievements and eagerly look forward to the future, brimming with new opportunities for innovation, growth and collaborations with experienced minds such as yourself who can contribute to our mission as Authors, Reviewers and/or Faculties. Together, let's foster a generation of nurses who are confident, competent, and prepared to succeed in a technology-driven healthcare system.

Mr Bhupesh Aarora
(Sr Vice President – Publishing & Marketing)
bhupeshaarora@cbspd.com| +91 95553 53330

Special Features of the Book

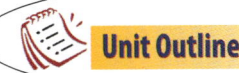

Unit Outline

After going through this unit the readers will be able to know:
- Introduction
- Health and administration
- Health system in India
- Panchayati Raj
- Agents of health care delivery in India
- Nursing services
- Aims of nursing service administration
- Current trends and issues in nursing
- Trends in nursing research

Every unit contains an outline to give a brief view of the contents covered in it.

The book is well illustrated with relevant figures.

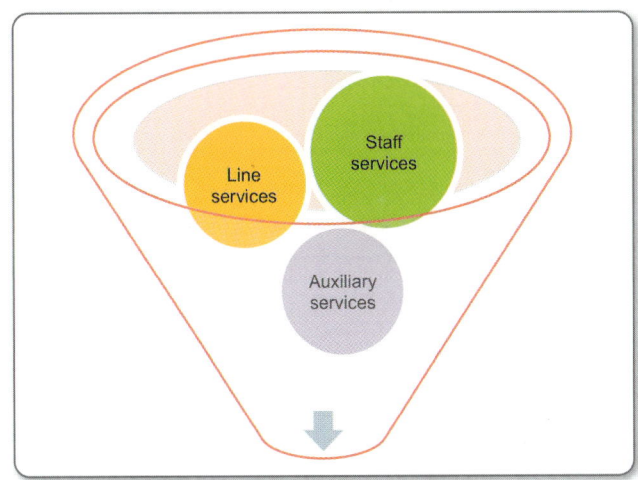

Fig. 7: Aspects of hospital services

TABLE 1: Organization of nursing services at center level

DGHS		
Additional DG	Additional DG (N)	Additional DG
	Deputy DG (N)	
Assistant Director General (ADG) (Community Nursing Service)	Assistant Director General (ADG) (Nursing Education and Research)	Assistant Director General (ADG) (Hospital Nursing Service)
Deputy Assistant Director General (DADG)	Deputy Assistant Director General (DADG)	Deputy Assistant Director General (DADG)

Numerous tables have been used in the chapters to facilitate learning in a quick way.

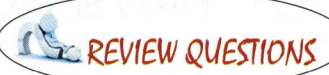 **REVIEW QUESTIONS**

1. Define health administration.
2. Explain the health administration system in India.
3. What are the agents of health care administration?
4. Explain current trends and issues in nursing.
5. Discuss the principles of health administration.

Important university level questions are enlisted at the end of every chapter to help students to assess their learning.

Additional reading sources to enhance the knowledge bed are enlisted in further reading.

Further Readings

1. Park K. Preventive and Social Medicine, 19th Edition: M/s. Banarasidas Bhanot Publishers, Jabalpur, 2007.
2. Goel SL. Healthcare System, and Its Management, Health Organization and Structure, 1st Volume, Deep and Deep Publishers, New Delhi; 2001.
3. Basavanthappa BT. Nursing Administration, 2nd Edition. Jaypee Brothers Medical Publishers (P) Ltd. New Delhi; 2008.
4. Goel SL, Kumar R. Management of Hospitals – Hospital Administration in the 21st century, Vol. 4, Deep and Deep Publication, New Delhi; 2002.
5. Ranga Rao SP. Administration of Primary Health Centers in India, 1st Edition: Mittal Publications, New Delhi; 1993.
6. Lucita M. Nursing: Practice and Public Health Administration. Current Concepts and Trends. B. I. Churchill Living Stone Pvt. Ltd. New Delhi; 2002.

Syllabus for BSc Nursing

NURSING MANAGEMENT AND LEADERSHIP

VI Semester
Course Outline

Theory: 60 hours (3 credits)

Unit	Time (Hrs)	Learning outcomes	Content	Teaching/learning activities	Assessment methods
I	1(T)	Explore the health care, development of nursing services and education in India and trends	**Health care and development of nursing services in India** • Current health care delivery system of India—review • Planning and development of nursing services and education at global and national scenario • Recent trends and issues of nursing service and management	• Lecture cum discussion • Directed reading and written assignment	• Short answer type • Assessment of assignment
II	2(T)	Explain the principles and functions of management applied to nursing Describe the introductory concepts of management as a process	**Management basics applied to nursing** • Definitions, concepts and theories of management • Importance, features and levels of management • Management and administration • Functions of management • Principles of management • Role of a nurse as a manager **Introduction to management process** • Planning • Organizing • Staffing • Directing/Leading • Controlling	• Lecture & Discussion	• MCQ • Short answer
MANAGEMENT OF NURSING SERVICES					
III	4(T)	Describe the essential elements of planning	**Planning nursing services** • Vision, Mission, philosophy, objectives • Nursing service policies, procedures and manuals • Functional and operational planning • Strategic planning • Program planning: Gantt chart & milestone chart • Budgeting—concepts, principles, types • Budget proposal, cost benefit analysis • Planning hospital and patient care unit (Ward) • Planning for emergency and disaster	• Lecture and Discussion • Visit to specific hospital/ patient care units • Demonstration of disaster drill in the respective setting	• Formulate Mission & Vision Statement for the nursing department/unit • Assessment of problem-solving exercises • Visit Report
IV	4(T)	Discuss the concepts of organizing including hospital organization	**Organizing** • Organizing as a process— assignment, delegation and coordination	• Lecture cum discussion • Comparison of organizational structure of various organizations	• Short answer • Assessment of assignment

Contd...

Unit	Time (Hrs)	Learning outcomes	Content	Teaching/learning activities	Assessment methods
			• Hospital—types, functions & organization • Organizational development • Organizational structure • Organizational charts • Organizational effectiveness • Hospital administration, control & line of authority • Hospital statistics including hospital utilization indices • Nursing care delivery systems and trends • Role of nurse in maintenance of effective organizational climate	• Nursing care delivery systems—assignment • Preparation of organizational chart of hospital/Nursing services	
V	6(T)	Identify the significance of human resource management (HRM) and material management and discuss its elements	**Staffing (Human resource management)** • Definition, objectives, components and functions **Staffing & scheduling** • Staffing—philosophy, staffing activities • Recruiting, selecting, deployment • Training, development, credentialing, retaining, promoting, transfer, terminating, superannuation • Staffing units—Projecting staffing requirements/calculation of requirements of staff resources, nurse patient ratio, nurse population ratio as per SIU norms/IPH norms, and patient classification system • Categories of nursing personnel including job description of all levels • Assignment and nursing care responsibilities • Turnover and absenteeism • Staff welfare • Discipline and grievances	• Lecture & discussion, role play • Games self-assessment, case discussion and practice session • Calculation of staffing requirements for a specified ward	• Formulate job description at different levels of care & compare with existing system • Preparation of duty roster
		Explain the procedural steps of material management	**In-service education** • Nature and scope of in-service education program • Principles of adult learning—review • Planning and organizing in-service educational program • Methods, techniques and evaluation • Preparation of report **Material resource management**	Visit to inventory store of the institution	• Preparation of MMF/records • Preparation of log book & condemnation documents • Visit report
		Develop managerial skill in inventory control and actively participate in procurement process	• Procurement, purchasing process, inventory control & role of nurse • Auditing and maintenance in hospital and patient care unit		

Contd...

Unit	Time (Hrs)	Learning outcomes	Content	Teaching/learning activities	Assessment methods
VI	5(T)	Describe the important methods of supervision and guidance	**Directing and leading** • Definition, principles, elements of directing • Supervision and guidance • Participatory management • Interprofessional collaboration • Management by objectives • Team management • Assignments, rotations • Maintenance of discipline • Leadership in management	• Lecture & discussion • Demonstration of record & report maintenance in specific wards/departments	• Assignment on reports & records maintained in nursing department • Preparation of protocols and manuals
VII	4(T)	Discuss the significance and changing trends of nursing leadership Analyze the different leadership styles and develop leadership competencies	**Leadership** • Definition, concepts, and theories • Leadership principles and competencies • Leadership styles—situational leadership, transformational leadership • Methods of leadership development • Mentorship/preceptorship in nursing • Delegation, power & politics, empowerment, mentoring and coaching • Decision making and problem solving • Conflict management and negotiation • Implementing planned change	• Lecture cum discussion • Self-assessment • Report on types of leadership adopted at different levels of health care in the given setting • Problem solving/conflict management exercise • Observation of managerial roles at different levels (middle level mangers-ward incharge, ANS)	• Short answer • Essay • Assessment of exercise/report
VIII	4(T)	Explain the process of controlling and its activities	**Controlling** • Implementing standards, policies, procedures, protocols and practices • Nursing performance audit, patient satisfaction • Nursing rounds, Documentation—records and reports • Total quality management—quality assurance, quality and safety • Performance appraisal • Program evaluation review technique (PERT) • Bench marking, activity plan (Gantt chart) • Critical path analysis	• Lecture cum discussion • Preparation of policies/protocols for nursing units/department	• Assessment of prepared protocols
IX	4(T)	Explain the concepts of organizational behavior and group dynamics	**Organizational behavior and human relations** • Concepts and theories of organizational behavior • Group dynamics • Review: Interpersonal relationship • Human relations • Public relations in the context of nursing • Relations with professional associations and employee unions	• Lecture & discussion • Role play/exercise-group dynamics & human relations	• Short answer • OSCE

Contd...

Unit	Time (Hrs)	Learning outcomes	Content	Teaching/learning activities	Assessment methods
			• Collective bargaining • Review—Motivation and morale building • Communication in the workplace—assertive communication • Committees—importance in the organization, functioning		
X	2(T)	Describe the financial management related to nursing services	**Financial management** • Definition, objectives, elements, functions, principles & scope of financial management • Financial planning (budgeting for nursing department) • Proposal, projecting requirement for staff, equipment and supplies for hospital & patient care units & emergency and disaster units • Budget and budgetary process • Financial audit	• Lecture cum discussion • Budget proposal review • Preparation of budget proposal for a specific department	• Short answer • Essay • Assessment of assignment
XI	1(T)	Review the concepts, principles and methods and use of nursing informatics	**Nursing informatics/Information management—review** • Patient records • Nursing records • Use of computers in hospital, college and community • Telemedicine & Tele nursing • Electronic Medical Records (EMR), EHR	• Review • Practice session • Visit to departments	• Short answer
XII	1(T)	Review personal management in terms of management of emotions, stress and resilience	**Personal management—review** • Emotional intelligence • Resilience building • Stress and time management—de stressing • Career planning	• Review • Discussion	
			Management of Nursing Educational Institutions		
XIII	4(T)	Describe the process of establishing educational institutions and its accreditation guidelines	**Establishment of nursing educational institutions** • Indian Nursing Council norms and guidelines—Faculty norms, physical facilities, clinical facilities, curriculum implementation, and evaluation/examination guidelines • Coordination with regulatory bodies—INC and State Nursing Council • Accreditation—Inspections • Affiliation with university/State council/board of examinations	• Lecture & discussion • Visit to one of the regulatory bodies	• Visit report
XIV	4(T)	Explain the planning and organizing functions of a nursing college	**Planning and organizing** • Philosophy, objectives and mission of the college • Organization structure of school/college • Review—Curriculum planning • Planning teaching and learning experiences, clinical facilities—master plan, time table and clinical rotation	• Directed reading—INC Curriculum • Preparation of organizational structure of the college • Written assignment—writing philosophy of a teaching department	• Short answer • Essay • Assessment of assignment

Contd...

Unit	Time (Hrs)	Learning outcomes	Content	Teaching/learning activities	Assessment methods
			• Budget planning—faculty, staff, equipment & supplies, AV aids, Lab equipment, library books, journals, computers and maintenance • Infrastructure facilities—college, classrooms, hostel, library, labs, computer lab, transport facilities • Records & reports for students, staff, faculty and administrative • Committees and functioning • Clinical experiences	• Preparation of master plan, time table and clinical rotation	
XV	4(T)	Develop understanding of staffing the college and selecting the students	**Staffing and student selection** • Faculty/staff selection, recruitment and placement, job description • Performance appraisal • Faculty development • Faculty/staff welfare • Student recruitment, admission, clinical placement	• Guided reading on faculty norms • Faculty welfare activities report • Writing job description of tutors	• Short answer • Activity report • Assessment of job description
XVI	4(T)	Analyze the leadership and management activities in an educational organization	**Directing and controlling** • Review—Curriculum implementation and evaluation • Leadership and motivation, supervision—review • Guidance and counseling • Quality management—educational audit • Program evaluation, evaluation of performance • Maintaining discipline • Institutional records and reports—administrative, faculty, staff and students	• Review—principles of evaluation • Assignment—Identify disciplinary problems among students • Writing student record	• Short answer • Assessment of assignment and record
XVII	4(T)	Identify various legal issues and laws relevant to nursing practice	**Professional Considerations** **Review—legal and ethical issues** • Nursing as a profession—Characteristics of a professional nurse • Nursing practice—philosophy, aim and objectives • Regulatory bodies—INC and SNC constitution and functions **Review—Professional ethics** • Code of ethics and professional conduct—INC & ICN • Practice standards for nursing—INC • International Council for Nurses (ICN) **Legal aspects in nursing:** • Consumer Protection Act, patient rights • Legal terms related to practice, legal system—types of law, tort law & liabilities • Laws related to nursing practice—negligence, malpractice, breach, penalties		

Contd...

Unit	Time (Hrs)	Learning outcomes	Content	Teaching/learning activities	Assessment methods
			• Invasion of privacy, defamation of character • Nursing regulatory mechanisms—registration, licensure, renewal, accreditation, Nurse Practice Act, regulation for nurse practitioner/specialist nursing practice		
XVIII	2(T)	Explain various opportunities for professional advancement	**Professional advancement** • Continuing nursing education • Career opportunities • Membership with professional organizations—national and international • Participation in research activities • Publications—journals, newspaper	• Prepare journal list available in India • Write an article—research/clinical	• Assessment of assignments

Contents

Unit 4 Organizing 53–75

Unit 5 Staffing (Human Resource Management) 77–124

Unit 6 Directing and Leading   125–141

Unit 14   Planning and Organizing of Nursing Educational Institutions   265–278

Unit 15   Faculty and Student Selection in Nursing Educational Institutions   279–296

Unit 16   Directing and Controlling Educational Institution   297–307

Unit 17   Professional Considerations   309–327

Unit 18   **Professional Advancement**   **329–339**

Unit

1

Health Care and Development of Nursing Services in India

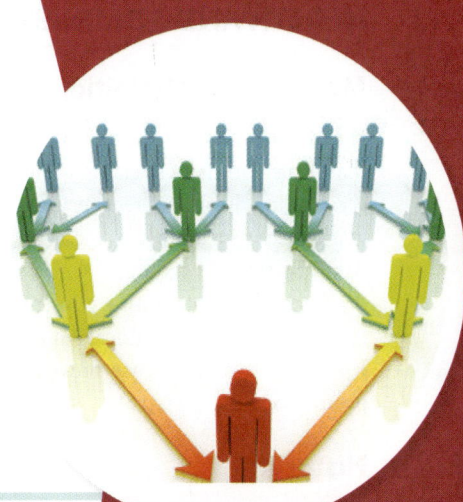

 Unit Outline

- Health and Administration
- Health System in India
- Panchayati Raj
- Agents of Health Care Delivery in India
- Nursing Services
- Current Trends and Issues in Nursing
- Trends in Nursing Research
- Issues Affecting Nursing Practice

INTRODUCTION

Constitutionally, every person in India has the right to avail health services to protect their fundamental right to be safe and healthy. The Indian government has developed machinery and structures for health administration to prepare, coordinate and provide healthcare services to the people living in all spheres of the country. The health care organization of India is established at a three-tier delivery system categorized as central, state and local to achieve health goals and deal with health subjects.

HEALTH AND ADMINISTRATION

Meaning and Definition

Health Administration is a division of public administration that deals with issues related to health promotion, preventive services, medical care, recovery, health service delivery, health workforce development, medical education, and training. Administration of public health is the science and art of organizing and integrating government agencies with the aim to enhance people's physical, emotional, and social wellbeing. It also focuses on disease prevention, protection, and health promotion.

History

Modern organization and administration of public health is designed to prevent illness, prolong life, and through coordinated group efforts to promote physical and mental performance. **During the period of independence**, there were two separate departments at the center such as the Director-General of Indian Medical Services and the Public Health Service Commission. Later on, after the independence of the Nation, these two departments were combined into the Directorate-General for Health Services, headed by the Director of Health Services.

Post-independence era (after 1947), a democratic regime was set up in India with a new concept aimed towards the establishment of a welfare state. The Bhore Committee (constituted in 1946 under the chairmanship of Sir Joseph Bhore) submitted a detailed report concerning the development of the Nation including the health care sector. These recommendations became the basis for most of the planning and measures adopted by the National Government. Few major milestones are mentioned below:

- 1947: Ministries of health were established at the center and states.
- 1948: India became a member of the WHO.
- 1949: The post of Registrar General of India was created in the Ministry of Home Affairs.
- 1950: The Government of India set up a planning commission to make an assessment of the material, capital, human resources of the country and to draft developmental plans for the most effective utilization of these resources. "The Planning commission was renamed as NITI Aayog in 2015".
- **Five-year plan:** Planning commission has formulated successive five-year plans to rebuild rural India to lay the foundation of industrial progress and to secure the balanced development of all parts of the country.

Objectives

- To increase the average length of human life
- To decrease the mortality and morbidity rates
- To increase the physical, mental, and social wellbeing of the individual
- To provide total healthcare to enrich the quality of life
- To increase the pace of adjustment of the individual to his environment
- To make provision of primary healthcare services to everyone
- To develop healthy manpower to provide proper services to the community
- To formulate health policies and their periodic revision from time to time

Principles

- Centralized director and decentralized activity.
- The administration must be based on sound economic consideration and practicable financial budgeting.
- A clear picture of the complete plan must be made before starting a program.
- A program of continuing staff education is essential and it should be scientific.
- Periodic appraisal of services rendered the effectiveness of the program, and evaluation of the results are the major responsibilities of the health administration.
- Provision must be made for desirable working conditions for all members of the staff.
- There should be sound national health policy including healthy administrative structures for the implementation of various health policies.
- There should be an integration of preventive and curative services at all administrative levels.
- Health should not be considered in isolation from other socioeconomic factors.
- Health opportunities need not be related to the purchasing power of the people.
- Health consciousness should be fostered through education and by providing opportunities for participation of people in the health programs.
- All the systems of medicine must be encouraged to provide decent health to people in a coordinated fashion.

HEALTH SYSTEM IN INDIA

India is a union of 28 states and 8* union territories. Under the constitution of India, the states are largely independent in matters relating to the delivery of health care to the people. Each state, therefore, has developed its system of healthcare delivery independent of the central government. The central responsibility consists mainly of policymaking, planning, guiding, assisting, evaluating, and coordinating the work of the state health ministries so that health services cover every part of the country and no state lags behind for the requirement of these services (Fig. 1).

Health Administration at the Central Level

The official organs of the health system at the national level consist of 3 units:
1. Union Ministry of Health and Family Welfare
2. Directorate General of Health Services
3. Central Council of Health and Family Welfare

1. **Union Ministry of Health and Family Welfare:** The Union Ministry of Health and Family Welfare is headed by a Cabinet Minister, a Minister of State, and a Deputy Health Minister. These are political appointments and have a dual role to serve political as well as administrative responsibilities for health. Currently, the union health ministry has the following departments (Fig. 2):

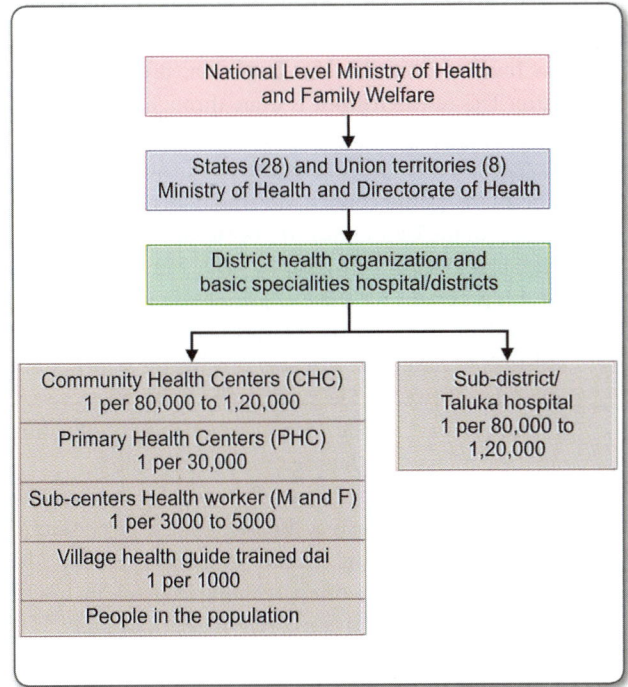

Fig. 1: Health system in India

---

*The merger of the former union territories of Dadra and Nagar Haveli and Daman and Diu came into effect on 26 January 2020.

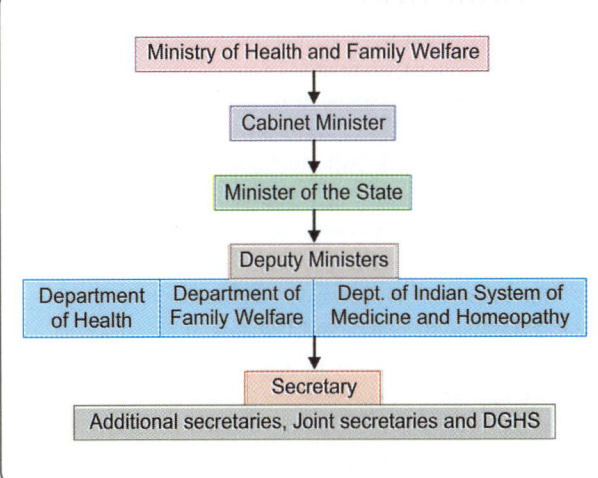

Fig. 2: Ministry of health and family welfare

■ **Department of Health:** It is headed by a secretary to the Government of India as its executive head, assisted by joint secretaries, deputy secretaries, and a large administrative staff. The Department of Health deals with planning, coordination, programming, evaluation of medical and public health matters, including drug control and prevention of food adulteration. The functions of the Union Health Ministry are set out in the seventh schedule of Article 246 of the Constitution of India under the Union list and Concurrent list.

Union list:
♦ International health relations and administration of port-quarantine
♦ Administration of central health institutes such as All India Institute of Hygiene and Public Health, Kolkata; National Institute for Control of Communicable Diseases, Delhi, etc.
♦ Promotion of research through research centers and other bodies
♦ Regulation and development of medical, nursing and other allied health professions
♦ Establishment and maintenance of drug standards
♦ Census, and collection and publication of other statistical data
♦ Immigration and emigration
♦ Regulation of labor in the working of mines and oil fields
♦ Coordination with states and other ministries for the promotion of health

Concurrent list: The functions listed under the concurrent list are the responsibility of both the union and state governments. The center and states have simultaneous powers of legislation. They are as follows:
♦ Prevention of extension of communicable diseases from one unit to another
♦ Prevention of adulteration of food
♦ Control of drugs and poisons

♦ Vital statistics
♦ Labor welfare
♦ Ports other than major
♦ Economic and social health planning
♦ Population control and family planning

■ **Department of Family Welfare:** It was created in 1966 within the Ministry of Health and Family Welfare. The secretary to the Government of India in the Ministry of Health and Family Welfare is in overall charge of the Department of Family Welfare. He is assisted by an additional secretary and commissioner, and one joint secretary. **Functions of the Department of Family Welfare are:**

♦ To organize the family welfare program through family welfare centers
♦ To create an atmosphere of social acceptance of the program and to support all voluntary organizations interested in the program
♦ To educate every individual to develop a conviction that small family size is valuable and to popularize appropriate and acceptable method of family planning
♦ To disseminate the knowledge on the practice of family planning as widely as possible and to provide service agencies nearest to the community
♦ To organize basic research of human fertility, genetics and population dynamics and the evolution of the easy and reliable method of contraception
♦ To study the social factors that affect fertility and to take such steps that will reduce the number of children in a family
♦ To coordinate the family planning program with child welfare and maternal health services throughout the country
♦ To organize the production of the contraceptive devices in adequate quantities to maintain the supply at all levels at a minimum cost
♦ To promote Indian System of Medicine through signifying the practice of AYUSH, proper training of professionals and research.

■ **Department of Indian System of Medicine and Homeopathy:** It was established in March 1995 and had continued to make steady progress. Emphasis was on implementation of the various schemes introduced such as education, standardization of drugs, enhancement of availability of raw materials, research and development, information, education and communication and involvement of ISM and Homeopathy in national health care. Most of the functions of this ministry are implemented through an autonomous organization called DGHS.

2. **Directorate General of Health Services:** The DGHS is the principal advisor to the Union Government in both medical and public health matters. He is assisted by a team of deputies and a large administrative staff. The Directorate comprises of Medical care and hospitals, Public health and

General administration. The general functions are surveys, planning, coordination, programming and appraisal of all health matters in the country. The specific functions include:

■ **International health relations and quarantine:** All the major ports in the country and international airports are directly controlled by the Director-General of Health Services. All matters related to the obtaining of assistance from international agencies and the coordination of their activities in the country are undertaken by the Director-General of Health Services.

■ **Control of drug standards:** The drug control organization is a part of the DGHS and is headed by the Drugs Controller. Its primary function is to lay down and enforce standards and control the manufacture and distribution of drugs through both Central and State Government offices. The Drugs Act (1940) vests the Central Government with the powers to test the quality of imported drugs.

■ **Postgraduate training:** The DGHS is responsible for the administration of national institutions. These institutions provide postgraduate training to different categories of health personnel.

■ **Medical education:** The DGHS is directly in charge of the medical colleges in India. Many medical colleges in the country are guided and supported by the Center.

■ **Medical research:** Medical research in the country is organized largely through the ICMR, founded in 1911 in New Delhi. The council plays a significant role in aiding, promoting and coordinating scientific research on human diseases, their causation, prevention, and cure. The research work is done through the councils, and several permanent research institutes, e.g., Cancer Research Center, TB Chemotherapy Center at Chennai. The funds of the council are wholly derived from the budget of the Union Ministry of Health.

■ **National Health Programs:** The various national health programs for the eradication of malaria and the control of tuberculosis, filariasis, leprosy, AIDS and other communicable diseases involve the expenditure of crores of rupees. The central directorate plays a very important part in planning, guiding and coordinating all the national health programs in the country.

■ **Central Health Education Bureau:** An outstanding activity of this Bureau is the preparation of education material for creating health awareness among the people. The bureau offers training courses in health education in different categories of health workers.

■ **Health intelligence:** The Central Bureau of Health Intelligence was established in 1961 to centralize collection, compilation, analysis, evaluation, and dissemination of all information on health statistics for the nation as a whole. It disseminates epidemic intelligence to states and international bodies.

- **National Medical Library:** The Central Medical Library of DGHS was declared the National Medical Library in 1966. The aim is to help in the advancement of medical, health and related sciences by collection, dissemination, and exchange of information.

3. **Central Council of Health and Family Welfare:** The Central Council of Health and Family Welfare was set up by a Presidential Order on August 9, 1952, under Article 263 of the Constitution of India for promoting coordinated and concerted action between the center and the states in the implementation of all the programs and measures about the health of the nation. The Union Health Minister is the chairman and the state health ministers are the members. The functions of the Central Council of Health are:

   - To consider and recommend broad outlines of policy concerning matters related to health in all its aspects such as the provision of remedial and preventive care, environmental hygiene, nutrition, health education and the promotion of facilities for training and research.
   - To make proposals for legislation in fields of activity related to medical and public health matters and to lay down the pattern of development for the country as a whole.
   - To make recommendations to the Central Government regarding the distribution of available grants-in-aid for health purposes to the states and to review periodically the work accomplished in different areas through the utilization of these grants-in-aid.
   - To establish any organization or organizations invested with appropriate functions for promoting and maintaining cooperation between the Central and State Health administrations.

Health Administration at the State Level

Historically, the first milestone in the state health administration was the year 1919, when the states (provinces) obtained autonomy, under the Montague-Chelmsford reforms, from the Central Government in matters of public health. By 1921-22, all the states had created some form of public health organization. The Government of India Act, 1935 gave further autonomy to the states. The state is the ultimate authority responsible for health services operating within its jurisdiction. At present, there are 28 states in India, with each state having its health administration. In all the states, the management sector comprises the State Ministry of Health and a Directorate of Health.

State Ministry of Health

The State Ministry of Health is headed by a Minister of Health and Family Welfare and a Deputy Minister of Health and FW. In some states, the Health Minister is also in charge of other portfolios. The Health secretariat is the official organ of the State Ministry of Health and is headed by a Secretary who is assisted by Deputy Secretaries and a large administrative staff.

Functions: Health services provided at the state level

- Rural health services through the minimum need program
- Medical development program
- Maternal and Child Health (MCH) family welfare and immunization program
- National Malaria Control Program (NMCP) (malaria) and National Filaria Control Program (NFCP) (filaria)
- National Leprosy Eradication Program (NLEP), Revised National Tuberculosis Control Program (RNTCP), National Treatment Elimination Program (NTEP), National Program for Control of Blindness (NPCB) prevention and control of communicable diseases like diarrheal disease, Kyasanur Forest Disease (KFD), Japanese encephalitis (JE)
- School Health Program, Nutrition Program, National Goiter Control Program.
- Laboratory services and vaccine production units
- Health education and training program, curative services, National AIDS Control Program

State Health Directorate

The Director of Health Services (DHS) is the chief technical advisor to the State Government on all matters relating to medicine and public health. He is also responsible for the organization and direction of all health activities. With the advent of family planning as an important program, the designation of DHS has been changed in some states and is now known as Director of Health and Family Welfare. The Director of Health and Family Welfare is assisted by a suitable number of deputies and assistants.

Health Administration at the District Level

The district is the most crucial level in the administration and implementation of medical/health services. At the district level, there is a district medical and health officer or CMO who is overall responsible for the administration of medical/health services in the entire district.

Bhore Committee (1946) recommended integrated services at all levels and the setting up of a unified health authority in each district. The principal unit of administration in India is the district under a collector. There are 640 districts in India (Census 2011). Each district has six types of administration areas.

1. Subdivisions
2. Tehsils (talukas)
3. Community development blocks
4. Municipalities and corporations
5. Villages
6. Panchayats

Most of the districts in India are divided into two or more **subdivisions**, each in charge of an assistant collector or sub-collector. Each subdivision is again divided into **tehsils** in charge of a Tehsildar. A tehsil usually comprises between 200 and 600 villages. Since the launching of the community development program in India in 1952, the rural areas of the district have been organized into blocks known as **community development blocks.** The block is a unit of rural planning and development and comprises approximately 100 **villages** and about 80,000 to 1,20,000 population in charge of a block development officer. Finally, there are the **village panchayats**, which are institutions of rural local self-government.

The urban areas of the district are organized into the following local self-government:

- **Town area committee**—(Population 5,000–10,000): The town area committees are like panchayaths. They provide sanitary services.
- **Municipal Boards or Municipality**—(Population 10,000–2,00,000): The municipal boards are headed by a chairman/president, elected usually by the members. The term of a municipal board ranges between 3 and 5 years. The functions of a municipal board are construction and maintenance of roads, sanitation, and drainage, street lighting, water supply, maintenance of hospitals and dispensaries, education, registration of births and deaths, etc.
- **Corporations**—(Population above 2,00,000). Corporations are headed by mayors. The councilors are elected from different wards of the city. The executive agency includes the commissioner, the secretary, the engineer, and the health officer. The activities are similar to those of the municipalities but on a much wider scale.

PANCHAYATI RAJ

The Panchayat Raj is a three-tier structure of rural local self-government in India linking the villages to the district. The three institutions are:
1. Panchayat—at the village level.
2. Panchayat Samiti—at the block level.
3. Zila Parishad—at the district level.

The Panchayat Raj institutions are accepted as agencies of public welfare. All development programs are channeled through these bodies. The Panchayati Raj institutions strengthen democracy at its root and ensure more effective and better participation of the people in the government.

AGENTS OF HEALTH CARE DELIVERY IN INDIA

In India, it is represented by five major sectors or agencies which differ from each other by health technology applied and by the source of fund available. These are:

- **Public Health Sector**
  - **Primary Health Care:** Primary health centers, Sub-centers.
  - Hospital/Health Centers, Community health centers, Rural health centers, District hospitals/health centers, Specialist hospitals, Teaching hospitals.
  - Health Insurance Schemes, Employees State Insurance, Central Govt. Health Scheme.
  - Other Agencies, Defense services, Railways.
- **Private Health Sector**
  - Private hospitals, polyclinics, nursing homes, and dispensaries.
  - General practitioners and clinics.
- **Indigenous Systems of Medicine**
  - Ayurveda
  - Siddha
  - Unani
  - Homeopathy
  - Naturopathy
  - Yoga
  - Unregistered practitioners.
- **Voluntary Health Agencies**
- **National Health Programs**

Public Health Sector

In 1977, the Government of India launched a rural health scheme, based on the principles of—Placing people's health in people's hands. As a signatory to Alma-Ata Declaration (1978), the government of India is committed to achieving the goal of the Health care approach, which seeks to provide universal health care at an affordable cost. Keeping in view the WHO goal of—Health for All by 2000 AD, the government of India evolved a National Health Policy in 1983. Keeping in view the Millennium Developmental Goals, the government of India revised the draft of the National Health Policy in 2002. Further, it was again revised keeping in view of the changes in the health context of the country. The National Health Policy 2017 aims to attain the optimum health for all through a promotive and preventive approach in all health care policies. It ensures universal access to health care services to all. It aims to achieve health for all by increasing access, lowering the cost of health care delivery and improving the quality of health services.

Primary Health Center: It is the backbone of the Indian health care system is based on principles such as:

- Equitable distribution
- Community participation
- Intersectoral coordination
- Appropriate technology
- Preventive in nature
- Manpower development.

Primary Health Centers (PHCs) are the cornerstone of rural health services. The first part of the call to a qualified doctor of the public sector in rural areas for the sick and those who directly report or referred from Sub-centers for curative, preventive and promotive health care. A typical Primary Health Center covers a population of 20,000 in hilly, tribal, or difficult areas and 30,000 population in plain areas with 4-6 indoor/observation beds. It acts as a referral unit for 6 sub-centers and refers out cases to CHC (30 bedded hospital) and higher-order public hospitals located at sub-district and district level. The PHC provides a wide range of services such as medical care, MCH care including family planning, MTP, management of STDs, Nutritional health, school health, immunization, disease surveillance, and many other necessary services.

Subcenters are set up under Primary Health Care centers to increase the accessibility of health services.

Community Health Centers: Health care delivery in India has been envisaged at three levels namely primary, secondary and tertiary. The secondary level of health care essentially includes Community Health Centers (CHCs), constituting the First Referral Units (FRUs) and the district hospitals. The CHCs were designed to provide referral health care for cases from the primary level and for cases in need of specialist care approaching the center directly. 4 PHCs are included under each CHC thus catering to approximately 80,000 population in tribal/hilly areas and 1, 20,000 population in plain areas. CHC is a 30 bedded hospital providing specialist care in Medicine, Obstetrics, and Gynecology, Surgery, and Pediatrics. These centers are, however, fulfilling the tasks entrusted to them only to a limited extent.

District Health System: It is the fundamental basis for implementing various health policies and delivery of healthcare, management of health services for the defined geographic area. The district hospital is an essential component of the District health system and functions as a secondary level of health care, which provides curative, preventive and promotive healthcare services to the people in the district. Every district is expected to have a district hospital linked with the public hospital/health centers down below the district such as Sub-district/Sub-divisional hospitals, Community Health Centers, Primary Health Centers, and Sub-centers. As per the information available, 734 district hospitals are present in India. However, some of the medical college hospitals or a sub-divisional hospital are found to serve as a district hospital where a district hospital as such (particularly the newly created district) has not been established. Few districts have also more than one district hospital. The overall objectives of district hospitals are:

- To provide comprehensive secondary health care (specialist and referral services) to the community through the district hospital.
- To achieve and maintain an acceptable standard of quality of care.
- To make the services more responsive and sensitive to the needs of the people of the district and the hospitals/centers from which the cases are referred to the district hospitals.

Health Insurance

There is no universal health insurance in India. Health Insurance is at present limited to industrial workers and their families.

- **Employees State Insurance Scheme:** It was introduced by an act of parliament in 1948. It covers employees drawing wages not exceeding Rs. 10,000 per month.
- **Central Government Health Scheme:** This scheme was introduced in New Delhi in 1954 to provide comprehensive medical care to Central Government employees. The schemes are based on the principles of a cooperative effort by the employee and the mutual advantage of both.

Other Agencies

- **Defence Medical Services**: Defence services have their organization for medical care to defense personnel under the banner Armed Forces Medical Services. The services provided are integrated and comprehensive.
- **Health Care of Railway Employees**: The Railways provide comprehensive health care services through the agencies of Railway Hospitals, Health Units, and Clinics.

Private Health Sector

In a mixed economy such as India's, private practice of medicine provides a large share of the health services available. There has been a rapid expansion in the number of qualified allopathic physicians to 7.5 lakhs in 2005; and the doctor population ratio is 1:1428. Most of them concentrate in urban areas. They provide mainly curative services. Their services are available to those who can pay. The private sector of health care services is not organized.

Indigenous Systems of Medicine

The practitioners of the indigenous systems of medicine provide the bulk of medical care to rural people. Ayurvedic physicians alone are estimated to be about 4.5 lakhs. Nearly 90% of ayurvedic physicians serve rural areas. To promote these indigenous systems, Indian government established Central Council of Indian Medicine in 1971. AYUSH is the new approach to this which encompasses Ayurveda, Yoga, Unani, Siddha, and Homeopathy.

Voluntary Health Agencies

A voluntary health agency may be defined as an organization that is administered by an autonomous board that holds meetings, collects funds for its support chiefly from private sources and expends money, whether with or without paid workers, in conducting a program directed primarily to promote public health by providing health services or health education or by advancing research or legislation for health, or by a combination of these activities. The voluntary health agencies in India are:

- Indian Red Cross Society
- Hind Kusht Nivaran Sangh

- Indian Council for Child Welfare
- Tuberculosis Association of India
- Bharat Sevak Samaj
- Central Social Welfare Board
- The Kasturba Memorial Fund

National Health Programs

Since India became free, several measures have been undertaken by the National Government to improve the health of the people. Prominent among these measures is the National Health Program which has been launched by the Central Government for control/eradication of communicable diseases, improvement of environmental sanitation, raising the standard of nutrition, control of the population and improving rural health. Various international agencies like World Health Organization (WHO), United Nations Children's Fund (UNICEF), The United Nations Population Fund (UNFPA), etc. have been providing technical and material assistance in the implementation of these programs.

NURSING SERVICES

Organization and Functions of Nursing Services

Nursing service administration is a complex of elements in interaction. It results in the output of clients whose health is unavoidably deteriorating, maintained or improved through the input of personnel and material resources used in an orderly process of nursing services. Nursing Service Administration is the system of activities directed toward the nursing care of patients and includes the establishment of overall goals and policies within the aims of health agency and provision for the organization, personnel, and facilities to accomplish these goals most effectively and economically through cooperative efforts of all members of the staff coordinating the services with other departments of the administration.

AIMS of Nursing Service Administration

The criteria for a well-organized Nursing service listed in 1965 by The National League for Nursing are the following:

- **A written statement:** Of the Philosophy, Purpose, and Objectives of the Nursing services.
- **A plan of organization:** Commonly diagrammed as an organization chart, the plan indicates areas of responsibility, to whom and for whom each person is accountable, and the major channels of formal communication.
- **Policy and administrative manuals:** Policies are established for the operation of the hospital and within the department to guide the nursing staff.

- **Nursing practice manual:** Written procedures are available as evidence standards of performance and have been established for safe, effective care, taking into consideration the best use of available resources and personnel.
- **Nursing service budget:** This is a statement of plans for the nursing service expressed in accounting terms.
- **A master staffing pattern:** This helps the director of the nursing service to visualize the equitable distribution of nursing personnel among the various nursing units.
- **Plans for appraisal of nursing:** In addition to the provision of supervision, there are one or more techniques for the continuous evaluation of nursing care such as ward conferences, nursing rounds, analysis of accident reports, patient and employee opinion polls, and the nursing audit.
- **Advisory committees:** Membership on standing committees provide for the active participation of staff members in problem-solving.
- **Adequate facilities, supplies, and equipment:** The director of nursing or his/her representative evaluates periodically the adequacy of facilities in terms of patient and personnel needs.
- **Written job descriptions and job specifications:** Help prevent duplication of functions.
- **Health services:** The plan of health care for employees is set.
- **In-service education of nursing personnel:** Programs are conducted that provide orientation to help the new employee adjust to a new environment and duties.

Planning and Organizing Nursing Service at Various Levels—Local, Regional, National, and International

A high power committee on nursing and nursing profession was set up by the Government of India in July 1987 under the chairmanship of Smt. Sarojini Vasadapan, an eminent social worker and former chairperson of Central Social Welfare Board with Smt. Rajkumari Sood, Nursing Advisor to Government of India, as the member secretary. The terms of reference of the committee were as follows:

- Looking into the existing working conditions of nurses with particular reference to the status of the nursing care services both in rural and urban areas
- To study and recommend the staffing norms necessary for providing adequate nursing personnel to give the best possible care, both in the hospitals and community
- To look into the training of all categories and levels of nursing, midwifery personnel to meet the nursing manpower needs at all levels of health service and education
- To study and clarify the role of nursing personnel in the healthcare delivery system including their interaction with other members of the health team at every level of health services management

- To examine the need for organization of the nursing services at the national, state, district, and lower levels with particular reference to the need for planning and implementing the comprehensive nursing care services with the overall healthcare system of the country at their respective levels
- To look into all other aspects which the committee may consider relevant concerning their terms of reference
- While considering the various issues under the above norms of reference, the committee will hold consultations with the state governments

Their recommendations on the organization of nursing services at central, state and district levels, and the norms of nursing service and education are given as follows.

- **Placement of nurses at the central level:** At the central level, there is a post of nursing advisor in the medical division of Directorate General of Health Services. The nursing advisor is directly responsible to the Deputy Director General (Medical). The nursing advisor is assisted by nursing officers and support staff for all his/her work. He/she advises the DGHS, Ministry of Health and Family Welfare as well as other ministries and departments, for example, railways, labor, Delhi Administration, etc. on all matters of nursing services, nursing education, and research. The nursing advisor also takes care of administrative aspects of Raj Kumari Amrit Kaur College of Nursing and Lady Hardinge Health School, Delhi. There is a post of deputy nursing advisor at the rank of Assistant Director General (ADG-Nsg) in the training division of Department of F. W. Presently the deputy nursing advisor deals with the training of ANMs, dais, health supervisor, etc. There is no direct linkage between the nursing advisor and deputy nursing advisor as they are independent posts (Table 1).
- **Placement of nurses at the state level:** There is no proper and definite pattern of nursing structure in the state directorates except the state of West Bengal. Usually, one or two nurses are posted with varying designations, e.g., in Tamil Nadu, there is one assistant director nursing who is responsible to Director, Medical Services, and Director, Medical Education. In Maharashtra, two nurses work, one each in the office of the Director of Medical Education, and Director of Health Services (Table 2).
- **Placement of nurses at the district level:** Nurses, public health nurses, lady health visitors, auxiliary nurse midwives, etc. have played a vital role in providing healthcare services at various levels in both urban and rural areas of the district. They have been the mainstream in providing primary healthcare services in the rural and urban areas from the very beginning. Today, the ANM designated as a multipurpose health worker is the key health worker rendering multipurpose healthcare services in rural areas. In this context, the professional nurses have a major role to play in providing support, guidance, supervision to ANMs

Multi Purpose Health Worker-Female (MPHW-F) and also in rendering direct comprehensive healthcare services that are beyond the competency of the ANMs (Table 3).

TABLE 1: Organization of nursing services at center level

DGHS		
Additional DG	Additional DG (N)	Additional DG
	Deputy DG (N)	
Assistant Director General (ADG) (Community Nursing Service)	Assistant Director General (ADG) (Nursing Education and Research)	Assistant Director General (ADG) (Hospital Nursing Service)
Deputy Assistant Director General (DADG)	Deputy Assistant Director General (DADG)	Deputy Assistant Director General (DADG)
Community Nursing Director	Principal tutor SON	Nursing Superintendent
PHN Supervisor	Senior tutor	Deputy Nursing Superintendent
PHN	Tutor	Assistant Nursing Superintendent
LHV	Clinical instructors	Ward sister
ANM	--------	Staff nurse

Note:
- The positions up to the DADG level are proposed to be at the office of the directorate general of health services. Positions below the level of DADG are to exist at the institutions governed by the central government.
- The principal of the College of Nursing will be equal to the rank of ADAG (N) and will be eligible for promotion to the post of DDG (N) and DG (N).

TABLE 2: Recommended organization at the state level for nursing services (union territory level)

Secretary (Health)		
Director, Nursing Services		
Joint Director, Nursing Services		
ADNS (Community Nursing Service)	ADNS (Nursing Education and Research)	ADNS (Hospital Nursing Service)
DADNS	DADNS	DADNS
District Nursing Officer	Principal SON	Nursing Superintendent
Public Health Nurse	Senior tutor	Deputy Nursing Superintendent
PHN at PHC	Tutor	Assistant Nursing Superintendent
LHV	Clinical instructors	Ward sister
ANM	--------	Staff nurse

Note: The Principal, College of Nursing will be equal to the rank of ADNS and will be eligible for promotion to the post of DDNS/DNS. The salary scales and structure of the staff of colleges of nursing will be as per norms of the Indian Nursing Council and the UGC.

Nursing Management and Leadership

TABLE 3: Recommended organization at the district level for nursing services

Director, Nursing Services	
Dy. Director, Nursing Services	
Asst. Director, Nursing Services	
Dy. Asst. Director, Nursing Services	
District nursing officer	
Assistant Dist. Nsg. Officer (Hosp. and Nsg. Edu)	Assistant Dist. Nsg. Officer (Community)
Nsg. Superintendent/Dy. Nsg. Suptd.	Dist. P. N. O.
Asst. Nsg. Supt.	P. N. Supervisor (CHC)
Ward sister	PN (PHC)
Staff nurse	LHV/HS
----------	ANM

The above recommended organizational set up needs the full administrative and financial support of the government. It looks after the overall nursing components, development of nursing standards, norms, policies, ethics, recruitment, selection and placement roles for both hospitals and community health nursing, development in specialty nursing, higher education in nursing, and research. These promote professional autonomy and accountability. The purpose of health administration at the center and local level is to improve the health status of the population. The scope of health services varies widely from country to country and is influenced by general and ever-changing national, state, and local health problems.

CURRENT TRENDS AND ISSUES IN NURSING

Nursing is one of the oldest arts but has recently developed into a profession. From the beginning, it has undergone many drastic modifications and updations, and currently, it is an unavoidable part of society. The recent trend analysis shows that future nursing will see significant advantages in multidimensional patient care, including promotive and preventive health. Nurses will be the most preferred healthcare providers in the coming time though there are challenges such as ethical considerations, rising health care costs, and quality of care. Healthier lifestyles, promotive environments, and continuity of quality care based on EBP are highlighted in nursing.

Nursing has a gigantic ability to change individuals. These requests require a broad learning base and essential reasoning capacities alongside able aptitudes. The focal point of nursing is moving towards perceiving patients as cooperative recipients as opposed to uninvolved beneficiaries of health care. Professional nursing is comprehensive as he/she will be effectively engaged with direct supervision, educating health care aspects, home care management, and OPD consultation.

The nursing profession continues to be challenged and rewarded by both new and changing opportunities and constraints, for all nurses, individually and collectively. Several forces that have affected the development of professional nursing and continue to affect significant issues, these include:

- Societal images and expectations of nurses
- Degree of the nursing profession's control over the quantity and quality of practitioners
- Impact of technology and theory on nursing practices, roles, and settings
- The professional self-image of nurses
- Sources of financing for health care services

Current Trends in Nursing in India

- **Reduction in the distance:** The introduction of modern communication techniques such as mobile phone, email, video conferencing has reduced the gap between patients and health care professionals/care providers. The introduction of different mobile applications has made the health care consultation available at the fingertips.
- **Computerization of patient care:** Gone are the days of manual data maintenance. The introduction of computer-based applications in the health care organizations has made the patient data digital from Outpatient Department (OPD) consultation/Admission to discharge and follow up. It includes computerized record-keeping, sharing of intra, and interdepartmental information about a patient (lab results, diagnostic reports, medical and surgical requirements). It also includes management and organizational aspects of an organization such as employee attendance, inventory management, inter-department communication, and so on.
- **Quality assurance in nursing:** In the changing health care environment, concerns over the quality of care are receiving more considerable attention than ever before. As consumers become more knowledgeable as a result of increased information available to them, much of the mystique surrounding health care is being dissipated.
- **Decentralized approach:** This approach makes the nurse accountable for the care of the allotted patient. It is appreciable and effective as it focuses on the satisfaction of the patient, quality of the health care, and smooth functioning of the department.
- **Continuing Nursing Education (CNE):** It is aimed at the motivation of the workers and to build up their skills and capacities according to their respective current/future designations. The health care system is highly dynamic, and it is imperative for a nurse to keep abreast of the changes. It can be achieved through attending conferences, seminars, workshops, presenting scientific papers, and so on. Generally, CNE should be regularly organized by educational and health care organizations.

- **Evidence-based Practice (EBP):** Nurses today should have a scientific bent of mind and a dynamic approach to patient care. Intensified researches and the application of the research findings in the clinical setting are yet another challenge.

Trends in Nursing Education

Currently, nursing is focused on Problem-based learning (PBL) and Evidence Based Practice (EBP) grounded with nursing research. Earlier the entry-level of profession was certificate level and diploma level. The specialization programs in nursing education are symbolical to this trend growth. Currently, in India, there are several educational programs such as;

- **Auxiliary Nurse Midwife (ANM)** is a two-year diploma program.
- **General Nursing and Midwifery (GNM)** is a 3-year diploma program in nursing.
- **BSc Nursing** is four years Bachelor's degree program
- **PBBSc (Post Basic BSc Nursing)** is two years additional qualification program offered to candidates after passing GNM.
- **MSc Nursing** is a master's degree program offered to candidates after successful completion of BSc(N)/PB BSc(N). Currently, MSc Nursing is offered in following specialties:
  - Medical Surgical Nursing
  - Child Health Nursing
  - Mental Health Nursing
  - Obstetrical and Gynecological Nursing
  - Community Health Nursing
  - Forensic Nursing
- **MPhil** is an additional qualification with a duration of 2 years.
- **PhD** is an additional qualification with a duration of 3–5 years. Some of the famous Universities currently offering PhD. Programs in Nursing are given below:
  - National Consortium for PhD in Nursing: Collaboration of Indian Nursing Council, New Delhi with Rajiv Gandhi University of Health Sciences, Bengaluru, Karnataka
  - All India Institute of Medical Sciences (AIIMS)
  - Jawaharlal Institute of Post Graduate Medical Education and Research (JIPMER), Pondicherry
  - Bharati Vidyapeeth Deemed University, Pune.
  - Dr D Y Patil University, Pune
  - Dr MGR Medical University, Chennai
  - SNDT University, Mumbai
  - Punjab University, Chandigarh
  - Baba Farid University of Health Sciences, Faridkot, Punjab
  - Manipal University
  - SRM University
  - Amity University

- Mahatma Gandhi Mission Institute of Health Sciences, Mumbai.
- **PG Diploma Courses:** Currently PG diploma courses are offered in following specialties:
  - Post Basic Diploma in Neonatal Nursing
  - Post Basic Diploma in Neurology Nursing
  - Post Basic Diploma in Psychiatric Nursing
  - Post Basic Diploma in Cardio-Thoracic Nursing
  - Post Basic Diploma in Orthopedic and Rehabilitation Nursing
  - Post Basic Diploma in Operation Room Nursing
  - Post Basic Diploma in Critical Care Nursing
  - Post Basic Diploma in Emergency and Disaster Nursing
  - Post Basic Diploma in Forensic Nursing
  - Post Basic Diploma in Geriatric Nursing
  - Post Basic Diploma in Oncology Nursing
  - Post Basic Diploma in Pediatric Nursing

The recent launch of Nurse Practitioner in Critical Care program by the Indian Nursing Council allows the graduate nurses to assume responsibility and accountability to provide competent care to critically ill patients and appropriate family care in tertiary care centers. On the contrary, the increasing demands of healthcare needs cause-specific issues in Nursing. A few of the problems faced by the nursing education are compromised students, the gap of theory and practice, underutilization of clinical facilities, inadequate facilities in educational institutions, lack of qualified teachers, and overall compromised education system.

The nursing service industry faces challenges such as compromised working conditions, biased staffing patterns, fewer wages, lack of practice guidelines, lack of proper research, and deficient in-service education programs. Most of the time, nurses need to focus on routine administrative/paperwork rather than bedside care.

Since the Nightingale era of nursing practice, the nursing profession has undergone numerous changes, and many faces have been responsible for this noble cause. From time to time, nurses have tried to develop better methods to cater the needs of the patient and his/her family. Certainly, the scientific knowledge and clinical expertise of nurses will result in better nursing care of patients. Being a dynamic profession, nursing accounts for several trends. Experimental and Evidence-based knowledge forms a strong base for the nursing profession like any other profession, and this knowledge creates innovations in nursing. The simple meaning of the trend is 'development in a specific course'. These trends are the cornerstones of the nursing profession for its dynamic nature.

Curriculum Innovations in Nursing Education

Nursing educational programs and its curricula are competencies put together, and it centers with respect to result and stress student support and obligation regarding learning. Accrediting bodies reexamine the educational program of nursing education every once in a while. Here the Indian Nursing Council, the autonomous body under the Ministry of Health and Family Welfare, responsible for uniformity of nursing education across the country, has made the following modification in the curriculum of different nursing programs in recent years.

- Revised the syllabus of the Auxiliary Nursing and Midwifery (ANM) course in 2006-07.
- Revised the syllabus of General Nursing and Midwifery (GNM) in the year 2005-2006. The course duration was extended to 3.5 years (including six months of internship).
- Revised syllabus for BSc Nursing and Post Basic BSc. Nursing was implemented from 2005-2006 in all Indian Universities. The syllabus revision was made in tune with the National Health Policy 2002.
- A national consortium for PhD in Nursing was constituted by Indian Nursing Council (INC) in collaboration with Rajiv Gandhi University of Health Sciences, Karnataka in the year 2005.

Technology and Nursing

- **Nursing informatics:** It empowers nurses to achieve good patient-centered health care. Nursing Informatics is defined as "science and practice (that) integrates nursing, its information, and knowledge, with the management of information and communication technologies to promote the health of people, families, and communities worldwide." (Amia.org, 2015).
- **Simulations in nursing education:** Simulation is the "process of designing a model of a real system and conducting experiments with this model for either understanding the behavior of the system and/or evaluating various strategies for the operation of the system" (Bradshaw and Lowenstein, 2009).
- **Technology and nursing education:** Technology influences nursing education to a greater extent, and it is an essential part of the teaching and learning process. The use of computers in patient management and student management have become common. The use of LCD projectors, smart classrooms, computer-based simulation models is now widely used by nursing teachers to educate nursing students. Students are familiar with the use of computers, smartphones, and different computer/mobile-based applications for learning and reading. The quality of nursing research increases with greater access to literature through the internet.
- **Animations and cinematic technology:** Animations are now widely used to enhance the learning experience. Video-assisted teachings with the help of animation for nursing procedures, physical examination, breath sounds, and stages of labor can be made clear and thorough with the help of this visual learning technologies.

Student's Population

- **Male nurses:** Nursing was predominantly considered as a female profession, especially in India. In recent decades, the trend is changing, and the numbers of male nurses have increased significantly.
- **Changing the demography of nursing students:** In earlier days, nursing care was provided by nuns, and many of the major hospitals were established by missionaries. Present-day nursing students represent a diverse population in terms of gender, age, and socioeconomic status.

Clinical Teaching-Learning Process

- **Evidence-based practice:** Evidence-based Practice (EBP) is defined as "a problem-solving approach to clinical care that incorporates the conscientious use of current best evidence from well-designed studies, a clinician's expertise, and patient values and preferences" (Fineout-Overholt, Melnyk and Schultz, 2005). Incorporating research-based evidence in nursing education enhances evidence-based practice. The quality of nursing practices improves in a more significant form by using evidence-based practices (D'Souza et al., 2014).
- **Advanced clinical, nursing education:** Apart from being care provider nurses perform independent roles like Nurse Specialist, Nurse-Midwifery Practitioner, and Nurse Anesthetist.
- **Supervised training by nurse educators:** According to INC standards, the teacher-student proportion is 1: 10. This guarantees the robust supervision of each student. Nursing institutions endeavor toward improving the clinical learning process. Teacher- practitioner model and faculty-student practice clinic are two newer concepts in clinical training.
- **Clinical instruction—training the trainers:** Over some time, more emphasis is given on clinical nursing education. Nursing faculty is now taking up responsibility and accountability of patient care, and they acknowledge the fact that clinical exposure of the student does not mean the clinical practice/learning. To overcome this dilemma faced by novice as well as experienced faculty, now clinical teaching is given more emphasis and training of all nursing faculty in the clinical area is mandatory in Indian settings.

Evaluation System

In recent years, the nursing education and its evaluation is brought under regulatory bodies. All the diploma courses are evaluated by the respective state nursing council or examination boards constituted by the respective State Governments. All the programs that are at the graduate level and above are reviewed by the Universities that are recognized by the University Grant Commission (UGC). Additionally, innovative evaluation methods, such as Objective Structured Clinical Evaluation' (OSCE), Rubrics, are now widely being used in nursing education.

Quality Assurance

Quality assurance is an inevitable part of every education system, especially nursing education. The emerging trends and scope of nursing give a flourishing stage of growth, and thus, it also tempts for dilution of the quality. Quality is the process of monitoring and evaluating the efficiency of the system. Accrediting agencies like International Organization for Standardization (ISO) has taken the initiative of accrediting colleges of nursing in India.

Knowledge Expansion

The last decade had witnessed a significant expansion in nursing literature. The CINAHL (Cumulated Index for Nursing and Allied Health Literature), Cochrane, PubMed databases serve as an excellent treasure for nurses and nursing students. Research has become a substantial area in the curriculum. Action research and the use of qualitative methodologies in research are getting full acceptance now.

Modes of Education

The recent trends in education such as distance education, E-learning/Online Education have brought about professional upgradation in the form of continuing nursing education and different certification programs. Many Universities in the world offer these courses. Few of them are IGNOU, Stanford, and so on. The programs that are offered through these modes are accelerated RN program, LPN to RN, and many other certifications and short term courses.

Trends are a kind of change that takes place and become vogue. The technological changes, changes in demographics, and health patterns have contributed to various trends in nursing education*.

Challenges in Nursing Education

- Independent Infrastructure for Nursing college
- Independence for Principal
- Acute Shortage of Qualified Teaching Professionals
- Lack of UGC status
- Underutilization of Clinical facilities
- Academic dishonesty
- Lack of discipline
- Workplace violence
- Student voices

TRENDS IN NURSING RESEARCH

Today almost all nursing leaders and nursing organizations offer rewards to professional nurses for doing nursing research. Research opportunities and needs await interested

*(Reference: Research article: Renjith Vishnu, G Renu and George Anice. (2015). Trends in Nursing Education. Indian Journal of Applied Research. 5. 496-498.)

professionals in nursing. To fulfill their professional obligations in the health care delivery system, nurses have to keep the following objective in mind

- Nursing research will be a core part of nursing education and nursing care service.
- Nursing practice will accomplish an environment equal to the evaluation of professional practice.

Challenges in Nursing Research

- Funding
- Acceptance from superiors
- Scarcity of resources
- Availability of nurse (nursing) expertise
- Appropriate research setting
- Non-availability of nursing research program

ISSUES AFFECTING NURSING PRACTICE

- **Demographical changes:** It includes the increased occurrence of illness at a younger age, increased poverty, lack of outreach of immunization and nutritional programs, compromised sanitation, cultural diversity, urbanization, etc.
  - Many older persons are healthy, but the likelihood of illness becomes more significant as age increases. It indicates that the nurse of the future should be equipped to work with the aged population.
  - Several people in our country and abroad are still living under the poverty line. For them, the priorities are focused on food, clothing, and shelter. Health care is always a luxury for them.
  - Immunization of children and pregnant women, provision of nutritious meals and other health maintaining aspects are still neglected though we have made some progress in it.
  - Preventive health care is not often focused. This is due to lack of education, increased population density, lack of sanitation and waste management techniques, etc.
  - The nursing profession is committed to provide care for people irrespective of sociocultural and economic factors. The cultural beliefs and practices of citizens are quite different. The nurse needs to understand these differences while planning the care.
  - Urbanization is a common phenomenon in society. People prefer to move from rural areas to the city. It causes many social issues such as homelessness, drugs, mental illness, violence, and crime. Nurses of the future should be equipped to confront health problems related to it.
- **Environmental changes:** They include issues such as natural as well as human-made calamities, pollution, overpopulation, etc. Major ecological tragedies such as nuclear power plant accidents, burning oil wells, tsunamis,

gradual decline in the purity of water, diminishing animal, and plant life lead to health problems. These are issues that the future nurse has to face.

- **Change in healthy practices:** Factors such as obesity, food habits, lack of exercise, stress, etc. Obesity is a significant reason causing risk for many illnesses among people. It contributes to hypertension, diabetes mellitus, Poly Cystic Ovarian Disease (PCOD), coronary artery diseases, cardiac abnormalities, and so on. The lifestyle and health habits such as sexual life, smoking/alcoholism habits contribute to HIV/AIDS, lung cancer, and liver diseases. In these conditions, nurses will have to play predominantly essential functions in educating the public regarding the health hazards of these lifestyles.

- **Emerging bioethical issues:** The ethical considerations such as prevention of conception, termination of pregnancy, fetal surgery, organ transplantation, genetic research, fetal research, selection between life and death, etc.

  - Issues such as prevention of conception, termination of pregnancy, test-tube conception, other artificial fertilization (artificial insemination, IVF) and contraception methods contribute to emotional changes in people.

  - The ethical considerations in this regard must be weighed against its outcome.

  - Issues related to life or death including the invention of life-saving apparatuses such as dialysis, ventilator, heart and the lung machine, new surgical procedures (organ transplant, fetal surgery) and new technologies (genetic research, fetal research) have all become necessary to redefine the terms of life and death.

- **Degree versus diploma for practice:** One of the major concerns in India is the lack of policies about nursing practice and the required professional training for intended designation. The distinction between the level of qualification and level of entry in service should be clearly defined. Recently, an attempt is made by the Govt. of India and Indian Nursing Council, adopting a policy to discontinue GNM (General Nursing and Midwifery),

and the level of entry to a health care organization as the nursing officer will be based on the graduation. (BSc Nursing/PBBSc Nursing).

- **Specialization in clinical area:** Currently, there are five clinical specializations in nursing education in India. The expanded role of the nurse based on these specializations is not in practice. The necessary policy and legal formulations have not yet been framed in this regard. Although few innovations in this regard have taken place in recent years such as the introduction of Nurse Practitioners in Critical Care, it is still in the primitive stage.

- **Nursing care standards:** Standards are "written formal statements" to describe how an organization or professional should deliver health service and are guidelines against which services can be assessed. Standards are directed at the structure, proces's, and outcome issues and guide the review of systems function, staff performance, and client care. The nurse has to be scientifically equipped for meeting the caring standards of patient's expectations.

- **Nurse patient ratio:** Staffing is an issue of both professional and personal concerns for nurses today. If staffing is inadequate, nurses contend and it further threatens patient's health and safety, results in greater complexity of care, and impacts their health and safety by increasing fatigue and rate of injury.

- **Long working hours:** Nurses are often required to work in long shifts. But in several cases, nurses have to work back-to-back or extended shifts. This work schedule makes them fatigued, and that could result in medical mistakes.

- **Workplace hazards:** Nurses face several workplace hazards each day while just doing their jobs. These hazards include exposure to bloodborne pathogens, injuries, and hand washing-related dermatitis and cold and flu germs.

The transition is a universal phenomenon, and nurses involved in the caring profession have to undergo it. Some techniques such as positive thinking, flexibility, organized and healthy personal life, and ideal mentor can help in the process of transition.

REVIEW QUESTIONS

1. Define health administration.
2. Explain the health administration system in India.
3. What are the agents of health care administration?
4. Explain current trends and issues in nursing.
5. Discuss the principles of health administration.

Further Readings

1. Park K. Preventive and Social Medicine, 19th Edition: M/s. Banarasidas Bhanot Publishers, Jabalpur, 2007.
2. Goel SL. Healthcare System, and Its Management, Health Organization and Structure, 1st Volume, Deep and Deep Publishers, New Delhi; 2001.
3. Basavanthappa BT. Nursing Administration, 2nd Edition: Jaypee Brothers Medical Publishers (P) Ltd., New Delhi; 2008.
4. Goel SL, Kumar R. Management of Hospitals – Hospital Administration in the 21st century, Vol. 4, Deep and Deep Publication, New Delhi; 2002.
5. Ranga Rao SP. Administration of Primary Health Centers in India, 1st Edition: Mittal Publications, New Delhi; 1993.
6. Lucita M. Nursing: Practice and Public Health Administration. Current Concepts and Trends. B. I. Churchill Living Stone Pvt. Ltd., New Delhi; 2002.

Unit
2

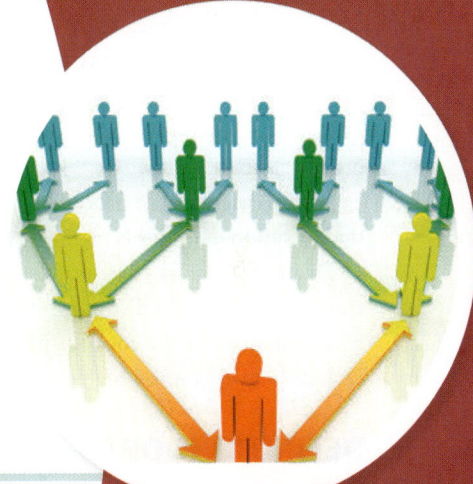

Management Basics Applied to Nursing and Management Process

Unit Outline

- ➡ Definitions of Management
- ➡ Definitions of Administration
- ➡ Levels of Management
- ➡ Management and Administration
- ➡ Nursing Management
- ➡ Nature of Administration
- ➡ Theories of Management
- ➡ Functions of Management (Management Process)
- ➡ Principles of Management
- ➡ Nurse Manager

INTRODUCTION

Management is a common term in our day to day life. Since the beginning of formation of groups among human beings to achieve those objectives that they could not achieve individually, managing has been essential to ensure the coordination of individual efforts. The word administer is derived from the Latin word "ad+ ministraire," which means to care for or to look after or to manage the affairs of the people.

Most of the time, words such as administration, management, and organization seem synonymous, but they are distinct in their meanings.

Administration is primarily the process of planning and stabilizing the broad lines of principles that govern action. The general lines are referred to as policies upon which the organization functions.

Management is the process or the agency through which the execution of policy is planned and supervised.

Organization is the process of dividing work into convenient tasks and duties. It includes a grouping of responsibilities in the form of posts, delegating authority to each job and appointing staff to perform that work as planned.

DEFINITIONS OF MANAGEMENT

"Management has been defined as the creation and maintenance of the internal environment in an enterprise where individuals working together in groups can perform efficiently and towards the attainment of group goals."

—Koontz and O'Donnell

"Management may be defined as the art of applying the environmental principles that underline the control of men and material in the enterprise under consideration."

—Kimball and Kimball

Management is defined as the art of securing maximum results with a minimum of effort to guarantee maximum prosperity and happiness for both employer and employee and give the public the best possible service. **—John Mee, 1963**

Management is a generic function that encompasses related essential duties in every field and civilization. Sometimes management and administration seem to be similar terms, but they are not so, though they are interdependent. Management is the other part of the same coin if we regard administration as one side of the coin. To transform any strategy into practice, individuals need an organizational structure. When there is a framework; there are some tasks to be done to achieve objectives, which is the operational element of the organization, and the management is responsible for it.

Distinct Meanings of the Management

- **Management as a discipline:** Discipline is a study with certain concepts and principles. Management when considered as a discipline; consists of many laws, ideas, and thoughts and it helps in the process of managing. From this point of view, management can be treated either as an art or science.
- **Management as a group of people:** Management is a group of people who performs the functions of a manager in the organization. The relationship between manager and labor in an organization may be compared to the relationship between people who are responsible for managerial tasks and those who are included in non-managerial personnel.
- **Management as a process:** It is considered as a process when there is a systematic method of handling activities. The process of management is complicated as it is the concept by which the flow of information is passed through different stages of analysis. The passing of tasks and information is regarded as the process of an organization. These tasks ultimately contribute to the achievement of desired goals.

DEFINITIONS OF ADMINISTRATION

The administration is the direction, coordination, and control of many people to achieve some purposes or objectives.

—Pfiffner and Prethus

The administration has to do with getting things done; with the accomplishment of defined objectives.

—Luther Gullick

The administration is the activities of the groups cooperating to accomplish common goals. **—Herbert A Simon**

Philosophy of Administration

What does a Philosophy need to do?
- Sharp focus-integrated elements, the system of a proper and unified relationship
- Principles are developed-valid guidelines for the future
- Both ends and means
- Provide a reliable tool to the executives
- Communicate spirit and rounded feelings and satisfaction

The administration is a moral act and also a moral agent. The philosophy of administration should be conceived in such a way that if not described relatively and provides a reliable tool to the executive, it constitutes a total that exceeds the sum of its parts.

- The administration believes in **cost-effectiveness:** In the management or administration of any enterprises or the organization, the quantity, the quality, timing and cost of the work necessary to reach the objectives of the enterprises are interrelated factors that must be given constant attention. If the resources of health work, in trained persons and finances, were unlimited, the need for constant attention to these factors would not be so great. But the limitation in the number of trained personnel and the lack of adequate financial resources are major obstacles to greatly improved health in the world today.

- The administration believes in **execution and control of work plans:** One of the greatest possible contributors to wastage of our precious resources, whether at the local or national level, is the failure of those at any level of administration, and at all stages in the management of the activity, to base all decision on verifiable facts.

- The administration believes in the **delegation of responsibility and authority:** The delegation of responsibility and authority is an important aspect of successful administration, to place the responsibility for decision at the lowest possible organizational level to attain decision as speedily as possible. No administration can do in detail all the work he is administering for; by definition of an administration manager the work of others. The responsibility and authority placed in each position must correspond to the responsibility which the position carries.

- The administration believes in **human relations and good morale:** The function of administration is to attain an established objective through the management of people, administration if deeply concerned with human relations. Good morale of the staff is essential to the success of any understanding and the morale is affected by both financial and non-financial factors.

- The administration believes **in effective communication:** Effective communications are essential for all aspects of effective administration. Staff must be adequately and correctly informed about plans, methods, schedules, problems, events and progress. The necessary instructions, knowledge, and information should be present to rule out any misinterpretations or misunderstandings. Proper and adequate communication is not just in one direction, it requires two-way passages. Communication must follow from the bottom to upwards as well as top to bottom.

Purposes of Administration

- Accomplishing the goals of the organization
- Maintaining the quality of service/ care within the financial limitations of the organization
- Encouraging the motivation of the employees and the clients in the area
- Increasing the ability of subordinates and peers to accept change
- Developing a team spirit and increased morale.
- Furthering the professional development of the personnel.

Scope of Administration

The scope of administration must then recognize the administration. The main form of applied administration based on its major functions is as follows:

- The political function of the administration includes the executive-legislative relationship, political-administrative activities of the cabinet or ministry and so on.

- The legislative function includes not merely delegated legislation, but the preparatory work done by the administrative officials and departments in connection with the drawing up of the bill to be introduced in the legislature and its passage through that body.

- The financial function includes the whole of financial administration from the preparation of the budget to its execution, accounting, audit, treasury, management.

- The defensive function covers the military administration.

- Educational function relates to educational administration in its broadest sense.

- Social administration includes the activities of the departments concerned with food, housing, health, social security, employment.

- Economic administration is concerned with the vast field of administration activities relating to protection and encouragement industries and agriculture, securing a prosperous and stable economy, encouragement and promotion of trade and commerce, and so on.

- Foreign administration includes the conduct of foreign affairs diplomacy, international cooperation, administration of the international agencies of various kinds, etc.

- Imperial administration covers the problems and techniques arising from the rules of one person or nation over another.

- Local administration is concerned with the activities of the local bodies.

LEVELS OF MANAGEMENT

There are three levels of management, top, middle and lower management (Fig. 1).

1. **Top/upper management:** Responsible for planning the process of execution. It thus provides a framework within which the entire enterprise works. Senior management is responsible for providing leadership, guidance, and supervision.

2. **Middle management:** Responsible for administrative work at the second tier, which certainly functions as the second-order to the top management.

3. **Lower level management:** Responsible for the execution of the plans, policies, and programs like the middle management. This level is directly involved in the operation of the job while the middle order management, the second tier, is indirectly responsible for execution.

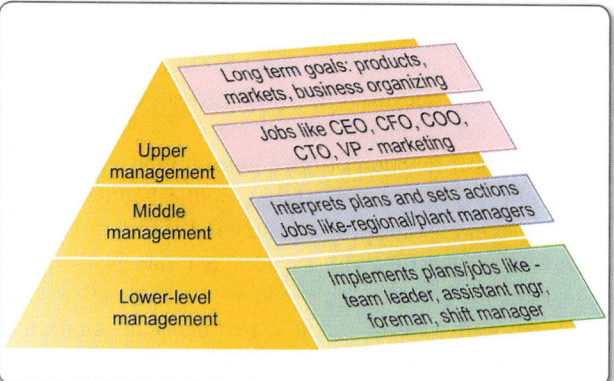

Fig. 1: Levels of management

MANAGEMENT AND ADMINISTRATION

Most often the two words management and administration are used interchangeably and synonymically even though they are different in terms of practice. According to Sukhothai Thammathirat Open University, Thailand, management is a term usually practiced in the private sector whereas administration is a word that is practiced in the public sector. Derek French and Heather Saward (authors of Dictionary of Management) supported this idea as management/administration is an act of acquiring the expected goal/objective.

According to Michel A Hitt (an American economist), management has a wider perspective comparing to administration. According to him, management involves the integration of resources to acquire the organizational goals based on four principles mentioned below and it is middle-level operation.

- Objectives
- Effectiveness
- Integration/Coordination
- Resources

Most of the time, administration is referred to as an executive-level of management.

NURSING MANAGEMENT

It is the process of working through nursing personnel to promote and maintain health, prevent illness and suffering. The role of the nurse manager is to plan, organize, direct, and control available resources to provide adequate economic care to groups of clients.

In reality, the management process is more complicated than the nursing process as it directly deals with the management of working with human beings, physical resources, organizational and psychological processes within a creative and innovative climate for the realization of organizational goals.

So, management is a dynamic process that is universal and can be used in a variety of settings and situations. Henry Fayol (1925) first identified the functions of management as:

- Planning
- Organization
- Command
- Control
- Coordination

Later, Luther Gullick (1937) added two more activities, namely Staffing and Directing. Hence, the services of management now include Planning, Organizing, Staffing, Directing, Coordinating, Reporting, and Budgeting (POSD-CORB). These were again reorganized by clubbing reporting and coordinating under the component of control.

NATURE OF ADMINISTRATION

Nature of Administration
- Universal
- Holistic
- It is intangible
- Continuous and Ongoing
- Goal oriented
- Social and Human
- Dynamic
- Creative or Innovative

- **It is universal:** because irrespective of nature and objectives of the organization, all essential elements of administration such as planning, organizing, staffing, directing, coordinating, reporting, budgeting can apply and contribute to the achievement of goals.
- **It is holistic:** the whole process of the administration considers the organization as a whole, and the developmental activities towards the growth of the organization are performed accordingly. The holistic administration considers all the members of the organization equally, and it also takes into account the strength, weaknesses, threats, and potential of the organization.
- **It is intangible:** The concept of intangibility in administration rose from the idea that administration is abstract but valued. The administration is not transferrable. So every organization has to develop its administrative style within the content of functional elements of administration.
- **It is the continuous and ongoing process:** The cycle of administration goes on continuously. It is a continuing process in the organization that is not time-bound.
- **It is goal-oriented:** The administration is always struggling to achieve the laid down goals and objectives of the organization.
- **It is social and human:** The administration requires human resources for its execution. Usually, the administration comprises of a group of people to achieve the objectives of

the organization. The success of an administration largely relies on the social contacts and interpersonal relationship present, in and out of the organization.

- **It is dynamic:** Administration has the elements of flexibility and adaptability and adjustability rising to the needs and demands of different situations.
- **It is creative or innovative:** The success of the organization largely relies on administrative policies. The administration should take into account the human resources of the organization, their creativity, and innovative approaches. The creativity and creative idea of the administrator will motivate and empower the workforce of the organization.

THEORIES OF MANAGEMENT

- **Scientific management theory:** The scientific management theory focuses on the observation of the organization and the measurement of outcome. The pioneers of scientific management are Frederick W. Taylor (1856-1915), Henry L. Gantt (1861-1910), Emerson (1853-1936) and Charles Babbage (1792-1871).

  Taylor is acknowledged as the "father of scientific management concept". He carried out research on Time-And-Motion among workers and analyzed their actions and laid their norms and standards. He conducted this study with the help of stopwatches to assess the time consumed for each activity. To determine the most efficient manner to achieve a job, he implemented the principles of observation, evaluation, and scientific review. The critical points of Taylor were:
  - Management responsibilities should be segregated from the worker's tasks.
  - Develop a comprehensive method to identify the most effective forms of production and deem the role of management to plan such as work description, selection, and preparation of employees, and so on.
  - Working circumstances or situations and techniques should be uniform and standardized to enhance output.
  - Introduce a compensation scheme such as incentives to reward employees at the rate of production to minimize dissatisfaction among employees.

  Gantt was concerned with problems related to efficiency. He contributed to scientific management by refining the previous work of Taylor than introducing new concepts.
  - The amount of work planned or completed on one axis was studied with the time required or taken to complete the task on the other axis.
  - Gantt also created a work and bonus scheme to provide employees with a secured daily wage plus a bonus according to the rate of production to boost greater efficiency.
  - Gantt suggested scientifically selecting employees and providing comprehensive directions for their duties.

- He advocated for a more managerial humanitarian strategy, emphasizing service rather than benefit goals.
- He acknowledged helpful non-monetary rewards such as work safety and the growth of employees.

Emerson's emphasis was on conservation and organizational goals and objectives. His theory explains about:
- Management can reinforce an organization's discipline by giving justice.
- Management must make decisions based on factual information and for it; they can consider credible data of equipment and human resources.
- The timing of production is suggested.
- The output should be facilitated by standardized plans, requirements, and published guidelines.
- "Efficiency bonuses" should be provided to complete the assignments successfully.

Charles Babbage, a scientist mainly interested in mathematics, contributed to the management theory by developing the principles of cost accounting and the nature of the relationship between various disciplines. He concentrated on production problems and stressed the importance of:
- Division and assignment of work based on skill.
- He emphasized the significance of replacing manual operations with automatic machinery.

- **Classic organizational theory:** Three pioneers of the Classic organizational theory were Henry Fayol, Max Webber, and James Mooney.

  Fayol was a French Mining Engineer and in " Management" he is referred as " Father of Management Process". He studied the functions of managers and concluded that management is universal
  - The organization should focus on the power structure, which is the hierarchy of authority.
  - The management should plan policies, procedures, and programs.
  - Concept of efficient direction to obtain an optimum yield from all employees.
  - Coordination represents a balance in the organization's operations and facilitates its work by monitoring the functionaries' mistakes.

  Max Webber was a German psychologist. He earned the title of the "father of organizational theory". His conceptualization was of bureaucracy, the structure of authority, which would facilitate the accomplishment of corporate objectives. According to him, the following are the basis for power:
  - Traditional authority is always accepted because people think that things have always been like this before. There is still a tendency of automatic obedience. For example, A King in a Monarchy.

- Charisma is a powerful character of influence that is possessed by the manager.
- The rational-legal authority is considered rational in the case of formal organizations because the person has demonstrated the knowledge, skills, and ability to fulfill the position.

Moony believed that management is the technique of directing people and organization based on four universal principles:

- Coordination and synchronization of actions should be done to accomplish the planned objective.
- The functional production and description of one's work are essential.
- The scalar method of arranging levels of command is also required.
- Arrange a structure of power such as hierarchy. Consequently, people from their place in the organization, get their right to control and command.

- **Human relation theory:** It focuses on the effect that the individuals have the success or failure of an organization. Classic organization and management theory concentrated on the physical environment, which failed to analyze the human element. Instead of focusing on the organizational structure, the managers should encourage workers to develop their potentials to help them meet their needs.

  - *Mary Parker Follett (1868-1933):* She was a renowned social worker, and authored many books on human relations and management. Her theory of management is commonly referred to as Follett's theory. She recognized every organization as a social system and suggested that every organization must function on the theory of "power with" and not "power over." She recognized the significance of reciprocal relationships on the growth of an organization. The concept of "power with" signifies mutual cooperation while the concept of "power over" signifies the concept of authority/ bureaucracy. She also indicated that legitimate power is produced by a cyclic behavior where superiors and subordinates mutually influence each other. A person does not take orders from another person but the situation.

  - *Kurt Lewin's theory (1890-1947):* He is considered as the "father of social psychology". The Change theory of Nursing was also contributed by Lewin. In the concept of management, he emphasizes the significance of group dynamics. According to him, every group has their own behavior and it is the sum of behavior of all members in that group. The group behavior concept also signifies the influence that exists on each other in a specified group. He also showed that group forces could overcome individual interests.

- **Behavioral science theory:** This theory indicates the importance of maintaining a positive attitude toward people, training managers, meeting the needs of the employees, and obtaining commitment through participation in planning and decision making.

- ***Douglas McGregor's Theory (1932):*** He developed the managerial implications of Maslow's theory. He noted that one's style of management is dependent on one's philosophy of humans. According to him, the method of management depends on two types of philosophies which he named "X" and "Y" (Table 1).

  According to theory X, the workers must be directed, controlled and threatened to achieve the goals of the organization. Managers who accept the assumption that theory X will do the thinking and planning with little input from staff associates will delegate little, supervise closely.

  According to theory Y, people do not inherently dislike the work, and that work can be a source of satisfaction. Workers have the self-direction and self-control necessary for meeting their objectives and will respond to the rewards for the accomplishment of those goals. Managers who believe in this Y theory will allow participation, and they will delegate.

- ***Rensis Likert's theory:*** He emphasized on a four-tier system of management which he explained as follows (Fig. 2):

  - *Exploitative-authoritative:* Managers show less confidence in staff associates and ignore their ideas.
  - *Benevolent-authoritative:* Staff associates' ideas are sometimes sought, but they do not feel free to discuss their jobs with the manager.
  - *Consultative system:* The manager has substantial confidence in staff associates, and their ideas are usually sought. They feel free to discuss their job with the manager.

TABLE 1: Douglas McGregor's theory of X and Y

	Human nature	Motivation/rewards	Work/job
X	People are passive and prefer to do nothing. They are immature.	Work itself is not satisfying. They need money, status, and rewards to keep them working. They are productive because of the fear of being terminated.	Jobs come first, and then people are selected. They need to be trained to achieve organizational goals.
Y	People are active and prefer working. They set goals and strive for them. They are mature.	Working keeps them satisfied. The Y people feel proud of achievements and establishing social contacts. The reason for productivity is the desire to achieve personal and social goals.	People come first; then the job is modified to seek self-realization. People are naturally integrated.

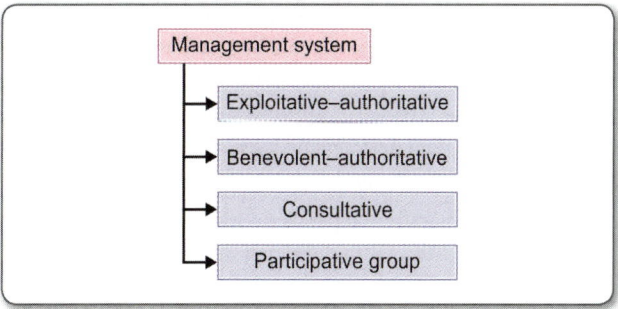

Fig. 2: Management system

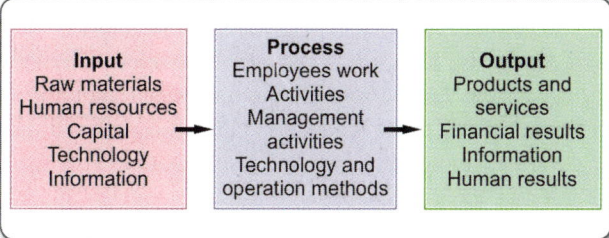

Fig. 3: Modern management theory

♦ *Participative group:* Participative group is the most effective performance. Managers have complete confidence in their staff associates.

● **Modern management theories:** Modern management theories can be further classified as the three streams such as (Fig. 3):

■ *Quantitative approach:* Management science refers to the application of quantitative methods to management. In this approach, the most important word is the Quantity or Output data. This approach purely depends on the statistical/mathematical output, which, if it is positive, then the management is excellent. It is present in all areas of management wherever output is measured in terms of data. For example, if a company manufactures some specific surgical instruments, someone has to statistically monitor the data that those devices are used for the particular procedures, and no defective devices are produced. This data is presented to the company for review and improvement.

■ *System approach:* According to system approach, the organization is the unified, purposeful systems composed of interrelated parts and also interdependent with its environment. The quantitative approach gives importance only to the output, whereas the system approach gives equal importance to the input, transformation/process, and the production. The environment influences the entire system. The output of the system is followed by feedback to modify/improve input.

■ *Contingency/Situational approach:* There is no set way to manage an organization. Contingency theory is the recognition of the extreme importance of an individual

manager's performance in the given situation. The manager's power and control are based on the type of situation and the uncertainty of the given job. Both quantitative and system approach does not consider any untoward occurrence or incidence in the management process. In a nutshell, the contingency approach explains the importance of the manager's ability to make the alternative plans of operations in times of failure of existing management policy. e.g. even the brand new car has a spare tyre to manage an unexpected breakdown.

The pioneers of modern management theories are:

● **Abraham H. Maslow:** He was the first psychologist to develop a theory of motivation based upon a consideration of human needs such as Physiological needs, Safety and Security needs, Need for love and Belongingness, Self Esteem and Self-Actualization (Fig. 4).

● **Herzberg's two-factor theory:** In 1959, Frederick Herzberg proposed a two-factor theory or the theory. He was a behavioral scientist. According to Herzberg, the opposite of "Satisfaction" is "No satisfaction". He considers two factors responsible for the functioning of the organization, hygiene factors and motivation.

Hygiene factors: Factors of hygiene are the job factors that are essential to productivity at work. This is not conducive to long-term optimistic fulfillment. The hygiene factors symbolized the physiological needs that people wanted to meet and expected. These factors can also be considered as unsatisfactory or maintenance factors. The hygiene factors focus on many aspects. The policies and administrative policies of companies should not be too rigid. The wage or job system in the same sector should be equitable and efficient. The status of the employees should be known and preserved within the company. Staff should have effective and reasonable interactions with their colleagues,

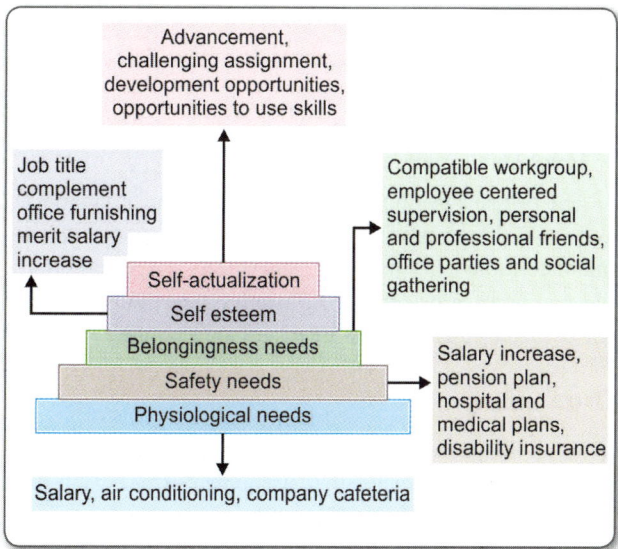

Fig. 4: Theory of motivation

supervisors, and subordinates. No dispute or dimension of embarrassment will occur. The work equipment should be well maintained and updated.

Job motivation: The hygiene factors cannot be considered as motivators, according to Herzberg. The factors that motivate people are pleased. These factors are working inherently. These factors are inherently worthwhile to employees. Employees need a sense of performance. In an organization, there must be opportunities for growth and progress to encourage employees. The workers will be kept responsible for the job. For the employee to perform and be motivated, the job itself should have meaning and challenging. Control should be minimized, but responsibilities should be retained.

FUNCTIONS OF MANAGEMENT (MANAGEMENT PROCESS)

Usually, the actions of the manager (planning, organizing, directing, coordinating, and controlling) are referred to as the functions of the management process. Henry Fayol explains the functions of management easily with the help of an acronym POS-D-CORB (Planning organizing, staffing, directing, coordinating, reporting and budgeting).

Planning

It is a process of making decisions in advance about the activities to be undertaken in the future. It is a highly sophisticated procedure that requires an acceptable level of intelligence as well as creativity. It is aimed to obtain the desired objectives. A good planning:

- Provides sensible organizational goals and creates alternative methods for achieving these goals
- Helps to remove or decrease potential confusion and opportunity
- Contributes to economic activities
- Lays the organizational basis
- Makes cooperation easier
- Helps monitoring easier

The primary planning operations are formulating policies and establishing goals. The strategy is the collection of policies that determine a health care organization's image and offer it the marketplace orientation. Objectives are the core of the whole management process in an authentic context

Organizing

Once all the goals are set through planning, the focus of the management must switch to the development of the organization worthy of fulfilling them. The notion of organizing could be described as the relationship between individuals and activities in such a manner that they are all mixed and interrelated into a system that can be oriented towards the organizational goals. The organization's most fundamental assumption is the division of labor either through **Horizontal differentiation** (Organization is divided into operational units for more effective and efficient performance) or **Vertical differentiation** (Hierarchy construction and division of work).

The formal organization depends on two basic principles:

1. **Responsibility:** All the working and available personnel in the organization share and take up the liability based on their functions and caliber. Efforts should be taken to avoid overlapping and gaps in accountability. Once the desired objective is achieved, the responsibility terminates or continues to the achievement of another target.
2. **Authority:** Authority is the other side of responsibility. A person can be responsible, only when authority is granted to make decisions, commitments, and use various resources to carry out his/her duties.

Staffing

The process of carrying out human resource activities (selection, induction, promotion, retention, and so on) is referred to as staffing. Every job or action in an organization requires appropriate personnel to perform the designated duties. The selection of a person for a job is based on the need and nature of the job, including its situation. The staffing helps to have an appropriate person for each type of employment. It prevents square peg in the round hole. Broadly, it consists of the following steps:

- Assess the current staff strength
- Foresee staff demand
- Understand and analyze staff turnover
- Plan work specifications along with job descriptions

Directing

Directing implies issuing orders, tasks, and guidelines that enable the trainee to comprehend what is anticipated of him, and guiding and supervising the trainee so that he can effectively and efficiently relate to the achievement of organizational goals. Directing involves the subsequent actions:

- **Giving commands:** Providing instructions is a crucial job in guiding. The command is the technical means of understanding the functions of a subordinate. The order should be clear, concise, and consistent to give sufficient information to ensure understanding. The tone of the order is fundamental. How the manager delivers the order has a great deal to do with its acceptance by the subordinate. It should be based on the apparent demands of a particular situation, and it seems logical to the subordinates and not just an arbitrary whim of the manager.
- **Supervision:** Supervision is the managerial function involved in the preparation and practice of the workforce.

It consists of monitoring to ensure that commands are executed promptly and adequately. Supervision is the practice of supervising, controlling and guiding others' jobs and conducting with power.

- **Leading:** Leadership is the capacity to encourage and impact others to help achieve their goals. Effective leadership is the consequence of a relationship in a specific organizational scenario between the manager and his subordinates.
- **Motivating:** Motivation corresponds to how the demands such as desires, different urges, and so on, regulate, guide, or justify human behavior. The manager should encourage the worker to follow directives or lead them to do so.
- **Communicating:** The transition of data from sender to receiver and its interpretation by the receiver is referred to as communication. Communication is essential to the management's leadership role; one method of visualizing this significance is to see the manager on one hand of a hurdle and the working group on the other. Communication is the tool for the manager or director to achieve job team operation through the obstacle.

Coordinating

The process of interfacing the individuals and functions to work efficiently in achieving organizational goals is termed as coordination. Coordination in the health care organization is essential because it is departmentalized functionally. Different corporate types involve varying levels of cooperation. Coordination methods usually include basic techniques such as:

- Corrective co-ordinations are those coordinating tasks that detect or correct an internal weakness or defect in the organization.
- Preventive coordination include those actions targeted at stopping or minimizing the effect of expected issues of improper coordination.
- Regulatory coordination is the maintenance of current functional and structural arrangements in the organization.
- Promotive coordination aims at the improvement of the existing coordination of an organization. It helps in the assessment of different functional areas of the organization for development.

Controlling

Controlling can be described as activity monitoring according to planned demands. The control mechanism includes four measures, irrespective of the area of application:

- Definition of standards
- Performance measurement
- The real outcomes are compared to the norms
- It helps in correcting standard deviations

Reporting and Recording

Reports are written or verbal information exchanges that are shared in several ways between caregivers or workers. A report outlines the individual, staff, and organization facilities. Reports are typically prepared and submitted on a daily, quarterly, monthly, or annual basis. Reporting is performed to:

- Demonstrate the type and quantity of services provided over a given period
- Demonstrate advancement in achieving objectives
- Use as a tool to help in the study of different conditions
- Plan the care
- Interpret the facilities that are rendered to the public and other accrediting agencies

Records and reports must be secret, operational, precise, total, existing, and structured.

Budgeting

Budgeting, although acknowledged mainly as a monitoring tool, becomes a significant component of any organization's planning method. It is reflected financially and is dependent on anticipated revenue and expense. The budget is the core of administration. It acts as a cooperation instrument and an instrument to eliminate wastage and duplication. Budget characteristics include:

- Must be versatile.
- Should be based on previous, current, and future.
- Must be the result of joint undertaking and co-operation of managers and other HoDs of different functional departments.
- It must be in the manner of a particular numerical and statistical norm.
- Senior and top managers must support the budgeting during the period of its planning and execution.

PRINCIPLES OF MANAGEMENT

They are the essential underlying factors that form the foundation of Management. Henry Fayol in his book "General and Industrial Management," in 1916, explains 14 principles of management.

1. **Division of labor:** In any administration, the manager cannot perform all the activities to achieve its objectives. So, there should be a division of work according to a job grouped according to departments.
2. **Authority, responsibility, and accountability**: If the person has to perform job assignments effectively according to their qualification and experience, there should be a delegation of authority and responsibility needed, which in turn helps to get accountability.
3. **Discipline:** The guidelines, laws, standards, etiquette, courtesy, the standard of ethics, and regard must be observed correctly to attain the goals. This needs the manager to implement it within the organization.

4. **Unity of command:** The supervision of each employee must be done by a single supervisor or manager to whom he/she ought to be responsible. It avoids confusion and improves the health of the organization.

5. **Unity of direction:** It is supplementary to the previous principle. A single manager must provide guidance and direction to the respective subordinates so that biased directions can be avoided.

6. **Subordination of individual interest to organizational interest:** The corporate interest always overlays the personal interest. The employee must overcome this narrow selfish conflict. A healthy way to achieve it is the placing and modifying of the individual interest along with organizational interest in a mutual achievement pattern for e.g., Collective Bargaining.

7. **Remuneration of personnel:** There must be a reasonable compensation system for staff that justifies the volume of work, work dangers, effectiveness, and quality of services.

8. **Centralization:** The power should be distributed according to the level of management. The top-level executives possess a higher level of authority.

9. **Scalar chain of command:** It means that from the highest level to the smallest level of employees in an organization, there remains a chain of hierarchy. It enables in the direction of authority and line of responsibility.

10. **Order:** Every administration must have an order and balance among employees, materials, supplies, and facilities. These systematic arrangements, in accordance with the requirements of particular organizational objectives, ease the process of administration.

11. **Equity:** The principle of equity emphasizes the importance of an impartial and fair approach to all workers. The administration must not consider the level of employee, designation, financial status during administration. All are considered to be equal as per the written policy of organization and job description.

12. **Stability of tenure of a personnel:** Organizations must create adequate attempts to maintain stable and continuous staff tenure, providing safety, and promoting growth. The application of this principle will help the growth of the organization as it enhances the dedication and efficiency.

13. **Initiative:** Every employee should be given freedom of expression and the best performance. This must be kept in consideration that the concept of freedom should be according to the level of employee.

14. **Esprit de corps (Team spirit):** It is the concept of togetherness. It creates a sense of belongingness. This fosters the team spirit, i.e., the spirit of working together to achieve objective effectively.

Management is a living science. From time to time, various thinkers of the subject have expressed their opinion on the principles. According to Urwick, Keith and Fayol, there are 15 principles.

1. **The principle of policymaking:** A practical management needs, bright and well thought out policy. The evolved systems should be such, which may be acceptable to all and should be based on the interest of the workers.

2. **The principle of improvement and adjustment:** An enterprise is a growing concern; it grows step by step steadily but inevitably. It should be flexible, able to accept improvement and adjust itself according to the dictate of the situation.

3. **The principle of balance:** The chief executives are required to go through all the details minutely, and they should also ensure that a proper balance between the duties, responsibilities, rights, and authority is well established.

4. **The principle of individual effectiveness:** Proper training, good wages policy, human relations, and healthy surroundings also help the enterprise in increasing the efficiency of an individual.

5. **The principle of the relationship between task and accomplishment:** To guarantee effectiveness and comprehension, everyone should be put in their allocated work as per their skills, expertise, aptitude, and experience.

6. **The principle of simplicity:** The principle of simplicity explains the ease of work. It includes the simplicity in the use of machines and instruments, simplicity in following standard operating policies and procedures, and simplicity in the calculation of performance appraisal. The concept of simplicity enables the employee to make fewer errors and improve efficiency.

7. **The principle of specialization:** Specialization is a scientific management focal point and is achieved through expertise. Specialization enhances efficiency. Product quality is improves owing to knowledge and specialization.

8. **The principle of standardization:** The systematic approach in management refers to the policy of standardization. It is of paramount significance to leadership in terms of manufacturing, advertising, oversight, and the most important use of accessible funds.

9. **The principle of financial incentives:** Financial incentives act as a key to motivation among employees. An appropriate and satisfactory compensation policy improves the cooperation of workers. This is directly linked to the growth and development of the organization.

10. **The principle of planning:** The smooth function of an organization depends on the extent of planned activities. Plans define what to do, when to do, how to do and, of course, who should do a job. Preplanned goals and thinking offer the expected level of success and accomplishment.

11. **The principle of control:** The efficiency and responsibility of a worker primarily rely on the code of conduct and discipline. The maintenance of discipline requires efficient supervision and control mechanisms. It helps in standardizing the jobs and helps in the control of men and materials.

12. **The principle of leadership:** The supervision and control mechanisms govern the leadership and direction of an organization. Efficient administration ensures the productive working of all men. The leader should be equipped with sound knowledge and expertise to guide and control the affairs and working of all his subordinates.

13. **The principle of cooperation:** Cooperation helps in ensuring mutual respect. Both cooperation and mutual respect are a must to the progressive functioning of an organization. The collaboration among employees creates confidence among them, and it facilitates the level of functioning.

14. **The principle of responsibility and authority:** It is essential to provide each worker and each segment of the company with a list of their duties and responsibilities to be fulfilled, and rights and authority to be enjoyed while carrying out the burden of their duties and satisfying their obligations.

15. **The principle of exception:** The principle of exception signifies the difference like job among top-level management. The top-level management should not be performing routine tasks; instead, they should focus on the growth of the organization. They must prepare policies, guidelines, assess the problems in the organization, and suggest a solution for it.

NURSE MANAGER

A nurse manager is a person who supervises, leads, and, directs the nursing staff of the health care organization. It requires critical thinking ability, organization capacity, and scientific knowledge about patient care as they monitor those who provide direct attention to the patients. Additionally, they need all other skills of an effective manager. They typically work in the health care organization in addition to ambulatory and long-term care area.

Managing the staff of nurses is a challenging career that requires nursing and managerial skills. A nursing management career starts with being a licensed practical nurse and working your way up through years of clinical practice and advanced education. They also participate in management training that addresses specific issues that deal with employees, behavioral standards, and handling of the legal problems that are associated with the supervision of the people working in the hospital environment.

Nurse managers are an inevitable component of any healthcare setting. They are accountable for the supervision of nursing care services in a health care setting. The surveillance includes monitoring of the nurses, assessing the effectiveness of patient care and budgeting of nursing services.

Roles of a Nurse Manager

A nurse manager has many responsibilities and wears many hats. Few of them are:
- Nurse managers are responsible for planning, organizing, and directing health services in their department to ensure that the goals and objectives are performed consistently and that the services provided to the patients are of the highest quality and standard.
- They select, mentor, motivate and direct the development and evaluation of the staff nurses. They are responsible for establishing and keeping track of quality improvement indicators and other information that concerns the patient care and services.
- They plan and execute in-service education to the staff in collaboration with the nurse educator.
- They participate, consult, and collaborate with interdisciplinary units and healthcare providers in developing long term plans for health care programs.
- Management of critical situations and support the patient and his family in times of escalated need.
- Official work of manager such as duty rotation planning, leave register of staff, and other records about the nursing workforce.
- They are also responsible for developing budget estimates and handle other information about financial concerns and requirements.
- Nurse manager also works as change agents as they work with other nurses to see the chance of improving the patient care delivery approach.
- Ensure the delivery of nursing services is under the norms of the regulatory bodies Centers for Disease Control and Prevention (CDC), Joint Commission International (JCI) and National Accreditation Board for Hospitals and Health Care Providers (NABH) hospital administration, and laws of the land.

Qualities of a Nurse Manager

Nurse managers should possess skills and traits beyond routine clinical works. They require leadership, business acumen, budgeting, and many other skills, including communication skills. The following characteristics are common among successful nurse managers:
- **Mutual respect for all:** A manager who does not respect his/her staff, especially in public will lose credibility and will not get respect in return. Autonomy should be promoted at all levels of professional practice irrespective of the hierarchy.

- **Creativity and flexibility:** A nurse manager should always be organized with all the rules and regulations but should be ready for flexibility if necessary. They should be able to adapt to the available resources of the organization to meet the organizational objectives.
- **Decision making:** All the nursing staff expect the nurse manager to make wise decisions in times of critical situations. At the same time, self-resolving problems should be promoted among the employees.
- **Empowering fellow staff:** The nurse manager should always find means to motivate the team. Participative decision making is necessary to drive the staff. The dispassionate or hopeless attitude of a nurse manager will de-motivate the staff.
- **Humor:** The sense of humor is the healthiest way to help the staff and the patients since nursing is one of the toughest and most stressful jobs around.
- **Honesty:** It helps to maintain trust among team members. Avoid lying and favoritism. Any type of double-dealing is not healthy for the relationship between the manager and staff.
- **Reliability and advocacy:** A nurse manager should have a good body of knowledge and clinical expertise. Sound experience and scientific expertise make the nurse manager more reliable. In some situations, the nurse managers may have to advocate for the staff members to smoothen the working environment and create a leap in productivity. Additionally, they may also have to support patients to make sure quality health care. They should not be afraid of using their voice and position.
- **Being available**. Despite the meetings and other managerial responsibilities, the manager should be available for the nursing staff when needed. Always make sure to acknowledge and incorporate staff suggestions to make them feel ease and accepted.
- **Communication skills:** Practical communication skills are necessary for all managers and leaders. It includes building effective rapport among all staff members from a higher level to a lower level of employment. The communication skills also must be extended to the patients, relatives, family members, and other significant members of society. Lack of communication leads to biased information and confusion.

- **Leadership quality:** Nurse managers must have leadership qualities. They should be able to strike a sufficient balance between nurses and other employees in the organization. They should be able to maintain the harmonious relationship between the workforce and administrators.
- **Participation:** The nurse manager must also balance patient care and business perspectives. The superior clinical skills of a nurse manager ensure the wellbeing and safety of the patients.
- **Mentoring:** The strength of a nurse manager relies on his/her staff members. The manager should not micromanage his/her staff. The encouragement, mentoring of the nurse and manager boosts the mindfulness and creativity of the staff members.
- **Maturity and professionalism:** The nurse manager should follow a moral compass and should not take partial decisions. They should face conflict and work healthy mechanisms out of it. Nurse managers should have honesty and integrity.

Future of Nurse Managers

The aging and retirement of current nurses and nurse managers will create new opportunities that can be explored by newly trained nurses and nurse managers. According to research, the retention of overall staff nurse primarily relies on the nurse manager rather than hospital administrators because they can create a healthy working environment and make the fellow workers feel the stability of the job. The rate of staff retention influences the quality of the work to a greater extent.

The active role of nurse managers has been linked with job satisfaction, decreased turnover, and quality patient outcome. A research conducted in 2014 says that nurse managers must be supported to resolve problems associated with the quality of the patient care and turnover of the staff members. The relationship between nurse managers and staff members should be cohesive and continuous. Continual changes in healthcare and a focus on costs are among the aspects a that make the role of a nurse manager challenging. The nurturing of future nurse managers requires proper planning and action. It is a great challenge today since the healthcare environment is fast-paced and continuously changing.

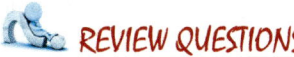 **REVIEW QUESTIONS**

1. Define nursing management. Explain the need and characteristics of management.
2. Explain the principles of management in detail.
3. Explain the scope and levels of management.
4. List the role of a nurse manager.
5. What are the qualities of a nurse manager?
6. List down the theories of management and explain modern management theories in detail.
7. Discuss management as a profession and explain the role of the nurse as a manager of a health care delivery system.
8. What are the functions of management?

Further Readings

1. Banerjee, Shyamal. Principles and Practice of Management. Oxford and IBM Publishing, New Delhi; 2000.
2. Basavanthappa BT. Nursing Administration. 2nd Edition: Jaypee Brothers Medical Publishers (P) Ltd., New Delhi; 2009.
3. Barrett, Jean. Ward Management and Teaching. Konark Publishers, Delhi; 1992.
4. Warren, Stevens F. Management and Leadership in Nursing. McGraw Hill Inc., New York; 1978.
5. Alexander et al. Nursing Service Administration. Mosby Publishers; 1962.
6. Goel SL. Healthcare System, and its Management, Health Organization and Structure, 1st Volume, Deep and Deep Publishers; New Delhi; 2001.
7. Basavanthappa BT. Nursing Administration, 1st Edition: Jaypee Brothers Medical Publishers (P) Ltd., New Delhi; 2002.
8. Lucita M. Nursing: Practice and Public Health Administration. Current concepts and trends. B. I. Churchill Living Stone Pvt. Ltd., New Delhi; 2002.
9. Sakharkar BM. Principles of Hospital Administration and Planning, 2nd Edition: Jaypee Brothers Medical Publishers (P) Ltd., New Delhi; 2009.
10. Patricia S Yoder-Wise. Leading and Managing in Nursing. 2nd Edition: Mosby Publication, US; 1999.
11. Douglass LM. The Effective Nurse: Leader and Manager. 5th Edition: Mosby Publication, US; 1996.
12. Trained Nurses Association of India, Nursing Administration and Management.
13. Chandorkar AG. Hospital Administration and Planning. 2nd Edition: Paras Medical Publisher, New Delhi; 2009.
14. Joshi DC, Joshi Mamta. Hospital Administration. 1st Edition: Jaypee Brothers Medical Publishers (P) Ltd., New Delhi; 2009.

Unit

3

Planning Nursing Services

Unit Outline

- Mission and Vision
- Philosophy/Value Statements
- Objectives of Nursing Services
- Policy: A Nursing View
- Nursing Protocols
- Nursing Manuals
- Nursing Procedures
- Standing Orders in Nursing
- Concept of Planning
- Planning Process
- Program Evaluation and Review Technique
- Gantt Charts (Activity Plan)
- Milestone Chart
- Basics of Budgeting
- Cost-Effectiveness and Cost Analysis
- Budget Proposal
- Hospital and Hospital Planning
- Planning in Emergency and Disaster Management

MISSION AND VISION

Mission statement describes the primary objectives of the organization. It primarily tries to explain the reason for the existence of any organization. It is the beginning of an organization's strategic planning. It tries to explain to the stakeholders the purpose of existence and what is the current performance of the organization. Mission statements support the achievement of the vision statements. It normally asks the following questions. What do we do? Whom do we serve? How do we serve them?

Vision statements are future-oriented and try to explain the prospects of the organization. It usually is a projected plan of functioning for the forthcoming years (normally 10–15 years). It is based on the purpose and values of the organization. For employees, it gives direction and understanding of the expected behavior in the organization. It usually asks questions such as; What are our hopes and dreams for the future?

In a nutshell, an organization through its mission statement tries to describe what the organization wants to do now and through a vision statement, it outlines the plans of the organization.

Mission statement	Vision statement
Organization: Fortis Health care "To be a globally respected healthcare organization known for Clinical Excellence and Distinctive Patient Care."	Organization: Fortis Health Care "Saving and Enriching Lives"

PHILOSOPHY/VALUE STATEMENTS

Philosophy or value statements are understood as a method of achieving the mission and vision. It briefs the ideologies, concepts, and principles of an organization. They are considered as the core belief of an organization that decides the pathway to achieve the mission/vision of the organization.

Philosophy of Nursing Service

The nursing service philosophy could be a statement of beliefs that is in agreement with the institution's philosophy. It should reflect the ideologies of the members of the nursing service and should be mutually agreeable.

Components

- **Nursing practice:** Nursing is a healthcare service based on scientific principles, and it has a body of knowledge. The services are provided as per the needs of the society and the individual. Primarily, the nurse manager should have expertise and know-how of the practical implications of the nursing theories, and it is an integral part of nursing practice philosophy. It also incorporates the principles of nursing education, nursing research, and nursing administration.
- **Patient/client:** The patient is the recipient of the nursing care services. They are the very existence of the organization, and hence, the patient's rights should be taken into utmost consideration. It also considers the policies and practices of the organization.
- **Nurses:** Nurses are the service providers in a hospital. The values and beliefs of the nurses who are employed in the hospital should be taken into consideration for the smooth functioning of the organization. These values and expectations should be on par with that of the professional organizations and other health professionals.

Philosophy of Nursing Education

These are the values, beliefs, attitudes, and ideas, which the faculty and students have collectively agreed upon about nursing education programs. It is a combination of the philosophy of education and nursing. It focuses on the overall development of student life. It may also be influenced by many factors such as institutional policies, availability of resources, health needs of the society, the cultural and ethical background of the student and faculty.

OBJECTIVES OF NURSING SERVICES

Objectives are vital in management because these are so important that lack of objectives or failure to keep these clearly in mind makes the task of management difficult. The common goals must be established so that the efforts are made towards the known ultimate objectives. Objectives are basic plans, which determine goals or end results of the projected action of an enterprise. By setting goals, objectives provide the foundation upon which the structure of the plan can be built.

"Objectives are goals, aims or purposes that organizations wish over varying periods of time."   —DE McFarland

Objectives are defined as the important ends towards which organizational and individual activities are directed.

—Weihrich and Koontz

Nature of Objectives

- **Objectives from hierarchy:** As the objectives range from the broad aim to specific individual objectives, right from top-level to an individual level, it may take a top-down or bottom-up approach for setting the objective. Both approaches have their own merits and demerits; thus a combination of the two is mostly followed.
- **The multiplicity of objectives:** As the organization may have multiple objectives, at each level there can be many goals. At any rate, the number of objectives depends on 'how much' the nurse administrators will do themselves and how much they will assign to subordinates, thereby

limiting their role to one among assigning, supervising and controlling.

- **Objectives have a time limit:** The objectives need to be framed keeping the time in mind. A quality without a time limit conveys no meaning.
- **Objectives are interrelated and interdependent:** All the objectives are interrelated and interdependent as per the management functions. Each objective cannot be achieved without considering the other one.
- **Objectives have different priorities:** The success of an organization depends on the approach to objectives and determination of priorities. It means that at a given time, the achievement of one objective may be relatively more important than another one.

Characteristics of Nursing Objectives

The characteristics of nursing objectives are given in Figure 1.

Formulation of Objectives in Nursing

All the organizations need to set up objectives in order to function effectively. The setting up of objectives in nursing is largely based on the few aspects mentioned below:

- Based on National Health Policy
- Based on the needs of the population
- Based on priority areas for improvement of basic Nursing and Midwifery
- Based on resources available
- Based on active participation
- Based on the philosophy of Nursing Services
- Based on the acceptance and approval of administrators

Classification of Objectives in Health Care

- **Levels of objectives:**
  - **Major/Organizational objectives:** Refer to the overall organizational objectives
  - **Departmental/Unit objectives:** About various departments in the organization
  - **Group objectives:** Refers to various groups formed in the organization

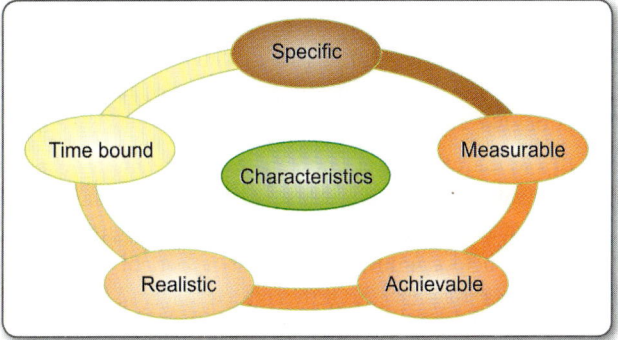

Fig. 1: Characteristics

- **Individual objectives:** Employee set/oriented objectives
- **Types of objectives:**
  - **Profit objectives:** These objectives are framed according to the owner's point of view, where profit return is the motto of having health or nursing services. Mostly this is seen in the private sector.
  - **Service objectives:** These are objectives that are prepared by keeping the patients' needs and interests in mind.
  - **Social objectives:** Made in light of the public interest.
  - **Personal objectives:** It is based on employees, individuals, economical, and psychological satisfaction.
- **Based on hierarchy:**
  - **Primary objectives:** The main primary objectives of hospital services are to provide curative services by ensuring patient care to indoor patients.
  - **Subsidiary objectives:** These objectives are based on managerial professional activities. For example, communication, human relations, teaching, research.

POLICY: A NURSING VIEW

A policy is an announcement or general understanding, which gives rules in making decisions to individuals of an association regarding any strategy. It is a human-made principle of a foreordained policy that is cultivated to the execution of work towards obtaining the aims of the organization. According to Joint Commission Accreditation (JCA, USA), the hospital policy should contain the essential elements:

- **Hospital philosophy:** The strategy /policy/ guidelines ought to have a short articulation that talks about the philosophy of the hospital.
- **Policy statement:** Write and depict what the strategy at which it applies and what it is expected to achieve.
- **Definitions of terms:** Define the relevant terms that are important and utilized inside the hospital such as Pharmacists, Direct caregivers, Key staff members, etc. to avoid unexpected results.
- **Patient contact algorithm:** Set forward rules for patient contacts:
  - **Initial patient contact:** The employees designated for initial communications such as receptionists, front office employees, call center employees should be set up for this experience whether it is reasonable or unforeseen and whether it is by phone, face to face or through an agent. Managing troublesome discussions and feelings is a communication and correspondence ability for which all staff individuals ought to get training.
  - **Directing the patient to the appropriate individual(s):** Based on the initial patient contact data and considering

the need and situation the staff should settle on the choice of the patient and their attendants whom to coordinate for further care and direction. A well thoroughly considered choice tree that is a piece of a policy/strategy rule will be advantageous to diminish staff wavering and perplexity amid critical situations.

- **Investigate unanticipated outcomes:** Complete root causes analysis if needed and review and communicate details of the investigation with appropriate staff members. It includes planning the disclosure discussion, disclosure of communication content, documentation and follow-up.

NURSING PROTOCOLS

These are detailed plans that describe particular patient care. It is essential to follow specific protocols when practicing patient care so that uniformity of care can be maintained. Nursing Protocol helps in quality control elements. Nursing tasks are always initiated by nurses. The nurses have a responsibility to make sure that the sick or ill people are given comprehensive and qualitative nursing care. Keeping all these elements in mind, the nursing protocols shall be developed. The nursing protocol is mainly divided into three parts:

1. Definitions and details such as etiology, objectives, and assessment of the condition.
2. The actual nursing care plan, including diagnostic studies, therapeutic methods, client education, counseling, follow up, and referral.
3. Scientific reasons to justify the nursing care plan, such as a proper reference to support the protocol.

Nurse Protocol is the written statement mutually agreed by a registered nurse and a licensed physician, by which a registered nurse is permitted to perform specific procedures, administration of certain medications, and other services. This may also be interpreted as a standing instruction.

NURSING MANUALS

The nursing manuals or procedure manuals provide guidelines to ensure adherence to consistently recognized standards of nursing practice. All the nursing procedures should be developed and performed based on current scientific knowledge and the upcoming technology. It is a good practice to compile all the rules/guidelines concerning the management and procedure in a manual that can be made available for reference. These directives generally fall under the following three headings:

1. Procedure issued by the administrative office and referring mainly to regulations. This is essential for maintaining discipline.

2. Procedure manuals, e.g., Lab procedure manuals, nursing procedure manuals.
3. Unit procedure outline the procedure to be used in the unit.

The contents of the manual, particularly concerning the specific procedure, will be more acceptable if compiled following a group discussion. The manual must be kept up to date and the old procedure should be removed when new materials are issued.

Functions of Nursing Manuals

- It provides a tool for a training program to enable new nursing service personnel to become acquainted with the standards of care to be followed.
- It works as a ready reference for the staff members who are already working.
- It helps in the standardization of procedures and equipment.
- It is a reference to evaluation.

NURSING PROCEDURES

Nursing procedures are standardized procedures used by nurses to achieve a high level of patient care. By creating routine responses to medical situations, nursing procedures keep nurses on task and allow them to ensure that patients are getting the care they need. Many hospitals have specific nursing guidelines which they expect their staff to follow, while other procedures are taught in nursing school. In both cases, the guidelines reflect years of experience and collaboration between doctors, nurses, and other medical personnel.

Benefits

- Having standard procedures is a critical part of medical care.
- Nursing procedures establish priorities of care so that nurses can work quickly to stabilize a patient, focusing on critical issues first and moving to less serious medical problems.
- They also act as a checklist, which can be used to confirm that every step necessary for the patient's wellbeing has been taken and that these steps have been followed in the right order.
- These procedures also dictate the number of patients a nurse can care for at once, the maximum hours in a day a nurse can work and how the nurse handles administrative duties like charting.

In a simple example of a nursing procedure, many hospitals require nurses to double-check the labels used on bags of intravenous medication, to confirm that the medication is correct before administering it to a patient. Dangerous medications may have brightly colored labels so that nurses are reminded that the contents of the bag could be dangerous to some patients.

While procedures for nursing are designed to standardize responses to situations to increase patient safety and make nursing more effective, nurses may at times be required to go outside procedural guidelines to deal with unique situations. A good nurse has sound judgment, which helps the nurse identify situations in which standard procedures do not apply, and he or she is not afraid to question actions and medical orders which could endanger a patient. When nurses start working at a hospital, they are typically given a nursing policy handbook, which provides information about working in that hospital. The handbook includes information about uniforms, hospital procedures, and expected standards of behavior, and it also includes a discussion of standard nursing procedures in that medical facility.

STANDING ORDERS IN NURSING

Standing orders are specific instructions regarding treatment for a condition that nurses and other health workers may encounter in the hospital, home, school, and industries where a doctor is not readily available. The standing order is intended to provide treatment only in emergencies and temporarily in the absence of a doctor, they should be limited.

Purposes of Standing Order

- To meet the emergency in a rural area
- To deliver care at home, school, community
- To provide temporary treatment in the absence of a doctor
- To promote health services in the community

Types of Standing Order

- **Institutional standing orders:** They are meant keeping in mind available resources, staff position and the objectives of a medical institution or hospital. E.g. Standing order of PHC can be different from those of district hospital.
- **Specific standing order:** These orders are meant for trained medical personnel, mainly the nurses, technical knowledge and specific skills are required to implement these orders. E.g. Giving care at home such as injections, oxygen therapy.
- **General standing order:** Owning to a large population, vast geographical area and the shortage of resources, some standing orders are used to propagate health care messages to the masses. E.g. Preventive measures against AIDS.

Roles of a Nurse in Standing Order

- The community health nurse should be skillful in recording history and in a physical examination to detect an abnormality.
- The community health nurse should be prompt in detecting appropriate action for a particular situation.

- The nurse should maintain a record of vitals and other care given to the patient.
- The nurse should have thorough knowledge to identify the actual problem of the patient and to plan appropriate nursing intervention.
- The nurse should intervene with services according to the given community standing orders.
- The nurse should develop a good therapeutic relationship with the individual and family.
- The nurse should use the referral system if it is possible.
- The nurse should inform the health officer immediately if there is a communicable disease.
- He/she should keep the medication safe and ready to follow standing orders.
- He/she should ensure a safe and healthy environment for the patient.
- Recording and reporting is an essential part of community health services.

Advantages of Standing Order

- Community standing orders provide timely treatment during emergencies.
- They enhance the quality and activity of health services.
- They provide a feeling of confidence and responsibility in the nursing staff and other health workers.
- They help to decentralize health responsibilities.
- They help to strengthen the primary services in the community.

CONCEPT OF PLANNING

Planning is understood as an intellectual method of creating selections or decisions, and it aims to attain a coordinated and consistent set of operations geared toward objectives for any work.

Planning is the function of the manager, which involves the selection among alternatives for the enterprise as a whole and each department within it.   —**Koontz and O'Donnell**

Planning is a process of determining the objectives of administrative effort and devising the means calculated to achieve them.   —**Millet**

Planning is a process of setting formal guidelines and constraints for the behavior of the firm.

—**Assoff and Brundinharg**

Planning means the determination of what is to be done, how and where is to be done, who is to do and how results are to be evaluated.   —**James Lundy**

Purposes/Objectives of Planning

- To diminish vulnerability and hazards and aid in decision making.

- To gives reasonable perspective without bounds anticipating the hierarchical achievement of the organization.
- To enable the organization to achieve its destinations.
- To provide excellent and affordable health services, cooperatively.
- To prepare professionals become skilled, empathetic, and moral health care providers, instructors, and pioneers.
- To build up an arrangement of the referral system and bridge the gap of health services in the community.
- To lead to the successful utilization of assets and monetary tasks.

Principles

- Planning must focus on purposes.
- Planning is a continuous and frequent process.
- Planning should be simple, and there should be provision for proper analysis and classification of actions.
- There should be good harmony with the organization and environment.
- Planning is hierarchical.
- Planning should be precise in its aims and scope and cover the entire organization with all its departments, sectors, and different levels of administration, and it should be balanced.
- Use all available resources.
- Planning should always be documented.

PLANNING PROCESS

- **Being aware of opportunities:** It is not a strict part of planning as the awareness of internal and external is the beginning step of the planning process.
- **Establishing objectives:** There is a need to develop general and specific purposes. This helps in determining the long-term as well as short-term range. It also determines the outcome of the planning process and its evaluation methods.
- **Developing premises:** It indicates the preparation of associated background features based on which the plan can form. Premises exists within and outside the company. Relevant internal premises are the skilled labor, machinery, methods of internal functioning, financial, and other abilities of the company. External premises include population growth, political stability, sociological factors, and government policies.
- **Determining alternative courses:** There may be many possibilities/courses of action to attain the desired objectives. Though all the plans may not always be equally effective and best, still, the planner must perform good homework to discover the most effective possibilities.

- **Evaluating alternative courses:** Here, the planner examines the merits and demerits of each course of action. This is followed by assessing the weight of merits and demerits to select one direction for the attainment of the desired objective.
- **Selecting course:** Based on the findings in the evaluation of the merits and demerits of all alternative courses, the manager decides the best course of action.
- **Formulating derivative plans:** It is the responsibility of the manager at the middle and the lower level to frame appropriate policies, associate programs, and day to day operations based on the selected broad course. It also includes the appropriate proposal of budget and its subunits for the smooth operations. This is commonly termed as a derivative plan.
- **Budgeting:** The final step in the planning process is budget. The budget becomes meaningful and standardized if the expected objectives are attained.

Types of Planning

- **Directional planning:** It is referred to as policy planning since it shows the generalized direction of the program. For example, state-level planning at directorate or secretarial of states or union. (center).
- **Administrative planning:** It is the implementation of desired or developed policies. It is done in conjunction with the mobilization and coordination of the personnel and material available in the administrative unit for the effectuation of the service. E.g., the Medical Superintendent of the major hospital is responsible for administrative planning.
- **Operational planning:** It is concerned with the actual delivery of the service to the community. Operational or short-range planning is undertaken by middle or supervisory level personnel. It involves planning for the short duration that may range from a few months to a year.
- **Strategic planning:** This is part of policy planning. It is broad and decides the primary goals or directions of the organization. The organization relies heavily on external information, i.e., estimates of costs, technological developments, etc. The top-level managers usually develop policies as per the challenges in the organization externally or internally.
- **Tactical planning:** It is the actualization stage of strategic planning. Here, the managers decide on the optimal utilization of resources that helps in achieving the strategic goals of the organization.

Distinction between Strategic and Tactical Planning

Strategic planning	Tactical planning
It is the overall planning that decides the objectives of the organization and the allotment of resources accordingly.	It is the practical application methods of strategic planning.
Done by top-level management and long-term in nature.	Done by middle and lower-level management and short-term in nature.
It takes into account the long-term forecast of technology, political environment, etc.	Based on the past performance of the organization.
Less detailed as it does not consider the day to day operations of the organization.	More detailed.

Advantages of Planning

- Planning leads to more effective and faster achievements of any organization.
- Planning gives strength to the business or service for its continuous growth and steady prosperity.
- Planning secures and ensures the unity of purpose, direction, and effort by focusing attention on objectives. It avoids duplication of services.
- Planning has a unique contribution to the efficiency of other managerial functions.
- Planning provides the basis for control in an organization.
- It is an integral part of administrative functions.
- It ensures order and control and determines the appropriateness and feasibility of actions in terms of cost-effectiveness and quality control.

Disadvantages of Planning

- It depends upon facts and information; reliable information is not possible.
- Planning may lead to internal inflexibilities and procedural rigidities.
- It is a time consuming and expensive process.

PROGRAM EVALUATION AND REVIEW TECHNIQUE

The program evaluation and review technique (PERT) was developed by the Special Projects Office of the U.S. Navy and applied to the planning and control of the Polaris Weapon system in 1958. It worked then, it still works, and it has been widely used as a controlling process in the business and industry.

Definition

"PERT is a network system model for planning and control under uncertain conditions. It involves identifying the key activities in a project, sequencing the activities in a flow diagram (critical pathways), and assigning the duration of each phase of the work."

The activities that cause the progress from one event to another are indicated by arrows, with the direction of the arrow showing the course of the workflow.

Steps for Accomplishing the PERT

The PERT also deals with the problem of uncertainty concerning time by estimating the time variances associated with the expected time of completion of the subtasks. It is a statistical method of time planning for a project/work. Three projected times are generally determined.

- **The optimistic time (O):** This occasionally happens when everything goes right. Optimistic time(t_o) estimates the completion time without complication.
- **The most likely time (M):** It represents the most accurate forecast based on standard developments. The most likely time(t_m) estimated the completion time with routine problems.
- **The pessimistic time (P):** This is estimated at maximum potential difficulties. Pessimistic time(t_p) determines the completion time given numerous problems.

The expected time of completion of a particular project by using beta probability distribution using the formula

$$(t_e) = \frac{t_o + 4(t_m) + t_p}{6}$$

Example: A nurse administrator is planning to set up a new ICU in a particular hospital. The Critical Path Method (CPM) is used to plan, coordinate, and control the activities of this project. The following subtasks are listed: (Fig. 2)

A: Meeting to finalize the idea of setting up an ICU.
B: Planning the infrastructure. (1 week)
C: Prepare the list of articles needed for the unit and put tender. (1 week)
D: Finalize the bid. (1 week)
E: Prepare the budget, both capital and operating. (1 week)
F: Draw the plan of ICU, and estimate the cost. (1 week)

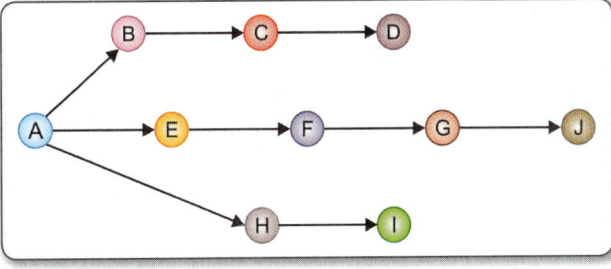

Fig. 2: Critical path method

G: Order for the articles. (1 week)

H: Give the work to the contractors to start the work. (1 week)

I: Get the materials like cement gravel tiles, electric and plumbing materials. (1 week)

J: Start the project.

PERT model indicates that subtask A should be done at first. Task C and D can be done only after the completion of task B. Task E is the predecessor of task F. Task A, B, C, D, E, and F must be completed before Task G. Finally Task J can be achieved after the completion of Task G and I. If the optimistic time is 8 weeks, the most likely time 10 weeks, and the pessimistic time 12 weeks, the expected time is,

$$t_e = \frac{8 \text{ weeks} + 4\,(10 \text{ weeks}) + 12 \text{ weeks}}{6} = \frac{60 \text{ weeks}}{6} = 10 \text{ weeks}$$

Using the critical pathways, one can also plan the time duration for completing each subtask, the sum of which can be the total expected time.

Advantages of PERT

- It encourages logical discipline in planning, scheduling, and control of the project.
- It encourages more long-range and detailed project planning.

- It provides a standard method of documenting and communicating project plans, schedules, and time and cost- performance.
- It identifies the most critical elements in the plan, thus focusing management attention, .i.e. most constraining on the schedule.
- It illustrates the effects of technical procedural changes on overall schedules.
- It is used for complicated and extensive projects.
- It is forward-looking.

GANTT CHARTS (ACTIVITY PLAN)

Early in this century, **Henry L. Gantt** developed the Gantt Chart as a means of controlling production/projects. It depicted a series of events essential to the completion of a project or program. It is usually used for production activities. It is typically a bar chart that explains a project schedule. It illustrates the start and finishes dates of the critical elements in a project. It is commonly used in combination with PERT as a medium to plot and represent the figures of PERT. PERT and GANTT CHARTS can be easily understood with the help of the same example as mentioned before (Fig. 3).

Example: A nurse administrator is planning to set up a new ICU in a particular hospital. The Critical Path Method (CPM) is used to plan, coordinate, and control the activities of this project. The following subtasks are listed (Table 1):

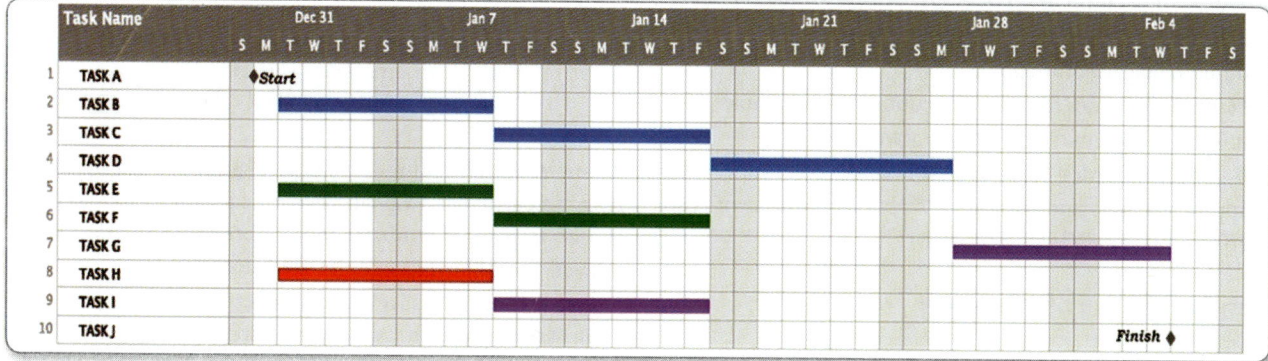

Fig. 3: Gantt chart

TABLE 1: Gantt chart

Sub task	Predecessor	Expected time
A: Meeting to finalize the idea of setting up an ICU.	Nil	0 days
B: Planning the infrastructure.	A (Start)	Seven days
C: Prepare the list of articles needed for the unit and put tender.	B	Seven days
D: Finalize the tender.	C	Seven days
E: Prepare the budget, both capital and operating.	A	Seven days
F: Draw the plan of ICU, and estimate the cost.	E	Seven days
G: Order for the articles.	D, F	Seven days
H: Give the work to the contractors to start the work.	A	Seven days
I: Get the materials like cement gravel tiles, electric and plumbing materials.	H	Seven days
J: Start the project.	G, I (Finish)	0 days

The PERT model indicates that subtask A should be done at first. Task C and D can be done only after the completion of task B. Task E is the predecessor of Task F. Task A, B, C, D, E, and F must be completed before Task G. Finally Task J can be achieved after the completion of Task G and I.

In the above table, there are ten tasks labeled from A to J. Some jobs can be done concurrently while others cannot be done until their predecessor task is complete. Additionally, each job has three-time estimates: the optimistic time estimate (O), the most likely time estimate (M), and the pessimistic time estimate (P). (Only the expected time is mentioned in the table which is calculated using PERT formula.)

Advantages of Gantt Charts

- It forces planning and shows how pieces fit together.
- It does this for all the nursing line managers involved.
- It establishes a system for periodic evaluation and control at critical points in the program.
- It reveals problems and is forward-looking.

MILESTONE CHART

A milestone is used to represent groups of activities or significant events or commitments in the project. A milestone chart shows a group of milestones in an organized way similar to a Gantt chart with one milestone per line vertically with a description on the left and the milestone located horizontally along a time scale showing when it occurs. Milestones differ from the bars in a Gantt chart in that they show only a single date and are usually depicted as a triangle instead of a bar. Milestone chart stones can be shown in various colors depicting the status of the milestone. Milestones can also appear on Gantt charts (Fig. 4).

A Milestone Chart focuses on planned significant events scheduled to occur at specific times in the program. Such events could be the initiation or completion of a particularly important or critical activity, equipment deliveries, reviews, or approval dates. Like the Gantt Chart, the milestone chart uses symbols imposed on a calendar to provide information about planned and actual completion dates and any revisions to the milestone schedule. There is no standard set of symbols for milestone charts. The Figure below shows examples of the symbols prescribed for reporting milestone information (Fig. 5).

In the early days of project management, project managers made up Gantt charts for their projects. These Gantt charts could be quite large when projects contained over one hundred activities. It was not practical for the project manager to duplicate the Gantt chart for his/her manager, and if the supervisor of the project managers had several project managers, it was not practical to display all of the projects' Gantt charts unless there was quite a lot of wall space.

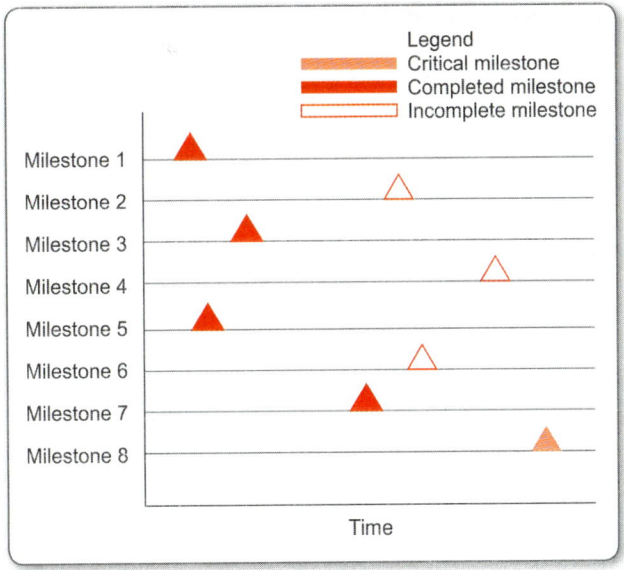

Fig. 4: Milestone chart

Standard symbols have been adapted for air force milestone schedules. The most common symbols used and their meanings are shown below.	
Basic symbol	**Meaning**
⇧	Schedule completion
⬆	Actual completion
◇	Previous scheduled completion—Still is future
◆	Previous scheduled completion—Date passed
Representative uses	**Meaning**
◇ ⇧	Anticipated slip—Rescheduled completion
◆ ⇧	Actual slip—Rescheduled completion
◆ ⬆	Actual slip—Actual completion
⬆	Actual completion ahead if schedule
⬆ ⇧	Time span action
⇧ ⇨	Continuous action

Fig. 5: Symbols

The milestone chart was devised to save space on the project managers' supervisor's walls. Each project manager collected related groups of activities in the project and assigned a milestone to each group. A milestone was placed on the project schedule representing the group. Another milestone was placed on the project managers' supervisor's milestone chart as well.

If there were changes in the schedule that affected the completion date of the milestone, the project manager had to visit the supervisor's office and move the milestone. In all likelihood, the project manager explained the schedule slide at this time as well.

Milestone schedules can be produced using today's project management software. They are created simply by listing the milestones as activities and giving them a duration of zero. Since they are being created on a Gantt chart, the length of the Gantt schedule bar for the milestone would have a zero-length and could not be seen. A triangle or another symbol is put on the chart instead. The symbol can be colored to show various statuses and conditions as needed.

Program Managers (PM) rarely use pure Gantt or milestone charts. Normally they integrate the information from these charts and display it in a combination chart. Such a chart can be useful in displaying the planned and actual duration of activities using the Gantt chart symbols and in monitoring the progress for completing key events in these activities using the milestone symbols.

BASICS OF BUDGETING

Budgeting, even though necessarily perceived as a gadget for controlling, turns into a remarkable piece of the planning. Each organization develops a plan that includes its anticipated volume of work, the cost of the work to be accomplished, and the expenses required to make that work a reality. In any organization, budgeting is done for indicating the expected results of the business and the possible future lines of action to be followed for the attainment of such outcomes (Fig. 6).

"Budget is a precise concrete picture of the total operation of an enterprise in monetary terms.   —(HM Donovan)

It is a plan for the coordination of resources and expenditures.

—(Merriam-Webster Dictionary)

Significance

- **Budget: A tool of effective administration:** When considering the budget as a tool of effective administration the executives will have requisite power and discretion in budgetary matters such as executive program, executive responsibility, and executive direction.

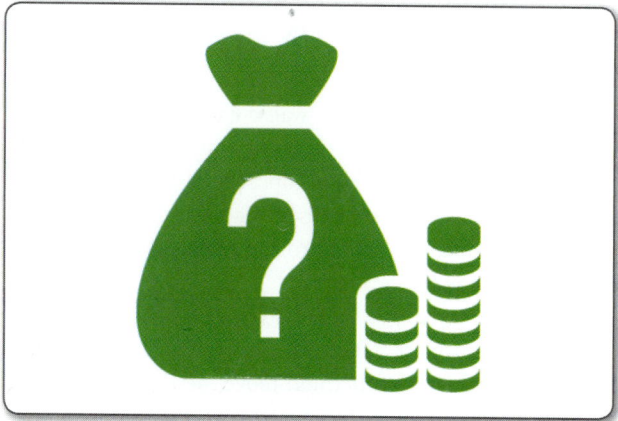

Fig. 6: Budgeting

- **Budget: A tool for legislative control:** The budget is the most important tool of legislature control over the money of the public. This control is extended not only to the creation of revenues but also covers the part of the expenditure. It brings publicity, clarity, comprehensiveness, and unity in the budget.
- **Budget: Integration role and functions:** A budget is a plan that uses numbers to predict the growth of the organization. The Nursing care budget accounts for 80% of the total expenditure of a health care organization. Hence, nurse managers must understand the concepts of financial planning so that they can be aware of their roles and responsibilities as a nurse manager.
- **Budget:** An instrument of Economic and social policies. The budget is used as a tool of progress by many disciplines. According to an Economist, budget is the key factor influencing the economical growth of the organization, whereas it is a tool of criticism for political parties. The administration uses the budget as an administrative tool to exercise discipline, coordination, and structure of the organization.

Purposes

- Budget supplies the instrument for deciphering financial year objectives into an anticipated month to month spending design.
- The budget improves financial arranging and necessary leadership.
- The spending plan/budget perceives controllable and wild cost zones.
- The budget offers a valuable arrangement for conveying financial destinations.
- The budget permits input/feedback on the use of the spending plan/budget.
- The budget gives to estimate and recording money related accomplishment with the targets of the establishment.

Principles

- The budget ought to give sound money related to administration by concentrating on the prerequisite of the establishment.
- The budget should center around the targets and strategies of the organization. It must spill out of goals and give reasonable articulation to the method for the practicability of such a purpose.
- The budget ought to guarantee the best utilization of rare money related and nonfinancial assets.
- The budget necessitates that program exercises arranged ahead of time.
- The budgetary process requires reliable designation for which settled obligations and duties are required to be distributed to administrators at another level for confining and executing the financial plan.

- The budget ought to incorporate activities of different offices, setting up a casing of reference for administrative choice, and giving specific criteria for assessing organizational execution.
- The budget is set up under the heading of the supervision of the organization or monetary/financial officer.
- The budget is to be readied and translated reliably all through the organization in the correspondence of the planning process.

Types of Budgets

- **Master and functional budgets:** A master budget is prepared for the entire organization incorporating the budget of different functions. For example, when we refer to the annual budget of the government of India, it includes the budget outlays of different ministries. In business organizations, the master budget incorporates various functions and units and their outlays. It generally includes sales, production, costs.

  A functional budget is prepared to incorporate a significant function and its sub-functions. Since an organization may have several functions, various operational budgets are prepared. For example, production budget, the cash budget for an organization.

- **Capital and revenue budget:** An activity at an organizational level includes two procedures, i.e., facilitation for different activities and actual performance activities. Creating facilities for carrying out activities include capital expenditure whose returns accrue over several years. For such exercises, the capital budget is readied, which is basically a rundown of what administration accepts to be beneficial activities for the procurement of new resources together with the evaluated cost of each task.

  On the contrary, the revenue budget is the formation of a target for a year or so for various organizational activities such as production, marketing, finance, etc. Thus, a revenue budget includes expenditure and earning for a specific period of one year.

- **Long-term and short-term budgets:** Many organizations integrate their yearly budgets with long-term projections of business activities and annual budgets; they prepare budgets for a more extended period of 2–3 years. When one budget period is over, budgets are ready for the next year and the subsequent 2–3 years.

  The short-term budget is for a year and is divided into many periods for effective implementation. For example, cash budgets are every year as well as on a monthly or quarterly basis to facilitate better cash management.

- **Fixed ceiling budget and flexible budget:** Generally, Fixed Ceiling Budget is prepared by organizations where there is no chance of modifying the budget according to the actual activity. It remains fixed/static for the specified period of time. When an organization's size of business can be predicted with a fair amount of precision, the fixed budget is satisfactory.

  A budget that is designed to change in accordance with the activities of the organization is known as a flexible budget. It considers several levels of activity and assumes that labor, material, or facilities used in production and hence cost varies with a known relationship to the actual activity.

- **Incremental budget:** It is prepared in reference to the previous years budget. Based on the current needs and previous performance some percentage of figures are added or subtracted to the previous year's budget to prepare Incremental Budget.

- **Open-ended budget:** A budget that does not close till the completion of all the transactions. It is in which each working director of each department shows an individual cost evaluation for each program in the unit, without demonstrating how the budget ought to be downsized if less income is available.

- **Rollover budget:** A type of budget where the credits and debts of a month roll over to another month. If there is overspending in a particular month, then the following month will begin with a negative count, but if the reverse happens, then the consecutive month will start with a positive count. To oblige customized that more prominent focus/target than the yearly budget cycle.

- **Sunset budget:** It is intended to "Self Destruct" inside a recommended day and age to guarantee the discontinuance of expense in by a foreordained date.

- **Sales budget and production budget:** This is the beginning stage in a budgetary process since sales are first initiates which offer shape to every single other action. Whereas, the production budget aims at maximizing, manufacturing and optimal utilization of available facilities.

Approaches to Budgeting

The Historical Approach

It is a traditional method of budgeting where the relationship between the volume of work and its required cost is calculated. Additionally, the nurse manager reviews and plans the budget accordingly based on the past experiences of the organization. Many diseases are seasonal and specific to certain geographic locations. A health care organization located in a rural hilly side shall be prepared in terms of manpower and materials to treat orthopedic patients with fractures. A clinical located near to an elementary school should be equipped with all the first aid materials required for the treatment of immediate injury to children while playing. This historical perspective helps to determine the number of supplies to stock and staffing patterns.

Standard Cost

Standard Costs may be developed to predict what labor and supplies should cost. A community health nurse can predict the standard number of visits done by each member of the family to choose and adopt birth control measures. Multiplying this number along with the cost of the birth control measures such as Pills, Condoms, others will help in the prediction of the inventory needed for the month/year along with its cost.

Zero-based Budgeting

Zero-based budgeting (ZBB) is a method of budgeting in which all expenses must be justified and approved for each new period. Developed by Peter Pyhrr in the 1970s, zero-based budgeting starts from a "zero base" at the beginning of every budget period, analyzing needs and costs of every function within an organization and allocating funds accordingly, regardless of how much money has previously been budgeted to any given line item.

Traditional budgeting calls for incremental increases over previous budgets, such as a 2% increase in spending, as opposed to a justification of both old and new expenses, as called for with zero-based budgeting. Traditional budgeting analyzes only new expenditures, while ZBB starts from zero and calls for a justification of old, recurring expenses in addition to new expenditures. Zero-based budgeting aims to put the onus on managers to justify expenses and aims to drive value for an organization by optimizing costs and not just revenue.

Suppose a company making medical equipment implements a zero-based budgeting process calling for closer scrutiny of manufacturing department expenses. The company notices that the cost of certain parts used in its final products and outsourced to another manufacturer increases by 5% every year. The company can make those parts in-house using its workers. After weighing the positives and negatives of in-house manufacturing, the company finds it can make the parts more cheaply than the outside supplier. Instead of blindly increasing the budget by a certain percentage and masking the cost increase, the company can identify a situation in which it can decide to make the part itself or buy the part from the external supplier for its end products. Traditional budgeting may not allow cost drivers within departments to be identified. Zero-based budgeting is a more granular process that aims to identify and justify expenditures.

Zero-based budgeting is known for accuracy, efficiency, reduction of wasteful spending and improved coordination and communication. At the same time, it is negatively influenced by bureaucracy, corruption, intangible justifications, managerial time, slower response time.

Periodic Budgetary Review

Managers must review the budget periodically and make necessary modifications if required. If the modifications are too frequent then the original budget becomes useless. One way to avoid this situation is to foresee the increased labor costs and inflations cost of materials in advance. When discrepancies are found between the actual and performing budget the managers must identify the cause for the same so that the necessary modification can be done to the future budget.

Supplementary Budget

Some budgetary flexibility may be obtained through a supplementary monthly budget. This is usually added to the basic minimal budget that is prepared annually.

Moving Budget

The moving budget is used when budget forecasting is difficult. The moving budget plans for a certain length of time such as a year. At the end of each month, another month is added to replace the one just completed. Thus the budgetary period remains the same.

COST-EFFECTIVENESS AND COST ANALYSIS

Cost-effectiveness analysis (CEA) is a type of financial examination that looks at the relative consumption (expenses) and results (impacts) of at least two strategies. Cost-effectiveness analysis is regularly utilized where a cost-benefit investigation is improper. Commonly the CEA is communicated in terms of a proportion where the denominator is the outcome of the activity, and the numerator is the cost of the action. E.g.

$$CEA = \frac{\text{The total cost of addressing a particular health problem using a specific intervention}}{\text{The total health gain}}$$

Cost is the aggregate sum of money that should be spent by an association or an individual or government.

Types of Costs

- **Fixed costs:** Fixed costs are those costs that stay the same regardless of the level of the activity. They are not related to volume. They remain constant as the volume increases and decreases over the period. Among fixed costs are deprivation of equipment and buildings, salaries, benefits, utilizes, interest on loans or bonds, and taxes. Example: Fixed costs are those which would exist even if the organization were "shut down."

- **Variable costs:** Variable costs are those cost that changes depending on the level of volume. They do relate to amount and census (patient-days). They include items such as meals and linen. The cost of supplies varies by patient registration, physician orders, and diagnosis. Example: the cost of surgical dressing increases when the patient's wound has drainage and dressings to be changed frequently.

- **Sunk costs:** Sunk costs are fixed expenses that cannot be recovered even if the program is canceled. Example: Advertising.
- **Accounting costs:** These are external costs are expressed in terms of money that is out of the specified bank account of the organization, and it is utilized for the functioning of the organization. These are the real costs of the working of an organization.
- **Economic costs:** These are costs that are both internal and external. These are values that are not necessarily registered in the account sheet, but they are assumed to be the cost of managing an organization.
- **Average cost:** "Full cost divided by the number of units of service or patients."
- **Direct costs:** Direct costs are those expenses that directly affect patient care, e.g., salaries for the nursing personnel who provide hands-on patient care is considered as a direct cost.
- **Indirect costs:** Indirect costs are the expenditures that are necessary but do not affect patient care directly. Ex: salaries for dietary or housekeeping personnel.

Cost Containment

The goal of the cost containment is to keep the cost within acceptable limits for volume inflation, and other adequate personnel. It involves the following:

- **Cost awareness:** It focuses on the employee's attention on costs. It increases organizational awareness of what prices are, the process available for containing them, how they can be managed, and by whom.
- **Cost monitoring:** It focuses on how much will be spent where, when, and why. It identifies reports and monitors costs. Staffing costs should be determined. Recruitment, turnover, absenteeism, and sick time are analyzed, and inventories are controlled.
- **Cost management:** It focuses on what can be done by whom to contain costs. Programs, plans, objectives, and strategies are essential. Responsibility and accountability for the control should be established. A committee can identify long and short-range plans and strategies.
- **Cost avoidance:** It means not buying supplies, technology, or services. Supply and equipment costs should be carefully analyzed. The values and effectiveness of disposable versus reusable items are compared.
- **Cost reduction:** It means spending less on goods and services. The amount of discount depends on the size of the agency, previous efficiency, skills of managers, and cooperation of employees.
- **Cost control:** It is a valid use of available resources through careful forecasting, planning, budget preparation, reporting, and monitoring.

Cost Analysis

It is the system of analyzing the relationship between the fixed and the variable cost.

Types of Cost Analysis

- **Cost-benefit analysis (CBA):** It is also called BCA benefit costs analysis (BCA) CBA is a measurement of the relative costs and benefits associated with a particular project or task. It is a procedure by which all the costs resulting from installing and operating a system are determined and converted to a money amount, and the ratio is calculated to reflect the relationship between costs and benefits. This approach has mainly two applications.
  - Understand the direction of investments or investment decisions.
  - How much is the weighting of benefits against the investments done?

    This provides guidelines for future investments. Cost-benefit analysis is often used in the public sector where there is no net income to serve as a guideline. To determine the ratio, it is necessary to assign a value to both the cost and the benefits in monetary terms. In practice, it is difficult to assign monetary values to health care outcomes. It is difficult to measure the value of life and even more difficulty in measuring the difference in health outcomes that do not involve life or death. There are two basic approaches to CBA such as;
  - **Ratio approach:** The ratio approach indicates the number of benefits (or outcomes) that can be realized per unit expenditure on a project. The upper side of the benefit-cost ratio (BCR) shows the profitability of the investment. As cost alter the benefit also alter.
  - **Net benefit approach:** The net benefits approach indicates the absolute amount of money saved or lost due to the use of technology against a comparator. In the net benefits formulation, a technique is cost-beneficial against a comparison if the net change in benefits exceeds the net change in costs.
- **Cost-benefit ratio (CBR):** It is the mathematical relationship between the value of the financial cost of a program and the importance of benefits. It is defined as the ratio of the value of the benefits of an alternative to the amount of alternative cost.

$$Z = \frac{\text{Present value of economic benefits}}{\text{The present value of economic cost}} \times 1000$$

- **Cost-of-illness analysis:** A determination of the economic impact of an illness or condition (typically on a given region, population, or country), e.g., of smoking, arthritis or bedsores, including the associated treatment costs.
- **Cost-minimization analysis:** A determination of the least costly alternative interventions that are assumed to produce equivalent outcomes.

- **Cost-utility analysis (CUA):** A form of cost-effectiveness analysis that compares costs in monetary units with outcomes in terms of their utility, usually to the patient, measured.
- **Cost-consequence analysis:** A form of cost-effectiveness analysis that presents costs and outcomes in discrete categories, without aggregating or weighing them.
- **Cost-effectiveness analysis (CEA):** It is a technique that measures the cost of alternatives that generate the same outcome. Cost-effectiveness analysis is the technique for choosing, from alternative courses of action, a preferred choice when objectives are not evident in such areas as sales, costs or profits or it is the desired effect of careful planning, or it means getting the most for your money or the product is worth the price. Cost-effective methods are those searches for the least costly way of achieving a defined result.

BUDGET PROPOSAL

A Budget Proposal is a formal document that is used to provide the financial budget plan for the company, a project, or a campaign. This proposal is very important because the accounting department will be based on this document to identify how much is needed by the company to continue the business. A budget proposal is essentially a detailed and research-supported cost pitch for a project or departmental operating period. Budget proposals are used in corporate, academic and non-profit enterprises. They are also good tools to help you understand the true scope of your project before you present it. Generally, the budget proposal comprises of the following;

- **Purpose or goal:** Clearly state your mission in the first section of the budget proposal. Your mission statement is a one or two-sentence description of the what, when, where, why and how of your budget's purpose or goal. For example: "This project is planned for the conduction of a National Conference in Jammu and Kashmir in the upcoming October-November. This will enable the creation of a great platform for the Teachers, Practitioners, Students, and Scholars to share their research and innovations in nursing education and practice. Sponsorships for this project will come in the form of grants from National agencies and Medical Book Publishers." Elaborate on the benefits to be derived from the project that the proposal represents or the operational continuance of your department. Explain how the benefits exceed the costs.
- **Direct costs:** The second section deals with the costs of conducting the conference. These are called direct costs because they directly relate to the benefit being created. It includes cost of arranging the resource persons, materials, equipment, travel, communications, research and so on.
- **Facilities and administration costs:** Most sponsorships and grants do not pay for facilities and administration costs, so list these costs separately in your budget proposal

if you are using it to request grants or sponsorships for a project. These are costs that are not directly identified with the project benefits, including facilities use, utilities, support staff and so on.

- **Anticipated revenue or benefit:** Finish your budget proposal with a section that details the expected benefits, such as revenue from registration fee, the non-monetary benefits of conducting the conference and so on. Remember the benefit must appear greater than the cost, so don't suddenly become conservative or modest in describing the benefit or you may not get your budget approved.

A Sample Budget Proposal: National Conference on (Nursing Education and Practices (NCNEP – 2020)

This proposal is planned for the conduction of two days National Conference in a particular Nursing College (Table 2).

NCNEP 2020 will focus on educational research directed toward its impact on clinical outcomes, through oral and poster presentations, educational workshop sessions, and influential plenary presentations. Attendees will be provided with the tools to enhance nursing education programs to make education more effective in Nursing and Healthcare practice.

Objectives

- This Conference is a platform for nursing students, faculty, deans, researchers, and leaders to collaborate on topics affecting nursing education.
- Attend prominent plenary sessions about relevant issues affecting Nursing and Healthcare.

Target Audience: (250–300 People)

- Deans/Professors
- Nursing Lecturers
- Nurses
- Nurse Practitioners
- Nursing Students

HOSPITAL AND HOSPITAL PLANNING

A Hospital is an integral part of a social and medical organization, the function of which is to provide for a population complete health care, both curative and preventive and whose outpatient services reach out to the family and its home environment. It also should have a provision for training and research. —**World Health Organization (WHO)**

A Hospital or Health Care Facility is a part of essential services. In satisfying this obligation, a hospital ought to be planned with specific generally recognized standards. The standards of hospital planning are equal for all types of hospitals at the national/state/local level.

TABLE 2: Budget proposal for NCNEP 2020

Sr. No.	Particulars	Estimated cost in INR
1	**DIRECT COSTS**	
A	Registration Kit for participants	15,000/-
B	Honorarium for invited Speakers	50,000/-
C	Printing and Stationery	65,000/-
D	Transportation	2,00,000/-
E	Accommodation	30,000/-
F	Accreditation Fee	10,000/-
G	Catering and Refreshments	3,00,000/-
2	**FACILITIES AND ADMINISTRATION COSTS**	
A	Rent/Charge for the venue	30,000/-
B	Decoration of the venue	30,000/-
C	Felicitation of Inaugural and Valedictory Function	30,000
D	Cultural Evening	20,000/-
E	Photography and Videography	50,000/-
	Total	8,30,000/-
3	**Anticipated revenue (Monetary)**	
A	Registration fee @ ₹4000/- per person 4000 × 300	12,00,000/-
B	Sponsorship expected from different sources (general)	2,00,000/-
4	**Anticipated revenue (Non-monetary)** Attendees can take advantage of opportunities to learn about the latest innovations in Nursing and Healthcare from a variety of oral and poster presentations. Meet and network with nurses ranging from students to deans, faculty, and researchers. Take advantage of opportunities to collaborate with nurses from around the country.	

Aims of Hospital Planning

- Update the current hospital facility with new offices/facilities.
- To cover more population and upgrade the utilization of hospitals.
- To modernize the hospital and enhance the maximum efficiency of the hospital.
- To reduce costs and increase the efficiency of services.

Classification of Hospitals

Hospitals, in general, are classified into two categories depending upon the agencies which finance them:

- **Government or public hospitals:** They are managed by government services, either central or state or federal, municipal, or departmental bodies that are managed from the overall budget for public services.
- **Non-government hospitals:** They are managed by individuals, charitable organizations, religious groups, industrial undertakings, etc. Based on ownership patterns, non-governmental hospitals are classified as:
  - Private (personal)
  - Partnership
  - Private (family) trust
  - Public charitable trust
  - Cooperative society
  - Private limited company

Detailed classification of hospitals is explained in the upcoming Units.

Principles in Hospital Planning

- Astounding Patient Care: It very well may be accomplished by the hospital by receiving or adopting the following measures:
  - Provision of suitable specialized types of equipment and supplies.

- A hierarchical structure that appoints obligation and requires responsibility for different capacities inside the association.
- A nonstop audit of the sufficiency of care and service given by doctors, nursing staff, and paramedical workforce.
- Effective Orientation to Community: This ought to be accomplished by adapting the following:-
  - A Governing board of people with administration capacity and those who are concerned with the community.
  - Policies that guarantee the accessibility of administrations to all individuals.
  - Participation in community projects to give preventive consideration.
- Sequential Planning: Systematic arranging ought to be accomplished by the hospital by following:-
  - Accept the responsibility of all planning with the consultation of all functional advisors such as financial, architectural, and so on.
  - Prepare short term plans for offices, staffing, material management, etc.
- Economic reasonability: It includes approaches such as:-
  - A corporate association that acknowledges an obligation regarding sound money related administration with regards to the quality of care.
  - An arranged program of development dependent on represented community needs.
  - A yearly budget that will allow the hospital to keep pace with times.
- Sound compositional/architectural arrangement: It can be accomplished by:-
  - Selection of a site adequately tremendous to oblige future improvement and accessibility of people.
  - Recognize and plan the internal traffic for staff, visitors, and patients, including their arrangements for transportation.
  - Create provisions to accommodate the future advancement in medical sciences and the public need.

Structural Hospital Planning Process

- **Conceptualization of hospital:** The originator of the idea takes the initiative to convert the innovative ideas into a plan. The design may include his/her dreams, knowledge, past experiences, reference to the clinics/hospitals in the country and abroad, etc. (Fig. 7).
- **Support groups:** Once the originator gets the bright idea of the conceptualization of the proposed health care setting, he/she seeks direction to get the backup of support groups. A health care organization at large scale comes to reality when the originator joins hands with other support people or groups who share the common interest.

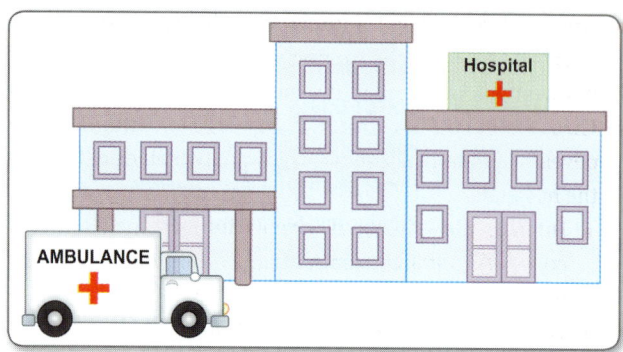

Fig. 7: Hospital planning

- **Temporary organization and securing funds:** A hospital trust duly registered with government is framed. It comprises of a chairperson and many members who perform different tasks as required. An unequivocal work out of the capital necessary for the hospital set up is also needed.
- **Geographical, ecological and random components:** Consider the geological and meteorological factors of the area including road transport, other means of transportation, type of land, rules for construction, building height limitations because of the closeness to air terminals. Assess the facilities for water, waste management, etc.
- **Hospital plan:**
  - **Bed planning:** The hospital will be used by people from the local, regional, state, national, and international levels. An ideal footfall of 85% of the bed strength is desirable.
  - **Hospital size:** As a large hospital of 1000 beds or more turns out to be to a high degree hastily to work, and a little hospital of 50 or less is not productive. Ideally, two 400-bedded-hospital is recommended than one 800-bedded-hospital. All establishments should have a provision for future expansion.
- **Land prerequisites:** Either urban or rural, the land must be available in abundance for the hospital enhancement. The property shall be well connected with other parts, and other facilities should be possible (Table 3).
- **Public utilities:** This fundamentally incorporates continuous power supply, water supply, sewage transfer framework, and different conveniences for extensive use.

TABLE 3: Land prerequisites

No. of beds	Storey of building	Land in acres
50 beds	Single floor	10 acres
100 beds	Single floor	15–20 acres
200 beds	Double floor	20–25 acres
500 beds	3–5 floors	55–70 acres
700 beds	4–6 floors	80–90 acres
1000 beds	6–9 floors	90–100 acres

- **Approval from local authorities:** All the constructions must be approved by competent authorities before the development of the desired structure.
- **Circulation courses/routes:** It decides the usefulness and development of the hospital. There are two kinds of flow in the hospital.-
  - **Interior flow/Internal circulation:** It includes the corridors, stairs, lifts, movement within different units/wards, etc.
  - **Outside flow/External circulation:** There ought to be separate gates for entry and exit. Both the entry and exit should be wide enough to accommodate the hospital traffic, movement of beds, wheelchairs, trolley, machines, etc. Separate entrance or retreat can be made for staff/employees.
- **Distances, parking and landscaping:** Minimize the gap between different departments and associated areas to increase the speed of accessibility by patients and staff.
- **Zonal conveyance and interrelationship of departments:** The OPD, Emergency and similar areas ought to be segregated from the primary inpatient territories and distributed zones nearer to the principal entrance as more people come to these areas.
- **Climatic consideration:** In an exceptionally warm and cold atmosphere hospital should be air-conditioned. This can be achieved through sound and advanced architectural planning and electrical facilities. There should be a sufficient ventilation facility.
- **Equipping a hospital:** Hospital equipment may be categorized as:
  - **Physical plant:** It incorporates necessary facilities such as lifts, air conditioning, central heating facility, incinerators, boilers, central oxygen supply, dietary facility, and so on.
  - **Hospital furniture and machines:** Patient beds, wheelchairs, stretchers, trolleys, bedside lockers, versatile/privacy screens, medicine/instrument trolleys, and so on.
  - **General-purpose furniture and apparatuses:** It incorporates office machines, office furniture, ceramics, etc.
  - **Therapeutic and demonstrative gear:** It includes equipment for general utilization, for example, BP apparatus, suction pumps, and so forth and gear for interacting with patients for diagnostic and therapeutic purposes. For example, X-ray, Ultrasound, Defibrillators, CT scan, etc.
- **Cost assessment of the development of hospital:** The most well-known technique for evaluating the expense is based on per bed cost. It will likewise change in accordance with the kinds of facilities provided by the hospital such as education, training and research.

Functional Planning of Hospital

Outpatient Department

The OPD is where all patients, aside from the individuals who are in an emergency, desire benefit in a hospital. It ought to be effectively open to the external individuals and has to be a different wing in the hospital, which is equally accessible from the main entrance of the hospital as well as the main public road. The span of OPD relies on the average footfall of the patients and services provided to them. It also relies on extended services like phlebotomy, diagnostic facility, blood bank, etc. too. The OPD has distinctive zones;

- **Functional zone:** This zone is for patients coming to OPD and relatives. It incorporates parking, entrance lobby, waiting area, "May I Help You" counter, registration, and other associated offices.
- **Administrative zone:** This zone is the part of a substantially larger hospital. It helps in the organization and coordination of the facilities provided in the OPD. It includes the offices such as In charge of OPD, Nursing Station, Billing/Cash counters, and MRD.
- **Diagnostic zone:** The different useful units are Clinical lab Imaging area such as X-ray/CT/MRI/Ultrasonography.
- **Ambulatory zone:** It is the meeting place of patients with significant health professionals such as consultants, nurses, and other paramedical staff. It comprises of Minor OT, Treatment Room, Pharmacy, etc.
- **Staff zone:** An area maintained exclusively for professionals. Entry to this area is limited to staff members. It comprises of stores, seminar/conference room, duty room, etc.

  OPD timings: Generally, the OPD of hospital functions for six days/week. The OPD timings are classified as morning shift (10 am to 2 pm), evening shift (3 pm to 6 pm) and extended/particular OPDs (6 pm to 8 pm). Congestion and waiting time for the patients and relatives must be limited. There ought to be an appropriate arrangement for record-keeping and advertising. However, the OPD timing largely depends on the hospital policy and the number of patients in OPD.

Inpatient Departments/Units

A crucial part of any health care organization where people stay for short term/long term observation/diagnosis/treatment/rehabilitation. It is also considered as a place meant for research, training, and education of health professionals. The main type of wards/departments/unit is explained below.

- **General wards/departments/unit:** A place of admission for patients with non-explicit diseases with less need for emergency management. The usual nurse-patient ratio is 1:3-5. The routine treatment and nursing care needs are met.
- **Special wards/departments/units:** The patients with severe sickness are admitted for profoundly advanced

and life-sparing treatment/diagnosing the reason. These incorporate patients kept for explicit consideration because of disease or social reasons. All types, specially qualified expert health professionals are available in these units, which gives the best treatment accessible. These Units additionally ought to have propelled technology and machinery to help the treatment and care of fundamentally sick patients. It incorporates Emergency Ward, OT, CCU, ICU, HDU, Burns Department and Pre and Postoperative units.

Ward/Department/Unit Planning

- **Physical parameters:** The size of the ward relies upon the kinds of the patient.
  - Ideally, every bed requires 100 to 120 sq.ft.
  - It is suggested to have small rooms with few beds, i.e., 2-4 in a room.
  - Each bed should be 5 ft far from the wall, and there should be a 2-4 ft distance between each bed.
  - The standard length and width of the bed shall be followed.
  - The size of rooms ideally followed are 125 sq.ft: single room, 160 sq ft/bed: two rooms, 320 sq ft/bed: 4 rooms, 120-150 sq ft/bed: Critical Units.
  - The estimations and details may shift as indicated by the hospital approach.
- **Supporting zone:** Nursing station/obligation room: It should be centrally located so that the minimum time will be taken to reach each patient's bed. The treatment room is furnished with an examination table, dressing material, spotlight, and an area to perform hand hygiene, and it is intended for examination of patients. The availability of a clean working area with adequate office furniture, the storage facility for equipment and supplies, sanitary facility, discussion room, are considered ideal.
- **Ward design:** It is to encourage health professionals to monitor the patients and see and hear everything in the ward. The patients can quickly call them when help is required.
  - **Nightingale ward:** The beds of patients are placed at either side of the hall. Side room may be constructed to create isolation. Duty Station will be at one end, and another end will be the sanitary area. It is a more common type of ward, but it reduces the concept of privacy and increases the movement of health professionals (Fig. 8).

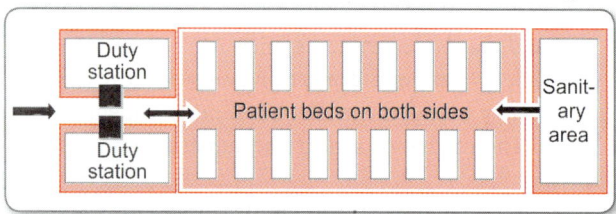

Fig. 8: Nightingale ward

- **Open ward:** In a spacious room/hall, beds are put in lines confronting one another and nursing station is in the focal/central point of the lobby. It is also referred to as modified Nightingale Ward.
- **Rigg's ward:** This was developed in 1910 in Rigg Hospital at Copenhagen. In this structure, a separate room or cubicle is structured. Each room consists of 3–4 beds, which are put parallel to the wall/windows. The room or cubicle may either be unilateral or bilateral. The duty station is located centrally. This type of ward design ensures the patient's privacy and minimizes the chance of cross-infection. The disadvantages of this design are that it reduces the staff's attention and communication to the patients (Fig. 9).
- **T-shaped ward:** Beds, including those of critical patients, are placed in front of the nursing station. Isolation Units are at either side of the centrally located duty station. Other facilities and services are behind the duty station giving the shape of "T" (Fig. 10).

- **Ward management:** It is a skill to use the ward and its materials for the maximum output in favor of the organization and patients. It incorporates:
  - **Strategic management:** These are generalized guidelines for the ward functioning. It formulates the policies and objectives of each activity in the ward. It also explains the plan of action in different types of situations.

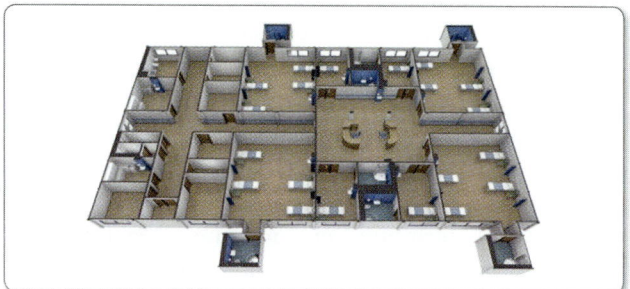

Fig. 9: Rigg's ward

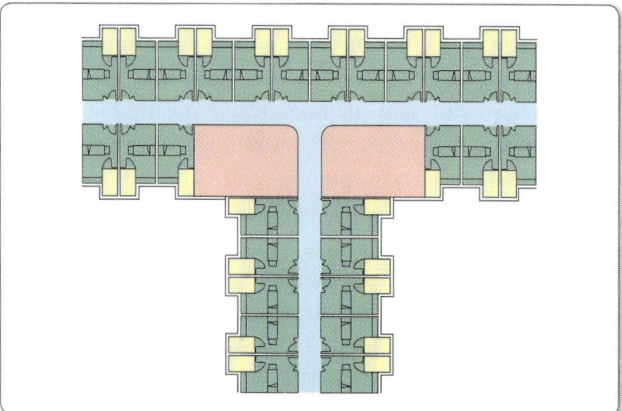

Fig. 10: T-ward

- **Operational management:** It explains the means and modes of achieving strategic plans. It rests with ward in-charges and staff members in the ward.

Central Sterile Supply Department (CSSD)

A CSSD is a division that outfits all provisions required for the nursing units and bureaus of a hospital such as wards, OPD, emergency unit, OT, etc. with sterile articles and kits prepared and accessible for prompt treatment of patients. These provisions incorporate clean cloths, clean units, working room packs, and other surgical and medical supplies. Likewise, the staff in this division clean, review, fix, collect, wrap, and disinfect/sterilize the trays used for a different type of treatment.

Laundry Services

The laundry helps in the control of cross-infection and helps in providing satisfaction to patients/clients. It is a part of public relations too. The laundry services can be classified as;

- In-house Laundry: Here, the hospital owns the laundry, and all the activities of laundry are within the hospital premises.
- Rented Laundry Service: It is an advanced system wherein the supplier of the linen takes the responsibility of laundry, including the replacement of worn-out/ damaged linen on a rental basis.
- Contract framework: An Indian practice wherein the hospitals have their linen and contract dhobies are arranged for laundry services.
- Cooperative framework: It is most useful to small-scale health care providers. Two or more hospitals share established laundry services.

Kitchen Services

A dietary facility of a hospital incorporates, in particular, a creation unit that changes over crude material into edible food. The readiness and dissemination of nourishment from the store to spoon have numerous difficulties for the organization, for example, legitimate arrangement, cost management, prevention of stealing, and wastage. The dietary services include services such as therapeutic diet, IPD services, nutrition advise, including the education of a healthy diet.

Laboratory Services

The essential capacity of the clinical lab is:

- To help specialists to affirm an analysis of the patient and to aid the treatment and follow up of patients.
- It creates reliable and prompt clinical reports of the patients and also stores them for future reference.
- It is useful in the training of health care professionals in various disciplines.
- Its services are always available as and when required.

The lab of a hospital comprises of following divisions:

- Hematology
- Microbiology
- Clinical chemistry/ biochemistry
- Histopathology
- Urine and stool analysis

Emergency Services

The department of emergency medicine must be created as a small hospital within the hospital, i.e., autonomous and independent in everyday working. It shall be located on the ground floor itself with complete accessibility to all needy people. This department will have a direct link with all emergency associated care facilities such as OT, Blood Bank, Intensive Units, etc. There should be provision for a store for wheelchairs, stretchers, etc., and the waiting area.

Medical Records

Legitimate maintenance of medical records is a high need in any health care organization. Appropriate documentation of the patient's case history with informed consent is essential. All medico-lawful cases, e.g., child abuse, assault, battery, mishaps, and so forth ought to be accounted for to appropriate experts, e.g., Police. The instances of AIDS and venereal illnesses shall be informed to competent authorities.

In addition to the above-mentioned facilities, the amenities such as Canteen, Gift Shop, Book Shop, Flower Shop, Stationery Shop and accommodation facilities for staff are also desirable.

PLANNING IN EMERGENCY AND DISASTER MANAGEMENT

A disaster is an occurrence that causes damage, ecological disruption, loss of human life, deterioration of health and health services on a scale, sufficient to warrant an extraordinary response from outside the affected community or area.

—**World Health Organization (WHO)**

Disaster Nursing is the application of professional skills of nursing care in meeting the health needs and other needs of persons affected by any disaster. "Disaster Nursing is nursing practiced in a situation where professional supplies, equipment, physical facilities, and utilities are limited or not available."

Types of Disasters

- Natural disasters are unavoidable. The impact can be compelling and can cause substantial, physical disruption, social disruption, and many secondary stressors such as loss of both home and income. Types of natural disasters are Hurricanes, Cyclones, Tornadoes and Typhoons, Snowstorms, Floods, Heavy Rain, Earthquakes, Landslides, Tsunami, and Epidemics.

- Man-made disasters are more deadly than natural. They are sudden in onset and produce a reaction of shock. Types of man-made disasters are Industrial accidents, Security related issues, Nuclear Warfare, Biological War, and so on.

Principles of Disaster Management Planning

- All departments and sectors of government should be involved in disaster management.
- The generally available resources should be utilized for disaster management.
- Organizations should work as an augmentation of their central business. To accomplish this amid calamities, associations ought to be utilized in a way that mirrors their everyday job.
- Individuals are in charge of their wellbeing and safety.
- Disaster management shall be planned on a considerable scale. It is simpler to downsize a reaction than upsizing according to the situation.
- There should be a separation between disasters and incidents.
- Recognize the role and involvement of NGOs in disaster management.

Disaster Management Phases

- **Disaster preparedness:** Disaster preparedness is an ongoing multispectral activity. This consists of strengthening the capacity of a country to manage efficiently all types of emergencies so that the resources should be able to provide assistance to the victims and bring back the life to normal. The preparedness should start from the community people because many times the external agency may not arrive for days to the affected area, especially if transportation and communication are affected. Preparedness should be in the form of money, human resources, and materials.
- **Disaster impact:** The number and severity of casualties in a disaster may vary according to its type. Much of the injuries take place during the impact phase, and hence, emergency service is required. The management in the impact phase may be further categorized as triage, provision of first aid, hospital reference, and search for more victims affected.

  Triage: It is the method of classifying the affected people in an emergency/disaster situation. It is based on the gravity of their injury, chance of survival, and need for medical intervention (Fig. 11).

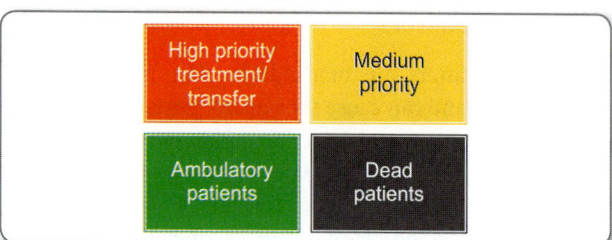

Fig. 11: Triage

- **Disaster response:** This is carried out in the following phases:
  - **Relief phase:** It commences when external assistance starts to reach the disaster area. The supplies can be categorized as primary and secondary. The primary is immediately after the disaster, and it includes health care materials for the treatment and prevention of any infectious diseases. The secondary type of supplies provides drinking water, food items, clothing, materials for preparing shelter, etc.
  - **Vaccination:** Mass vaccination is required in public, followed by a disaster. The political people may pressurize the health professionals for the same. The standard vaccination programs done are usually against cholera, typhoid, and tetanus.
  - **Nutrition:** The disaster causes nutritional problems, and it may be the result of disturbances in the food chain. It is an area of grave concern that requires the attention of authorities as well as community health professionals.
- **Rehabilitation phase:** It starts on the day of the disaster. The approach and pattern steadily move from emergency management to primary health care. All the services should be carefully planned and structured as per the need. The priorities shift from curative services to preventive and promotive services along with modifying the environmental factors.
- **Disaster mitigation:** It is aimed to decrease the impact of a disaster. It includes strict adherence to building/construction rules, especially for schools, colleges, hospitals, etc., improves and monitors public health services (safe water, waste disposal, etc.) and so on.

Facilities Required in Hospital for Disaster Management

- **An examination cum treatment room:** It can be preferably arranged in the emergency department. There should be sufficient tables/beds and facilities for emergency procedures such as first aid, CPR available. Here the procedures like bandaging, dressing, catheterization, suturing of minor wounds can be performed.
- **An observation area:** Depending upon the patient load, 4-8 beds may be placed in this area. Patients waiting to be evaluated can be placed here.
- **Storage space:** This includes space for the storage of extra linen, consumables like drugs, dressing material, IV fluids, etc. There also should be space for the disposal of biomedical wastes.
- **Fixtures:** These are facilities such as electrical connections, extra power facilities, oxygen, and suction line spots, etc.
- **Other support services:** This includes clinical laboratory, diagnostic facilities, blood bank, operation theater, etc.

Disaster Drill

Disaster Drill is an activity in which individuals re-enact the conditions of a debacle with the goal that they have a chance to rehearse their reactions. Catastrophe drills can run from earthquake drills in schools to multi-day practices which may be extended to the entire community, including point by point reenactments and an opportunity to work with similar objects or types of equipment which would be used in a calamity.

Hospital Disaster Manual

A hospital disaster manual is a written statement of a disaster plan, which is implemented during a disaster. It includes the following:

- Introduction: This should consist of the disaster alert code, general principles of conduct, and a brief synopsis of the complete plan. When the alert is given, all personnel must report to duty and take over their assigned jobs.
- Distribution of responsibilities: Duties of each individual and department are put on an action card. These cards describe in detail the duties and actions to be taken by every member of the hospital staff, starting from the hospital administration to stretcher-bearers and ward boys.
- Chronological action plan. The action should be listed in chronological order.
  - Initial Alert: This may be received through the casualty itself or telephones or authorities like the police. On receipt of this information, the concerned person must gather information regarding the place, time and type of emergency, and the estimated number and type of casualties.
  - Activate hospital Plan: The designated hospital staff activates the disaster plan. All the departments and people involved get into readiness to attend to casualties and depending upon the nature and number of injuries, crisis expansion of hospital beds is undertaken, utilizing additional space by discharging minor cases and transfers to other hospitals.
  - Formulation of command nucleus: The command nucleus should be formed immediately and located in the casualty department.
  - Management of casualties: The next phase in the hospital will involve further treatment of patients and the collection of information for the administration.

Roles of Nurse in Disaster Management

- They are the immediate care providers.
- They participate in government and voluntary relief organizations.
- Nurses protect human rights.
- Maintain social justice and equality.
- Prepare the society and identify and update the records of the susceptible population within.
- Understand the available resources in a community.
- Nurse function as a member of the appraisal team and is involved in continuous reconnaissance.
- Provision of health education, psychological support, and appropriate referrals as and when required.

REVIEW QUESTIONS

1. Differentiate mission, vision, and philosophy.
2. What are the objectives of nursing? Explain the characteristics and classification of objectives in nursing science.
3. Define planning and list characteristics of planning.
4. Describe the principles of planning.
5. Explain the types of planning and differentiate strategic planning and tactical planning.
6. Explain significance of procedures and manuals in nursing practice.
7. Explain the Gantt Chart and its significance.
8. Explain Milestone Chart.
9. Explain PERT.
10. Define Budget, and brief the types of budget.
11. What are the principles of budgeting?
12. Explain approaches to budgeting and cost-benefit analysis.
13. What is the budget proposal? Prepare a sample budget proposal.
14. Define the hospital and explain the objectives of a hospital.
15. Hospital Planning Process: Explain the structural and functional planning of hospitals.
16. Explain the types of wards in the hospital.
17. What are the principles of hospital planning?
18. Explain the functions of emergency care in the hospital.
19. Describe the site, area, and design of emergency departments.
20. Explain the hospital disaster manual and the role of a nurse in disaster management.
21. Brief the planning process in emergency and disaster.

Further Readings

1. Banerjee, Shyamal. Principles and Practice of Management. Oxford and IBM Publishing, New Delhi; 2000.
2. Basavanthappa BT. Nursing Administration. 2nd Edition: Jaypee Brothers Medical Publishers (P) Ltd., New Delhi; 2009.
3. Barrett, Jean. Ward Management and Teaching. Konark Publishers, Delhi; 1992.
4. Warren, Stevens, F. Management and Leadership in Nursing. McGraw – Hill Inc, New York; 1978.
5. Alexander et al. Nursing Service Administration. Mosby Publishers, US; 1962.
6. Park K. Preventive and Social Medicine, 19th Edition: M/s. Banarasidas Bhanot Publishers, Jabalpur; 2007.
7. Basavanthappa BT. Nursing Administration, 1st Edition: Jaypee Brothers Medical Publishers (P) Ltd., New Delhi; 2002.
8. Goel SL, Kumar R. Management of Hospitals – Hospital Administration in the 21st century, Vol. 4, Deep and Deep Publication, New Delhi; 2002.
9. Ranga Rao SP. Administration of Primary Health Centers in India, 1st Edition: Mittal Publications, New Delhi; 1993.
10. Lucita M. Nursing: Practice and Public Health Administration. Current Concepts and Trends. B. I. Churchill Living Stone Pvt. Ltd., New Delhi; 2002.
11. Sakharkar BM. Principles of Hospital Administration and Planning, 2nd Edition: Jaypee Brothers Medical Publishers (P) Ltd., New Delhi; 2009.
12. Patricia S Yoder-Wise. Leading and Managing in Nursing. 2nd Edition: Mosby Publication, US; 1999.
13. Bessie L. Marquis and Carol J. Huston. Leadership Roles and Management Functions in Nursing: Theory and Application. 5th Edition: Lippincott Williams and Wilkins, New York; 2006.
14. Linda Roussel. Management and Leadership for Nurse Administrators. 4th Edition: Jones and Bartlett Publication, USA; 2006.
15. Wehrich H, Koontz H. Management A Global Perspective. 11th Edition: Tata McGraw-Hill Publishing Company, Ltd., New Delhi; 2005.
16. Marquis BL, Huston CJ. Leadership and Management Functions in Nursing- Theory, and Application. 5th Edition: Lippincott Williams and Wilkins, Philadelphia; 2006.
17. Douglass LM. The Effective Nurse: Leader and Manager. 5th Edition: Mosby Publication, US; 1996.
18. Trained Nurses Association of India, Nursing Administration, and Management.
19. Samson Rebecca. Leadership and Management in Nursing Practice and Education 1st Edition: Jaypee Brothers Medical Publishers (P) Ltd., New Delhi; 2009.
20. Kunders GD. Designing for Total Quality in Health Care, Prism Book Pvt. Ltd., Bangalore; 2002.
21. Chandorkar AG. Hospital Administration and Planning. 2nd Edition: Paras Medical Publisher, New Delhi; 2009.
22. Joshi DC, Joshi Mamta. Hospital Administration. 1st Edition: Jaypee Brothers Medical Publishers (P) Ltd., New Delhi; 2009.
23. Eleanor J Sullivan, Philip J Decker. Effective Leadership and Management in Nursing. 4th Edition: Published by Addison Wesely; 2011.
24. Kulkarni GR. Financial Management for Hospital Administration, Jaypee Brothers Medical Publishers (P) Ltd., New Delhi; 2009.

Unit

4

Organizing

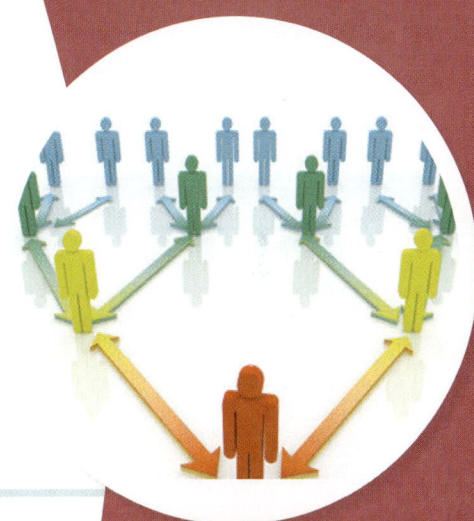

 Unit Outline

CONCEPT OF ORGANIZATION

The organization is "a group of people working together and with each other towards the achievement of the common goals." An organization does not exist in a vacuum. An organization exists in association with its environments which provide resources and limitations. An organization must continuously adapt to its environments which are constantly changing. The environment determines the future resources and the constraint that will be placed on the organization. The following are the various fundamental elements of an organization.

- **People:** The very first element of an organization is its people. Unless people of the organization interact and do assigned jobs, there would be no organization.
- **Physical resources:** The manufacturing organization must have the raw materials to make their products.
- **Climate:** The climate affects the location of the operations of the organization.
- **Economic and market conditions:** The governmental monetary and fiscal policies are of profound effects.
- **Attitude:** The social, religious, political, and cultural attitudes are of significant importance in an organization's environment.
- **Legal constraints:** The rules and regulations of the land influence the functioning of an organization.

Characteristics of an Organization

- Group of people with common goals or objectives.
- There is a division of work.
- Vertical and horizontal relationship (It is the relationship between supervisor and subordinates or the relationship between different departments and divisions).
- Chain of command with laid down channels of communication. (flow of authority from the higher to the lower levels of management in the hierarchy).
- Group dynamics – It is the interactions that take place between the individuals and groups within the organization, based on their values, needs, sentiments, attitudes, beliefs, and interests. It is a social, self-generating, and dynamic interactive process that gives rise to an informal group.

Organizing is a common term synonymic to the division of labor in the context of management. Once a plan has been created, a manager can begin to organize. Organizing involves assigning tasks, grouping tasks into departments, delegating authority, and allocating resources across the organization. During the organizing process, managers coordinate employees, resources, policies, and procedures to facilitate the goals identified in the plan. Organizing is highly complex and often involves a systematic review of human resources, finances, and priorities. Before a plan can be implemented, managers must organize the assets of the business to execute the plan efficiently and effectively. According to Henry Fayol, "The specialization of the workforce according to the skills of a person, creating specific personal and professional development within the labor force and therefore increasing productivity, leads to specialization, which increases the efficiency of labor. By separating a small part of the work, the workers' speed and accuracy in its performance increases." This principle applies to both technical as well as managerial work.

Organizations can be structured in various ways, with each structure determining how the organization operates and performs. An organization's structure is typically represented by an **organization chart** (often called simply an "org chart") and it is a diagram showing the interrelationships of its positions. This chart highlights the chain of command or the authority relationships among people working at different levels. It also shows the number of layers between the top and lowest managerial levels. Organizational structure also dictates the **span of control** or the number of subordinates a supervisor has. An organization with few layers has a wide span of control, with each manager overseeing a large number of subordinates; with a narrow span of control, only a limited number of subordinates report to each manager. The structure of an organization determines how the organization will operate and perform. The structure of the organization may be structural, functional or matrix in nature. Organizing follows the following steps:

- **Identifying the work:** The obvious first step in the process of organizing is to identify the work that has to be done by the organization. This is the ground level from which we will begin. Identification of the work helps to avoid miscommunication, overlapping of responsibilities and wastage of time and effort.
- **Grouping of work:** For the sake of a smooth flow of work and smooth functioning of the organization, similar tasks and activities should be grouped. It is essential to create departments within the organization and divisions within each department. Such an organization makes the functioning of work smooth and systematic. The grouping depends on the size of the organization and the volume of work.
- **Establish hierarchy:** It is the process to establish the reporting relationships for all the individual employees of the company. The manager establishes the vertical and horizontal relationships of the company. This enables the evaluation and control over the performances of all the employees promptly.
- **Delegation of authority:** Authority is the right of an individual to act according to his wishes and extract obedience from the others. So, when a manager is assigned certain duties and responsibilities, he must also be delegated authority to carry out such duties effectively. If we only assign the duties, but no authority he will not be able to perform the tasks and activities that are necessary.
- **Coordination:** The manager must ensure that all activities carried out by various employees and groups are

well coordinated. Otherwise, it may lead to conflicts between employees, duplication of work and wastage of time and effort. He must ensure all the departments are carrying out their specialized tasks and there is harmony in these activities. The ultimate aim is to ensure that the goal of the organization is fulfilled.

HOSPITAL

A hospital is a residential establishment that provides short-term and long-term medical care consisting of observational, diagnostic, therapeutic and rehabilitative services for persons suffering or suspected to be suffering from a disease or injury and for parturients. It may or may not also provide services for ambulatory patients on an out-patient basis.

—**WHO Expert Committee, 1963**

The hospital is an integral part of a social and medical organization, the function of which is to provide complete healthcare, both curative and preventive for people, and whose outpatient services reach out to the family in its home environment; the hospital is also a center for the training of health workers and biosocial research.

—**WHO Expert Committee, 1956**

Classification of Hospital

- **Based on objective:**
  - **General hospitals:** General hospitals are meant to provide a wide range of various types of healthcare, but with limited capacity. They care for patients with various-disease conditions for both sexes to all ages, medical, surgical, pediatrics, obstetrics, eye and ear, etc. Usually, general hospitals are devoid of super-specialist medical care.
  - **Special hospitals:** They limit their service to a particular condition, orthopedics, maternity, pediatrics, geriatrics, oncology, etc.
  - **Teaching cum research hospital:** College is attached for medical/ nursing/ dental/ pharmacy education. The main objective is to provide medical care and teaching and research are secondary.
- **Based on administration, ownership, control or financial income:**
  - **Governmental or public:** They are owned, administered and controlled by the government. They provide free care for patients. The government hospitals are owned by The Ministry of Health, Central or State Governments, local governments and so on. A public hospital or government hospital is a hospital that is owned by a government and receives government funding. In some countries, this type of hospital provides medical care free of charge, the cost of which is covered by government reimbursement.

- **Non-governmental or private:** Privately owned or controlled by an individual or group of physicians or citizens or by a private organization. e.g. Apollo Hospital, Narayana Hospital and so on. The purpose is to provide services for profit-making.
- **Semi-government hospital:** Hospitals run both by the government and private entities. Corporate hospitals are public limited companies formed under the companies' act.
- **Voluntary agency hospitals:** Hospitals run by Red Cross, HOPE Foundation, CARE and so on.
- **Based on length of stay:**
  - **Short-term or short-stay hospitals (Stay less than 30 days):** These are hospitals where over 90% of all patients admitted stay less than 30 days.
  - **Long-term or long-stay hospitals: (Stay more than 30 days):** These are hospitals where over 90% of all patients admitted stay 30 days or more, i.e., mental hospital.
- **Depending on the type of medical staff:**
  - **Closed-staff hospital:** Physicians are held responsible for all medical activities in the hospital including the diagnosis and treatment of patient, fee-paying and emergency. Only affiliated staff can work in this hospital.
  - **Open-staff hospital:** This type of hospital permits other physicians in the community to admit and treat patients to the hospital and treat them. Open medical staff, which means any physician can request to practice at the facility, regardless of their hospital affiliation.
- **Based on bed capacity (size)**
  - Small hospital (Up to 100 beds)
  - Medium hospital (More than 100 to less than 300 beds)
  - Large hospital (More than 300 beds)
- **Based on the type of care:**
  - **Primary care:** Primary care is the day-to-day healthcare given by a health care provider. Typically, this provider acts as the first contact and principal point of continuing care for patients within a healthcare system and coordinates other specialist care that the patient may need. It provides the most basic health care. It is generally regarded as the 'gateway' to receiving more specialist care. It is a 10–20 bedded hospital.
  - **Secondary care:** This is the first level of referral services and more complicated services and care is dealt with and this care is beyond the capacity of the primary level. This level is assigned to provide specific care to certain specialties such as medical, surgical, obstetrical, accident and trauma and so on. These are usually 50–200 bedded hospital.
  - **Tertiary care:** This provides highly specialized services provided at regional or central-level hospitals. Such hospitals include District and Regional Hospitals and Central Hospitals such as AIIMS, PGI and so on.
- **Based on teaching affiliation:**
  - **Teaching hospital:** A hospital upgraded for training and teaching of health professionals such as doctors, nurses, dentists, and other paramedical and medical students.

■ **Non-teaching hospital:** A hospital that does not provide the facility of training and education for health care professionals.
- **Based on the system of medicine:**
  - Allopathic hospital
  - Ayurvedic hospital
  - Homeopathic hospital
  - Unani hospital
  - Siddha hospital
- **Based on regionality:**
  - **Regional:** In India, regional hospitals are those which are specialized to provide comprehensive and specialized health care to people. These hospitals may belong to government (AIIMS, PGI) or private/corporate sector (NH, Apollo, Fortis and so on).
  - **District:** These are District and Taluk Hospitals. It also comprises of multi-specialty services for people of all kind.
  - **Community clinics:** This generally comprises of Primary Health Centers and Community Health Centers hospitals. It can provide general medical services to all at the first hand but usually lack the specialized care services.
- **As per WHO classification:**
  - **Regional hospital:** In India regional hospitals are those which are specialized to provide comprehensive and specialized health care to people. These hospitals may belong to government (AIIMS, PGI) or private/corporate sector (NH, Apollo, Fortis and so on).
  - **Intermediate/District hospital:** These are District and Taluk Hospitals. It also comprises of multi-specialty services for people of all kind.
  - **Rural hospital:** This generally comprises of Primary Health Centers and Community Health Centers hospitals. It can provide general medical services to all at the first hand but usually lack the specialized care services.

Functions of the Hospitals

Hospital functions may generally be termed as Intramural (Services within the wall of the hospital) and Extramural (Services outside the wall of the hospital (Fig. 1).
- The intramural services generally include Therapeutic, Preventive, Education, and Research.
- The extramural services include Outpatient services, Home care, Community outreach and so on.

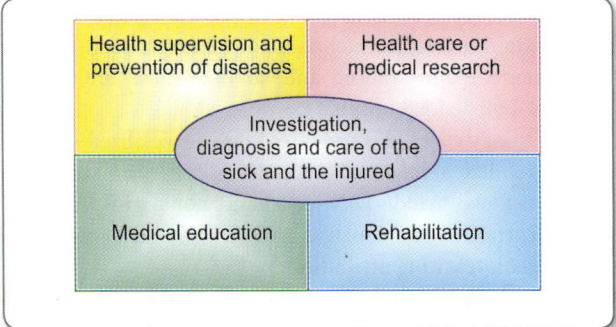

Fig. 1: Functions of the hospitals

Another way of classifying the hospital functions are:
- **Preventive function:** It is also one of the major significant functions of the hospital to provide preventive health care services to people through a community approach. This includes the prevention of communicable and non-communicable diseases, maternal and child health, Nutritional Health, Occupational Health and Health Education.
- **Curative function:** It is the primary function of the hospital to provide care and treatment to the people who are ill. It includes all the diagnostic, therapeutic, curative and rehabilitative aspects of health care.
- **Training function:** It is concerned with providing training and education courses for health care professionals and technicians who provide health services to the people. (Physician, Nurses, Dentists and so on)
- **Research function:** It is a secondary function and concerned with conducting health-related researches that focus on the improvement of the health and/or prevention of diseases.
- **Rehabilitative function:** The Rehabilitation Services is dedicated to providing high quality, individualized, and effective interventions aimed at promoting both patient safety and a return to independent function. Services include Physical Therapy, Occupational Therapy, and Speech-Language therapy, etc. with compassion and empathy in a patient and family-centered care environment.

According to another method of classification, the Hospital administration functions can be classified into three broad categories:
1. **Medical:** Involves the treatment and management of patients through the staff of physicians.
2. **Patient support:** Relates directly to patient care and includes nursing, dietary diagnostic, therapy, pharmacy and laboratory services.
3. **Administrative:** Concerns the execution of policies and directions of the hospital governing the discharge of support services in the area of finance, personnel, materials and property, housekeeping, laundry, security, transport, engineering and board, and the maintenance.

ORGANIZATION OF HOSPITAL SERVICES

- **Administrative office:** Directs and supervises the activities and functions of administrative units to effectively deliver quality support services.
- **Personnel section:** Development and administration of a comprehensive manpower development program, which includes recruitment and selection, promotion, training, employee welfare and benefits, manpower planning and research.
- **Property and supply section:** Procurement, storage, inventory, distribution and disposition of hospital supplies, materials and equipment.

- **Housekeeping section:** Develop and maintain a clean, safe and sanitary environment for patients and hospital personnel.
- **Linen and laundry section:** Ensure an adequate supply of clean linens for patients and hospital units.
- **Engineering and maintenance section:** Installation, operation, and maintenance of electrical, mechanical and communication equipment and allied facilities including buildings and vehicles.
- **Motor pool section (transport):** Transport patients, hospital officials, and personnel to their destination.
- **Security force:** Ensure the safety of hospital patients, facilities and personnel, maintain peace and order, and enforce hospital rules and regulations.
- **Medical social service:** The Medical Social Service Function is to see to it that patients attain emotional equilibrium as they are assisted with other needs that interfere in hospitalization and treatment.
- **Medical records:** Process, maintain, analyze and safely keep all medical records created in this hospital; prepares hospital statistical reports; and formulate and develop effective policies, systems, and procedures for the efficient operations of the section.
- **Pharmacy section:** Ensures a continuous supply of drugs and medicines to patients by maintaining an adequate quantity in stocks of those approved by the Pharmacy Therapeutic Committee. Dispenses, compound drugs for in and outpatients. Controls the purchasing, requisitioning, safekeeping and issuing of drugs. Maintains records and files of dangerous drugs and other pharmaceuticals as required by law.
- **Dietary service:** Maintain or enhances the health of the patients and personnel by providing them with high quality and nutritious food through an efficient Dietary Service. Provides or serves safe, nutritious and attractive food through careful planning, wise procurement and proper preparation of balanced and satisfying meals within budgetary limits. Implements diet prescription in coordination with physician and nurse. Provides nutrition consultation and education services to patients as well as in-service training to both dietary personnel and other related fields. Promotes and maintains cooperation with other departments in the hospital towards total patient care.
- **Accounting section:** Systematic recording of all financial transactions, preparation of financial statements and relevant reports, and maintenance and safekeeping of the hospital's Book of Accounts.
- **Budget service:** Prepares the work and financial plan and provision of fund estimates for hospital programs and projects.
- **Cashier service:** Receipt, deposit, custody, and disbursement of cash/collection of the hospital (Cash Management).

- **Medicare and billing section:** Admits, classifies Pay and Medicare Patients, orients patients concerning privileges, obligations, responsibilities during the course of confinement. Prepares statements of account on service and bills rendered to the patient. File records, bills and statement of account.
- Public information center.

Functions of the Nursing Service

The functional areas of the hospitals which are mentioned above have specific roles and responsibilities to perform. The responsibilities of different key functional areas of the hospitals may be organized as follows:

- Plans, organizes and directs the overall nursing service activities in all clinical and special areas in the health fields of maternal and child nursing, medical and surgical nursing.
- Defines the philosophy, goals, objectives, and policies of the hospital, and interprets them to the nursing staff, patients, and the community.
- Develops the basic, functional and position organization chart that will allow for open communication horizontally and vertically to ensure smooth operations of the service.
- Formulates qualification standards, job specifications and job descriptions of various categories of nursing personnel in line with the hospital policies and Civil Service Commission rules and regulations and the Nursing Law.
- Delegates assignments with commensurate authority to ward supervisors and follows this up.
- Determines and makes recommendations concerning hospital wards' facilities, equipment and surgical supplies affecting nursing care, and plans for allocation and utilization of space and equipment to ensure a safe environment for patients and working personnel.
- Formulates and implements nursing care policies and standards operating procedures as guides for the nursing personnel and initiates periodic revision of some as the need arises.
- Determines the staffing needs based on patients' conditions ranging from the minimally-ill, moderately-ill or critically-ill to ensure smooth operations of the service.
- Makes general nursing rounds weekly and as the need arises and looks into patients' nursing needs and ward conditions to ensure a safe environment and safe care.
- Cooperates in providing referral systems between the hospital and community health centers and other agencies. Assigns and re-assigns nursing personnel periodically to meet the needs of the nursing service. Provides opportunities for growth and development of personnel-recognizes personnel and professional abilities, maintains a continuing staff development program. Develops and carries a guidance and counseling program.
- Cooperates with individuals/groups in other departments or services in carrying forward the work of the hospital as a whole.

- Supervises and coordinates activities of nursing personnel engaged in specific nursing services such as Obstetrics, Pediatrics, Surgical or Medical, or from two or more clinical nursing divisions.
- Supervises Senior Nurse in carrying out the responsibilities in the management of nursing care. Evaluates the performance of Senior Nurse and nursing care as a whole. Inspects clinical nursing division to verify that patient needs are met.
- Plans and organizes orientation for clinical nursing division staff members and participates in guidance and education programs. Interviews pre-screened applicants and make recommendations for employing or for terminating employees.
- Visit clinical nursing divisions to oversee nursing care and to ascertain the condition of patients. Gives advice for treatment medications, and narcotics, by medical staff policies in the absence of a physician. Arranges for emergency operations and relocations of personnel during emergencies. Admits or delegates admissions of new patients.
- Assigns duties to professional and ancillary nursing personnel based on patients' needs, available staff, and service needs. Supervises and evaluates work performance in terms of patient care, staff relations and efficiency of service.
- Provides for nursing care and cooperates with other members of the medical care team in coordinating patients' total needs. Identifies and studies nursing service problems and assists in their solutions. Observes nursing care and visits patients to ensure that nursing care is carried out as directed and treatment is administered as per physician's instructions and to ascertain needs for additional or modified services. Maintains a safe environment for patients. Operates or supervises the operation of specialized equipment assigned to the unit and provides assistance and guidance to the nursing team as required.
- Accompanies physicians on rounds to answer questions, receives instructions and notes patients' care requirements. Reports to replacement on the next tour on condition of patients or any untoward or unusual actions taken. May render professional nursing care and instruct patients and members of their families in techniques and methods of home care after discharge.
- Collects clinical data through the process of interviewing observations using all senses and clinical instruments and utilization of diagnostic examination reports.

Functions of Training Service

- Provides qualified individuals with practical and scientific knowledge in the diagnosis and treatment of diseases.
- Installs a sense of responsibility, discipline, and compassion in the management of surgical patients.
- Develops adequate administrative ability and leadership qualities.

- Trains qualified individuals to practice various clinical disciplines in areas where their expertise is needed within the context of the national dispersal program.
- Develops and implements a strict training and a fair selection process for the admission of resident physicians.
- Maintains a good atmosphere for teaching and learning in the different clinical departments.

ORGANIZATION DEVELOPMENT

"Organization Development is an effort for planned, organization-wide, and managed from the top, to increase organization effectiveness and health through planned interventions in the organization's 'processes,' using behavioral-science knowledge." —**Beckhard**

Organization development is a response to change a complex educational strategy intended to change the benefits, attitudes, values, and structure of organizations so that they can better adapt to new technologies, markets, challenges and dizzying rate of change itself. —**Bennis**

Organizational development is focused on Planned Change and Action Research. Change means the new state of things that is different from the old state of things. Change is everywhere; change will be one of the few constants during the end of this century and into the next. Change has different facets, for example, it can be deliberate or accidental. Its magnitude can be large or small. It can affect many elements of the organization or only a few. It can be fast or slow. The new state of things can have an entirely different nature from the old state of things or the new state of things can have the same nature modifications. Action research is the process of systematically collecting research data about an ongoing system relative to some objective, goal or need of that system. Feeling these back into the system, taking actions by altering selected variables within the system based both on the date and on hypotheses and evaluating the results of actions by collecting more data.

Characteristics of Organizational Development

- It focuses on culture and processes.
- It encourages collaboration between organization leaders and members.
- It is important for accomplishing tasks.
- It focuses on the human and social side of the organization.
- Participation and involvement in problem-solving and decision making by all levels of the organization are hallmarks of OD.
- OD focuses on total system change and views organizations as complex social systems.
- OD takes a developmental view that seeks the betterment of both individuals and the organization.

Components of Organizational Development

Organizational development has three basic components. They are:

- **Diagnosis:** Diagnosis represents a continuous collection of data and data analysis about the total system, its subunits, its processes, and its culture. There are two areas of the diagnosis; the diagnosis of the various subsystems such as top management, the production department, or research group, middle management, or the workforce that make up the organization; and the diagnosis of the organization processes that are occurring. The organization process includes communication patterns and styles, the relationship between interfacing group, the management of conflict, the setting of goals and planning methods.

- **Action:** It consists of all the activities and interventions designed to improve the functioning of organization. OD intervention is a set of structured activities in which selected organizational units engage in task or sequencing task with the goal of organizational improvements and individual developments. Intervention constitutes the action thrust of organization development. It comprises of a set activity, large diagnostic and problem-solving activities that ordinarily occur with the assistance of a consultant who is not a regular member of the particular system or sub-system. According to Robert Blake and Jane Mouton, the interventions may be categorized as:

  - **Discrepancy intervention:** This calls attention to a contradiction in action or attitudes that then leads to exploration.
  - **Theory intervention:** Where behavioral science knowledge and theory are used to explain the present behavior assumption underlying the behavior.
  - **Procedural intervention:** This represents a critiquing of how something is being done to determine whether the best methods are being used.
  - **Relationship intervention:** Which focuses the attention on interpersonal relationship and surfaces the issues for exploration and possible resolution.
  - **Dilemma intervention:** In which two different action plans are tested for their consequences before a final decision is made.

- **Program management:** It encompasses all activities designed to ensure the success of the program. Almost all the OD intervention and their desired effects can be specified on some elements such as Conceptual, Behavioral, Procedural, Structural, Intrapersonal, Intra-group, Interpersonal, Inter-group, and Organizational changes. For example, a team-building intervention would have the subgroup, as a target and the content area of change would be either interpersonal or intergroup. With such a classification system in mind, a researcher can design a data collection method better and can start to test for the effects of various interventions on the different faces and elements of the group change.

Importance of Organizational Development

Organizational development is the use of organizational resources to improve efficiency and expand productivity. It can be used to solve problems within the organization or as a way to analyze a process and find a more efficient way of doing it. Implementing organizational development requires an investment of time and money. But when you understand its importance, you can justify the costs. Few of them are:

- **Organizational change:** The process of organizational development identifies areas of company operations where change is needed. Each need is analyzed, and the potential effects are projected into a change management plan. The plan outlines the specific ways in which the change will improve company operations, which will be affected by the change and how it can be rolled out efficiently to employees. Without organizational development as part of change management, a company would have a difficult time developing effective change management programs.

- **Growth:** Organizational development is an important tool in managing and planning corporate growth. An organizational development analysis brings together sales projections and consumer demand to help determine the rate of company growth. This information is used to alter the company business plan and plan the expansion and use of company resources such as personnel and the distribution network to accommodate future growth.

- **Work processes:** When a company is involved in organizational development, it analyzes work processes for efficiency and accuracy. Any quality control measures required to attain company standards are put in place. Evaluators analyze the duplicate process or processes that can be combined for greater efficiency, and develop and implement detailed plans on how to improve company methods.

- **Product innovation:** Product innovation requires the analysis of several kinds of information to be successful. Organizational development is critical to product innovation because it can help analyze each element of product development and create a method for using it effectively. Some of the processes that come together in organizational development to assist in product innovation are competitive analysis, technology development, consumer preferences, target market research, manufacturing capabilities, analysis and patents, and trademarks.

ORGANIZATIONAL STRUCTURE/ CLASSIFICATION OF ORGANIZATION

An organizational structure is a system that outlines how certain activities are directed to achieve the goals of an organization. These activities can include rules, roles, and responsibilities. The organizational structure also determines how information flows between levels within the organization. For example, in a centralized structure, decisions flow from the top down, while in a decentralized structure, decision-making power is distributed among various levels of the organization. Having an organizational structure in place allows organizations to remain efficient and focused.

Types of Organizational Structures

- **Functional structure:** This is also referred to as a bureaucratic organizational structure and breaks up a company based on the specialization of its workforce. Most small-to-medium-sized businesses implement a functional structure. Dividing the firm into departments consisting of marketing, sales, and operations is the act of using a bureaucratic organizational structure.
- **Divisional or multidivisional structure:** The second type is common among large companies with many business units. Called the divisional or multidivisional structure, a company that uses this method structures its leadership team based on the products, projects, or subsidiaries they operate. A good example of this structure is Johnson and Johnson. With thousands of products and lines of business, the company structures itself so each business unit operates as its own company with its president.
- **Flatarchy structure:** Flatarchy, a newer structure, is the third type and is used among many startups. As the name alludes, it flattens the hierarchy and chain of command and gives its employees a lot of autonomy. Companies that use this type of structure have a high speed of implementation.
- **Matrix structure:** The fourth and final organizational structure is a matrix structure. It is also the most confusing and the least used. This structure matrixes employees across different superiors, divisions, or departments. An employee working for a matrixed company, for example, may have duties in both sales and customer service.
- **Formal organization:** These are organizations that have an established framework concerning the responsibility, delegation, authority, and accountability of the members. This primarily relies on the philosophy of the organization. Based on the philosophy, the formal structure may be rigid or loose.
- **Informal organization:** The Informal organization is an authoritative structure that sets up the relationship based on the preferences of officers without thinking about the principles, directions, and methodology.
- **Vertical/Tall organization:** This refers to the increase in the length of the organization's hierarchical chain of command.
- **Horizontal/Flat organization:** This refers to a broader structure; there are fewer levels in the organizational hierarchy of such organizational structures, with a relatively large span of control.

Factors Influencing Organizational Structure

- **Size of the unit:** Size indicates the scale of operation. Typically there are three scales of activity such as small, medium, and large. Size is an important fact governing cost, efficiency, and profitability.

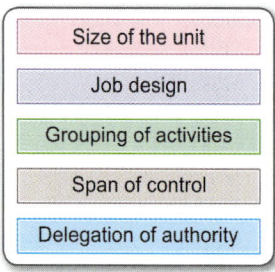

- **Job design:** The bricks that built up an organization structure are jobs. The jobs to be done in an organization are decided by the top boss.
- **Grouping of activities:** The designed jobs have to be formed into groups according to the nature of the action. The cluster of events is essential to achieve coordination.
- **Span of control:** Another factor that determines the organizational structure is the number of persons to be managed by each manager.
- **Delegation of authority:** If the span is more, there will be more authority levels, and the top management has to delegate authority to each level.

ORGANIZATIONAL CHART

The organizational charts and manuals explain the structure of the organization. An organization chart is a diagrammatic representation of the framework or structure of an organization.
—**J Batty**

An organization chart is a diagrammatical form that shows the essential aspects of an organization including the significant functions and their relationship, the channels of supervision and the relative authority of each employee who is in charge of each function.
—**Terry**

Contents of Organization Charts

- Basic organization structure and flow of authority
- Authority and responsibilities of various executives
- The relationship between the line and staff officers
- Positions of various office personnel
- Ways of promotion
- The requirements of management development

Types of Organization Charts

All use a spatial relationship (i.e., a distance between) to illustrate differences in rank, authority, or status.
- **Basic (vertical chart):** The fundamental relationship is that between superior and subordinate, and usually this is shown vertically. The lines of command flow from upward to downward in vertical lines. This vertical chart is in the form of a graph. This type is followed in companies.

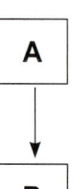

- **Horizontal chart:** the line of command flows horizontally. Here, the supervisor is on the left side of the structure and followed by subordinates on the right side or vice versa. This is not observed in any organization.
- **Master and supplementary chart:** A chart that shows the entire organization is called a master chart. It gives a clear picture of the organization and significant sections or divisions in the organization. A diagram that shows a particular part or division of the organization is called a supplementary or unit chart. It shows the details of the relationship, authority, and duties within the specified area. The gangplank relationship is also observable.
- **The 'T' chart:** The job task pyramid idea becomes a little clearer if we use a "T" chart, the most widely used and accepted map/workflow chart/organizational chart of the organization. In its most basic form, it consists of a series of inverted letter "T"s (taking a ruler, we can quite quickly draw a pyramid shape around the chart.) There are many ways of setting out relationships, and we are at liberty

to combine "T" charts with wheel chart (or any other variety) (Fig. 2). This kind of organizational chart is called **Modified T Chart.**
- **Scalar chain:** Henry Fayol produced what he called the "Scalar Chain or Chain of Grades or Steps," and his chart looked like a triangle without a connecting baseline.

This chart looks odd to our eyes: as we have seen, we do not often meet a situation where nearly every manager (i.e., B, C, D, E, F and L, M, N, O, P) has only one subordinate. However, it would appear Fayol's chart was even more abstract than the type of charts we use commonly today (Fig. 3).
- **Wheel chart:** Sometimes, it is more useful to indicate, in addition to a superior/subordinate relationship, a geographical one. We could envisage such an organization as a wheel with the group production director (A) in the center, and the subordinates at the ends of the various spheres (Fig. 4).

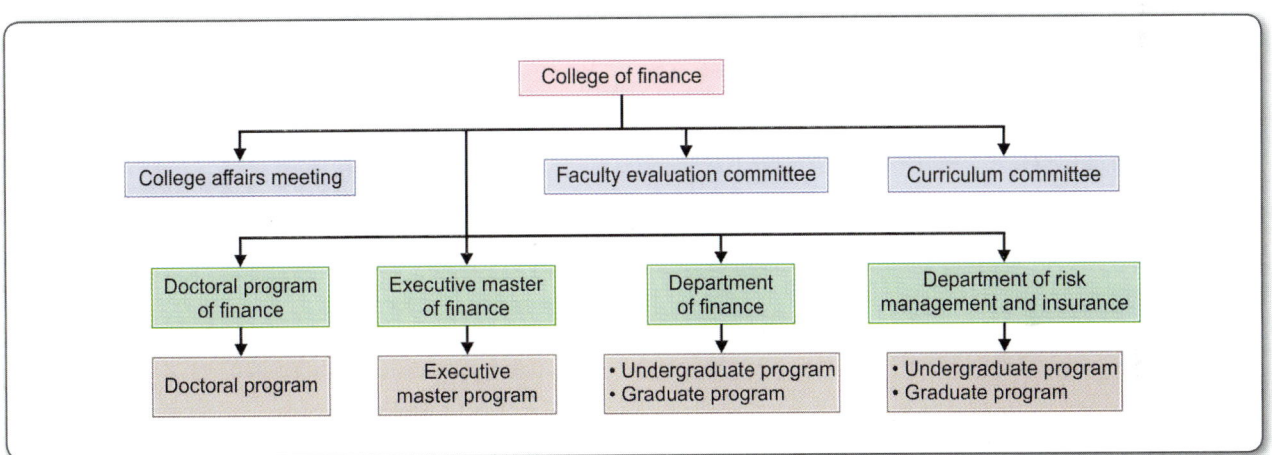

Fig. 2: T-chart

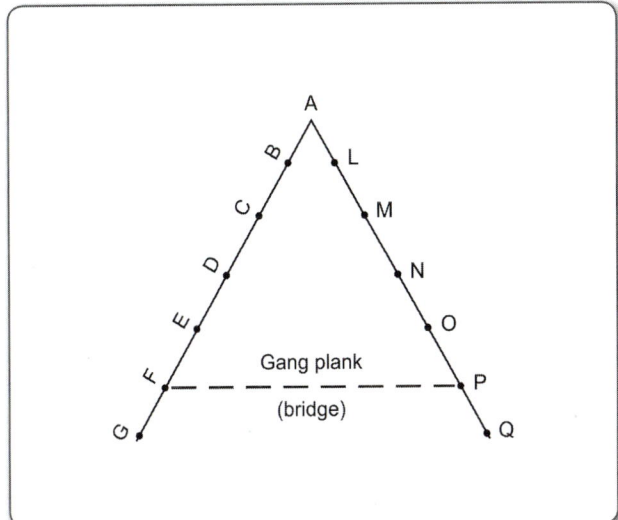

Fig. 3: Scalar chain

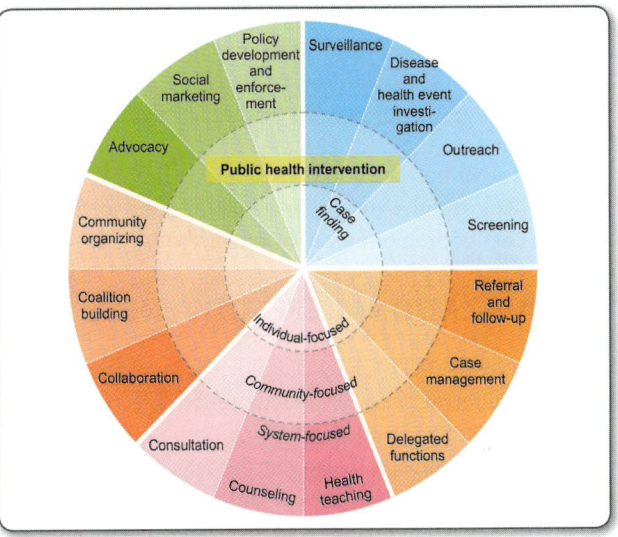

Fig. 4: Wheel chart

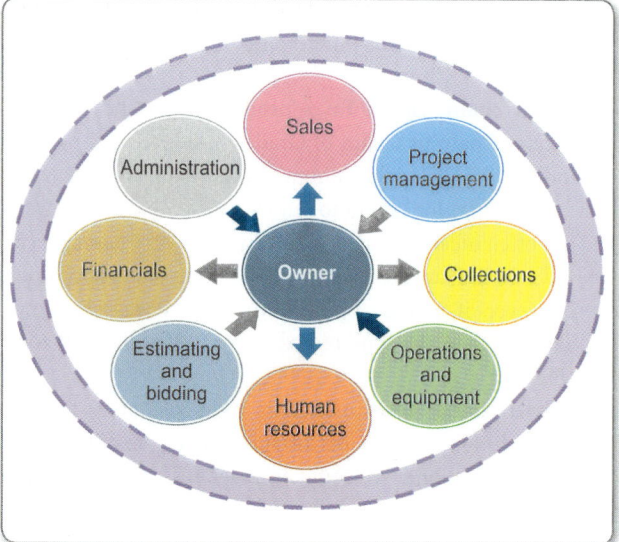

Fig. 5: Circular concentric chart

- **Circular concentric chart:** Here we place the top person in the center and jobs at different levels are shown in concentric circles surrounding the central role. The position of the senior executive is shown in the center of the chart. The subordinates of this senior executive are shown in all directions outward from the center. It explains the status of different levels of assistants and shows clearly each person's responsibility. It is the best representation of the relationship existing among the employees in an organization structure (Fig. 5).

Advantages of Organization Charts

- They give a clear picture of the organization efficiently.
- They show the levels of authority and relationship prevailing among employees at a glance.
- Dual reporting relationships and overlapping positions come to light in the preparation of the organization chart.
- Instructing work is simplified.
- Newly hired personnel can understand their role in the organization and behave accordingly.
- The strengths and weaknesses of an organization are evaluated.
- It acts as authoritative sources of information.
- The lines of authority shown are definite and formal.
- The lines of promotion can be understood.

ORGANIZATIONAL EFFECTIVENESS

Organizational effectiveness is defined as an extent to which an organization achieves its predetermined objectives with the given amount of resources and means without placing undue strain on its members. It also may be referred to as meeting organizational objectives and prevailing societal expectations soon, adapting and developing in the intermediate future, and surviving in the distant future.

Sometimes efficiency and effectiveness are used as synonyms. However, there exists a difference between the two concepts. Therefore, it is important to explain the difference between the concepts of effectiveness and efficiency to understand why organizations may be effective but not efficient, or efficient but not effective. Effectiveness is a broad concept and takes into account a collection of factors both inside and outside an organization. It is commonly referred to as the degree to which predetermined goals are achieved. On the other hand, efficiency is a limited concept that pertains to the internal working of an organization. It refers to several resources used to produce a particular unit of output. It is generally measured as the ratio of inputs to outputs. Further, effectiveness concentrates more on the human side of organizational values and activities whereas efficiency concentrates on the technological side of an organization.

The product or output of an organization is termed as organizational effectiveness. There should be a relationship between organizational effectiveness and organizational performance. Nurse managers define the goals and provide the resources for both organizational effectiveness and organizational performance. The goals have many dimensions, which include the following:

- Patient satisfaction with care
- Family satisfaction with care
- Staff satisfaction with work
- Staff satisfaction with rewards, intrinsic and extrinsic.
- Staff satisfaction with professional development: career, personal and educational.
- Staff satisfaction with the organization
- Management satisfaction with staff
- Community relationships
- Organizational health

Approaches to Organizational Effectiveness

However, the concept of organizational effectiveness is not simple because there are many approaches to conceptualizing this term. Such approaches can be grouped into the following five approaches:

1. **Goal approach:** Goal attainment is the most widely used criterion of organizational effectiveness. In goal approach, effectiveness refers to the maximization of profits by providing an efficient service that leads to high productivity and good employee morale. Several variables such as quality, productivity, efficiency, profit, turnover, accidents, morale, motivation, and satisfaction help in measuring organizational effectiveness. However, none of the single variables has proved to be entirely satisfactory. The main limitation of these approaches is the problem of identifying the real goals rather than the ideal goals.
2. **Functional approach:** This approach solves the problem of the identification of organizational goals. The vital question in determining effectiveness is how well an organization is

doing for the super-ordinate system. The limitation of this approach is that when organizations have the autonomy to follow its independent courses of action, it is difficult to accept that the ultimate goal of the organization will be to serve society. As such, it cannot be applied for measuring organizational effectiveness in terms of its contributions to the social system.

3. **System Resource approach:** The system-resource approach of organizational effectiveness emphasizes on inter-dependency of processes that relate the organization to its environment. The interdependence takes the form of input-output transactions and includes scarce and valued resources such as physical, economic and human for which every organization competes. The limitation of this model is that an acquisition of resources from the environment is again related to the goal of an organization. Therefore, this model is not different from the goal model.

4. **Constituencies approach:** Effectiveness is the ability to satisfy multiple strategic constituencies both within and outside the organization. An effective organization is one that satisfies the demand of those constituencies in its environment from whom it requires support for its continuous existence. It seeks to appraise only those in the environment who can threaten the organization's survival.

5. **Competing values approach:** The competing value approach is the criteria you value and use in assessing organization effectiveness. The common competing values are Return on investment, New product innovation, Market share, and Job security.

Thus, the discussion of organizational effectiveness leads to the conclusion that there is no single indicator of effectiveness. Instead, the approach should focus on operative goals that would serve as a basis for assessment of effectiveness. Managerial effectiveness is a causal variable in organizational effectiveness. It has been defined in terms of organizational goal-achieving behavior, i.e., the manager's behavior contributes to the achievement of organizational goals.

Factors Affecting Organizational Effectiveness

Likert has classified the factors affecting organizational effectiveness into the following three variables:

1. **Causal variables:** Causal variables are those independent variables that determine the course of developments within an organization and the objectives achieved by an organization. These causal variables include only those independent variables, which can be altered by the organization and its management. Causal variables include organization and management's policies, decisions, business and leadership strategies, skills and behavior.

2. **Intervening variables:** Intervening variables according to Likert are those variables that reflect the internal state

and health of an organization. For example, loyalties, attitudes, motivations, performance goals and perceptions of all the members and their collective capacity for effective interaction, communication, and decision-making.

3. **End-result variables:** End-result variables are the dependent variables that reflect the achievements of an organization such as productivity, costs, loss, and earnings.

Determinants of Organizational Effectiveness

There are various determinants of organizational effectiveness. They are listed below:

- Managerial characteristics
  - Strategies, policies, and practices of the institution.
  - The standards of the organization and its objectives.
  - Leadership skills of the manager.
  - Decision-making ability of the manager.
  - Communication skills of manager.
  - Human resource management tactics such as attraction, retention, and motivation of the workforce.
  - Staff training and development.
  - Rewards and Incentives.
- Organizational characteristics
  - Structural design of the organization such as specialization, departmentalization, a chain of command, a span of control, concept of centralization and so on.
- Size of the organization.
- Environmental characteristics
  - Internal aspects such as resources, raw material, budget, etc.
  - The complexity of the organization refers to heterogeneity and the range of the activities and its relevance to the operations.
  - Public opinion of the organization.
- Employees characteristics
  - Individual goals of the employee.
- Skills of the employee.
- Motives, attitudes, and values of the employee.

HOSPITAL ADMINISTRATION

As a hospital administrator, one has to carry out management functions of planning, organizing, staffing, directing, controlling and coordinating. The management applies to all kinds of organizations, whether government or non-government, small or big hospitals, profit-making hospitals or charitable hospitals. Administration applies to an administrator at all organizational levels, whether lower level or top level. The aim of all administrators is the same that is to maximize the output. It is concerned with productivity that implies effectiveness and efficiency.

Role of Hospital Administrators

General Roles

The hospital administrator like any other manager performs various roles; the managerial roles as described by Mintzberg can be grouped as follows, which are equally relevant for hospital administrator also (Fig. 6).

Specific roles: By virtue of serving a healthcare organization the hospital administrator performs some specific roles which are described below.

- The hospital administrator ensures that the hospital runs effectively and efficiently.
- The role of hospital administrators varies, depending upon the nature and complexity of the hospital.
- Various roles can be grouped as role towards patients, towards hospital organization, towards the community.

Role Towards Patients

The hospital administrator has a great responsibility to understand and appreciate the emotional aspects of the patient care, his responsibility is to understand the specific needs of certain groups of patients, i.e., patients on wheelchairs, stretchers, geriatric group of patients, pediatric patients, neonates, serious cases, foreign nationals, etc. Some of the aspects of patients are the Creation of a friendly environment, Understanding the patient's physical needs, Patient's emotional needs, Patient's clinical needs, Patients' satisfaction, Patients' education, and the Patient's communication needs.

Role Towards Hospital Organization

To handle the hospital resources for maximizing the output is one of the fundamental roles of the administrator. The role of administrator is more of coordination in nature instead of controlling, he is a coordinating officer. It includes strategic planning, environmental influence on the hospital. Operational management, management of hospital staff, materials management, financial management, hospital information, communication, public relation, risk management, law, ethics and code of conduct, marketing of health services and quality management.

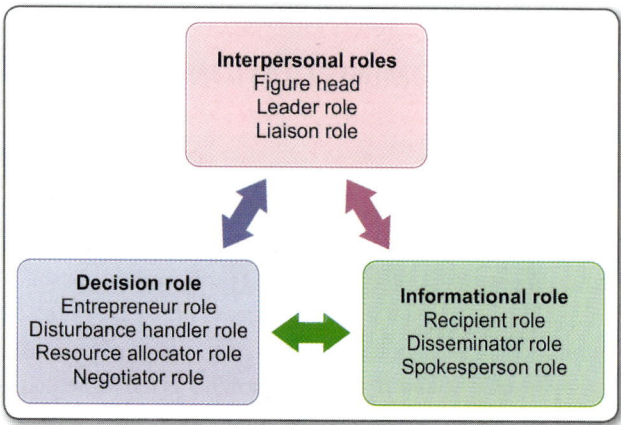

Fig. 6: Role of hospital administrators

Role Towards Community

- Integrating with primary health care.
- Integrating hospital with other healthcare organizations.
- Community participation in the planning of services and also for the utilization of hospital services.
- Outreach program: outreach program like health camps, camp surgery, immunization camps, etc.

HOSPITAL ORGANIZATION/LINE OF AUTHORITY/CONTROL

Hospitals are formal institutions developed by the society for patient care. It is intended to meet the complex health needs of its members. Hospital is a place where sick or injured individuals have access to centralized medical knowledge and technology. It protects the family from many of the disruptive effects of caring for the ill in the home and making the problems less disruptive for society as a whole. Currently, the hospital is a place for the diagnosis and treatment of human ills and restoration of health and well-being of those temporarily deprived of these. Professionally and technically skilled people apply their knowledge and skill with the help of complicated equipment and appliances - to provide quality care for the patient.

A hospital is a multifaceted organization comprising many committees, departments, types of personnel, and services. It requires highly trained employees, efficient systems and controls, necessary supplies, adequate equipment and facilities, and, of course, physicians and patients. It is a business as well as a caring, people-oriented institution and it has a similar structure and hierarchy of authority as any large business.

- **Board of trustees:** The "board of trustees," or governing board, operates the hospital in trust for the community and has a fiduciary duty to protect the assets of the hospital through efficient operation. The trustees are responsible for establishing the hospital's mission and establishing its bylaws and strategic policies. Trustees select the administrative leader of the hospital and delegate the hospital's daily operations and budgeting to the appointed executive.
- **Executive administration:** The chief executive officer (CEO) reports to the governing board and provides leadership in implementing the strategic goals and decisions set by the Board. The CEO also represents the hospital to the external environment and the community. In these tasks, the CEO must coordinate the collective effort of the hospital's personnel.
- **The medical staff:** The physician is the leader of the clinical team and the major agent working for the patient. The physician's responsibility is to diagnose the patient's condition accurately and to prescribe the best and most cost-effective treatment plan. The medical staff is a formally organized self-governing unit within the hospital, primarily comprised of physicians, but may also include other doctoral-level health care professionals such as dentists or psychologists.

- **Nursing services:** Nursing services employees are responsible for carrying out the treatment plan developed by the physician. Nursing services also called patient care services are the largest component of the hospital.
- **Allied health services:** Several departments perform functions that help with diagnosis and treatment. The clinical laboratory is a diagnostic center that performs a variety of functions, including autopsy, clinical cytology, and clinical pathology. Medical technologists, radiology department and rehabilitation services also come under allied health services.
- **Clinical support services:** The hospital pharmacy purchases and dispenses all the medications used to treat patients in the hospital. The pharmacist works directly with the medical staff in establishing a formulary, the listing of drugs chosen to be included in the pharmacy.
- **Administrative support services:** Non-medical administrative services are necessary for the hospitals business and physical plant management. The CEO leads these administrative services and is directly responsible for the day-to-day operations of the facility. Business services manage the hospital's admitting and discharge functions, record charges to a patient's account, and handles accounts receivables with third-party payers such as insurance companies. The finance department advises the CEO on financial policy and long-range planning, establishes procedures for accounting functions, receives and deposits all money received by the hospital, and approves the payments of salaries and other expenditures.
- **Accounting:** It is central to the hospital's financial business. Detailed and sound accounting practices are fundamental to maintaining important organizational statistics for administrative decision-making.
- **Admitting services:** This service is used when the patient first contacts the hospital. The sensitivity and efficiency of this department can greatly influence the patient's perception of the quality of care received.
- **Information services and medical record maintenance:** They are core functions of hospital management.
- **The human resources department:** It interacts with all departments in the hospital to ensure the quality and motivation of personnel working at the hospital.
- Other important administrative and business functions may include marketing and planning, public relations, plant and materials management, fund-raising, housekeeping, and security.

Aspects of Hospital Services

Aspects of hospital services have been given in Figure 7.

Line Services

- **Emergency services:** Diagnosis and treatment of illness of an urgent nature and injuries from accidents.
- **Out-patient services:** Provision of diagnostic, curative, preventive and rehabilitative services.

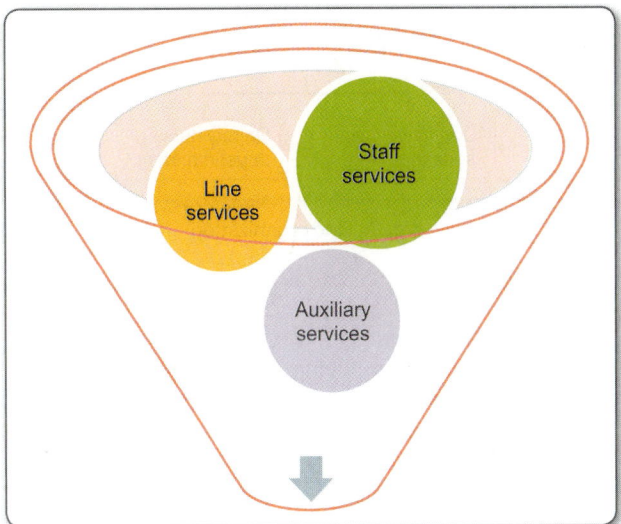

Fig. 7: Aspects of hospital services

- In-patient services (Wards).
- **Intensive care unit:** Those who need acute, multidisciplinary and intensive observation and treatment.
- **Operation theatres:** Should have a preanesthesia room and sterilization room and a scrub room for doctors and nurses.

Supportive (Staff) Services

- Central sterile supply services management
- Diet management (catering department)
- Pharmacy services management
- Laundry
- Laboratory facilities
- Radiology

Auxiliary Services

- Registration and indoor case records
- Stores
- Transport
- Mortuary
- Dietary services
- Engineering and maintenance services
- Hospital security

Levels of Organization

- **Line organization:** The oldest and purest form. The entire organization is headed by a chief executive. The supreme authority rests on the top or the highest levels of management, and the quantum of power decreases in a stepladder fashion for the subsequent levels of management in the hierarchy (Fig. 8).

Merits of Line Organization

- **Fixed responsibility:** Responsibilities are well defined, and persons are accountable to someone in the line form.

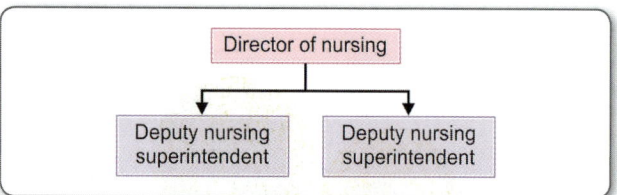

Fig. 8: Line organization

- Simplicity.
- Unity of control.
- Better discipline.
- **Prompt decision:** Being the chief and having the possession of supreme power, unified control, and fixed responsibilities, rapid and timely decision making is possible.
- **Flexibility:** There is the enjoyment of autonomy and freedom within their defined sphere of activities by respective employees.

Demerits of Line Organization

- **Its lack of specialization:** This system does not provide any scope for employing specialists.
- **Overloading or overreliance:** The departmental head is all in all of his department/division in this type of organization.
- **Inadequate communication:** It occurs as there is no down to upward communication in this type of organization.
- **Favoritism:** Since one man is the decision-maker and also opinion maker, he/she may be influenced by a few people.
- **Functional organization:** Underline organization, the person-in-charge finds it challenging to supervise all the activities efficiently. The reason is that the person does not have enough capacity and requires training. In a functional organization, the technical departments are framed to address the problems at each successive level. Although the expert and specialized services are mainly concentrated on the top, every section or unit can make use of their services. The functions of this type of organization may be classified as purchasing, marketing, production, research and development, finance, office management, personnel, etc. in a business enterprise. Functional departments of patient care services, pharmaceutical services, laboratory services, etc. in a hospital setting (Fig. 9).

Merits of Functional Organization

- **The benefit of specialization:** Under the functional organization, each work is performed by a specialist. It helps to maintain the efficiency of the organization. Each task is divided among the workers scrupulously.
- **Reducing the workload and improving efficiency:** Each person is expected to look after only one type of work. Hence the quality of work and effective control over the work is achieved.
- **Adequate supervision:** Each staff member is in charge of work. So he can devote enough time to supervise the workers.
- **Economy:** Each specialist is responsible for the performance of the work. Wastage in the production can be avoided, and the expenditure could be considerably reduced.
- **Flexibility:** Any change in the organization can be introduced without any difficulty.

Demerits of Functional Organization

- **Complicated relationship:** A single worker is working under many specialists; it is challenging for the worker to be responsible to all persons. This results in a conflict between workers and specialists.
- **Discipline:** It is challenging to maintain control among the workers when a single worker has to serve many masters.
- **Overspecialization:** There might be overlapping of authority and divided responsibility.
- **Ineffective coordination:** The extent of the authority of a specialist is not correctly defined. It creates problems while getting the cooperation among the specialists.
- **Speed of action:** When the control of a worker is divided among the specialists, the rate of work of the workers may be hampered.
- **The line and staff organization:** To strike a balance between the line and functional organization, it is believed that the best system to adopt in any progressive and elite organization is the line and staff organization. The power of making decision and execution of the decisions to meet the organizational objectives are entrusted with the line officers. Each functional unit will have line officers, and they are assisted by a large number of supportive staff (general and technical staff). This method has benefits for both line and functional organization (Fig. 10).

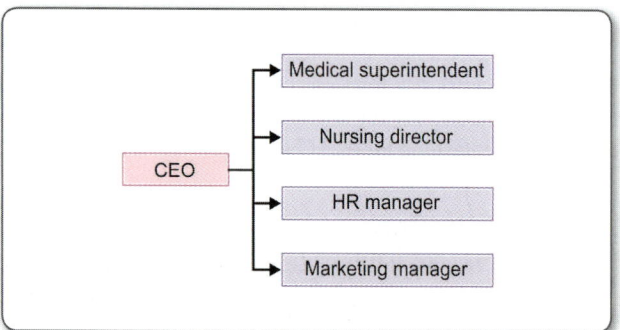

Fig. 9: Functional organization

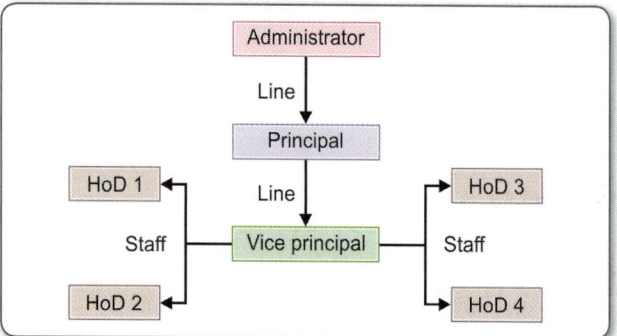

Fig. 10: Line and staff organization

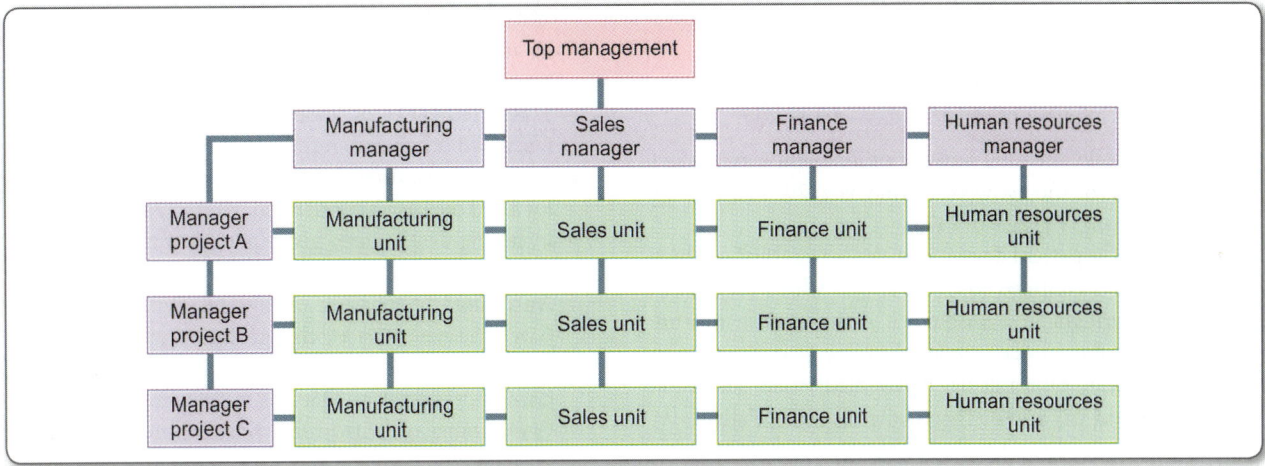

Fig. 11: Matrix organization

Demerits of Line and Staff Organization

- Staff tends to assume line authority and thus may become a cause of friction between the two.
- Sometimes the staff does not give sound advice because the team is not accountable for the implementation of the information.
- Staff steals credit, although the direction and planning are done by the manager through sheer hard work and intelligence.
- Staff fails to see the whole picture as they lack the mind of relating advice to the task and objectives of the enterprise.
- **Matrix organization:** Matrix structures are characterized by teams built directly into the organizational structure. These teams are coordinated both vertically (within the hierarchy) and horizontally (among the groups involved). The team has formal authority to make and enforce decisions. Matrix structure requires less rigid adherence to rules and procedures. Freeform organizational structures are called matrix organizations. The matrix organization design enables timely response to external competition and to facilitate efficiency and effectiveness internally through cooperation among disciplines (Fig. 11).

HOSPITAL STATISTICS

Information obtained from hospital indoor and outdoor facilities regarding the quality of care, utilization of services, quantity of services delivered, workload and other hospital-related administrative and logistic affairs is called Hospital Statistics.

Uses of Hospital Statistics

- The measure of evaluation of the quality of care
- It helps with planning.

- Allocation of resources in different areas.
- Identify deficiencies at various levels; i.e., input, process and outcome of services.
- Evaluate the effectiveness and efficiency of the administration.

Hospital Utilization Statistics

Admission: The formal acceptance by a hospital or other inpatient health care facility of a patient who is to be provided with room, and continuous nursing service in an area of the hospital or facility where patients generally reside at least overnight.

Discharge: Discharge from the hospital is the point at which the patient leaves the hospital and either returns home or is transferred to another facility such as one for rehabilitation or to a nursing home. Discharge involves the medical instructions that the patient will need to fully recover.

Hospital Beds: WHO defines a hospital bed as a bed that is regularly maintained and staffed for the accommodation and full-time care of a succession of inpatients and is situated in wards or a part of the hospital where continuous medical care for inpatients is provided. The total number of beds excludes bed compliments of the hospital for normal, healthy new-born babies in the maternity ward; but includes incubators used for premature babies.

Sanctioned bed is the official bed capacity of the hospital.

Functional bed is the actual functional status of beds in a hospital.

There are many types of hospital statistics. It is broadly classified into the following:

- **Reports related to hospital beds includes:**
  - **Daily census:** In a hospital setting, the total number of patients admitted to the facility by midnight, or sometimes at another time of the day or evening.
  - **Average daily census (ADC):** Average number of patients in the hospital at a given time per day in a

hospital over a given period of time. IPD and OPD patients are counted separately.

$$ADC = \frac{\text{Total patient days}}{\text{Number of calendar days in a period.}}$$

For example, the total number of inpatient service days provided for the 1st week of May is 1729. The average daily census is 1729/7 = 247.

- **Bed days or patient days:** A bed-day is a day during which a person is confined to a bed and in which the patient stays overnight in a hospital. It is the unit of measure denoting the services rendered to one in-patient day in the hospital. One full day is counted when admission before mid-day and discharge after mid-day. Patient-day should not include data for healthy newborn infants.
- **Total patient days care:** Determine total inpatient days of care by adding the daily patient census for 365 days. Then determine the total bed available by multiplying the total number of beds (inpatient beds) by 365. Divide the total inpatient days of care by total beds available.
- **Average bed occupancy:** Average number of days during which the bed is occupied by a patient in the course of a given period of time.
- **Bed occupancy rate (BOR):** BOR is the average occupancy of hospital beds in percentage. It is the ratio between beds used and beds provided. The bed occupancy rate is calculated based on the midnight bed census at each hospital. [For example, the BOR for Monday is based on the bed census taken at 0000 hrs Tuesday].

$$\frac{\text{Number of patient's day (service days) in a year}}{\text{Number of Beds} \times 365} \times 100$$

80–85% BOR is ideal for good quality of patient care. 15–20% beds are vacant for an emergency, maternity, isolation, intensive care (dead space beds). 100% occupancy means over-utilization. Occupancy of less than 80% is uneconomical. Example: In the month of June, 4000 inpatient days were served in a hospital with 150 beds. Given, the Total number of inpatient days = 4000. Available beds = 150. June has 30 days. So, number of days in the period = 30 BOR = Total number of inpatient days for a given period × 100/Available beds × Number of days in the period = 4000 × 100/150 × 30 = 400000/4500 = 88.889%

- **Bed turn over interval:** Average length of time (in days) that elapses between the discharge of one inpatient and the admission of the next inpatient to the same bed. It is the average period in days, that a bed remains empty. Calculation of turnover interval (TOI): TOI = (Available staffed bed days – Occupied bed days)/Inpatient discharges. Inpatient discharges include deaths, transfers out to other specialties/significant facilities and transfers out to other hospitals. Interpretation: Negative TOI indicates a scarcity of beds

and over-utilization. Long positive TOI is indicative of under-utilization because of defective admission procedures or poor-quality medical care. Short positive TOI is indicative of optimum utilization. TOI is 'zero' when bed occupancy rate is 100%.

- **Bed turnover rate:** Average number of patients cared for a bed during a given period. BTR = (No of discharges including deaths for a given period of time ÷ Average bed count for that period of time) x 100. Indications: An important measure of hospital utilization indices. Gives the net effect of changes in occupancy rate and average length of stay (ALOS) Example: In a particular hospital, there were 2358 discharges in the year 2009. The number of beds in that hospital in 2009 was 300. Hospital Bed turnover rate = 2358/300 = 7.86.
- **Vacancy rate:** Vacancy rate = 100% - Bed occupancy rate.
- **Reports related to admission/discharge/death admission:**
  - **Average length of stay (ALOS):** Length of stay is a term which is used to calculate a patient's day of admission in the hospital till the day of discharge i.e., the number of days a patient stayed in a hospital for treatment. The formula for calculating average length of stay: (total days of care (cumulative) for a specific period/number of patients during the period (admissions). The average length of stay in hospitals (ALOS) is often used as an indicator of efficiency. All other things being equal, a shorter stay will reduce the cost per discharge. For example:

Number of patients = 4

Total Length of stay = 6 + 11 + 5 + 8 = 30 days

$$\text{Average length of stay} = \frac{\text{Total length of stay}}{\text{Total number of admissions}}$$

$$= \frac{30}{4}$$

$$= 7.5 \text{ days.}$$

  - **Discharge:** It may be measured by counting the daily discharges or calculating the total discharges over a specified period of time.
  - **Deaths:** It includes the daily number of deaths, Total deaths over a period, Total deaths over 48 hours and total deaths under 48 hours.
  - **Gross death rate:** Ratio of total deaths to total discharges including deaths. In the general hospital, it should not exceed 3%.

$$\text{Gross Death Rate} = \frac{\text{Total death in a period}}{\text{Total discharge including the deaths}} \times 100$$

  - **Net death rate:** A death rate, also known as the institutional death rate, does not include deaths, which occur within 48 hours of admission (24 hours of admission in some countries).

- **Anesthetic death rate:** (No of deaths due to anesthesia ÷ No of patients anesthetized during that period) × 5000. It should be <1 in 5000.
- **Postoperative death rate:** (Deaths within 10 days of surgery ÷ Total operations during that period) × 100 Usual value is 1–2% (Depending on nature of surgery).
- **Workload statistics:**
  - **The total number of outputs:** This is a part of analyzing the productivity of the hospital using the data envelopment analysis (DEA) technique. Here the comparison is made in terms of the input and output of the hospital. The input of a hospital is budget allocation, number of doctors, number of nurses, number of other technical and non-technical staff including the supporting staff. The input also includes the expenditure of running the hospital such as the operational costs (salary, drugs, equipment, maintenance, other articles used for functioning.) The output is measured in terms of Number of IPDs, OPDs, Bed occupancy, number of surgeries, and other productive outputs of the hospital.
  - **New cases/Repeat cases**
  - **Total number of operations**
  - **Total number of X-rays**
  - **Average OPD patients per day:** Average number of OPD patients in the hospital at a given time per day in a hospital over a given period of time.
  - **Cesarean section rate:** (Total CS performed ÷ Total live-births during that period) × 100. The normal value is 3–4%.
- **Hospital care evaluation statistics:**
  - **Hospital acquired infection (HAI) rate:** HAI is an infection that develops as a result of medical care. The most common infections associated with healthcare can be divided into four categories: catheter-associated urinary tract infections, bloodstream infections, surgical site infections, and pneumonia. To determine HAI rates, divide the number of new cases of infection for a period of time by average census or patient population and multiply by 100. Hospital-wide prevalence of HAI varies from 5.7% to 19.1%, with a pooled prevalence of 10.1%.
  - **Postoperative complication rate:** It is calculated by dividing the numbers of postoperative complication in a specific period of time by the total number of surgeries conducted in that particular period and multiplying it by 100.
  - **Autopsy rate:** Autopsy rate = (Number of pathological autopsies performed ÷ Number of deaths during that period) × 100. Patients who are dead on arrival (DOA) at the hospital and fetal deaths are excluded from both the numerator and the denominator. Autopsy rate of more than 15–20% indicates inquiry.
  - **Gross result of treatment:** It includes the total number of patients treated, recovered, not improved or dead during a given period of time.
- **Indices related to the population at risk.**
  - **Admission rate:** Number of hospital admissions per person per year. It is calculated by dividing the total number of admissions in a year by the total population of the target area and multiplying it by 100. e.g. A hospital has 30000 admissions per year. It is serving a population of 300,000. Then the admission rate is 30000/300,000 × 100
  - **Bed supply rate:** Bed supply rate (Bed to population ratio) BSR = (Number of beds available ÷ Number of the population served) × 1000
- **Other types of classification:**
  - **Patient movement statistics:** Admission, discharge, deaths.
  - **Morbidity statistics:** Patients under various diagnoses.
  - **Administrative statistics:** Manpower, material, money-finance

NURSING CARE DELIVERY SYSTEMS

As nursing has evolved over a period, nursing is still focused on caring. Rapid technologic advances, knowledge explosion, emphasis on quality, cost-effectiveness, accessibility of health care and increased demand by the patients for advanced alternative health care modalities present many challenges for the nursing profession. How are nurses responding to these challenges? So how can we best utilize professional nurses across various practice settings? The answer to this question is that it is possible by reshaping organizational (administrative) policies and developing such a system of nursing care delivery as best suited to client needs.

A system may be defined as a whole made up of integrated or joined and interrelated parts. Although each component of the system has its specific function, yet all of them work harmoniously for the common outcome. The nursing care delivery system means 'the process of delivering care to the client by combining various aspects of nursing service, which will fit various patient care settings to produce a common outcome of delivering quality care and meeting the needs of clients.' There are various types of nursing care delivery systems including case method, functional method, team nursing, primary nursing, modular nursing, nursing care management, patient-focused care.

Principles of Nursing Care Delivery

- A holistic approach is used to identify nursing care needs: physical needs, mental and social needs, and spiritual needs.
- Nursing care is based on a helping relationship.
- It is the unique function of the nurse to provide nursing care according to the client's needs.
- The aspect of patient care has to be initiated and controlled by the nurse.
- There should be a justification for selecting each delivery system.
- Before planning care organizational policies to be considered.

Factors Influencing Nursing Care Delivery

- Availability of adequate staff in wards or units.
- Patient census.
- Extend of staff deficiency.
- Organizational policies regarding its practice.
- Patient's preferences for care.
- Availability of skilled staff.
- Opportunities for continuing and in-service education to the staff.
- The budget of the organization.
- Socio economical condition of the patient.
- The organization's mission.
- Patient and community needs.

Means of Organizing Nursing Care Patient Assignments And Nursing Responsibilities

Nursing is an integral part of any health care organization, which goes for fulfilling the nursing needs of the patients/society. In nursing administrations, the nurse works with individuals from partnered disciplines, for example, dietetics, therapeutic social service, drug store and so on in providing a far-reaching project of patient care in the organization. As indicated by the WHO master advisory committee, the nursing care/services are characterized as part and parcel of the total health care delivery system. The most outstanding methods for providing nursing care to patients in the health care organization are:

- **Case method:** It was one of the first types, and here, the nurses accept the total accountability for addressing every need and necessity of allocated patients amid their time of duty. It includes the task of mapping one or more than one patient to a nurse for a specific timeframe of the assignment. This model is utilized in places such as CCU, labor department, etc., wherein one nurse thinks about one patient's aggregate needs. Initially, this method was considered as part of home care services. With the introduction of health care organizations, this method's fame got diminished, and nowadays it is referred to as private duty nursing. The nurse duty incorporates providing medications and other required nursing procedures with the planning of total nursing care.

Merits

- The nurse can attend to the total needs of clients due to the adequate time and proximity of the interactions.
- Good client nurse interaction and rapport can be developed.
- The client may feel more secure.
- RNs were self-employed.
- The workload can be equally divided by the staff.
- Nurse's accountability for their function is in built.
- It is used in critical care settings where one nurse provides total care to a small group of critically ill patients.

Demerits

- Cost-effectiveness.
- The more considerable disadvantage to case nursing occurs, when the nurse is inadequately trained or prepared to provide total care to the patient.
- The nurse may feel overworked if most of her assigned patients are sick.
- She/he may tend to neglect the needs of the patient when the other patients' problems or needs demand more time.

- **Functional nursing:** Here, health care is categorized by different sectors or functional areas such as personal hygiene, medication administration, etc. Separate nurses perform various functions. Ordinarily, a shift in charge allocates available nursing staff as indicated by their capabilities, their specific capacities, and assignments to be finished during the same shift of duty. There will be a shift in charge and under her diverse nurses.

Merits

- Each person becomes very efficient at specific tasks, and a significant amount of work can be done in a short time (time-saving).
- The best utilization can be made of a person's aptitudes, experience, and desires.
- The organization benefits financially from this strategy because patient care can be delivered to a large number of patients by mixing staff with a large number of unlicensed assistive personnel.

Demerits

- Client care may become impersonal, compartmentalized, and fragmented.
- Continuity of care may not be possible.
- Only parts of the nursing care plan are known to personnel.
- Patients get confused as so many nurses attend to them, e.g., head nurse, medicine nurse, dressing nurse, temperature nurse, etc.

- **Team nursing:** Team nursing depends on the theory in which the team of expert professionals and non-professional staff cooperate to recognize, plan, actualize, and evaluate the extensive customer-focused care. It is where the nurse leads a group made out of different professionals and support staff. The colleagues or members of the team give direct coordinated patient care under the guidance of the leader. The leader nurse or team leader is a professional nurse. She holds a group of 4–6 members in her team, and they would be taking care of 15–25 patients. The supervisor doles out assignments, plans care, and trains team leaders and colleagues. To enable the exchange of information and enhance the care planning among the fellow workers, a meeting is arranged at the beginning and at the end of each shift. Complex patients and nursing care are attended by the team leader herself/himself and take an active part in the evaluation of the teamwork.

Advantages

- High-quality, comprehensive care can be provided to the patient.
- Each member of the team can participate in decision making and problem-solving.
- Improved patient satisfaction.
- Division of labor allows members the opportunity to develop leadership skills and share workload.

Disadvantages

- Establishing a team concept takes time, effort, and constancy of personnel. Merely assigning people to a group does not make them a group or team.
- An unstable staffing pattern makes team nursing difficult.
- All personnel must be client-centered.
- There is less individual responsibility and independence regarding nursing functions.

- **Modular nursing:** It is an altered form of team nursing where the team of nurses is divided based on the geographical area of patients in the ward. It follows the principle of forming a smaller group of nurses for taking care of a smaller group of patients. It is aimed to make the nurse accountable for arranging and planning the care. The ward has many cubicles/regions/modules, and the patients are admitted accordingly. A group of nurses, along with a leader, is assigned a module for care. The group head is responsible for the complete attention, and it is a collective responsibility of all team members. The achievement of modular nursing depends extraordinarily on the authority capacities of the group leader.

Merits

- The client can identify personnel who are responsible for his care.
- Continuity of care is improved when staff members are consistently assigned to the same module.
- Feelings of participation and belonging are facilitated with team members.
- The workload can be balanced and shared.

Demerits

- Costs may be increased to stock each module with the necessary patient care supplies (medication cart, linens, and dressings).
- Establishing team concepts takes time, effort, and constancy of personnel.
- An unstable staffing pattern makes the team difficult.
- There is less individual responsibility and autonomy regarding nursing function.

- **Progressive patient care:** It is a technique of creating different levels and dimensions of care. It is based on the principle of the optimum and effective use of all facilities, including the human resources for useful and comfortable care of patients. First of all, the patients are evaluated for the intensity of care that they require and are placed in a category or unit. As they become well, the levels are changed/updated, or the patients are shifted to the next level/units, which are purely based on the type of care required. The nursing care is provided by the staff of designated groups at different levels. According to this, the patient care assignment is classified to the following types such as

- **Intensive care:** For example, ICU and intermediate care, e.g. cardiac ward.
- **Self-care:** For example, Other general areas
- **Long-term care:** For example, Cancer patients and home care. e.g. Mentally retarded
- **Ambulatory care:** For example, Follow up facilities.

Merits

- Efficient use is made of personnel and equipment.
- Clients are in the best place to receive the care they require.
- The use of nursing skills and expertise are maximized.
- Clients are moved towards self-care; independence is fostered where indicated.

Demerits

- There may be discomfort to clients who are moved often.
- Long term nurse/client relationships are challenging to arrange.
- Great emphasis is placed on a comprehensive, written care plan.

- **Primary care nursing;** Here, one nurse takes up the complete care of a patient or more than a patient within 24 hours. The nurse accounts for the total responsibility of the said patient/s and collaborates with other professionals and departments for providing better care to him/her from admission to leaving the hospital. If in case the said nurse is not accessible for some time, the associated members may take up the role. The nurse remains as the primary nurse of the said patient during the whole stay of the patient in the hospital. All communications about the patient shall be passed through the primary nurse. The nurse-patient ratio in the case of primary nursing depends on the type of care required by the patient. This kind of nursing care can likewise be utilized in hospice nursing or home nursing.

Advantages

- Primary Nursing Care System is suitable for long-term care, rehabilitation units, nursing clinics, geriatric, psychiatric, burn care settings where patients and family members can establish a good rapport with the primary nurse.
- Primary nurses are in a position to care for the person- physically, emotionally, socially, and spiritually.
- High patient and family satisfaction.

Disadvantages

- More nurses are required for this method of care delivery, and it is more expensive than other methods.
- Level of expertise and commitment may vary from nurse to nurse, which may affect the quality of patient care.
- An associate nurse may find it difficult to follow the plans made by another nurse if there is disagreement or when a patient's condition changes.
- It may be cost-effective, especially in specialized units such as the ICU.

- **Case management:** The caseworker or case manager has been appointed with the duty of assisting a patient from diagnosis of the disease, admission to the hospital, process of treatment and rehabilitation and finally returning to home care. Usually, case managers are external persons designated by a company or any other third party such as an insurance company to assist and verify the cases of treatment or any other claim in case of serious illness such as renal transplantation, cardiac conditions, etc. The case managers provide the necessary guidance and counseling to the clients.

Merits

- Case management provides a well-coordinated care experience that can improve the care outcome, decrease the length of stay, and use multiple disciplines and services efficiently.
- It provides comprehensive care for those with complex health problems.
- It seeks the active involvement of the patient, family, and diverse health care professionals.

Demerits

- Nurses identify significant obstacles in the implementation of this service, financial barriers, and lack of administrative support.
- The nurse is client-focused and outcome-oriented.
- Facilitates and promotes coordination of cost-effective care.

Factors Influencing the Quality Patient Care

Many variable factors influence the number of nurses needed in a unit or ward to render a high quality of patient care.

- The total number of the patient to be nursed
- The degree of illness of patients (physical dependence)
- Type of service: medical, surgical, maternity, pediatrics, and psychiatric
- The number of nursing aides and other nonprofessional available, the amount and quality of supervision available
- The experience of the nurses who are to give patient care
- The number of non-nurses who involve in patient care, the quality of their work, their stability in-service
- The physical facilities

- Methods of performing nursing procedures
- The standards of nursing care

ORGANIZATIONAL CLIMATE

Organizational Climate is about the perceptions of the climate and about absolute measures. The 'Climate' may be regarded in absolute terms and measured by instruments but is 'felt' differently by individuals. The absolute climate may suit one person and not another. All organizational theoreticians and researchers unanimously agree that a social climate is extremely important for the ultimate achievement of organizational goals. Organizational climate though abstract in concept, is normally associated with job performance and job satisfaction and morale of the employees' climate.

Organizational climate is defined as a set of characteristics that describes an organization, distinguishes it from other organizations, is relatively enduring over time and can influence the behavior of people in it.

—**Forehand and Gilmer, 1964**

Organizational climate is a normative structure of attitudes and behavioral standards that provide a basis for interpreting the situation and act as a source of pressure for directing activity.   —**Grego Poulos, 1970**

The organizational climate is the personality of an organization, the perceptions, and feelings shared by members of the system. It can be formal, relaxed, defensive, cautious, accepting, trusting and so on. It is the employer's subjective impressions or perceptions of the organization. Practicing nurses create or at the very least, contribute to the creation of the climate perceived by the patients. The manager creates a climate in which practicing nurses work. If managers trust them, practicing nurses will provide their managers with good information to keep their managers informed.

It is the identity of an association, the discernment, and sentiments shared by individuals of the framework. It may be formal, loose, protective, careful, tolerating, trusting, etc. It is the business's emotional impressions or view of their association. Nurses make or at any rate, add to the making of the organizational climate seen by the patients. It is the responsibility of the manager to make the same for nurses' work. If there is mutual trust, then there will be a good flow of communication that enhances the organizational climate.

Sociological Dimensions of Organizational Climate

- The clarity in specifying certification of the organization's goals and policies. This is facilitated by a smooth flow of information and management support of the employee.
- Commitment to goal achievement through employee involvement.
- Standards of performance that challenge, promote, provide and improve individual performance.

- Responsibility for one's work fostered and supported by managers.
- Recognition for doing good work.
- Teamwork—a sense of belonging, mutual trust and respect.

Dimensions of Organizational Climate

- Orientation to the obedience of established rules and obtaining objectives.
- Interpersonal Relationship of the members of the organization.
- The extent of supervision and style of supervision.
- Attitude towards mistakes, its tolerance, and management of mistakes.
- Conflict management techniques of the organization as it is a precursor of threat.
- Communication and its efficiency and channel.
- Decision making and development of trust.
- Management of rewards
- Opportunities for innovations and change.

Factors Influencing Organization Climate

- **Organizational Context:** The climate is said to be highly favorable when the organizational techniques are harmonized with the principles of the organization.
- **Structure:** It is the framework that establishes formal relationships and defines power as well as functional responsibility.
- **Process:** Communication, decision making, and control are some of the significant procedures through which the organization carries out its goals.
- **Physical environment:** The external conditions of the environment, the size, and location of the building in which the staff works, the size of the town, climate conditions, noise in the workplace, etc. affect the organizational climate.
- **System values and norms:** It refers to certain types of behavior that are rewarded as well as motivated. It includes the reward system, promotion, etc.

Roles of Nurse Manager in Maintaining the Organizational Climate

- **Organizational communication:** Communication is the basic pillar of any organization and one of the main areas for improvement. It is essential for coordination between departments and within the department itself, knowing the opinions of patients and fellow workers and knowing the aims and development of each person and/or department. The most common and useful practices in this area include opinion polls, evaluation tools (performance and competencies), activities to propose ideas to promote innovation, interdepartmental breakfasts/tea, sessions to share best practices, ideas and suggestions boards, etc. There should be some times in the week reserved to speak about own family, children and other non-official aspects of life. It encourages familiarity and communication.

- **Job recognition:** Recognition in the working environment is a practice that can take place through several people: a direct supervisor, the general management of the company, our colleagues, patients, students and so on. The actions that we may be recognized for include: A job well done, helping a co-worker, good patient service, working at the organization for several years (seniority), improving internal processes, contributing new ideas to improve the organization, etc. The recognition includes monetary compensation, extra days' holiday, gifts, extra activities (trips, celebrations, breakfast with the head of the organization, etc.), internal promotions, both publicly (bulletin boards, thank-you notes, corporate e-mails, events, etc.) and/or privately.

- **Reconciliation between work and private life:** To reconcile work and private life, we see practices such as flexible working hours, summer working hours, continuous workdays on Fridays, continuous workdays on the days before public holidays, day or afternoon off on birthdays, extended maternity/paternity leave, work meetings with limited start and end times, permission to take time off for school meetings/tutoring, etc. Social benefits that can also help reconciliation include worker support services for formalities for employees, subsidized meals, refreshments, gift vouchers and so on.

- **Leaders:** One of the main jobs of leaders is to ensure that there is a good organizational climate in the company. More than just demanding results, these professionals should motivate employees, and spark the necessary energy to carry out excellent work. So, when it's time to hire leaders for your company, try to find professionals who can awaken the individual and collective potential, in others and who know how to foster teamwork.

- **Physical environment:** The physical environment of the workplace has a huge impact on the organizational climate. Professionals who work in a place that stimulates creativity is comfortable and makes all the tools available for daily tasks, often give much better feedback. This may seem obvious, but numerous organizations simply don't pay attention to this aspect. It's not about providing a luxurious office to employees, but making it a space that is favorable for people to do their activities. Ergonomics, equipment, colors, how the furniture is arranged, all of this directly affects the employees' experience.

- **A good relationship among employees:** Teamwork, when utilized correctly, generates much more than results: it helps to build a richer organizational climate.

Activities to Promote Positive Organizational Climate

- Developing statements of the organization's mission, philosophy, vision, goals, and objectives with input from practicing nurses, including their personal goals.

- Establishing trust and openness through communication that includes prompt and frequent feedback and stimulates motivation.
- Providing opportunities for growth and development, including career development and continuing education programs.
- Promoting teamwork.
- Asking practicing nurses to state their satisfaction and dissatisfactions during meetings and conferences and through surveys.
- Marketing the nursing organization to the practicing nurse, other employees and the public.
- Following through on all activities involving practicing nurses.
- Analyzing the compensation system for the entire nursing organization and structuring it to reward competence, productivity, and longevity.
- Promoting self-esteem, autonomy, and self-fulfillment for practicing nurses, including feelings that their work experiences are of high quality.

- Emphasizing programs to recognize practicing nurses' contributions to the organization.
- Assessing unneeded threats and punishments and eliminating them.
- Providing job security and an environment that enables the free expression of ideas and exchange of opinions. (threats and recriminations, which may occur as downscaled performance reports, negative counseling, confrontation, conflict or job loss, are not part of a positive organizational climate).
- Being inclusive in all relationships with practicing nurses.
- Helping nurses overcoming their shortcomings and develop their strengths.
- Encouraging and supporting loyalty, friendliness, and civic consciousness.
- Developing strategic plans that include decentralization of decision making and participation by practicing nurses.
- Being a role model of performance desired for practicing nurses.

 ## REVIEW QUESTIONS

1. Define organization. Classify the organization and explain the factors influencing organizational structure.
2. Enlist and explain the levels of the organization.
3. What is a functional organization? What are its merits and demerits?
4. Explain the principles of the organization.
5. Define organizational behavior.
6. Explain the theories of organization/organizational behavior.
7. Define an organization chart. Explain its types in detail.
8. Define the hospital and explain the types of hospital.
9. Explain organization of Hospital Services.
10. What is organizational development? Explain its components and importance.
11. Explain organizational effectiveness.
12. Explain different hospital utilization indices with relevant examples.
13. What is a patient assignment? Differentiate case method and functional nursing.
14. Define the patient assignment system and explain various types of patient assignment system.
15. Discuss team nursing and discuss the advantages and disadvantages in detail.
16. Role of nurse in maintaining organizational climate.

Further Readings

1. Banerjee, Shyamal. Principles and Practice of Management. Oxford and IBM Publishing, New Delhi; 2000.
2. Basavanthappa BT. Nursing Administration. 2nd Edition: Jaypee Brothers Medical Publishers (P) Ltd., New Delhi; 2009.
3. Barrett, Jean. Ward Management and Teaching. Konark Publishers, Delhi; 1992.
4. Warren, Stevens, F. Management and Leadership in Nursing. McGraw – Hill Inc, New York; 1978.
5. Alexander et al. Nursing Service Administration. Mosby Publishers, US; 1962.
6. Park K. Preventive and Social Medicine, 19th Edition: M/s. Banarasidas Bhanot Publishers, Jabalpur; 2007.
7. Basavanthappa BT. Nursing Administration, 1st Edition: Jaypee Brothers Medical Publishers (P) Ltd., New Delhi; 2002.
8. Goel SL, Kumar R. Management of Hospitals – Hospital Administration in the 21st century, Vol. 4, Deep and Deep Publication, New Delhi; 2002.
9. Ranga Rao SP. Administration of Primary Health Centers in India, 1st Edition: Mittal Publications, New Delhi; 1993.
10. Lucita M. Nursing: Practice and Public Health Administration. Current Concepts and Trends. B. I. Churchill Living Stone Pvt. Ltd., New Delhi; 2002.
11. Sakharkar BM. Principles of Hospital Administration and Planning, 2nd Edition: Jaypee Brothers Medical Publishers (P) Ltd., New Delhi; 2009.
12. Patricia S Yoder-Wise. Leading and Managing in Nursing. 2nd Edition: Mosby Publication, US; 1999.
13. Bessie L Marquis, Carol J Huston. Leadership Roles and Management Functions in Nursing: Theory and Application. 5th Edition: Lippincott Williams and Wilkins, New York; 2006.
14. Linda Roussel. Management and Leadership for Nurse Administrators. 4th Edition: Jones and Bartlett Publication, USA; 2006.
15. Wehrich H, Koontz H. Management A Global Perspective. 11th Edition: Tata McGraw-Hill Publishing Company, Ltd., New Delhi; 2005.
16. Marquis BL, Huston CJ. Leadership and Management Functions in Nursing- Theory, and Application. 5th Edition: Lippincott Williams and Wilkins, Philadelphia; 2006.
17. Douglass LM. The Effective Nurse: Leader and Manager. 5th Edition: Mosby Publication, US; 1996.
18. Trained Nurses Association of India, Nursing Administration, and Management.
19. Samson Rebecca. Leadership and Management in Nursing Practice and Education 1st Edition: Jaypee Brothers Medical Publishers (P) Ltd., New Delhi; 2009.
20. Kunders GD. Designing for Total Quality in Health Care, Prism Book Pvt. Ltd., Bangalore; 2002.
21. Chandorkar AG. Hospital Administration and Planning. 2nd Edition: Paras Medical Publisher, New Delhi; 2009.
22. Joshi DC, Joshi Mamta. Hospital Administration. 1st Edition: Jaypee Brothers Medical Publishers (P) Ltd., New Delhi; 2009.
23. Eleanor J Sullivan, Philip J Decker. Effective Leadership and Management in Nursing. 4th Edition: Published by Addison Wesely; 2011.
24. Kulkarni GR. Financial Management for Hospital Administration, Jaypee Brothers Medical Publishers (P) Ltd., New Delhi; 2009.

Unit
5

Staffing (Human Resource Management)

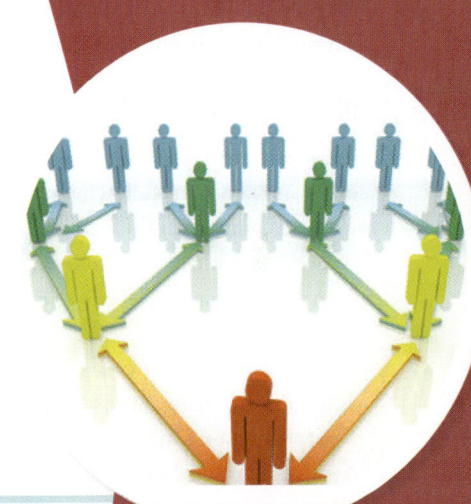

 Unit Outline

- Staffing
- Staffing Methods/Scheduling/ Procedure/Modules in Clinical Setting
- Recruitment
- Selection
- Placement
- Promotion
- Retention
- Superannuation
- Deployment
- Training and Development
- Training
- Credentialing
- Transfer
- Termination
- Human Resource Management in Hospital and Community
- Projecting Staffing Requirements: Staffing Study

- Norms of Staffing According to Staff Inspection Unit
- Staffing Norms: Indian Public Health Standards (IPHS)
- Patient Classification System
- Staffing Formula
- Categories of Nursing Personnel and their Job Description in a Hospital
- Patient Assignments and Nursing Responsibilities
- Absenteeism
- Employee Turnover
- Staff Welfare
- Discipline
- Grievance
- In-service Education
- Adult Education/Learning (Distance Learning)
- Material Management
- Nursing Audit and Maintenance

STAFFING

Staffing is undoubtedly one of the significant issues of any nursing association, regardless of whether it is a clinic, nursing home, home services, mobile care organization, or any another setting.

Staffing is a deliberate and systematic process with a particular purpose to decide upon the number and type of manpower (nursing) required to deliver nursing care and service in a particular health care setting to the needy in accordance with the pre-determined standards and protocols. The ultimate purpose of staffing is to ensure the right type of staff to cater the needs of the patients in the hospital.

Philosophy of Staffing in Nursing

Nurse administrators of a hospital nursing division should accept and adopt the following philosophy.

- Nurse administrators trust that it is conceivable to coordinate a worker's knowledge and aptitude in patient care, in a way to streamline work fulfillment and care quality.
- Nurse administrators believe that the specialized and humanistic care needs of chronic sick patients are perplexing or complicated, and hence, all the skilled care must be given by proficient nurses.
- Nurse administrators suggest that the health education recovery needs of constantly sick patients are involved to the point that demands the need for expert and specialized nurses.
- The Master Plan of staffing and policies/strategies associated with staffing shall be developed by the Heads/Supervisors of the health care setting and the same may be executed by the Unit Heads in collaboration with fellow workers keeping a focus on the workload and work process.

Objectives of Staffing in Nursing

- Provide expert nursing staff in different areas of requirement. E.g. Intensive care unit (ICU), OT, Emergency.
- Provide adequate staff to allow a 1:1 nurse-patient proportion for each shift.
- Provide adequate nursing staff in Medical, Surgical, Obstetrics, Pediatric, and Mental Health units to allow a 1:5 nurse-patient proportion during the day. This nurse-patient proportion may be modified during the night shift as 1:10. (The percentage may change according to the authoritative arrangements).
- Inform each nursing professional that solicitations for particular get-away occasion time will be regarded inside the cutoff points forced by patient's care and work contract necessities.

- Based on the seniority, facilitate employees for long-term services by providing special duty hours.

Factors Affecting Staffing

- The policies and philosophy of the hospital, such as duty roaster, weekend policy, and off-duties.
- The kind of patients (regardless of whether paid or free).
- The number of patients and the seriousness of their disease.
- The learned skill and different qualities of nursing staff concerning patient care needs.
- The design of the different nursing units and assets accessible inside the division, for example, sufficient hardware, supplies, and materials.
- Budget including the sum distributed to pay salary, incidental advantages, supplies, materials, and gear.
- Professional exercises, for example, inclusion in different professional associations, formal instructive improvement, and interest in research and staff advancement.
- Expected working hours per annum for each employee. This is affected by the 40–48 hrs/week, which is the permitted working hours per week according to the Factories Act 1948, Govt. of India.
- Patterns of work routine; 5 days weekly - 8 hrs/day off 4 days weekly – 10 hrs/day and 3 days off; or 3½ days duty per week with continuous 12 hours duty every day and followed by 3 ½ days off every week.

Staffing Policies

A policy is a foreordained and acknowledged course of considerations and activities built up as a guide towards accepted objectives and goals. These are generally encircled by the governing body or the higher administration while strategies are prepared by other senior officials.

Personal policies fill in as a guide toward hierarchical purposes and help with avoiding choices as opposed to its goal. It is an aggregate responsibility of the association/organization to act in predetermined ways. **The process of creating personal policies includes the consideration of the following elements:**

- Identification of the reason and targets, which the associations wish to achieve with respect to its employees.
- Analysis of the considerable number of components under which the association's workforce strategy/policy will function.
- Examining the conceivable options in every zone in which the personnel policy is fundamental.
- Implementation of the policy through the advancement of strategies adjusted to the whole organization.
- The ongoing revision of the policy to face newer trends and challenges.

STAFFING METHODS/SCHEDULING/PROCEDURE/MODULES IN CLINICAL SETTING

Cyclic Scheduling

It is a standout amongst other methods for staffing to meet the necessities of impartial circulation of long periods of work and time. An essential time design for a specific number of weeks is built up and afterward rehashed in cycles. This is the least complicated strategy for planning the staff by scheduling equal rotations. The critical components of this strategy are;

- Once created, it is a generally perpetual timetable requiring just impermanent changes.
- Nurses will not have the anticipation of their off-duty as it is scheduled in advance for a more extended period.
- Personal plans might be made ahead of time with a reasonable level of reliability.
- Modifications can be done ahead of time with the least deviations.
- It tends to be utilized with rotating, permanent or mixed shifts and can be changed to permit settled days off and uneven work periods, in light of individual needs and work period inclinations.
- It very well may be altered to fit known or foreseen times of overwhelming workloads or substantial workloads and can be briefly balanced on account of cyclic planning moderately resolute; it works just with a staff that rotates by policy and personal choice.

The staff who requires adaptable planning to meet their own needs do not acknowledge it. A limitless number of essential cyclic examples can be created and customized to suit the necessities of every unit. Examples ought to reflect the approach, workload, and staff inclinations. Nursing staff may utilize a staffing board to build up an example and cycle acceptable to them. The staffing board is used to demonstrate the quantity of diverse nursing workforce required for every day of the week for about a month and a half.

Self-scheduling

Self-scheduling is a method that may make staff more joyful, firmer, and more dedicated. It should be arranged precisely on a unit premise or according to units. Planning may utilize either a self-coordinated workgroup or a quality circle strategy approach. Self-scheduling matches the staff's inclinations. It has been found to abbreviate scheduling time; increment staff retention and self-satisfaction; and decrease clashes, disease time, willful truancy and turnover.

Self-scheduling leads to more responsible employees. It meets personal goals such as family, social life, education, childcare, and commuting. It is an example of participatory management with decentralized decision making. The rules should be minimal to meet legal and professional standards. This method becomes successful when every staff functions with responsibility.

Modified Approaches to Nurse Staffing and Scheduling

A wide range of ways to deal with nurse staffing and planning is being attempted with an end goal to fulfill the requirements of the employees and meet workload demands of patient care. These incorporate adjusted work-filled weeks such as10 or 12 hours shifts, group rotation, premium day, weekend staffing, etc. Such methodologies should bolster the objectives and philosophy of the organization. The division of nursing care should be precisely mentioned in the policy statement and staffing philosophy.

- **Modified workweek:** The utilization of 10- and 12-hour shifts are ordinary. Nurse administrators should create work routines that are satisfying the staffing logic and arrangements, especially concerning productivity. Such modified schedules should not be forced on the nursing staff but rather should demonstrate common advantages to Patient, Employee and Employer.

  One change of the worksheet is four 10-hour shifts for every week in composed time increments. One issue with this model is time covers of 4 hours for every 24-hour day.

  A second alternative is a 12-hour move in which nurses work even shifts, in which nurses work seven shifts in about fourteen days: three on, four off, four on, three off. They operate an aggregate 84 hours and are paid for extra time. Twelve-hour shifts and adaptable staffing have been accounted for to have enhanced care monetary profit since nurses can more readily deal with their home and individual lives.

- **The weekend alternatives:** Nurses work two twelve-hour moves/shifts and are paid for 40 hours in addition to benefits. They can utilize the weekdays for continuing nursing education (CNE) or other individual needs. The end of the week booked has a few varieties. Nurses working Monday through Friday have off on all weekends.

- **Premium day weekend:** It is a design where the nurse opts for an additional day off, called the premium day when he/she initiates working an extra weekend past the scheduled requirement. This strategy does not add straight to clinic costs.

- **Premium vacation night:** It is the same principle as the previous one but with the difference of long-term benefits. E.g. It is giving five days of vacation (working days) for those who opt night shifts for some time, such as 3–6 months.

- **Other modified approaches:** Team rotation: It is a type of cyclic staffing where a team of the nurse is rotated as a unit. This is based on a team nursing modality.

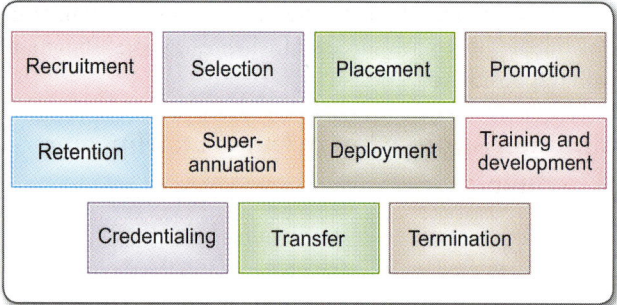

Fig. 1: Activities of staffing

Activities of Staffing (Human Resource Management)

Human resource management is an essential part of an association. It guarantees sufficient supply, an appropriate amount, and quality compelling the use of HR. The management will decide its labor needs when there is a deficiency and after that, discover the sources from which the necessities will be met. This may be described as under (Fig. 1).

RECRUITMENT

Recruitment is a vital capacity of organizations, which decides; regardless of whether the required will be accessible at the work spot, when an occupation is really to be embraced. It incorporates the procedure and the techniques by which openings/vacancies are projected, published/advertised, applications are received and screened, interviews are directed, and offer of appointments are made.

"Recruitment is defined as the process of searching for prospective employees and stimulating them to apply for a job in the organization."

According to IGNOU Module: "It is a process in which the right person for the right post is procured."

Types of Recruitment

There are three types of recruitment:
1. **Planned:** It is preplanned and is based on the revision of the organizational recruitment policy.
2. **Anticipated:** Though not preplanned, these are expected due trends and challenges faced by the organization both internally and externally.
3. **Unexpected:** These are unexpected, and it may arise as a result of the transfer, severe illness of some staff, accidents, etc.

Objectives of Recruitment

- To draw in individuals with multi-dimensional abilities and encounter who suit the present and future organizational strategies.
- To welcome newcomers and outsiders who are talented to lead the organization.
- To implant new blood at all levels of the association.
- To build up an organizational culture that pulls capable individuals into the organization.
- To devise approaches for surveying mental qualities.
- To search out the non-conventional advancement of ability.
- To scan for talents universally and not merely inside the organization.
- To foresee and discover individuals for new positions.

Principles of Recruitment

- Termination and production of any post should be finalized by capable officers.
- Only the empty positions should be filled and neither less nor more ought to be employed.
- A job profile/work examination should be made before recruitment.
- Procedure for recruitment has to be prepared by experts, it has to be from internal and external sources, and it should be based on set standards and required qualifications.
- Promotion policy has to be set.

Sources of Recruitment

The origins of recruitment are:
- **Internal sources:** Internal sources include present employees, employee referrals, a former employee, and previous applicants.
    - **Present employees**: Transfers and promotions from among the current workers can be a decent wellspring of recruitment. Transfers are frequently critical in furnishing workers/staff with a broad-based perspective of the association, vital for the future.
    - **Employee referrals:** This is the excellent wellspring/source of internal recruitment. Staff can grow excellent prospects for their families and companions by familiarizing with the upsides of occupation with the organization, promoting acquaintance and supporting them with the application. This is exceptionally compelling because much-qualified personnel comes up with little to no effort.
    - **Former employees:** Some staff might be ready to come back to the organization after the superannuation. They may work full time or part-time. The leverage of these sources is that the execution of these individuals is as of now known.
    - **Previous applicants:** Although not genuinely an inner source, the individuals who have already connected for employment can be reached via mail, a snappy and reasonable approach to fill an unforeseen opening.

- **External sources:**
  - **Professional or trade associations:** Numerous associations give recruitment services to individuals who are registered with them. These administrations may comprise incorporating job seekers' points of interest and providing access to its individuals who require them, Naukri.com, Shine.com, and so on. The professional organization in India such as the Trained Nurses Association of India, also aids the nurses in overseas employment. It is helpful when the specialized individuals for a specific assignment are not locally accessible in the market.
  - **Advertisements:** These constitute a well-known technique to reach for employees as many recruiters suggest this as an excellent method because of its broad reach. For exceedingly specific volunteers/professionals, the ads might be put in proficient/business journals and newspapers. The daily newspaper is the most widely recognized medium.
  - **Employment exchange:** Employment exchange has been set up everywhere throughout the nation according to the provisions of the Employment Exchanges (Compulsory Notification of Vacancy) Act, 1959. The Act applies to every single organization having 25 laborers or more. This Act requires all the organizations to advise the opportunities to Employment Exchange before they are filled. The job aspirants should enlist themselves with the closest Employment Exchange with their qualifications.
  - **Campus recruitment:** It covers all the educational and technical training organizations such as Universities, IIT, IIM, Colleges, etc.
  - **Walk-ins, Write-ins, and Talk-ins:** It is one of the conventional methods of recruitment. The job seeker directly walks in or writes a letter to the HR department or talks to the executives about the availability of any vacancy. The recruiter also can initiate this process. Most of the organizations where there are massive human resources involved follow this pattern as the other methods would be expensive. E.g. Corporate Hospitals.
  - **Internship:** It is a newer form of recruitment. Many organizations sponsor internship programs for intern students of different institutes in their organization with some stipend allowance. After the period of the internship, the organization recruits those who was excellent during the period of internship. This is a unique method to hire outstanding performers.
  - **Consultants:** These are agencies specially established for the recruitment of different categories of human resources to a different organization that is in need.
  - **Contractors:** They usually recruit casual workers in bulk and employ them in the respective work sites of own or provide human resources supply to others who are in need.
  - **International recruiting:** It is recruitment across the borders of the country. This is significant in those countries where there is a scarcity of trained professionals or workers. It is also done in case of the need for extraordinary talent. E.g. Indian nurses recruitment to the Middle East and European Countries.
  - **Tele recruitment**: Organizations advertise job vacancies through the internet, television, radio, etc.

Recruitment Process/Steps

Recruitment process is aimed at creating a pool of job applicants with the desired qualification by identifying and attracting them. This is carried out in five interconnected stages

1. **Planning:** It includes identifying the need for recruitment and other aspects such as the number of posts to be filled.
2. **Strategy development:** This involves developing the appropriate method of recruitment.
3. **Searching:** This may vary according to the method of recruitment.
4. **Screening:** According to the planned strategy, the candidates are screened and finalized.
5. **Evaluation and control:** Final stage of offering the order of appointment.

Factors Affecting Recruitment

All associations, regardless of whether vast or small, take part in recruitment, however, not to a similar degree. This contrasts with:

- The size, area of the association, and the work conditions.
- The impacts of past recruitments, which demonstrate the association's capacity to find and keep great performing individuals.
- Working conditions, for example, compensation/salary and advantage bundles offered by the association, which may impact turnover and requires future selection.
- The rate of development of the association/organization.
- The level of the regularity of tasks and future development and generation programs.
- Cultural, economical and legal factors, etc.

SELECTION

Selection begins when applications are screened in the workforce office. The selection procedure incorporates meeting, the business' offer, acknowledgment by the candidate, and marking of an agreement or composed offer.

Those candidates who appear to meet the job prerequisites are sent offer letters and are directed to top them off and send back to the employer for further proceedings. The job application form is a standout amongst the essential part of the job determination procedure.

"It is the process of choosing the best-qualified individuals among the applicants. It includes interviewing, the employer's offer, acceptance by the applicant, and signing of a contract or written offer."

Steps in Selection (Education)

- **Application forms:** The issue and receipt of application forms is the responsibility of the administration department, and a significant part of the primer work is taken care of by the administrative staff under the supervision of the managerial leader of the school/college. The data contained in the application form and reports, regarding them, should be organized and documented.
- **Selection committee:** A selection panel involving the head of the school/college, a faculty, delegates of representations from statutory bodies, educational psychologists and a clinician is responsible for the investigation of applications, and after that, the suitable candidates are chosen.
- **Orientation program:** After confirmation of the admission, an introduction program is organized to make the students mindful of the college structure, clinical training areas, labs, school/college rules, and inn/hostel. The introduction should be given by the senior staff of the school/college of nursing. The introduction program may take three to five days.
- **Development of master plan:** When a specific batch is conceded, the class instructor may draw a comprehensive strategy known as master plan as indicated, by which the entire program is arranged. Date of examinations and occasional assessment and so on are detailed.
- **Parent-teachers association:** All guardians are selected in the parent-teacher association, and this helps in establishing contact between the parents and teachers. This enhances the organization. Gatherings of PTA are held often, and the guardians are kept educated about the students' advancement. When students' distress happens, PTA individuals are called before taking any disciplinary actions. Therefore, guardians are additionally associated with the administration of the organization.

Steps in Selection (Service)

- **Interviewing by Personnel Department:** Interviewing is the primary strategy to assess a candidate's appropriateness for a post. This is the most mind-boggling and troublesome piece of the determination procedure. The principle destination of an interview is to get all the data about the

possibility to choose the reasonableness for the post, to give the candidates an entire picture of the activity as well as that of the organization.

- **Pre-employment tests written/oral/practical:** It guarantees the determination of the most appropriate candidate for different posts. Interviews should be led deliberately and pre-employment checks should be held methodically wherever essential and conceivable. These tests can comprehensively be divided into four sorts:
  - **Tests of general ability:** These tests provide a helpful sign for the applicant's psychological score. It has been seen that for different professions, there is an ideal level of I.Q. while choosing people which includes ideal range IQ, not higher or lower.
  - **Tests of aptitude:** It measures whether an individual has the limit or latent capacity to take in another activity if given sufficient preparation. These tests measure skills and capabilities that have the potential for later improvement in the individual.
  - **Personality tests:** These are utilized to survey specific identity attributes. These tests are being used in choosing the possibility for deal employments, supervisory occupation, administration dazes, and so because specific identity qualities are essential to prevail in such employment.
- **Interview by the departmental head:** In few clinics, the choice/selection panel comprises one individual from the workforce office/HR (Human Resources), the office head/chief of the concerned division/NS (Nursing Superintendent) and one agent of the hospital administration. After talking to every one of the applicants, the committee presents its suggestions for endorsement to the head of hospital administration.
- **The decision of administrator to accept or reject:** The Hospital Administrator/Head of HR may like to talk with every one of the candidates by himself for the key occupations and leave the same to the selection committee for less significant appointments. If there is an appointment of HoD, then an external expert is also included. The administrator has the discretion to accept or reject the offer of appointment to any candidate.
- **Medical examination:** The medical scan of a planned staff is a guide both to the staff and to the administration. The choice of the correct kind of staff who can put forth a valiant effort and be glad requires accurate information about his/her physical limits and disables. The restorative examination will take out a candidate whose wellbeing is beneath the standard or one who is therapeutically unfit.
- **Joining report by the employee:** When new workers/staff report for joining, he/she ought to be given an offer letter, his expected set of responsibilities, and handbook of the hospital/organization. He should be requested to forward his joining report.

PLACEMENT

Placement is a credit-bearing element of a degree course, and all placements are discretionary. On the off chance that a student quits a placement or there is no placement facility accessible, it implies placement is not ensured. Placement is characterized as the condition of being set or orchestrated.

Placement is a process of assigning a specific job to each of the selected candidates. It involves assigning a specific rank and responsibility to an individual. It implies matching the requirements of a job with the qualifications of the candidate. Placement is understood as assigning jobs to the selected candidates. Assigning jobs to employees may involve a new job or a different job. Thus, placement may include the initial assignment of a job to the new employee, on transfer, promotion or demotion of the present employees. Placement involves assigning a specific job to each one of the selected candidates. However, placement is not so simple as it looks. Instead, it involves striking a balance between the requirements of a job and the qualifications of a candidate.

Definition

Placement may be defined as "the determination of the job to which an accepted candidate is to be assigned, and his assignment to that job. It is a service provided by the educational organizations or any other agencies for finding a suitable job for students or any other aspirant. This also includes the assessment of a person as what he/she can do as per the demands of the required job. The process of placement is further extended to the financial incentives, promotional possibilities, collegial relationship and so on.

Proper placement of a worker reduces employee turnover, absenteeism and accident rates, and improves morale.

"Placement refers to the allocations of people to the job. It includes the initial assignment of new employees and promotion transfer or demotion of present employees."

Placement can also be defined as the internal filling of vacancies as distinguished from external recruitment. Placement is a process of assigning a specific job to each of the selected candidates. It involves assigning a specific rank and responsibility to an individual. It implies compression of the requirements of a job with the qualifications of the candidate.

Significance of Placement

- It improves employee morale
- It helps in reducing employee turnover
- It helps in reducing absenteeism
- It helps in reducing accident rates
- It avoids the misfit between the candidate and the job
- It helps the candidate to work as per the predetermined objectives of the organization.

Placement Team/Cell

The team of Placement Cell comprises a Chairperson, Coordinator, four faculty/trainers each with desirable knowledge and qualification of the placement area and few student representatives. The Placement Cell is constituted in all educational organizations to foster the placement of passing out students. This team will bolster the young aspirants all through the preparation of the placement process.

Problems of Placement

The difficulty with placement is that we tend to look at the individual but not at the job. Often, the individual has not worked independently. Whether the employee works independently or is dependent, depends on the type of jobs. Jobs in this context may be classified into three categories:

- **Independent jobs:** In certain cases, jobs are independent, for example, postal service or field sales. Here, nonoverlapping routes or territories are allotted to each worker.
- **Sequential jobs:** In sequential jobs, activities of one worker are dependent on the activities of a fellow worker.
- **Pooled jobs:** Where jobs are pooled in nature, there is high interdependence among activities. The final output is the result of the contribution of all the workers. Project teams, temporary task forces, and assembly teams represent pooled jobs.

Independent jobs do not pose great problems in placement, for each employee needs only to be evaluated relative to the comparison between his or her capabilities and interests, and those required on the job. But independent jobs are becoming rarer and rarer, as most jobs are dependent (sequential or pooled).

Process of Placement

- Collect details about the employee
- Construct his or her profile
- To which subgroup profile does the individual's profile best fit?
- Compare subgroup profile to job family profiles
- To which job family profile does the subgroup profile best fit?
- Assign the individual to job family
- Assign the individual to a specific job after further counseling and assessment

Importance of Placement

The importance of placement lies in the fact that proper placement of employees reduces employee turnover, absenteeism, accidents, and dissatisfaction, on the one hand, and improves their morale, on the other. Placements are also important for employment agencies, especially executive search firms, a type of employment agency that specializes in recruiting executive personnel for companies in various industries.

Benefits of Placement

- Employing a placement or work experience student can be viewed as part of the interview process for future company employees.
- Gain an intelligent, motivated, cost-effective labor resource with valuable skills, knowledge and fresh ideas.
- Projects which otherwise would not be done due to a shortage of resources can be moved forward.
- Offer a solution to short term staff shortages.

Placement is understood as the allocation of people to jobs. If the number of individuals is large concerning the available jobs, only the best-qualified persons can be selected and placed. Once we establish this unique profile for each individual, people and jobs can be matched optimally within the constraints set by available jobs and available people.

PROMOTION

A change for better prospects starting with one occupation then onto the next activity is considered by the employee as an advancement or promotion. An employee thinks about advancement/promotion as an expansion in the pay, increment in eminence, upward development in the chain of command of occupation/job, extra supervisory duty, and a superior future.

Nature and Scope of Promotion

- Seniority versus merits: There has been a great deal of controversy over the relative values of seniority and excellence in any system of promotion. Seniority will always remain a factor to be considered, but there should be a more significant opportunity for efficient personnel based on the merits, irrespective of their rank, to move up speedily if merit is used as the basis for promotions. There has been a lot of contention over the relative estimations of position and legitimacy in any arrangement of promotion. Rank/seniority will dependably remain a factor to be considered. However, there should be significantly more outstanding open door/opportunity for proficient faculty, independent of their position, to climb expediently if merit is utilized as the reason for promotion.
- The nature of work is more critical in the lower positions as in the higher.

Promotion Policy

The promotion strategy is a standout amongst the most disputable issues in each association. The administration, as a rule, favors promotion based on merits, and the associations energetically inverse by saying that the administration turns to

partiality. In any case, by and by, both position and legitimacy/merit criteria ought to be mulled over. Placement strategy may incorporate the following aspects:

- Charts and graphs demonstrating work connections and steps of advancement should be readied. Those graphs and charts recognize each activity and associate different occupations with lines and bolts, demonstrating the channels to promotion.
- There should be some distinct framework for making a holding up list after identification and determination of those applicants who are to be promoted as and when openings/vacancies happen.
- All opportunities inside the association should be projected with the goal that every single potential competitor/employee may compete.
- The advancement should be founded on merit, seniority, and so forth. In a few examples, it might be conceivable to utilize a pre-work test, to decide qualification for the vacant position.
- All promotion should be for some time for testing. On the off chance that the promoted individual is not discovered fit for taking care of the activity type, amid this time for testing, he draws pay at the higher pay-scale, however, it should be particularly clarified to him in composing that if his execution is not found up to the mark, he will be returned to his previous post at the last scale.

Advantages of a Sound Promotion Policy

- It gives an impetus and inspiration to the employees to work increasingly and demonstrate enthusiasm for their work, which builds efficiency. They put in their best efforts and plan for promotion inside the association.
- It creates reliability and occupation fulfillment among the workers because a sound promotional policy guarantees them of their advancements if they are found fit.
- A sound promotion policy holds capable workers and gives them plentiful chances to rise further and builds the adequacy of an association.

RETENTION

Retention may be stated as the process where a staff chooses to stay for long periods within the organization at the request of the employer or mutually agree on conditions. It is usually practiced when a suitable person or persons are not available for the expected vacancy, or the employee is outstanding in his/her performance.

With not a single end to be seen for the country's nursing lack, hospitals and other clinical settings are setting more noteworthy accentuation on holding their present RN staff. It is a complicated procedure, requiring the top to bottom learning of the necessities and needs of the nursing staff and bunches of inventiveness.

TABLE 1: Principles of staff retention and activities to actualize the principles

Principles	Activities
Deferential collegial correspondence and conduct	• Team introduction • Presence of trust • Respect for assorted variety
Correspondence rich culture and responsibility	• Open and trusting • Role desires are characterized • Everyone is responsible
The nearness of sufficient quantities of qualified nurses	• Ability to give quality care to meet customer/understanding needs • Work and home life adjust
The nearness of expert, equipped stable, apparent leadership	• Serve as a backer for nursing practice • Support shared basic leadership • Allocate assets /responsibilities to help to nurse
The consolation of expert practice and proceeded with development/ improvement.	• Continuing instruction/accreditation is upheld/energized. • Active membership in professional organizations

Importance of Staff Retention

- Essential aptitudes, thoughts, learning, and experience stay inside your association.
- Client connections and systems are likewise protected in conjunction with all the pay that these territories produce.
- Losing your key workers exposes the likelihood that these individuals will expect to part with your immediate rivals. Subsequently, those priceless aptitudes, thoughts, information, experience, connections, and systems are altogether exchanged by another association.
- The cost of supplanting such an individual incorporates publicizing, enrollment/recruitment, office expenses and the time spent leading the whole interview process.

Although a component of employee turnover is both inescapable and robust, it is all things considered precise that maintenance conveys generous advantages to the organization.

Principles to Help Foster Staff Retention

The principles of staff retention and activities to actualize the principles are given in Table 1.

SUPERANNUATION

A kind of retirement plan set up by an organization for the advantage of its staff. These kinds of programs utilize reserves kept by the organization (characterized by advantage/benefit plan) or by the team (described commitment/contribution plan), with the assets developing in an incentive until the point when the worker resigns or retires. It is likewise called a pension plan. Superannuation is a method for gathering monetary resources amid your working life with a specific end goal to support a wage stream in your retirement.

Advantages

- **For employees:** The superannuation system will help the employee with all the financial benefits of managing the rest of life effectively after retirement.
- **For government:** The amount that is deducted from the employee during their period of service will help the government to carry out the development of the nation. E.g. CPF fund, EPF Fund, etc.

Disadvantages

- **Lump sums:** Lump sums withdrawn from superannuation either in accumulation or pension cause various problems, particularly when people suddenly have access to a comparatively enormous amount of money that can be quickly exhausted leaving the person to live in poverty or fall back on Center link (after a while).

DEPLOYMENT

Deployment is the development of staff starting with one task then on to the next to address operational issues. The arrangement may appear as work assignments inside the present place of employment, parallel exchanges, migration, or impermanent assignments.

It is not an arrangement or appointment inside. Deployment is the movement of a worker starting with one position then onto the next that does not constitute advancement and does not change the individual's time of work from a predetermined term to uncertain. The arrangement of staff empowers the realignment of HR to new work assignments or occupation obligations to meet changing business needs or to give chances to pick up new abilities and experience.

Guidelines for Good Deployment

- Managers must make deployments in a manner characterized by fair and transparent employment practices, and respect for employees.
- Deployments are to be made with the consent of the person being deployed, unless agreement to being deployed is a condition of employment of the person's current position; or it is found, after investigation, that the person has harassed another person in the course of his/her employment.
- A deployment takes effect on the date agreed to in writing, or, if consent is not required, on the date fixed by the delegated person.
- The deployed employee becomes the substantive incumbent of the position to which he or she is deployed, and assumes the classification level and any terms and conditions of employment of the new location. He/she ceases to be the incumbent of the post to which he/she previously occupied.

TRAINING AND DEVELOPMENT

Training is important, not only for the organization but also for the employees. It gives them greater job security and an opportunity for career advancement. A skill acquired through training is an asset for the organization and the employee. The benefits of training stay for a very long time.

TRAINING

Training is often looked upon as an organized activity for increasing the knowledge and skills of people for a definite purpose. It involves systematic procedures for transferring technical know-how to the employees to increase their knowledge and skills for doing specific jobs with proficiency.

According to Flippo, "Training is the act of increasing the knowledge and skills of an employee for doing a particular job". Training can become obsolete only when there is a complete elimination of the desire for that skill and knowledge, which may happen because of the technological changes. In general terms, the need for training can arise because of the following reasons:

- **Changing technology:** Technology is changing at a fast pace. Be it any industry, technological changes are taking place every where. Newer machines are being used for automation of the processes. Computers have made the controls very easy. Advances in information technology have enabled a greater degree of coordination between various business units, spread far across the globe. To keep themselves abreast of the changes, the employees must learn new techniques to make use of advances in technology. Training needs to be treated as a continuous process to update the employees in new methods and procedures.
- **Demanding customers:** As free markets become stronger, customers are becoming more and more demanding. They are much more informed about the products. They have many sources of information. Intensified competition forces organizations to provide better and better products and services to them. Added to the customer consciousness, their requirements keep on changing. To satisfy the customers/patients and to provide the best of the quality of products and services, the skills of those producing them need to be continuously upgraded through training.
- **Thrust on productivity:** In competitive times, organizations cannot afford the extravaganza of lethargy. They have to be productive to survive and grow. Continuous upgradation of the employees' skills is an essential requirement for maintaining high standards of productivity. Productivity in the present times stems from knowledge, which has to be relearned continuously.
- **Improved motivation:** Training is a source of motivation for the employees as well. They find themselves more updated while facing challenging situations at the job. Such

skill development contributes to their career development as well. Motivated employees have lesser turnover, providing an organization with a stable workforce, which has several advantages in the long run.

- **Accuracy of output:** Trained workers handle their job better. They provide service much more safely and are experts in using different machines. They achieve greater accuracy in whatever job they do. This reduces accidents in organizations. Quality reduces wastage and ensures better customer satisfaction.
- **Better management:** Training can be used as an effective tool for planning and controlling. It develops skills of the workers for the future and also prepares them for promotion. It helps them in reducing the costs of supervision, wastage and industrial accidents. It also helps increase productivity and quality.

Objectives of Training

- To increase the knowledge of workers in doing specific jobs.
- To systematically impart new skills to human resources so that they learn quickly.
- To bring about change in the attitudes of the workers towards fellow workers, supervisor and the organization.
- To improve the overall performance of the organization.
- To make the employees handle materials, machines, and equipment efficiently and thus to check wastage of time and resources.
- To reduce the number of accidents by providing safety training to employees.
- To prepare employees for higher jobs by developing advanced skills in them.

Training, Development, and Education

No longer do the organizations talk of training in isolation. It is usually addressed along with development. While referring to the conjugation of the two processes, Dale Yoder has observed: "The use of the terms training and development in today's employment setting is far more appropriate than 'training' alone since human resources can exert their full potential only when the learning process goes far beyond simple routine". Although the terms training and development are used together, they are often confused. Training means learning the basic skills and knowledge necessary for a particular job or a group of jobs. In other words, training is the act of increasing the knowledge for doing a particular job. But development refers to the growth of an individual in all respects (Table 2). An organization works for the development of its executives or potential executives to enable them to be more effective in performing the various functions of management. The distinction between training and development is shown below.

TABLE 2: **Distinction between training and development**

Training	Development
Training means learning skills and knowledge for a particular job and increasing the skills required for a job.	Development refers to the growth of an employee in all respects. It is more concerned with shaping attitudes.
Training generally imparts specific skills to the employees.	Development is more general in nature and aims at the overall growth of the executives.
Training is concerned with maintaining and improving current job performance. Thus, it has a short-term perspective.	Development builds up competencies for future performance and has a long-term perspective
Training is job centered in nature.	Development is career centered in nature.
The role of the trainer or supervisor is very important in training.	All development is 'self-development' and the executive has to be internally motivated for the same.

Training is also different from education in the following respects:

- Training is concerned with increasing knowledge and skills in doing a particular job. The major burden of training falls upon the employer. But education is broader in scope. Its purpose is not confined to developing the individuals, but it is concerned with increasing general knowledge and understanding of the total environment.
- Education generally refers to formal learning in a school or a college, whereas training is vocation oriented and is generally imparted at the workplace.
- Training usually has a mere immediate utilitarian purpose than education.

Significance of Training

Fostered by technological advances, training is essential for any human resource development exercise in organizations in the rapidly changing times of today. It is an essential, useful and productive activity for all human resources working in an organization, irrespective of the job positions that they hold. It benefits both employers and employees.

Benefits of Training to Employers

- **Faster learning of new skills:** Training helps the employers to reduce the learning time of their employees and achieve higher standards of performance. The employees need not waste time in learning by observing others.
- **Increased productivity:** Training increases the skill of the new employee while performing a particular job. An increased skill level usually helps in increasing both the quantity and quality of output. Training can be of great help even to the existing employees. It helps them to increase their level of performance on their present job assignments and prepares them for future assignments.

- **Standardization of procedures:** Training can help the standardization of operating procedures, which can be learned by the employees. Standardization of work procedures makes high levels of performance rule rather than the exception. Employees work intelligently and make fewer mistakes when they possess the required know-how and skills.
- **Lesser need for supervision:** As a generalization, it can be stated safely that trained employees need lesser supervision. Training does not eliminate the need for supervision, but it reduces the need for detailed and constant supervision. A well-trained employee can be self-reliant in his/her work because s/he knows what to do and how to do.
- **The economy of operations**: Trained personnel will be able to make better and economical use of the materials and the equipment and reduce wastage. Also, trained employees reduce the rate of accidents and damage to machinery and equipment.
- **Higher morale:** The morale of employees is increased if they are given proper training. A good training program molds employees' attitudes towards organizational activities and generates better cooperation and greater loyalty.
- **Managerial development**: The top management can identify the talent, who can be groomed for handling positions of responsibility in the organizations. Newer talent increases the productivity of the organization.

Benefits of Training to Employees

- **Increasing confidence:** Training creates a feeling of confidence in the minds of employees, who feel comfortable while handling newer challenges. It gives a feeling of safety and security to them at the workplace.
- **New skills:** Training develops skills, which serve as a valuable personal asset of a worker. The skills remain permanently with the worker himself.
- **Career advancement:** The managers can develop their skills to take up higher challenges and work in newer job dimensions. Such an exercise leads to the career development of the employees, who can move up the corporate hierarchy faster.
- **Higher Earnings**: Higher earnings are a consequence of career development. A highly trained employee can command a high salary in the job market and feel more contended.
- **Resilience to change:** In the fast-changing times of today, training develops adaptability among workers. The employees feel motivated to work under newer circumstances and they do not feel threatened or resist any change. Such adaptability is essential for the survival and growth of an organization in the present times.
- **Increased Safety:** Trained workers handle the machines safely. They also know the use of various safety devices in the factory, thus, they are less prone to accidents.

CREDENTIALING

Credentialing is a formal process that utilizes an established series of guidelines to ensure that patients receive the highest level of care from healthcare professionals who have undergone the most stringent scrutiny regarding their ability to practice medicine, nursing or any other profession. Credentialing also assures the patient that he or she is being treated by providers whose qualifications, training, licensure, and ability to practice medicine are acceptable. Credentialing also ensures that all healthcare workers are held to the same standard.

Credentialing is the process of establishing the qualification of licensed professionals, organizational members or organizations, and assessing their background and legitimacy. Many health care institutions and provider networks conduct their own credentialing, generally through a credentialing specialist or electronic service, with review by medical staff or credentialing committee. It may include granting and reviewing specific clinical privileges and medical or allied health staff members.

Definition

Credentialing is the process by which selected professionals are granted privileges to practice within an organization. In health care organizations this process has been largely confined to physicians. Limited privileges have been granted to psychologists, social workers and selected categories of nurses, such as nurse anesthetists, surgical nurses, and midwives.
—Russell C Swansburg

A credential is an attestation of qualification, competence, or authority issued to an individual by a third party with a relevant or de facto authority or assumed competence to do so.

Purposes of Credentialing

- To prevent a problem before it happens.
- To research the qualifications and backgrounds of individuals and companies.
- Credentialing is also the process of reviewing and verifying information.

Credentialing and Privileges in Healthcare

In the current era of medical practice, all healthcare institutions have the onus of ensuring patient safety and delivering an acceptable standard of care. While employing excellent medical staff is vital for success, the healthcare institution must have medical bylaws that define the required minimum credentialing and privileging requirements to validate the competency of healthcare providers. In the past, only hospitals used to perform credentialing, but today almost all healthcare facilities, ambulatory care centers, long-term care institutions, and even urgent care clinics perform credentialing. Credentialing is a vital process for all healthcare institutions that must be performed to ensure that those healthcare workers who will be providing the clinical services are qualified to do so. There are ample cases reported in the literature about healthcare workers who worked in hospitals with bogus certificated and falsified experience. Over the past 20 years, the credentialing process has become complex and onerous primarily due to the expansion of the provider scope of practice, accrediting bodies, and requirements of third-party payers like insurers.

Health care credentialing is a system used by various organizations and agencies to ensure that their health care practitioners meet all the requirements and are appropriately qualified. The credentials may vary depending on the specified area of the practitioner. For example, an X-ray technician may have different credentialing forms than an osteopathic physician.

Process of Credentialing

- Healthcare institutions should have staff bylaws that guide administrative processes to ensure that healthcare workers provide competent and safe care.
- All healthcare workers should understand that practicing clinical medicine is a privilege and it goes hand-in-hand with first being credentialed.
- After the individual is credentialed, the next step is to address the privileges of practice, which depend on the evaluation of the provider's clinical qualifications, training, and overall performance.
- For privileges and credentialing, the bylaws should address the following:
  - The pre-application process to screen if a healthcare professional satisfies the basic criteria for working in the hospital.
  - Establish grounds for denying applications after the pre-application process.
  - Establish a process where the rejected healthcare worker can re-apply after the initial denial.
  - Have a process for rapid credentialing for locums, emergency staff, and short-term employment.
  - Have steps in place to limit the practice of medicine for those healthcare workers who do not follow guidelines or the standard of CARE IS NOT SATISFACTORY.

Significance of Credentialing

- **Legal issues:** All healthcare institutions that develop written policies that govern credentialing and privileges must consult with legal counsel to ensure that the policies abide by state laws, professional organizations and federal requirements.

- **Identification of the applicant:** With every application, the healthcare worker must supply some type of government-issued identification and a photograph. Many hospitals now require that the photograph is stamped and notarized. When the hospitals request references, they should send the applicant's photo identification together with the request to ensure that the applicant has not been misusing someone else's identification.
- **Background check:** Today most healthcare institutions perform a background check on all applicants. A background check may reveal any criminal or domestic violence at both the state and federal levels. Some states recommend that hospitals also request that applicants provide a copy of the police report.
- **Clinical significance:** All healthcare institutions are responsible for ensuring that their medical staff is competent through a bona fide credentialing process. Today the credentialing process is not only tied to the demonstration of proper education and training but also maintains accreditation standards reimbursement requirements, and satisfies state and federal laws.

TRANSFER

Transfer means a change in job assignment. It refers to a horizontal or lateral movement of an employee from one job to another in the same organization without much change in his status or pay package. Transfer causes a shift of individual from one job to another without there being any marked change in his responsibilities, skills and other benefits. Sometimes they may involve a change in pay also. For example, in permanent personnel transfers, an employee normally receives the rate of pay on the job to which he is transferred. Transfers are an important source for internal recruiting. Often the most suitable candidate for an existing opening maybe someone already working in one or the other department of the working organization. The transfer of such an employee to fill the job is preferred by managers of the organization.

Definition

A transfer, "is a change in job where the new job is substantially equal to the old in terms of pay, status, and responsibilities".

—**Edwin Flippo**

The transfer is defined as "a lateral shift causing movement of individuals from one position to another usually without involving any marked change in duties, responsibilities, skills needed or compensation". —**Yoder and Associates**

Objectives of Transfer

- **To fulfill organizational needs:** Arising out of change in technology, the volume of production, production schedule, quality of the product, etc., an employee can be transferred.
- **To satisfy employee needs:** Sometimes employees themselves demand transfer due to their problems like ill health, family problems native attractiveness and so on.
- **To adjust the workforce:** Excess or surplus employees in one department can be transferred to another department or section where there is a shortage of workforce.
- To reduce monotony and to make the employees versatile
- **For effective use of employees:** If the management feels that the service of the able employee should be used in different branch of the same organization, then such employee is transferred.
- **To punish employees:** If employees are found indulged in undesirable activities like fraud, bribery, duping, etc., such employees are transferred to remote places as a disciplinary action.
- **To give relief to the employees:** Employees who are overburdened and doing complicated or risky work for a long period are relieved from such work by transferring such employees to a place of their choice.
- **To improve employees' backgrounds:** By placing them in different jobs of various departments and units.

Principles of Transfer

- In a usual phenomenon, a transfer causes some disturbance to the transferee. Hence, a minimum period between transfers and the frequency of transfer must be decided by the HR department and made known to all the employees.
- Authorities of the manager who will handle transfer must be earmarked and responsibilities must be defined. In an organization, the authority to handle transfers should be centralized to ensure uniformity in practices.
- Transfers on individual employees' requests should be based on a documented transfer system.
- Transfer orders must specify whether the transfer is of permanent or temporary in nature.
- Before transfer, the performance of an employee needs to be assessed. The assessment helps management to assign new tasks to the employee as per the job description.
- While developing the transfer policy, the interest of the organization must always be remembered.

Types of Transfer

Aswathappa (2006) proposed the following five types of transfers:

1. **Production transfer:** Employees are posted in different departments, based on their interests and qualifications. This also depends on the workload that a

department possesses. However, this load keeps fluctuating, and the demand for manpower keeps changing with time.

2. **Replacement transfer:** When an employee leaves a department for a particular reason, the department needs a replacement. In such scenarios, especially in demanding situations, a senior employee might have to function in place of the junior employee, till the time a replacement is found.

3. **Versatility transfer:** Some organizations believe that the workforce needs to have multiple skills capable to perform multiple tasks. People can achieve multiple skills only by working in different departments. In learning organizations such as ordnance factories, banks, and many private companies, people get the scope of working in different departments and can learn different systems, procedures, and rules and regulations.

4. **Shift transfer:** To enhance capacity utilization, industrial organizations operate in multiple shifts generally morning, evening, and night shifts. Some organizations allow employees to staggered shifts as well. Employees are engaged in all the shifts on a rotational basis.

5. **Remedial transfer:** After induction, employees are placed in a department and jobs are assigned to him/ her, and their performance and behavioral dispositions are recorded. Some employees may emerge as good performers, while many others may emerge as underperformers. The objective of remedial transfer is therapeutic in nature, that is, to rectify the wrong placement.

Transfer Policy

A sound personnel policy requires that there is a clear policy regarding transfers. If there is arbitrariness in the policy, the superiors can misuse the "transfer" of subordinates for their reasons. Similarly, subordinates can also misuse the policy by asking for transfers on trivial issues. A sound transfer policy must be based on the following elements:

- In the case of production and replacement transfers operations in different departments must be sufficiently similar.
- Jobs to which transfers are contemplated should be indicated with the help of job description and job analysis.
- Responsibility for initiating and approving transfer decisions should be clearly defined and properly located. Such decisions may originate from the first-line supervisor subject to the review and approval of the foreman or the personnel department.
- The area or unit within which transfers are to be made should be decided.
- It should be made clear if the seniority to the credit of the employee before his transfer will remain to his credit even after the transfer.
- The rate of remuneration for the employee on the new job (to which he is transferred) must be decided.

- The basis for transfers should be properly chosen. This problem is of particular importance when more than one employee requests for transfer to the same job or same shift.

TERMINATION

Employee termination is the process by which an organization ends an individual's employment against his or her will. Termination means the removal of the employee from employment by his employer mainly due to the expiratory of employment contract period between employee and his employer, due to the ill-health of the employee.

Termination of employment is an employee's departure from a job and the end of an employee's duration with an employer. Termination may be voluntary on the employee's part, or it may be at the hands of the employer, often in the form of dismissal (firing) or a layoff. Dismissal or firing is usually thought to be the fault of the employee, whereas a layoff is usually done for business reasons (for instance a business slowdown or an economic downturn) outside the employee's performance.

Causes of Termination

- Poor job performance
- Lack of fit with the organization
- Inability to perform job responsibilities
- Conflict with managers and other employees
- Misconduct
- Many instances of employment separation
- For poor performance, including lack of punctuality, absenteeism, or failure to desired results
- For resisting change
- For negativism
- For insubordination
- For not conforming to company values
- For questionable character or ethical lapses
- For criminal acts
- Absenteeism and tardiness
- Unsatisfactory performance
- Lack of qualifications or ability
- Challenged job requirements
- Gross misconduct, which might involve drug abuse, stealing
- Breaches of the company or public policy

Termination Types

There are two main termination types:

1. **Voluntary:** The employee elects to end employment such as giving resignation or notice of resignation.
2. **Involuntary:** The organization elects to end the employment relationship with the employee due to multiple reasons mentioned above.

Process of Termination

The termination of an employee is always the last option to select and a human resource manager has to be honest, genuine, and steady in this decision. Few aspects mentioned below should be considered during the process of initiating the termination process against an employee.

- **Write down everything:** Documentation is a must during the process of termination as it is the key to the whole procedure. If sufficient documentation is not done, it can be argued that a particular incident or the cause of termination had never occurred. Hence, though time-consuming documentation is considered as the key to the termination.

- **Communicate expectations:** Most of the time the employee fails to recognize the expectation of the organization and it may lead to the termination. For every job, there should be a job description. Even if an organization doesn't have any formalized job description, still the employer should clearly explain the roles, responsibilities, and expectations to each employee as it is what takes employees to be successful in each role. It must not be assumed that the employee may know everything as people come with their perspectives that do not always match the perspective of the employer. Each role should be clearly defined. This makes it easier to pinpoint and correct problems. Additionally, a progressive discipline policy should already be established, outlining how corrective action and termination should take place. This helps ensure every issue is handled consistently and fairly.

- **Be a good coach:** Both new and existing employees should be coached. This is informal feedback and consists of what's right as well as what's wrong. The employees need this feedback to understand how they are doing well before you get to the point of considering disciplinary action or termination.

- **Initiate a performance improvement plan (PIP):** The PIP should articulate specifically what the problem areas are and give detailed goals for what is expected to correct them. In some cases, verbal counseling might be the better way to go. This must be used in addressing things like attendance, communication, and other behavioral issues. Document the conversation and plan. The employees should sign an acknowledgment form to confirm that they understand verbal counseling. It is also suggested to send a follow-up email to the employee.

- **Conduct written counseling:** If things are getting egregious, there may be a need to move to written counseling. Written counseling is somewhat similar to the PIP. It should outline areas that employees need to correct. Again, in writing, detail specifically what needs to improve and how this should be accomplished. The counseling form should also express that improvement needs to be immediate, marked (noticeable) and sustained. Employees should sign this form after the discussion.

Despite all of the efforts, if the quality is not improved the only option left is to sever the relationship. However, by now, there will be sufficient documentation to prove the underperformance of the employee. Performance-based terminations should never come as a surprise to the employees. Before terminating an employee, it should be made sure to review all associated documentation. Also, contact the legal counsel or HR representative to ensure the case is supported, justified and sound. In releasing employees, honesty is the best policy as no organization intends to make anyone feel bad.

HUMAN RESOURCE MANAGEMENT IN HOSPITAL AND COMMUNITY

Human Resource Management is a part and parcel of every organization irrespective of its domain of operation. Human Resource Department (HRD) ensures the recruitment and selection of right persons for right places. The HRD decides the work needs of an organization as projected by the respective department heads. The HRD must meet all the existing and future manpower needs of the organization.

Functions of HRM in Community and Hospital Services

- Creating the policy of human resource management in the organization, which is acceptable to the top management and beneficial to the organization.
- Recognize the human resource needs of the organization.
- Informing and educating other significant members of the organization regarding the human resource policy of the organization.
- Applying research in the policy-making of the organization.

Human Resource in Hospital Services

Regardless of the type/category, every hospital or health organization should have a sound human resource management policy and a team for carrying out the functions of HRM. This may vary according to the hospital policies, the type of human resources required, and sectors of service. Every organization has a separate department of human resource, which performs the functions in collaboration with other departments and top-level officers/managers.

Category of Manpower in a Hospital

- **Administration team:** Consists of Medical Superintendent, Nursing Superintendent, and other managerial members.

- **Medical team**: Consists of specialists, consultants, medical officers, medical residents, and medical students.
- **Nurses:** They are qualified and registered nurses and midwives. There are staff nurses, ward in-charges, shift in-charges, nursing managers, etc. They provide direct patient care or perform extended duties such as supervision, clinical nurse specialist, nurse practitioner, advanced nurse practitioner, etc.
- **Social workers:** They are those who are trained specially in social service (MSW; master in social work). Their primary role is to provide psychological, financial, and emotional support to the individuals and families affected with some illness or disability.
- **Dietitian:** They help in meal planning as per the requirement of the patients and their diseases. The nutritional needs of each patient are different, and a healthy diet is an inevitable component in the treatment and recovery of ill patients.
- **Physiotherapist:** They help the patients in achieving range of motion (ROM) and assist in the rehabilitation of patients by delivering different therapeutic approaches.
- **Pharmacists:** They deal with purchasing, storage, and distribution of medicines and other surgical equipment as per the requirement of the hospital.
- **Lab Technicians:** They carry out all the investigations of body fluids and other substances for diagnostic purposes.
- **Other technical staff**: They include X-ray and other imaging technicians, receptionists, central sterile supply department (CSSD) staff, OT staff, hospital marketing department, human resource department, sanitary staff, etc.

Human Resource in Community Health Services

Community health is a focus of health service beyond the curative concept of health care. It focuses on preventive, therapeutic and rehabilitative health services provided either as an institutionalized service or deinstitutionalized service.

Category of Manpower in Community Health Services

- **Medical officer:** A person who plans, organizes, coordinates, and evaluates the functions of Health Centers. It may be at the primary level or the block level. The overall purpose of the health centers such as Outpatient department (OPD) services, Inpatient department (IPD) services, maternal and child health care services, national health programs, and implementation of all health policies.
- **The medical team:** Consist of Consultants, Medical residents, specialists of AYUSH.
- **Community health nurse:** Provides direct patient care at Community Health Center (CHC), Primary Health Center (PHC), Sub centers. They perform various functions, such as patient care, health education, advocate, supervisor, etc.

- **Female/male health worker:** Provides direct patient care at CHC, PHC, Sub centers.
- **Pharmacist:** They deal with purchasing, storage, and distribution of medicines and other surgical equipment as per the requirement of the hospital.
- **Social workers:** Their central role is to provide psychological, financial, and emotional support to the individuals and families affected by some illness or disability.
- **ASHA workers:** Conducts home visiting and helps in the implementation of National health programs.
- **Others:** They include drivers, peons, cleaning staff, etc.

Human resource management is the organizational function that decides the overall functioning of any organization. It helps in fostering the knowledge, skills, and values among employees so that their efficiency performance can be increased.

PROJECTING STAFFING REQUIREMENTS: STAFFING STUDY

A staffing study should accumulate information about natural factors inside and outside the association that influence staffing necessities. According to Frank Aydelotte, a renowned educator, four techniques are used to measure the work of nurses, all of which include the idea of the time required for execution.

1. Time study and task frequency
   - Tasks and task elements (procedure)
   - Point and time started
   - Point and time ended
   - Sample size
   - Average time
   - Allowance for fatigue, personal variation, and unavoidable standby.
   - Standard time = step 1.e + step 1.f
   - Frequency of task × standard time = volume of nursing work.
2. Work sampling is be the statistical method of understanding the need for the time required by workers for performing the different tasks. The procedure is as follows:
   - Identify major and minor categories of nursing activities. Both activities need to be calculated separately.
   - Make the elements of the task, and this should be done according to the broken-down steps of a complicated task.
   - Determine the number of observations to be made. This may be done statistically.
   - Observe a random sample of nursing personnel performing activities. It may be informed to the whole group priorly.
   - Analyze observations: Frequency occurring in a specific category of work and percentage of total time spent in that activity.

     Most work sampling studies sample direct care and indirect care to determine the ratio.

3. Continuous sampling (variation of task frequency and time). The technique is the same as for work sampling except:
   - Observer follows one individual in the performance of a task.
   - The observer may observe work performed for one or more patients if they can be seen concurrently.
4. Self-reporting (variation of task frequency and time)
   - The individual records the work sampling or continuous sampling on himself or herself.
   - Tasks are logged using time intervals or time tasks start and end.
   - Logs are analyzed.

On the other hand, there are three cardinal principles for assessing staff necessity in an organization. It incorporates:
- Staffing projections on past staffing history; information such as the history of illness, extra time, occasion, and leisure time.
- Review current staffing levels.
- Review of tentative future arrangements for the organization.

Clinical nurses who are engaged in staffing plans will believe in the ideas. These staffing studies can be made with electronic spreadsheets.

NORMS OF STAFFING ACCORDING TO STAFF INSPECTION UNIT

Norms are set standards that lead, control, and direct people and society. For arranging human nursing resources, we need to abide by a few or all of the rules. The nursing standards are suggested by different committees (High-power Committee, Bajaj Committee, Staff Inspection Committee, Trained Nurses' Association of India (TNAI), and Indian Nursing Council (INC). The criteria and norms have been prescribed considering the workload anticipated in the wards and other territories of the hospital.

All the above committees and Staff Inspection Unit (SIU) have prescribed the standards for ideal nurse-patient proportion, for example, 1:3 for Non-Teaching Hospital and 1:5 for the Teaching Hospital. The Staff Inspection Unit (SIU) is the unit that has prescribed the nursing standards in the year 1991-92. According to this SIU standards, the present nurse-patient ratio is planned in all Central Govt. Hospitals. The Staff Inspection Unit was set up by the Ministry of Finance, Government of India in 1964 to scrutinize the economy of staffing in government organizations.

Recommendations of SIU

- The posts of the head nurse or senior nursing officers and staff nurses are clubbed to calculate the staff privilege for performing nursing care work, which they will keep on functioning even after the promotion.
- Based on the entitlement, working with regard to the norms, 30% of the posts might be authorized as the head nurse/senior nursing officer. This would additionally

enhance the current proportion of 1 head nurse to 3.6. staff nurses settled by the administration in a settlement with the Delhi Nurse Union in May 1990.
- The assistant nursing superintendent (ANS) is suggested in the proportion of 1 ANS to each 4.5 head nurse. The ANS will play out the obligation to perform the duty of the Head Nurses, even in shifts.
- The posts of Deputy Nursing Superintendent may proceed at the level of 1 deputy nursing superintendent (DNS) per every 7.5 ANS.
- There will be a post of Nursing Superintendent for each clinic having bed strength of 250 and above.
- There will be a post of 1 Chief Nursing Officer for each clinic having at least 500 beds.
- It is suggested that 45% of posts included for the region of 365 days working including 10% leave hold (maternity leave, earned leave, and days off as nurses are entitled to 8 days off every month and 3 National Holidays every year while in three-shift duties.

The majority of the hospitals today are following the SIU standards. In this, the posts of the Nursing Sisters and the Staff Nurses have been clubbed together and crafted by the ward sister, remain the same as staff nurse even after advancement. The Assistant Nursing Superintendent and the Deputy Nursing Superintendent need to do the obligation of one classification beneath their rank.

Nurse-Patient Ratio as per the SIU Norms

Nurse-patient ratio as per the SIU norms is given in Table 3.

TABLE 3: Nurse patient ratio in hospital as per SIU norms

Sr. No	Area/Wards	Ratio of Staffing
1	General	1:6
2	Special - (Child Health, Skin, and burns, Neuro Surgery, Cardio-Thoracic, Neuro Medicine, Emergency units attached to Casualty)	1:4
3	ICU/CCU/ITU	1:1
4	Labor Room	1:1 per table
5	Operation theater	Major - 2:1 per table Minor - 1:1 per table
6	OPD: Blood bank, Eye, ENT, Vaccination, Medical, Dental, Central sample collection center, Orthopedic, Microbiology, Psychiatry, etc.	One each
	OPD: Pediatric Immunization, Family planning, Venereal Disease center, Chemotherapy, Neurology, Orthopedic, Gynecology, X-ray, Skin, Burns	Two each

Notwithstanding the 10% reserve according to the rules, 45% of posts might be included where administrations are accommodated 365 days in a year/24 hours. According to the Trained Nurses Association of India and Indian Nursing Council in 1985, the acceptable nurse-patient ratio in the hospital is as given below:

- **Chief Nursing Officer:** 1 for every 500 beds.
- **Nursing Superintendent:** 1 for every 400 beds or above.
- **D.N S.:** 1 for every 300 beds and one extra for every 200 beds.
- **ANS:** 1 for 100-150 beds or 3-4 wards.
- **Ward Sister:** 1 per 25-30 beds or one ward. 30% leave hold.
- **Staff Nurse:** 1 for three beds in Teaching Hospitals and 1 for five beds in Non-Teaching Hospital. Additionally, there should also be a provision for +30% staff to leave hold.
- Other nursing staff to be accommodated for carrying out departmental research work.
- **For OPD and Emergency:** 1 staff nurse for 100 patients (1: 100) + 30% leave save.
- **For Intensive Care unit:** (ICU) – 1:1 or (1:3 for each move) +30% leave hold.
- It is proposed that for 250 bedded hospitals, there ought to be one Infection Control Nurse (ICN).

STAFFING NORMS: INDIAN PUBLIC HEALTH STANDARDS (IPHS)

(*Source:* www.nhm.gov.in, National Health Mission, Ministry of Health and Family Welfare, GoI)

National Rural Health Mission (NHM) was launched in the year 2005 to strengthen the Rural Public Health System and has since met many hopes and expectations. The Mission seeks to provide effective health care to the rural populace throughout the country with a special focus on the States and Union Territories (UTs), which have weak public health indicators and/or weak infrastructure. Towards this end, the Indian Public Health Standards (IPHS) for Sub-Centers, Primary Health Centers (PHCs), Community Health Centers (CHCs), Sub-District and District Hospitals were published in January/February 2007 and have been used as the reference point for public health care infrastructure planning and up-gradation in the States and UTs. IPHS is a set of uniform standards envisaged to improve the quality of health care delivery in the country. The staffing at sub center, primary health center, community health center, sub-divisional hospital and district hospital are given in Tables 4, 5, 6, 7 and 8 respectively.

Staffing at Subcenter

TABLE 4: Staffing pattern in sub center as per IPHS norms

Type of sub-center	Sub-Center A		Sub-Center B (MCH sub-center)	
Staff	Essential	Desirable	Essential	Desirable
ANM/Health Worker female	1	1	2	
Health Worker male	1		1	
Staff Nurse				1
Safai-Karamchari	1		1	

Staffing at Primary Health Center

Type A PHC: PHC with a delivery load of fewer than 20 deliveries in a month, Type B PHC: PHC with a delivery load of 20 or more deliveries in a month.

TABLE 5: Staffing pattern in primary health center as per IPHS norms

Type of PHC	PHC Type A		PHC Type B	
Staff	Essential	Desirable	Essential	Desirable
Medical Officer MBBS	1		1	1
Medical Officer AYUSH		1		1
Accountant cum Data Entry Operator	1		1	
Pharmacist	1		1	
Pharmacist AYUSH		1		1
Nurse Midwife (Staff Nurse)	3	1	4	1
Health Worker female	1		1	
Health Worker male	1		1	
Health Assistant/Lady Health Visitor	1		1	
Health Educator		1		1
Laboratory Technician	1		1	
Cold Chain and Vaccine Logistic Assistant		1		1
Multi-skilled Group D worker	2		2	
Sanitary worker cum watchman	1		1	1
Total	13	18	14	21

Staffing at the Community Health Center

TABLE 6: Staffing pattern in community health center as per IPHS norms

Personnel	Essential	Desirable	Qualification
Block Medical Officer/ Medical Superintendent	1		Senior-most specialist/ GDMO preferably with experience in Public Health
Public Health Specialist	1		MD (PSM)/MD (CHA)/ MD Community Medicine/ or PG with MBA/DPH/MPH
Public Health Nurse (PHN) #	1	1	
Specialty Services			
General Surgeon	1		MS/DNB, (General Surgery)
Physician	1		MD/DNB, (General Medicine)
Obstetrician and Gynecologist	1		DGO /MD/DNB
Pediatrician	1		DCH/MD (Pediatrics)/ DNB
Anesthetist	1		MD (Anesthesia)/DNB/ DA/ LSAS trained MO
General Duty Officers			
Dental Surgeon	1		BDS
General Duty Medical Officer	2		MBBS
Medical Officer - AYUSH	1		Graduate in AYUSH
Nurses and Paramedical			
Staff Nurse	10		
Pharmacist	1		
Pharmacist AYUSH	1		
Lab Technician	2		
Radiographer	1		
Dietitian	1	1	
Ophthalmic Assistant	1		
Dental assistant	1		
Cold Chain and Vaccine Logistic Assistant	1		
OT Technician	1		
Community-Based Rehabilitation worker	1	1	
Counselor	1		
Administrative Staff			
Registration Clerk	2		
Statistical Assistant/ Data Entry Operator	2		
Account Assistant	1		
Administrative Assistant	1		
Group D Staff			
Dresser	1		**(certified by Red Cross/Johns Ambulance)**
Ward Boys/Nursing Orderly	5		
Driver	1		
Total	46	52	

Staffing at Sub-divisional Hospital

TABLE 7: Staffing pattern in sub divisional hospital as per IPHS norms

Staff	31-50 bedded		51 to 100 bedded	
	Essential	Desirable	Essential	Desirable
Hospital Superintendent	1		1	
Medicine Specialist	1	1	1	1
Surgery Specialist	1		1	1
OBG specialist	1	1	1	1
Dermatologist/Venereologist	1	1	1	
Pediatrician	1		1	1
Anesthetist (Regular/trained)	1		1	1
ENT Surgeon	1		1	
Ophthalmologist	1		1	
Orthopedician	1		1	
Radiologist	1		1	
Casualty Doctors/General Duty Doctors	7 (3 lady MOs)		9 (4 female MBBS)	
Dental Surgeon	1		1	
Public Health Manager	1		1	
Forensic Expert				1
AYUSH Physician	1		1	
Pathologist			1	
Psychiatrist				1
Total	20	23 (Essential + Desirable)	24	31 (Essential + Desirable)
Staff Nurse	18	2	30	
Sister In-charge			5	
General Duty Attendant/hospital workers	6		11	
Ophthalmic Assistant/Refractionist	1		1	
ECG Technician	1		1	
Audiometrician	1		1	
Laboratory Technician (Lab + Blood storage)	4		5	
Laboratory Attendant (Hospital Worker)	2		3	
Radiographer	1		2	
Pharmacist	3		4	
Dietitian		1		1
Dental Assistant/Dental Technician/ Dental Hygienist	1		1	
Physiotherapist/occupational therapist/ rehabilitation therapist	1		1	
Counselor			1 female	1 male
Multi Rehabilitation worker	1		2	

Contd...

Staff	31-50 bedded		51 to 100 bedded	
	Essential	Desirable	Essential	Desirable
Statistical Assistant	1		1	
Medical Records Officer/Technician	1		1	
Electrician	1		1	
Plumber	1		1	
Cold Chain and Vaccine Logistics Assistant	1		1	
Total	45	48 (Essential + Desirable)	73	75 (Essential + Desirable)

Staff			31-50 beds	51 -100 beds
Administrative Staff				
Office Superintendent			1	1
Accountant			2	2
Computer Operator			4	6
Driver			1	2
Peon			2	2
Security Staff			2	2
Operation theater				
Staff Nurse			2	5
OT Assistant			2	6
Safai Karamchari			1	3
Blood Storage Unit				
Staff Nurse			1	1
Attendant			1	2
Blood Bank/Storage Technician			1	3
Safai Karamchari			1	2

TABLE 8: Staffing pattern in district hospital as per IPHS norms

Specialty	100 beds	200 beds	300 beds	400 beds	500 beds
Manpower–Medical					
Medicine	2	2	3	4	5
Surgery	2	2	3	3	4
OBG (Obstetrics and Gynecology)	2	3	4	5	6
Paediatrics	2	3	4	4	5
Anaesthesia	2	2	3	3	4
Ophthalmology	1	1	2	2	2
Orthopedics	1	1	2	2	2
Radiology	1	1	2	2	2
Pathology	1	2	3	3	4
ENT (Ear Nose and Throat)	1	1	2	2	2
Dental	1	1	2	3	3
Medical officer	11	13	15	19	23
Dermatology	1	1	1	1	1
Psychiatry	1	1	1	1	1

Contd...

Specialty	100 beds	200 beds	300 beds	400 beds	500 beds
Microbiology	1	1	1	1	1
Forensic	1	1	1	1	1
AYUSH	1	1	1	1	1
Total	32	37	50	58	68
Manpower: Nursing and Paramedical					
Staff Nurse	45	90	135	180	225
Lab Technician	6	9	12	15	18
Pharmacist	5	7	9	11	13
Storekeeper	1	1	2	2	2
Radiographer	2	3	5	7	9
ECG/ECO Technician	1	2	3	4	5
Audiometrician	0		1	1	1
Ophthalmic Assistant	1	1	2	2	2
EEG Tech	0		1	1	1
Dietitian	1	1	1	1	1
Physiotherapist	1	1	2	2	3
OT Technician	4	6	8	12	14
CSSD Assistant	1	1	2	2	3
Social Worker	2	3	4	5	6
Counselor	1	1	2	2	2
Dermatology Technician			1	1	1
Cyto-Technician			1	1	1
PFT Technician					2
Dental Technician	1	1	2	2	3
Darkroom Assistant	2	3	5	7	9
Rehabilitation Therapist	1	1	2	2	3
Biomedical Engineer	1	1	1	1	1
Total	76	132	201	261	325
Manpower Administration					
Administrator	1	1	1	2	2
Housekeeper	1	2	3	4	5
Medical records officer.	1	1	1	1	1
Medical record assistant	1	2	3	3	3
Accounts/Finance	2	3	4	5	6
Administrative officer	1	1	1	1	1
Office assistant Grade I	1	1	2	2	2
Office assistant Grade II	1	1	2	3	4
Ambulance Services (1 driver + 2 Technician)	1	1	2	3	3
Total	12	15	21	26	29

Abbreviations: CSSD: Central Sterile Supply Department; ENT: Ear Nose and Throat; OBG: Obstetrics and Gynecology; OT: Operation Theater; MO: Medical Officer; PFT: Pulmonary Function Tests

PATIENT CLASSIFICATION SYSTEM

Patient classification system (PCS), which evaluates the nature of the nursing care, is fundamental to staffing nursing units of every clinical care setting. PCS is used as an essential element of staff scheduling in hospitals. It is also used to calculate the number of nursing/ non-nursing staff required to manage each schedule. In choosing or actualizing a PCS, a committee of nurse managers can incorporate a delegate from medical practitioners or hospital authority, which would diminish incredulity about the PCS. The primary focus of PCS is the readiness to react to the constant change in the care of the patients as per his/her need.

Purposes

- The framework will build up a unit of measure for nursing, that is, time which will be utilized to decide numbers and sorts of staff required.
- It will help in program costing and plan of the nursing budget.
- It will track changes in the patient's needs. It assists the nurse administrator's capacity with moderating and control conveyance of nursing administration.
- It will determine the estimations of the profitability conditions, including assurance of value.

Grouping Patient's Categories

It is a strategy for gathering patients as per the complexity and need of the nursing care required, including the need for time and expertise. It helps in deciding the measure of nursing care required, for the most part within 24 hours and the class of nursing workforce who ought to give that care (Table 9).

NCH = Nursing Care Hours

The ratio of patients' allocation at various levels of care is different as per the types and standards of hospitals. The table given below illustrates the patient distribution according to the categories in a 100-bedded hospital (Table 10).

While calculating the quantity of nursing staff required, the nursing manager should guarantee that there is adequate staff to cover all shifts, off-duties, leaves, and public holidays and make up the work of the team who are absent. It also should make provisions and time frames for equal opportunity to staff development programs. The 40–48 hours of work every week is rehearsed in India. Let us compute the total number of working and nonworking hours for nurses in a year (Table 11).

The requirement of relievers for those staff who are on leave can be calculated by dividing the total number of leaves (CL + EL + PH + SL + CNE) by the number of working days per year per employee/nurse.

TABLE 9: Classification of patient's categories and nursing care hours

Category	Description	Ward
Category I Able to perform self-care. Require minimum support. —Nursing Care Hours 1.5/patient/day —Ratio 55:45	• Patients can eat, bath self and can perform their own ADL. • Patients who are ready for discharge. • This category also includes newly admitted patients who do not have any unique signs and symptoms. • Patients admitted for observation only.	Medicine ward
Category II Patients who require moderate or intermediate care and support—NCH 3/patient—Ratio 60:40	• Require little assistance with basic needs. • May have slight emotional needs. • Periodic treatments and observations are required.	Surgical Ward Obstetrics Prof: Non-Prof Ratio 60:40
Category III Patients who require total or complete nursing care—NCH 4.5 hrs/patient/day—Ratio 65:35	• They are completely dependent. • Unconscious or conscious. • Have marked emotional needs. • Have different tubes of drainage. • Under oxygen therapy. • Require continuous observation every 30 minutes for emergencies such as hemorrhage, cardiac arrest.	Intensive Care Unit Professionals: Non-Professionals Ratio 70:30
Category IV Patients who require critical and highly specialized care. NCH is 6–9 or even more per patient per day. Ratio 70:30 or 80:20	• Require active nursing service, preferably at a rate of 80:20. • Require continuous observation and treatment such as medications, IV infusions, and monitoring, etc. • We are monitoring every 15-30 minutes.	Critical Care Unit Prof: Non-Prof Ratio 80:20

Abbreviation: ADL, Activities of daily living

TABLE 10: Estimation of patient's allocation as per level of care

Hospital Category	Hospital (Primary level of Care) In %	Hospital (Secondary level of care) In %	Hospital (Tertiary level of Care) In %
Category I	70%	65%	30%
Category II	15%	30%	45%
Category III	15%	05%	15%
Category IV	–	–	10

TABLE 11: Distribution of privileges and working hours in Hospital (May change as per the policy of the organization)

Privileges for Nurses per Year	Working Hours per Week (48 hours)
Casual Leave (CL)	10
Earned Leave (EL)	20
Off-duties (as per rule)	96
Public Holidays (PH)	10
Sick Leave (SL)	10
Continuing Education Program (CNE)	03
Total Days per Year (nonworking)	149
Total Days per Year (working)	216
Total Hours per year (working)	216 x 8= 1728 hours.

No. of Reliever = 53/216= 0.25 per person. (48 hours weekly duty) If we multiply the given value (0.25) by the computed number of nursing staff, then we will get the total number of relievers required.

STAFFING FORMULA

The staffing formula is used to understand and calculate the total number of Nursing and Non-Nursing staff required for a hospital. An example of this formula is described below to calculate the requirement of the nursing workforce in a 100-bedded hospital;

- Categorize the patients according to levels of care needed

> 100 × 0.30 = 30 persons/patients needing minimal care
> 100 × 0.45 = 45 persons/patients needing moderate care
> 100 × 0.15 = 15 persons/patients needed intensive care
> 100 × 0.10 = 10 persons/patients need highly specialized nursing care
>
> **Total: 100 patients**

- Find the number of nursing care hours (NCH) needed by patients at each level of care per day.

> 30 patients × 1.5 hrs (Category I, NCH) 45 hours NCH/day
> 45 patients × 3.0 hrs (Category II, NCH) 135 hours NCH/day
> 15 patients × 4.5 hrs (Category III, NCH)67.5 hours NCH/day
> 10 patients × 6.0 hrs (Category IV, NCH) 60 hours NCH/day
>
> **Total: 307.5 NCH hours per day**

- Find the total NCH needed by 100 patients per year. 307.5 × 365 (days per year) = 112237.5 NCH hours per year
- Find the actual working hours rendered by each staff per year.
  8 (working hours per day) × 216 (working days per year) = 1728 working hours per year.
- Find the total number of nursing personnel needed.
  Total NCH per year/individual working hours per year
  = 112237.5/1728 = 64.95 (65)
  Add the number of relievers; Number of Relievers = computed reliever per person × total number of staff = 0.25 × 65 = 16.25 (16)
  Total number of Nursing Personnel = 65 + 16 = 81.
- Categorize nursing staff into professional and non-professional as per the ratio 60:40 or 70:30, 80:20.
- Distribute by shifts: The staff can be distributed as per the schedule of duty in the hospital.

Note: The above-given calculation is for illustration only. The actual number of staff may differ according to the organizational policy, hospital layout and ward pattern, geographical location, internal quality policies, availability of human resources, number of other categories of professionals available, etc.

New Methods/Formula for Calculating Staffing Needs

Estimating staffing requirements is a component of the planning of human resources. It may be expressed as the process of evaluating and recognizing gaps and surpluses in staffing. Different equations are used to measure and forecast staffing requirements based on past and estimated performance information such as sales and manufacturing figures from the company. HR planning concentrates on staffing the organization with the correct amount of staff with the necessary abilities when necessary, to fulfill short-and long-term company goals.

- **Rule of Thumb Method**: It is based on a particular structure of the enterprise. For example, if the organization has established its structure to have one shift in-charge per 5 staff nurses, then the short term planning will include the maintenance of the same pattern for the appointment of each shift in-charge uniformly during all time. As part of long term planning, every shift in-charge added will have five staff nurses under her/him. This is not an in-depth method of staffing, but it helps to maintain the structure of the organization.
- **Employing the Delphi Technique**: The Delphi Technique is based on the fact that staffing in an organization should be found on the input of senior experts. Usually, a group of experts comprising of senior managers, stakeholders of the organization and senior officials sit together and discuss the staffing pattern after discussion. The group may not have physical proximity but may be coordinated with the help of a facility manager.

- **Understanding Ratio Methods**: It comprises of two methods. Human resource forecasting is based on the number of senior officials and the number of junior officials under them. It is calculated based on a fixed ratio such as 1:5, 1:10, and so on. Every recruitment of senior or junior officials is based on these ratios. The productivity ratio is maintained with relevance to the number of human resources and the rate of productivity.
- **Statistical Regression Analysis**: Analysis of statistical regression equates relations between staff required and the relevant past data. This analysis may include the staffing done during a particular period and the rate of sales or service gain during the same period.

CATEGORIES OF NURSING PERSONNEL AND THEIR JOB DESCRIPTION IN A HOSPITAL

There is a definite need for job description because it is learned through some studies that most workers function mechanically and are not conscious of the role assigned to them. Providing job description becomes the primary responsibility of the management as it highlights the details of work, the primary purpose of employment, nature of work, kind of communication maintained as per hierarchy levels and expected job performance from every worker.

The job description is defined as the specification of roles and functions of the nature of the job of each individual who has to deliver effectively to be retained in the institution.

Purposes of Job Description

- Job analysis and categorization
- To enlist the staff
- Delegation of responsibilities
- Staff development
- Staff appraisal

The Nursing Superintendent/Director of Nursing

Qualification: MSc in Nursing, PhD Nursing is desirable. Administrative skills are also beneficial. Should be registered with the State Nursing Council.

Experience: A minimum of 10–15 years of experience out of which 3–5 years shall be in administration and teaching.

Job Summary: He/She is in charge of the running and supervision of a nursing division. Contingent upon the span of the office, she may control auxiliary offices, for example, housekeeping. The Nursing Director shall report to the Director of the hospital or Medical Superintendent.

Roles and Responsibilities

- Participates in general policymaking and especially those which are of the hospital.
- Determines objectives, goals, and strategies of the nursing service.
- Budgeting of Nursing Department.
- Supervising the nursing department and conduct recruitment of nursing as well as other associated staff for the hospital.
- Quality maintenance of nursing service and make appropriate decisions as and when required.
- Conducts nursing rounds.
- Participates meetings and conferences in and out of the hospital as and when required.

Joint/Deputy Nursing Superintendent/Nursing Superintendent Grade I

Each hospital with a bed strength of 200 ought to have one Joint/Deputy Nursing Superintendent/Nursing Superintendent Grade I. 1 Nursing Superintendent Grade I for 2 to 4 Nursing Superintendent Grade II.

Qualification: MSc/PBBSc/BSc Nursing. Higher qualification is desirable.

Experience: A minimum of 7-10 years of experience out of which three years in administration and teaching. She/He should have worked as Nursing Superintendent Grade II.

Roles and Functions

- Implements hospital strategies and principles through different nursing units.
- Decides and suggests the workforce and materials prerequisite for running different nursing departments.
- Interviews and recruitment nursing staff.
- Ensures the protected and effective care is rendered in different nursing units of the hospital.
- Conducts nursing rounds.
- Checks the standard of care provided and ensure that the patients are kept in a safe and comfortable condition.
- Member of condemnation board for hospital supplies.
- Plans duty list and ensures leaves and allowances of the nursing staff.
- Gives advising and direction to the subordinate staff and maintains the code of conduct among staff members.
- Takes part in conferences and meetings and plans staff development programs etc.

Assistant Nursing Superintendent/Nursing Superintendent Grade-II

Qualification: MSc/PBBSc/BSc Nursing

Experience: A minimum of 5–7 years experience of which two years in administration/education.

Roles and Responsibilities

- Assists in arranging work plans, deciding human resources and supplies for each unit.
- Discussion of potential issues, work obstructions, plan challenges, and so forth with higher specialists. Help with going around/settling such issues as required.
- Maintains contact with different offices, i.e., Purchasing, Accounting, Engineering, and so on as required.
- Complies and prepare nursing statistics.
- Conducts and takes care of the departmental and interdepartmental gatherings/meetings from time to time.
- Making nursing rounds.
- Acts as Liaison officer with other departments and the general public.
- Reports to Nursing Superintendent Grade I and officiates in the absence of Nursing Superintendent Grade I.

Senior Staff Nurse

Qualification: BSc/GNM Nursing.

Experience: Minimum of 5 years of experience as a Staff Nurse.

Job Summary: Senior staff nurse is a first dimension nursing supervisor who is responsible for the nursing care of a unit or ward or a unit allocated to her/him. She/he reports to the Nursing Superintendent Grade II for her/his ward/unit. She or he takes full charge of the ward and appoints work for different classes of nursing and non-nursing staff working with her/him. She or he is in charge of the security and solace of the patients in her/his ward.

Roles and Responsibilities

Patient Care

- Ensure legitimate admission and discharge of patients.
- Plans nursing care and makes patients' assignments according to their nursing needs.
- Assists in the immediate consideration/gives care to patients as and when required.
- Ensures the appropriate perception of records of the patients and relevant data conferred to the concerned specialists/doctors/seniors.
- Makes rounds with specialists/doctors, helping them in diagnosing and treatment of patients.
- Implements specialists guidelines concerning the treatment of the patient.
- Coordinates with other departments such as diagnostic, dietary department, billing section, etc. for patient care.

Supervision and Administration

- Ensures a safe and clean condition for the ward/unit/ special division.
- Preparation of duty list and work assignment.

- Identifying and acquisition of ward supplies and types of gear and keep records.
- Does standard stock checking of his/her ward/unit.

Educative Function

- Organizes introduction programs for new staff.
- Organizes formal and casual ward education such as incidental health education to staff, patients, and relatives, including a demonstration.
- Encourages staff improvement/development program in her/his ward/unit.

Staff Nurses

Qualification: BSc Nursing/PBBSc Nursing/GNM with enrolment with State Nursing Council.

Job summary: Staff Nurse is a first dimension health professional who gives care to patients who are doled out to her/him amid his/her duration of duty. She also assists in other routine activities of the wards/units. She/He straightforwardly reports to Senior Staff Nurses or nurses who are in charge of the ward or Nursing Superintendent Grade II.

Patient Care

- Carries out the procedure of admitting and discharging the patient.
- Maintains individual cleanliness and solaces of the patient.
- Attends to the nourishing needs of the patient and feeds the vulnerable patients.
- Maintains perfect and safe conditions for the patient.
- Implements and keeps upward strategies and schedules.
- Coordinates patient care with other team members.
- Takes round with the specialists/doctors and follow their orders.
- Performs different specialized procedures related to nursing care, such as medication administration, diagnostic procedures, specimen collection, recording vital signs, other nursing procedures as and when required.

Ward/Unit Management

- Helps the in charge to do her/his work.
- Makes sure the general tidiness of the ward and the sanitary area.
- Supervises the obligations of Group "D" representatives and aides them and reports accordingly.
- Maintains diet register and ensure sound distribution of diet to patients.
- Maintenance of records.

PATIENT ASSIGNMENTS AND NURSING RESPONSIBILITIES

Nursing is an integral part of any health care organization for fulfilling the nursing needs of the patients/society.

In nursing administrations, the nurse works with individuals from partnered disciplines, for example, dietetics, therapeutic social service, drug store and so on in providing a far-reaching project of patient care in the organization. As indicated by the WHO master advisory committee, the nursing care/services are characterized as part and parcel of the total health care delivery system.

Note: The Patient Assignments and Nursing Responsibilities are explained in detail in Unit 4.

ABSENTEEISM

Absenteeism refers to the worker's absence from his regular work when he is normally scheduled to work.

It is defined as the failure of the worker to report for work when he is scheduled to work. **—Labor Bureau**

Absenteeism is defined as a condition that exists when a person fails to come to work when he is properly scheduled to work. **—Filippo**

We can say absenteeism signifies the absence of an employee from work, i.e., unauthorized, un-explained, avoidable and willful. As per the above definitions, the following causes of absence cannot form part of absenteeism

- Absence due to strike or lock-out
- Employee reports for duty in later half schedule
- The employee takes Casual leave, Earned leave, Medical leave.
- When his name is removed from the list of active employees Absenteeism is calculated as:

$$\frac{\text{Number of persons days lost}}{\text{The average number of person X number of working days}} \times 100$$

Classification: Kerr classified absenteeism in the following categories:

- **Total absenteeism:** Absenteeism of workers at a given time who are scheduled to work but remain absent for any reason whatsoever excluding lay-off and lock-out.
- **Excused absenteeism:** Absence of work due to a bonafide cause, like self-illness or accident due to employment.
- **Un-excused absenteeism:** Absence as a habit and not a necessity.
- **Chronic absenteeism:** Habit of remaining on un-excused absence and normally increases the rate of absenteeism.

There are essentially two kinds of absences: Culpable and innocent/non-culpable.

Causes

- Nature of work
- Poor working conditions
- Absence of regular leave arrangement
- Accidents
- Poor Control
- Absence of transport facility
- Lack of interest
- Miscellaneous Causes

Effects

- Normal work-flow is disturbed.
- The difficulty is faced in executing the orders in time.
- Casual workers are employed to deliver orders in time.
- Extra pressure on employees who are present for the work, may disappoint them.
- Loss of wages for unauthorized absence from work.

Measures to Control Absenteeism

- Proper selection and proper orientation
- Better working conditions
- Provision of transport and housing facility
- Incentive bonus for regular employees
- Disciplinary actions
- Effective supervision
- Employee counseling

EMPLOYEE TURNOVER

Employee turnover is the movement of members across the boundary of an organization. Employee turnover refers to the number or percentage of workers who leave an organization and are replaced by new employees. Measuring employee turnover can be helpful to employers who want to examine reasons for turnover or estimate the cost-to-hire for budget purposes.

$$\text{Turnover} = \frac{\text{Number of staff leaving per year}}{\text{The average number of staff}} \times 100$$

Types of Turnovers

- **Involuntary employee turnover:** Employee termination for poor job performance, absenteeism or violation of workplace policies is called involuntary turnover, also referred to as termination, firing or discharge. It is involuntary because it is not the employee's decision to leave the company.
- **Voluntary employee turnover:** When an employee leaves the company of her own volition, it is called voluntary termination. Employees give several reasons for leaving their jobs. They may be accepting employment with another company, relocating to a new area or dealing with a personal matter that makes it impossible to work. When an employee voluntarily terminates the employment relationship, she generally gives the employer verbal or written notice of intent to resign from her job.

- **Desirable and undesirable turnover:** Turnover often has a negative connotation, yet turnover is not always a negative event. For example, desirable turnover occurs when an employee's performance falls below the company's expectations and is replaced by someone whose performance meets or exceeds expectations. It is desirable because poor job performance, absenteeism, and tardiness are costly than replacing a poor performer with an employee whose job can improve the company's profitability. Desirable turnover occurs when replacing employees infuses new talent and skills, which can give an organization a competitive advantage. Conversely, undesirable turnover means the company is losing employees whose performance, skills and qualifications are valuable resources.
- **Functional and dysfunctional turnover:** Functional turnover occurs when people leaving the firm are underperformers. Dysfunctional turnover is the exact opposite of functional turnover, as the best employees leave. This can happen for a variety of reasons, but a common cause is a low potential to advance.
- **Avoidable and unavoidable turnover:** Avoidable turnover is when an employee leaves and it is something you as an organization could have prevented. The exit could have been avoided. The issue is in your control, it is not an issue with the employee and their performance. Unavoidable turnover is the turnover that you have no control over. For example, if you require employees to be present in the office, and one of your employees is moving to take care of an aging parent.

Consequences of Employee Turnover

- **Negative**
  - Recruitment and selection costs
  - Training and development costs
  - Operational disruption
  - Demoralization of organizational membership
- **Positive**
  - Increased performance
  - Reduction of entrenched conflict
  - Increased mobility and morale
  - Innovation and adaptation

Reasons for Turnover

- Monetary factors
- Lack of good working conditions
- No flexible work schedules
- Lack of respect
- Very few supportive colleagues
- The organization is highly business-oriented
- Increase favoritisms
- Lack of appreciation

- Lack of challenges
- Stress from overwork and work-life imbalance
- Loss of trust and confidence in senior leaders

STAFF WELFARE

Employee welfare is a comprehensive term including various services, facilities, and amenities provided to employees for their betterment. It generally includes those items of welfare that is provided by statutory provisions or required by the customs of the industry or the expectations of employees from the contract of service from the employers. The basic purpose is to improve the lives of the working class. The purpose of providing welfare amenities is to bring about the development of the whole personality of the worker-his social, psychological, economic, moral, cultural and intellectual development to make him a good worker, a good citizen and a good member of the family. Employee welfare is a dynamic concept. These facilities may be provided voluntarily by progressive and enlightened entrepreneurs from their side out of their realization of social responsibility towards labor, or statutory provisions may compel them to make these facilities available, or these may be undertaken by the government or trade unions if they have the necessary funds for the purpose. Employee welfare measures are also known as fringe benefits and services. 'Labor Welfare' is a very broad term, covering social security and such other activities as medical aid, crèches, canteens, recreation, housing, adult education, arrangements for the transport of labor to and from the workplace.

Meaning and Definition

Employee welfare means "the efforts to make life worth living for workmen". According to Todd, "employee welfare means anything done for the comfort and improvement, intellectual or social, of the employees over and above the wages paid which is not a necessity of the industry."

The objectives of employee welfare are: Employee welfare is in the interest of the employee, the employer and the society as a whole. The objectives are:

- It improves the loyalty and morale of the employees.
- It reduces labor turnover and absenteeism.
- Welfare measures help to improve the goodwill and public image of the enterprise.
- It helps to improve industrial relations and industrial peace.
- It helps to improve employee productivity.

Agencies of Employee Welfare

- **Central government:** The central government has made elaborate provisions for the health, safety and welfare under Factories Act 1948, and Mines Act 1952. These acts provide for canteens, crèches, restrooms, shelters, etc.

- **State government:** Government in different states and Union Territories provide welfare facilities to workers. The state government prescribes rules for the welfare of the workers and ensures compliance with the provisions under various labor laws.
- **Employers:** Employers in India, in general, looked upon welfare work as fruitless and barren though some of them indeed had done pioneering work.
- **Trade unions:** In India, trade unions have done little for the welfare of workers. But few sound and strong unions have been pioneering in this respect. E.g. Ahmedabad textiles labor association and Mazdoor Sabha, Kanpur.
- **Other agencies:** Some philanthropic, charitable and social service organizations like—Seva Sadan Society, YMCA., etc

Types of Employee Welfare

- **Intramural:** These are provided within the organization like:
  - Canteen
  - Restrooms
  - Crèches
  - Uniform
  - Drinking water
  - Washing and bathing facilities
  - Provision of safety measures like fencing and covering machines
  - Fire extinguishers
  - Provision of Pension, Provident Fund, Fringe benefits
- **Extramural:** These are provided outside the organization like:
  - Housing
  - Education
  - Child welfare
  - Leave travel facilities
  - Interest-free loans
  - Workers cooperative stores
  - Vocational guidance, etc.
- **Statutory welfare work:** Comprising the legal provisions in various pieces of labor legislation.
- **Voluntary welfare work:** Includes those activities, which are undertaken by employers for their voluntary work. Different ways of Social Security Provision in India.
  - **Social Insurance:** The common fund is established with periodical contributions from workers out of which all benefits in terms of cash or kind are paid. The employers and state prove a major portion of finances. Benefits such as PF, Group Insurance, etc. are offered.
  - **Social Assistance:** Benefits are offered to persons of small means by govt out of its general revenues. Eg- Old age pension Social Security Employee Welfare, Medical care benefit, Maternity benefit, Accident benefit, Survivor's benefit and so on.

Role of Management in Employee Welfare

- Organizations provide welfare facilities to their employees to keep their motivation levels high. The employee welfare schemes can be classified into two categories, viz. statutory and non-statutory welfare schemes.
- The statutory schemes are those schemes that are compulsory to provide by an organization as compliance with the laws governing employee health and safety. These include provisions provided in industrial acts. The statutory welfare schemes include drinking water, facilities for sitting, first aid appliances, canteen facilities, spittoons, lighting.
- The non-statutory schemes differ from organization to organization and from industry to industry. It includes personal health care, flexi-time, employee assistance programs. Various assistant programs are arranged like external counseling service so that employees or members of their immediate family can get counseling on various matters.

Impact of Welfare on Productivity

- The welfare measures are aimed at integrating the socio-psychological needs of employees, the unique requirements of a particular technology, the structure and processes of the organization and the existing sociocultural environment.
- It creates a culture of work commitment in organizations and society which ensures higher productivity and greater job satisfaction to the employees.
- Due to the welfare measures, the employees feel that the management is interested in taking care of the employees that result in the sincerity, commitment, and loyalty of the employees towards the organization.
- The employees work with full enthusiasm and energetic behavior, which results in the increase in production and ultimately the increased profit.

DISCIPLINE

Discipline can act as a natural control by which a worker brings his or her conduct into a concurrence with the organization's legitimate conduct code, or it tends to be an administrative action to implement worker consistency with office principles and directions. It alludes to working as per certain perceived principles, instructions and traditions, regardless of whether they are composed or understood in character.

Discipline is defined as training or molding of the mind and character to bring about desired behaviors.

Discipline is the practice of making people to obey rules or standards of behavior, and punishing them when they do not.

—**Collins Dictionary**

Aims and Objectives of the Discipline

- To get an acknowledgment of the principles, directions, and strategies of an association with the goal that authoritative objectives can be accomplished.
- To bestow a component of assurance, despite a few contrasts in casual personal conduct and other related change in an association.
- To build up tolerance and adjustment among employees.
- To make a climate of regard for human identity and human relations.
- To increment the working effectiveness and confidence of the workers/representatives with the goal that their efficiency is ventured up, the expense of generation is cut down, and quality is increased.

Types of Discipline

- **Self-controlled discipline:** For the situation of Self-controlled discipline, the worker brings her or his conduct into a concurrence with the associations' authentic conduct code, i.e. the worker controls their very own exercises for the benefit of all of the association. Therefore, individuals are acquainting with work for a pinnacle execution under Self-controlled discipline.
- **Enforced discipline/control:** Here, an administrative activity authorizes worker consistency with the association's tenets and directions, i.e., it is a typical control forced from the higher level. Here, the supervisor practices his power to urge the workers to carry on with a specific goal in mind.

Approaches to Discipline

- **Traditional methodology:** It accentuates correction/punishment for unfortunate conduct. The reasons for conventional order are punishment for wrongdoing, implement an adjustment to custom, and fortify the power of the old over the youth.
- **Developmental methodology:** It accentuates discipline as a shaper of attractive conduct. The reason for formative discipline is to shape behavior by giving excellent results to the correct functioning and severe modifications for the wrong conduct; and shirking of physical punishments, defend the privileges of the blamed and swap for individual discretionary decisions of the blame.
- **Positive approach:** It depends on the presumption that a good worker with a sense of pride, regard for power, and enthusiasm for the activity will stick to brilliant work benchmarks; and when an intrigued, conscious and self-regarding employee briefly strays from his/her typically exclusive expectations, an amicable reminder/update is sufficient to divert their endeavors in the ideal bearing.

Indiscipline of an Employee

- Changes in behavior
- Absenteeism
- Apathy
- Go slow at work
- Strikes and agitations
- Increase in number and severity of grievances, persistent and continuous demand for raises, allowances, lack of concern for performance

Causes of Indiscipline

- Delay in administering discipline.
- Ignoring rule violation in the hope that it is an isolated event.
- Accumulations of rule violations, causing irritated supervisors to become outrageous.
- Failure to administer progressively severe sanctions.
- Failure to document disciplinary actions accurately.
- Imposing discipline disproportionate to the seriousness of the offense.
- Disciplining inconsistently.

Principles of Disciplinary Action

- **Have an inspirational frame of mind:** The supervisor's demeanor is imperative in averting or amending unwanted conduct. Individuals will, in general, do what is anticipated from them. Subsequently, the administrator must keep up an uplifting frame of mind by anticipating the best from the staff.
- **Investigate cautiously:** If staff nurse is restrained unreasonably or superfluously, the consequences for the whole staff members might be severe and hence the administrators must continue with an alert. They should gather certainties, check charges, and even approach the blamed representatives for their side of the story.
- **Be prompt:** If the disciplinary action is postponed, the connection between the corrective measures and the mistakes turns out to be less precise.
- **Protect privacy:** Disciplinary activities influence the sense of self of the staff nurse. Talking about the circumstances in private causes less hatred and a more possibility for future co-activity.
- Focus on the mistake or act but not the employee as the action was not acceptable, not the worker.
- **The consistency of rules:** It diminishes the likelihood of bias, advances uniformity, and cultivates acknowledgment of punishments.
- **Be adaptable:** Individuals and conditions are never the equivalents. Punishment should be resolved merely after the whole record is looked into.
- **Take remedial, reliable action:** The administrator should make sure that the staff nurse comprehends that the conduct was in opposition to the association's prerequisites.

- **Follow up:** The supervisor ought to unobtrusively explore to decide if the staff nurse's conduct has changed. If not, the administrator ought to determine the explanation behind that mentality.

Punishments/Penalties

- **Oral reprimands:** It is recommended in case of minor faults due to any reason. An oral warning will be given by the Nurse Manager but add the same in the anecdotal record with nature of the event, time, and place.
- **Written reprimands:** It is advised in times of serious faults. A notice may be issued by the supervisor to prevent the same in the future. It should include the name of the worker and the supervisor, the idea of the issue, the punishment, and the outcomes of future redundancy. The worker needs to sign it, to demonstrate that the worker has perused it. A duplicate should be given to the person who is getting punished and one held for the staff record. On the off chance that again, the terms are not met, different punishments will most likely be vital.
- **Other punishments:**
  - Financial punishments may be initiated, such as deducting salary, etc.
  - Loss of benefits may incorporate exchange to a less attractive position and loss of inclination for nursing assignments.
  - Demotion is a sketchy arrangement. It makes hard emotions, which might be infectious and more probable spots for wrongdoers in a situation of low grade.
  - Suspension from the employment for a timeframe, withholding an appraisal/salary hike.
  - Termination (rejection): perpetual end of employment in the organization.

Advantages of Discipline

- Discipline establishes a pattern for acceptable conduct and performance. It provides a code of conduct for all the students and employees.
- It promotes individual growth, develops human efficiency, and enhances the will power to perform higher.
- It creates an environment under which individual excellence gets a boost, group performance is improved, and harmonious working evolves.

GRIEVANCE

A grievance is any dissatisfaction or feeling of injustice having a connection with one's employment situation which is brought to the attention of management. Speaking broadly, a grievance is any dissatisfaction that adversely affects organizational relations and productivity. To understand what a grievance is, it is necessary to distinguish between dissatisfaction, complaint, and grievance.

Dissatisfaction is anything that disturbs an employee, whether or not the unrest is expressed in words.

A complaint is a spoken or written dissatisfaction brought to the attention of the supervisor or the shop steward.

A grievance is a complaint that has been formally presented to a management representative or a union official.

According to Michael Jucious, 'grievance is any discontent or dissatisfactions whether expressed or not, whether valid or not, arising out of anything connected with the company, which an employee thinks, believes or even feels to be unfair, unjust or inequitable'.

Classification of Grievance

Grievance can usually be classified as:

- **Those caused by misunderstanding:** Grievance caused by a misunderstanding usually stem from circumstances surrounding the grievance, a lack of familiarity with the contract or an inadequate labor agreement.
- **Those caused by intentional contract violations:** Intentional violation of a contract is usually an effort to capitalize on ambiguous contract language or past practices.
- **Those caused by symptomatic problems outside the scope of the labor agreement:** Symptomatic grievances are simply a means for the employee to show dissatisfaction or frustration and stem from the human element in management/labor relationship.

Causes of Grievance

- **Work environment:** It may be undesirable or unsatisfactory conditions of work. For example, light, space, heat, or poor physical conditions of the workplace, defective tools and equipment, poor quality of material, unfair rules, and lack of recognition.
- **Supervision:** It may be objections to the general methods of supervision related to the attitudes of the supervisor towards the employee such as perceived notions of bias, favoritism, nepotism, caste affiliations, and regional feelings.
- **Economic:** Employees may demand individual wage adjustments. They may feel that they are paid less when compared to others. For example, late bonus, payments, adjustments to overtime pay, perceived inequalities in treatment, claims for equal pay, and appeals against performance-related pay awards.
- **Organizational change:** Any change in organizational policies can result in grievances. For example, the implementation of revised company policies or new working practices.
- **Employee relations:** Employees are unable to adjust with their colleagues, suffer from feelings of neglect and victimization and become an object of ridicule and humiliation, or other inter-employee disputes.

- **Miscellaneous:** These may be issues relating to certain violations in respect of promotions, safety methods, transfer, disciplinary rules, fines, granting leaves, medical facilities, etc.

Effects of Grievance

Grievances, if not identified and redressed, may adversely affect workers, managers, and the organization. The effects are the following:

- **On the production:**
  - Low quality of production
  - Low productivity
  - Increase in the wastage of material, spoilage/leakage of machinery
  - Increase in the cost of production per unit
- **On the employees:**
  - Increase in the rate of absenteeism and turnover
  - Reduction in the level of commitment, sincerity, and punctuality
  - Increase in the incidence of accidents
  - Reduction in the level of employee morale
- **On the managers:**
  - Strained superior-subordinate relations.
  - Increase in the degree of supervision and control.
  - Increase in indiscipline cases
  - Increase in unrest and thereby machinery to maintain industrial peace

Grievance Process

The following steps comprise the typical grievance process:

- **Step 1:** The employee talks informally with her or his direct supervisor, usually as soon as possible after the incident has occurred. A representative or a bargaining agent is allowed to be present. A written request for the next step is given to the immediate supervisor within ten working days. The employee, supervisor, and agent will be present for any discussion.
- **Step 2:** If the response to step 1 is not satisfactory, a written appeal may be submitted within 10 working days to the director of nursing. The employee, agent, grievance chairperson, and the top nursing administrator or designs can be provided in 5 working days after these meetings.
- **Step 3:** The employee, agent, grievance chairperson, nursing administrator, and director of human resources meet for discussion. The 10 and 5 day time limits for appeal and answer are again observed.
- **Step 4:** The final step is arbitration, which is invoked when no solution suggested is acceptable. An arbitrator who is a neutral third party is selected and is present at these meetings. The submission of grievance may be required within 15 days after step 3 is completed.

Grievance Hearing

In the grievance hearing, remember the following key behaviors:

- Put the grievant at ease. Do not interrupt or disagree.
- Listen openly and carefully.
- Discuss the problem calmly and with an open mind.
- Get the story straight. Get all the facts to ask logical questions.
- Consider the grievant viewpoints
- Avoid snap judgments. Do not jump to conclusions.
- Make an equitable decision, and then give it to the grievant promptly.

IN-SERVICE EDUCATION

It is characterized as an ongoing program given by the respective employers or their representatives by specialized educators to employees. It is aimed at the motivation of the workers and to build up their skills and capacities according to their respective current/future designations. It is a sort of training that is given to the representatives while they are at work to enhance their working limits and effectiveness. The idea of in-service training is in the maturing structure in India, while in western nations, it has developed completely and has turned into a fundamental prerequisite for the expert development of a nurse.

In-service education is understood as learning experiences provided in the work setting to assist staff in performing their assigned functions in that particular agency. It is a continuous program of education provided by the employing authority, to develop the competences of personnel in their functions appropriate to the position they hold, or to which they will be appointed in the service. It is a planned instructional or training program provided by an employing agency in the employment setting and designed to increase competence in a specific area.

Definitions

In-service education and training may be in the most general sense taken to include everything that happened to the teacher from the day he takes up his first appointed to the day he retires, which contributes directly or indirectly to how he executes his professional duties.　　　**—Henderson**

Planned education activities intended to build upon the educational and experimental basis of the professional nurse for the enhancement of practice, education, administration, and research or theory development aimed at improving the health of the public.　　**—The American Nurses Association**

Characteristics of In-service Education

- It helps to improve the employee's performance and meets organizational goals.

- All staff, as lifelong learners, shares personal responsibility for individual and organizational growth through in-service education.
- Training is planned, systematic, and sustained, or sometimes it may be incidental.
- Internal resources are valued and used effectively for arranging training programs.
- Collaboration and trust are essential to the success of the program.
- Programs include rigorous evaluation and communication of results to all concerned.

Aims of In-service Education Program

- It helps in the acquisition of newer knowledge.
- It improves performance.
- It helps in the development of the specific skill required for practice.
- It improves the staff member's chances of promotion.
- The employee develops the right concept for client care.
- It helps in the maintenance of a high standard for nursing.
- It helps to observe and bring change in staff behavior.

Need and Scope of In-service Education

The nurses and other health care professionals should be expertly equipped to get by the stream of the health care industry, which is consistently evolving. The health care recipients are highly informed about their rights, and hence, there is a need for updating themselves in terms of knowledge, attitude, and practice. Research has investigated the learning skyline of the nursing sciences, and graduates have to update themselves continuously to maintain the competency and keep pace with the changing concepts of delivery of nursing services to the patient.

A graduate nurse who is competent today may not be considered competent five years later if he/she has not updated himself or herself with the changing knowledge or skills. Four avenues have been identified as the primary means for examining the competence of nurses. They are peer review, practice audits, re-examination, and continuing education. In-service education is another area of concern that has gained popularity in the corporate sector of health care to maintain the competency of the nurses.

We live in a period of knowledge explosion with rapidly changing healthcare technology. New research findings, emphasis on evidence-based practice, and use of sophisticated technology are necessities for in-service education or staff development so that the staff can perform better with the latest knowledge and skills. Educational preparation of the nurses varies (ANM, GNM, BSc Nursing), which depends on the quality of facilities in the educational institutions, and most of the time majority of the students fail to achieve/develop the required knowledge and skill to practice nursing, thus requiring in-service education. The success

of a healthcare organization depends on the educational level and competency of the personnel; therefore, properly educating employees will help to provide nursing care with high productivity and minimized errors. In this era of cost containment, organizations cannot afford the cost caused by negligence and malpractice of the incompetent nurses. Increased public awareness, quality assurance demands and efficient and competent nurses are required to fulfill patient expectations.

It includes the following;

- Maintenance of familiarity with new knowledge and subject matter so that the members of the profession regularly update themselves of the relevant expertise. It is partially the part of regulatory bodies since they have framed norms regarding the credits and credit hours required by each practicing professional during their course.
- Increased skills in providing service, which makes each professional unique in the health care system.
- Improved attitudes and skills as in-service education frequently re-emphasizes the idea that curriculum improvement is primarily a consequence of the development of the people.
- More considerable skill in utilizing community resources and in working with adults. An important task of modern education is the development of intelligent civic loyalties and understanding.
- Development and refinement of shared values and goals.

Types/Approaches to In-service Education

There are three types approaches to in-service education (Fig. 2)

Centralized approach: In this case, the whole process of in-service education/training is planned and implemented by the central administration department that consists of nurse managers and other senior officials. The learners do not participate in the planning process but are expected to attend the training program organized by the central department.

Advantages

- Budget control.
- Evaluation of the program can be facilitated.
- There is a prior decision on resources of the education program, who will attend it, where will it be held and other aspects of the program.

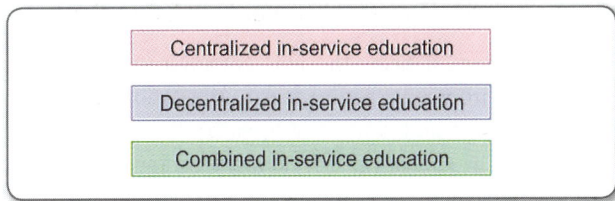

Centralized in-service education

Decentralized in-service education

Combined in-service education

Fig. 2: Approaches to in-service education

- Committees are directed to work on specific problems identified by the administration.

Disadvantage

- It may lead to reducing spontaneous, interested participation, and enthusiasm of learners.

Decentralized Approach: This is in reverse to the centralized approach. It is arranged by and directed for the nurses at different departments. The workers are relied upon to keep the organization educated of their exercises and potentially counsel with the organization when help is required, yet the representatives are required to create and coordinate their very own learning aspects. In this methodology, control in making arrangements is an obligation of workers, and the characteristics which are esteemed more are self-course, activity, and participative collaboration.

Advantages

- The individuals work in the same unit.
- As it is provided mutually, the common confronted problems and needs of the staff can be easily recognized.
- Share the responsibilities for meeting the in-service needs.
- The proper contribution of the participants is expected.

Disadvantages

- Lack of leadership
- Conflicts
- Inefficiency
- Lessor no budget

Coordinated/Combined Approach: It is a trade-off between the above approaches. Here the responsibility of planning and participation is mutual. The central department frames the broader guidelines, whereas the recipients decide the execution of the plans. This approach helps both the nursing officers and the administration in meeting their expectations and need.

Advantages

- Mutual coordination and assistance to central administration are improved.
- Duplication is avoided.
- The unity of efforts is maintained.

Components/Types of In-service Education

- **Orientation:** It helps the new employee to adjust to a new environment and duties. Orientation influences the structure and content of learning of various nursing groups. The goal of the orientation program is to enhance the competencies of nursing service personnel so that employees may continuously improve the quality of care

provided to patients. It is also aimed to introduce newly inducted staff to get added to the system in terms of practices, policies, and protocols of the organization.
- **Skill Training:** It provides employees with the skills and attitude required for the job and keeps them abreast of changing methods and new techniques.
- **Leadership and Management Development:** It equips a selected group of employees to shoulder growing responsibilities and new positions. Staff should have skills in leadership and management to guide new employees in outpatient care.
- **Continuing Education:** It helps an employee keep abreast of new concepts and increase knowledge, understanding, and competency with the number of additional educational programs and activities.
- **Staff Development Programs:** It includes all the workshops, seminars, webinars, self-instruction, short term courses, online courses such as MOOC, scientific paper presentations and other methods, which are also part of in-service education.

ADULT EDUCATION/LEARNING (DISTANCE LEARNING)

The training of adults or grown-ups is a multifaceted, complicated procedure, which incorporates many subjects and intrigue territories. It is comprehensive and shifted as those it serves. It includes Adult Basic Education (teaching essential learning and survival skills to the undereducated), Continuing education endeavors for individual and enrichment activities for the highly educated. It is intended for individual expertise improvement, for upgraded professional openings, or satisfaction. It can include a brief length of time or quite a long while of exertion.

Grown-up training is where grown-ups who have never gain to school, or do not go to class on a standard or, full-time premise, or school dropouts who attempt consecutive and composed instructive exercises in different subjects, for example, health and family welfare, agriculture and animal husbandry and so on. This is proposed to realizing changes in learning, mentality, and expertise for the motivation behind identifying and taking care of individual or community issues. Grown-up training grasps all types of educative encounters required by people as per their fluctuating advantages and necessities at their different dimensions of appreciation and capacity and in their changing jobs and duty all through life.

Definitions

The Exeter Conference 1969 defines it as the process whereby persons who no longer attend school regularly (unless full-time programs are specially designed for adults) undertake sequential and organized activities within a conscious

intention of bringing about changes in information, knowledge, understanding, skills, appreciation, and attitudes, for identifying and solving personal or community problems.
—**Liveright and Haygood, 1969**

Adult Education is part-time or full-time education for men and women of all ages either organized by themselves or provided by schools, learning centers, or other agencies which enables them to improve their general or professional knowledge, skills and abilities by either continuing their education or resuming their initial or incomplete education of previous years. —**Reddy, 2000**

Objectives of Adult Education

- Improves the quality of life of an individual and enables him/her to realize his/her potential for self-realization.
- The standard of living of the families, communities, societies, and nations will be raised.
- Helps in promoting communal harmony and peace in the multi-cultural global village.
- Contributes directly to the growth of the nation; improves the welfare of the international community.
- Imparting literacy of diverse types such as basic literacy, scientific literacy, economic literacy, technological literacy, legal literacy, computer literacy, and so on.
- Generating awareness on various matters/subjects such as awareness about one's self, community, society, and the nation.
- Promoting functionality of individuals for addressing the felt needs, for solving the problems, for promoting more extensive public participation in various activities and so on.

Adult Education in India

Adult education has achieved great success in the western nations. India has done very little in the field of Adult education and must address the issue more earnestly and systematically. Adult education brings new hope for the illiterate masses who failed to get an education during their school years.

A well-defined adult education program will help the illiterate people to take part in the daily activities of the country. The National Adult Education Program (NAEP) which was launched in 1978 by the government, is the first nationwide effort to eradicate illiteracy. It was a vast program to educate 100 million non-literate adults in the 15–35 years age group within a five-year time frame.

Most individuals make the error of looking adult education from a narrow view of the notion. But it is like any other literacy program conducted in a nation to eradicate illiteracy among grown-up people. Adult education has come a long way as a discipline, and it is not limited to literacy. On a broader connotation, Adult Education refers to any form of the learning process that engages mature men and women beyond the confines of a traditional learning environment.

Also termed as continuing education, it includes everything from learning the three basic R's (reading, writing, and arithmetic) to learning for personal accomplishment and goes to the extent of enabling a person to attain a higher degree. To have a better understanding of adult education, it becomes necessary for us to trace its beginning and know how it has evolved over the years. Adult Education theory evolves by the different concepts such as:

- **Fundamental education:** It is the minimum and general education aimed at helping kids and adults who do not have the benefits of formal education to comprehend the issues of their surroundings and their rights and responsibilities as citizens and people.
- **Out-of-school education:** It was first proposed by Lauren Resnick in 1987. It is aimed to overcome the difficulties in learning, the development of different talents, increasing the interest in education, and strengthening the communities and individuals. It is beneficial for improving the opportunities of an individual in the real world.
- **Lifelong education:** It is voluntary, ongoing, and self-motivated. Lifelong education is a process aimed at active learning throughout life that comprises all ages, all levels of teaching, all forms of education, and all educational policies.
- **Continuing education:** Continuing education seems to have reference to some retraining when needed, for example, in a new job.

Forms of Adult Learning

- **Vocational education:** It is defined as a kind of training given for improving the present career and upgrading technical education called the career technical education or vocational training. It enables adults to engage themselves in any skill or craft. It may be offered as full time or part-time. It can be applied at the secondary or post-secondary level for further education. In India, the main vocation education programs provided by the government are UDAAN, National Urban Livelihood Mission, Training Programs based on Modular Employable Skill, Aajeevika Mission of National Rural Livelihood, Craftsmen Training Scheme and so on.
- **Education for family and society:** This kind of education helps the adults in the family to improve their status and quality. In India, many schemes such as Samagra Shiksha, Rashtriya Ucchatar Shiksha Abhiyan (RUSA) are intended to make the people literate, and thus they will be able to raise their standard of living.
- **Personal enrichment:** This includes provisions for attending seminars, workshops, and conferences that help the students to improve knowledge.
- **Remedial education:** It helps the people to compete with the latest technological expectation and become active members and efficient and productive citizens of India. E.g. Computer skill training, Training in different software, and so on.

Characteristics of Adult Learners

- Usually, adults want to take more control of their learning than young people.
- More than young people, adults draw on their experiences as a resource in their reading attempts.
- In learning circumstances, adults tend to be more driven than adolescents. Higher motivation is associated with the voluntary nature of most adult teaching.
- Young people are less pragmatic in learning compared to adults.
- Many adults lack confidence in their learning.
- It is more difficult to bring changes in adults with regard to learning. Learning demands change in our attitude and behavior.
- In terms of age, adults differ from one another as learners and experience much more than traditional-age learners.
- Adults need to work hard to learn with regard to the learning age.

Principles of Adult Learning

Principles of adult learning are essential for the successful deployment of the in-service education program. Adult learning theory was proposed by *Knowles*, which emphasizes that children and adults learn differently. *Malcolm Knowles* suggested that there are fundamental conceptual differences between adult and child education. According to him, the basic principles of adult learning are:

- It is a self-directed learning process where the adults decide their learning needs.
- It comprises of an amalgam of learning and experience, and it makes the current learning much more meaningful. They possess vast experience. The newly learned knowledge and skills are readily practiced.
- Reinforcing or rewarding for better performance motivates the learner to learn further in a better way and perform well.
- Adult Education can be successfully implemented by teamwork; wherein all department teachers cooperate with the students in achieving the goals and philosophy of the adult education.
- They are highly motivated and concentrate more on task-centered learning.
- The learning needs of adults arise from real-life situations.
- In adult learning, the trainer should focus more on problem-solving as they are much concerned about practical situations.
- The learning situations/facilities should be respectful and friendly for adults.
- It should be well planned within the time frame, and there should be a provision for physical needs such as coffee, snacks, and break time.

Adult education is a multidisciplinary, process-oriented program to favor lifelong education for all, as well as efficient learning throughout life. It aims to provide the knowledge that improves professional qualifications and to achieve civic, social, moral, and cultural attitudes and skills for performing responsibilities and progress in all spheres of life. It attempts to prepare individuals so that they may perform multiple functions participating in the presence of their community. The various kinds of clientele deriving benefits of Adult Education would indicate its scope, which is children outside school, the unemployed youth, people with disabilities and women and girls and elderly citizens. Adult education brings new hope for the illiterate masses who failed to get an education during their school years. Though a well-defined program of Adult Education, the illiterate adults can hope to take part in the day to day activities of their country.

Organizing the In-service Education Program/ Planning for In-service Education

The literature explains the number of models and methods to organize in-service education that ranges from simple to complex (Fig. 3). Here we discuss a standard model of in-service education based on the system approach. It comprises of five stages as mentioned below.

Stage 1: Analysis of the Learning Needs of the Employees/Need Assessment

No training program is developed from thin air. All the training programs are based on some needs. The learning needs are identified systematically, and it is based on the gap of knowledge or practice. The difference between knowledge and practice is caused by time and technological advancements supported by the research element and evidence-based learning. These needs may be identified by consultation with advisory groups, analysis of quality improvement data, professional standards of practice, communication with employees, analysis of records and reports, and changes within and outside the organization.

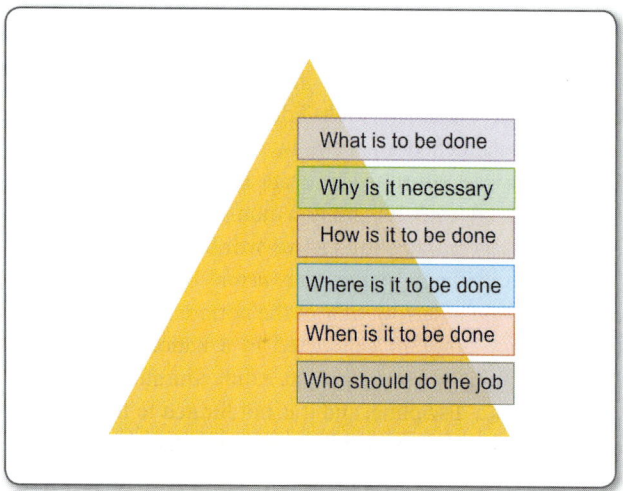

Fig. 3: Planning process

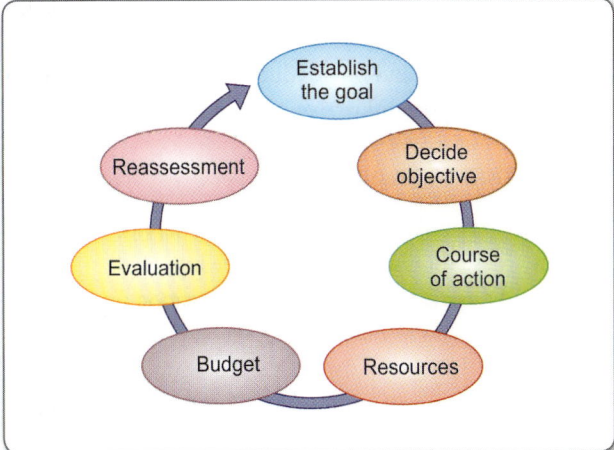

Fig. 4: Planning and designing the program

Stage 2: Plan and Design the In-service Education Program

In this stage, the program coordinator or managers decide on the overall plan and design of the program (Fig. 4). The whole planning and designing of the in-service program includes the following:

- *Training approach*: The nature of training, especially the type of skills to be taught, decides whether it has to be done at a classroom, laboratory, or an advanced method of simulation. Therefore, the program coordinator has to decide about the training approach that will be suitable for specific learning objectives and available resources. The process of evaluation of the learning is also decided by the coordinator.
- *Learning objectives*: As mentioned before, the learning objectives are framed before the commencement of training to make measurable results.
- *Measurement of performance*: Evaluation of all in-service training programs helps in identifying the ability/capacity of the employee to reproduce the newly learned knowledge and skills. It suggested following an experimental approach such as pre-test and post-test design to improve its effectiveness.
- *Develop program specification*: The program coordinator has to determine the time, venue, topics, and the teaching-learning strategies for each item and the program schedule is based on the available data.

Stage 3: Development of Resource Materials and Media

In the first part, there is a need to prepare a broader outline of the curriculum, and it should be the foundation for building of further training programs. The lesson plan and various educational media for training programs also should be developed.

Stage 4: Implementation of the Program

It involves bringing together educators, learners, and the materials and methods needed for education. It includes implementation of the training plan, conduction of actual training sessions, formative evaluation at regular intervals, and documentation of training results.

Stage 5: Evaluation

It is aimed to identify the components of the program that needs improvement as well as to streamline the effectiveness of the instructor and other facilities. It includes the conduction of summative evaluation, analyzing information collected and initiating corrective actions for deficiencies explored.

Evaluation of In-service Education

Staff development is considered a vital component of improving the organization and its services. The growth of the organization primarily relies on improvements in its human resources. This has to be realized by the organization, the workers, and everyone associated with the functioning of the hospital. In-service education is aimed at the development of the participants as well as the recipient of the care. Hence, it is highly significant to measure the extent of transfer of learning. It may very well be assessed through an extensive review process or any other scientific evaluation techniques. The result of the evaluation will contribute to the overall success of the organization.

Evaluation is the process of finding out how the development or training process has affected the individual, team, and organization.

- Questionnaire and Inventories: The advantage of pencil-paper responses procured sometime after training is roughly parallel to those written immediately after training. They have the added benefit of relatively systematic planning and coverage.
- Interviews: Talking with group members or co-workers sometime after the training either individually or in groups elicits valuable and thorough data, which is helpful because it differs from answers received to a systematic pre-planned set of questions.
- Observation of behavior in the in-service education program: One of the most effective methods of evaluation wherein, the employee is observed for the performance improvement as desired or planned in the training program. It elicits the actual behavior rather than the verbal data of the employee.

Problems Related to In-service Education Program

- Lack of incentives, motivation, and interest
- Lack of trainers/educators

- Organizational problems
- Inadequate evaluation technique

Benefits of Ongoing In-service Education

- Knowledge, skill, and attitude of the employees are improved
- Improved attitudes of the employees toward learning
- Employees are better prepared to manage change
- More effective in their roles
- Maximum use of resources
- Staff feels valued and show commitment to lifelong learning
- Quality assurance or quality control
- Professional enhancement and growth

Factors Influencing In-service Education

Generally, the in-service education program is influenced by all those factors that influence society, such as financial aspects, social aspects, therapeutic, technological advancements, etc. Few are briefed below:

- **Healthcare cost:** In-service education improves the knowledge and skills of professionals, thus updating the health care delivery. At the same time, it also accounts for the additional financial expense. The additional expense on the planning and implementation of in-service education may be a burden for any organization.
- **Human resources:** The training programs demand the availability of trained and skilled professionals as instructors. The in-service training and education should be provided by experts within the organization or by an external expert. It needs to be organized regularly. It may cause additional financial as well as manpower burden for the HR department.
- **Change in practice:** Learning is an ongoing process, and it may bring considerable changes in the health care delivery system that may cause inconvenience to the recipients and may also account for lack of consistency. The changes and modifications in the health care services may not be welcomed by all.
- **Existing standards and principles:** of nursing practice In-service education aims to upgrade knowledge and skill, and it is evidence-based. There may be occasions where the current protocols need to be revised. The resistance to change and doubt of the result may influence the practice of professionals.
- **Structure, mission, philosophy, and aim:** These aspects of the organization and the nursing department, including the personal preferences of the higher officials of the organization influence the in-service education. The higher authority in the organization makes the final decision regarding the provision of in-service education.
- **Laws, rules, and norms:** The government's laws, rules and norms are related to the organizational growth. It is

mandatory in some countries to have in-service education in health care organizations. In India, it compulsory to attend in-service and other educational programs to keep the nurses' registration active.

Preparation of Report

Reports are essential documents of an in-service education program. These should be prepared showing;

- Date and duration of the in-service education program.
- Coordinator and resource persons.
- Purpose of the topic of in-service education.
- Group of individuals with the necessary qualifications and the number of individuals in the group.
- Plan of the in-service education program.
- Evaluation report related to change in knowledge, attitude, and practices based on the program.
- A summary of all this should be recorded in the report and submitted to a higher authority.

MATERIAL MANAGEMENT

Material management is a scientific technique, concerned with Planning, Organizing, and Controlling of the flow of materials, from their initial purchase to destination.

Material management is concerned with providing the drugs, supplies, and equipment needed by health personnel to deliver health services.

Purposes

- To gain an economy in purchasing.
- To satisfy the demand during the period of replenishment.
- To carry reserve stock to avoid stock out.
- To stabilize fluctuations in consumption.
- To provide a reasonable level of client services.
- Increase the efficiency of healthcare systems.
- Provide materials in the required quantity and quality as when needed.

Basic Principles of Material Management

- Effective management and supervision; it deals with the material; functions of planning, organizing, staffing, controlling, reporting and budgeting.
- Sound purchasing method with skillful and hard poised negotiation.
- Simple inventory control program.

Process of Material Management

The process of material management involves planning, review, and control of materials (Fig. 5).

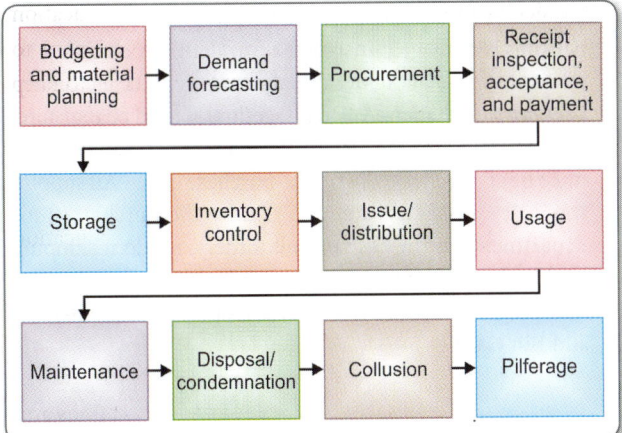

Fig. 5: Process of material management

1. **Budgeting and material planning:** Based on the data of past levels of performance and on anticipated/plans, capital equipment, consumables, and supplies to be procured during the year ahead can be projected department wise. This is the material budget that should be prepared annually. At periodic intervals, budgetary appraisals and determines should be carried out the variance between the accruals and the budget.

   Important in budgetary control and reduction of material cost is the concept of standardization. This involves grouping together similar items depending on their specification/use/application to choose one of these more universally acceptable for the purpose.

   Related to standardization, there is something equally important, and it is referred to as value analysis. It examines all the facts of the function and cost of a product/item in use to determine whether the cost can be reduced while retaining all the futures of performance or quality of the product/item. Value analysis attempts at addressing the following issues:
   - What is the item/component?
   - What does it intend to do?
   - What does it cost?
   - What else can do the same job?
   - What is the suggested alternative cost?

   Introduction of non–disposable, autoclavable, plastic syringes instead of easily breakable, more expensive glass syringes is based on the value analysis principle.

2. **Demand forecasting:** Estimation of the right amount of each material is the most crucial factor for maximizing availability with minimum wastage. The main methods of forecasting are:
   - **Last period demand:** Forecasting for the next period is done based on the level of demand that occurred in the previous period (the past year's demand is considered).
   - **Arithmetic average:** An average of all past demands is taken for forecasting demand. Arithmetic means is found out by averaging over a while.

   - **Moving average:** The moving average method is the one used more widely. A moving average strictly corresponds to the middle of the time over which it is calculated. It serves as a forecast of the immediate next period in the time serves, there is a time/lag equivalent to half the time/span.

3. **Procurement:** An effective procurement system aims at purchasing items of acceptable quality, in the appropriate quantities, at the minimum price and within the available time. Purchases may be made by the respective department of the hospitals or by a single purchase department. Centralized purchasing has the advantages in that quantity discounts are possible because of standardization and bulk orders.

   Objectives of the procurement system:
   - Acquire needed supplies as inexpensively as possible
   - Obtain high-quality supplies
   - Assure prompt and dependable delivery
   - Distribute the procurement workload to avoid the period of idleness and overwork
   - Optimize inventory management through scientific procurement procedures

   The methods in procurement process and negotiation strategies are:
   - **Open tender:** It is public bidding and thus results in low prices. Usually, the bid is published in newspapers. Quotations must be sent in the specific forms that are sold, before the time and date mentioned in the tender form. Technically two packets or two bins system is followed, and it includes technical bid and financial bid. The technical bid is opened first and shortlisted, which is supported by the opening of the financial bid of selected companies. Delayed tenders and late tenders are not accepted.
   - **Restricted or limited tender:** It is a form of procurement whereby the bid is open to selected firms, suppliers, or contractors. It is also called as limited bidding. It is less time consuming, and the preferred quality of the products is assured. The organizations usually open these types of tenders to those vendors who are already registered with them.
   - **Negotiated procurement:** The buyer approaches selected potential suppliers and bargain directly. The buyer generally invites a particular firm, suppliers, and service providers according to the procurement needs. It is preferred in the cases of long-time supply contracts.
   - **Direct procurement:** Here, the procurement is done from a single supplier at his quoted price. In these cases, the costs may be high. It is done in case of reserved for proprietary materials or low priced, small quantity and emergency purchases.
   - **Rate contract:** Firms are asked to supply stores at specified rates during the period covered by the agreement.

- **Spot purchase**: It is done by a committee, usually called a purchase committee constituted by the competent authority of the organization. The committee includes an officer from stores, accounts, and purchasing departments. The purchase committee surveys the market and makes a comparison on quality and prices and places the order for those materials which meet the criteria of the needs of the organization.
- **Risk purchase:** If the supplier fails, the item is purchased from other agencies, and the difference in cost is recovered from the first supplier.

4. **Receipt, inspection, acceptance, and payment:** While taking delivery from the road transporters, railways, customs, check containers for deficiency, and damages. If packing is damaged, insist on open delivery, checking the number of packages, individual items, weights, etc. against packing slip/challan. Any damage/loss should be registered immediately through a claims statement. All the materials must be cross-checked with the purchase order. All supplies should be inspected and certified by the purchase/stores department. In the case of bulk orders, random sampling may suffice. All necessary documentation, a daybook of receipt, goods inward note, stock ledger, purchase register, and Bin Card.

Material Receipt Register Format

Date	S. No.	Supplier's Name	PO order details	Challan details	Quantity received	Quantity accepted	Quantity rejected	Remarks	Sign

Procedure for payment: On accepting the goods and certifying correctness, send the bills to the accounts department for payment. Before releasing the amount, the accounting department should ensure that the bills bear proof of receipts of goods, certification of acceptance, and completion of purchase documentation.

5. **Storage:** Storage and preservation are an essential part of the storekeeping function. When materials remain idle in the store, these materials should be taken care of and looked after properly. Actions to protect the materials from various adverse effects:

- The store must be of adequate space.
- Divide the store into homogenous sections with separate areas mark for different groups of items, e.g., stationery, furniture, etc.
- No material should be stocked on the floor as it may be affected by dampness, white ants, etc.
- Categorize items in a group based on their generic name/application, store similar items together E.g. Stationery, Electrical, Civil Engineering, Cleaning, and related articles may be stocked in the steel racks.
- Medicine items may be stocked in the fridge.
- Keep heavy items as low and as near to the door as possible for easy retrieval. Light items may be placed on top shelves.
- Daily and monthly verification of stock should be carried out to ensure the correctness of stock.
- Hazardous materials should be segregated and stocked in a separate storehouse away from other storehouses.
- Safety precautions should be taken, and safety appliances should be provided.
- Follow two bins or double shelf system to avoid stockouts.

Codification and preparation of bin card: Based on the nature of the material and based on its generic name application, each item purchased and stocked should be given a code or identifying the number. It should be unique for each item and must be marked out in the Bin Card of the item and at its permanent locations.

Bin Card is also called as Cardex, Tag Card, etc. The detailed information about the materials is contained in the Bin Card. Typically Bin Card consists of the info like Quantity Received, Quantity Issued, Minimum Stock Level, Maximum Stock Level, Reorder Level, Re-Order Quantity, Closing Stock, Opening Stock, etc. Maintenance of the Bin Card System is part of the perpetual inventory accounting system.

Stock register: Stock Register is a register maintained by the stores in charge to record all the receipts and issues of the stock items. The given format is a typical stock register format giving all the details of inward and outward of the materials for a given period of the register. This is a summarized report of all the stock items to help the stores in charge to keep better control of the movement of the materials. Maintenance of Stock Register ensures effective inventory control.

Stock records for month/year: _____   Record holder: _____

Date	Material ID	Material Name	Opening stock	Invoice No. & Date	Received	Total Qty	Issue receipt no.	From department	Qty /U.O.M	Closing stock	Sign.	Remarks

- **Inventory control:** It is the process of having the necessary equipment and supplies available at the appropriate time. It means stocking an adequate number and kind of stores so that the materials are available whenever required and wherever required. Scientific inventory control results in optimal balance. There are different methods of inventory control. Various ways are commonly used depending upon the objective of control. The principles of selective inventory management recognize that it is impossible to manage and control every item in inventory holding in the same way.

   The functions of inventory control are to provide maximum supply service, consistent with maximum efficiency and optimum investment and to provide a cushion between forecasted and actual demand for the material.

6. **Control of Inventory Cost**
   - **Cyclic system:** This is a periodic inventory system where the physical stock position is reviewed at regular fixed intervals, and orders are placed depending on the stock on hand and rate of conception. The time interval to be chosen depends on the lead time for the procurement of the item, critically out the cost, degree of control required, etc.
   - **Two bin system:** This is a perpetual inventory system where conceptually the stock of each item is held in two bins, one larger bin contains sufficient stock to meet the demands during the interval between the arrival of order and placing of next order, the other bin contains stocks large enough to satisfy probable requirements during the period of replenishment. In the cyclic system, the ordering interval is fixed. But the quantity order varies each time. In contrast, in the two-bin system, the order quantity is fixed but the time for placing orders is not at definite intervals.

- **Lead time:** This is the time required to obtain the supply once the need is determined, i.e., it is the average number of days between placing an order and receiving the material. Lead time is composed of administrative lead time or bias time and delivery lead time or supplier's time.
- **Minimum stock or safety stock or buffer stock:** This amount of stock should be kept in reserve to avoid stock out in case of conception increases unexpectedly or in case the lead time turns out to be longer than usual. It is also the level at which fresh supply should generally arrive.

Methods of Inventory Control

Economic Order Quantity

- It is the quantity for which the cost of ordering the annual requirement of an item and the inventory carrying cost is equal. It seeks to strike a balance between purchase costs and the costs of holding inventory. Economic order quantity aims to determine the optimum amount that should be ordered such that both the ordering costs and holding cost have lowest **EOQ** = Average Monthly Consumption X Lead Time [in months] + Buffer Stock/Stock on hand. Fixation of order quantity through economic order quantity is subjected to availability of space for storage and cost, variation in the pattern of consumption, the likelihood of obsolescence, lead time for delivery, government regulations, convenience possible through reduction of work and seasonal availability.

ABC Analysis

ABC analysis helps us in segregating the items from one another and tells us how much value the things are and controlling it to what extent is in the best interest of the organization.

Class A: High-value items, which account for a significant share of annual inventory value. Class A items are controlled and purchased only on an as-required basis to minimize carrying a cost. Higher-level control is exercised, these being high-value items.

Class B: Medium value items, which do not belong to either of the classes and not so strict control procedures need to be followed regarding the items in this group. Class B items come in between A and C on the degree of control.

Class C: Low values items, but are required in large quantities and consists of various types and varieties of clips, washers. It needs only a simple and inexpensive system of control in which some of the routines may be relaxed. Class C items can be purchased in bulk for the requirement of the entire year, being of low value.

- "A" approximately 10% of items or 66.6% of the value.
- "B" approximately 20% of items or 23.3% of the value.
- "C" approximately 70% of items or 10.1% of the value.

When carrying out an ABC analysis, inventory items are valued (item cost multiplied by quantity issued/consumed in period) with the results then ranked. The results are then grouped typically into three bands. These bands are called ABC codes.

Advantages of ABC Analysis

- It helps to segregate those items which should be given priority to maximize results.
- The usefulness of this management tool is that, by focusing on the A category items, 70% of results can be achieved with just 5% effort.
- Once category items are identified, it is possible to devote more attention to these items to minimize purchase costs and exercise control over consumption in a more effective manner.
- Proper use of valuable time for store personnel.
- Simple and no confusing formulas are involved.

Disadvantages of ABC Analysis

- When several items run into several thousand, it is not convenient to compute and carry out this analysis.
- More chances of deterioration in storage exist since class C items are purchased in bulk and inventory on these piles up.
- Lose control over C may result in shortages.
- ABC focuses on monetary value and not on the functional importance of such items, resulting in shortages of critical items.
- ABC does not take into account the variation of prices of items as time goes.
- ABC ignores market conditions, market availability, competitions, seasonal variations, etc.

VED Analysis

In VED analysis, the inventory is classified as per the functional importance of the following three categories:

Vital (V) Items without which treatment comes to a standstill: i.e., unavailability cannot be tolerated. The vital items are stocked in abundance; it is required daily.

Essential (E): The unavailability of these items can be tolerated for 2–3 days because similar or alternative items are available. Essential items are stocked in average amounts; the purchase is based on rigid requirements and reasonably strict watch.

Desirable (D): Items whose unavailability can be tolerated for an extended period. Desirable items are stocked in small amounts, and the purchase is based on usage estimates.

In a manufacturing organization, several items are very vital or critical in production. Their availability must be ensured at all times for smooth production, so they need to be strictly controlled. Essential items follow vital items in their hierarchy of importance. Desirable items are the least important in terms of functional considerations, which are loosely controlled at the lower level.

Control of VED Items

- **Category I items:** these items are the most important ones and require monitoring by the administrator himself.
- **Category II items:** these items are of intermediate importance and should be under the control of the officer in charge of the stores.
- **Category III items:** these items are of least importance which can be left under the control of the storekeeper.

FSN Analysis

Fast-moving, Slow-moving, Nonmoving. Fast-moving items are used at a rapid rate, items that have moved at least once a month/day. Slow-moving items are used consistently but at a slow rate, items that have moved at least once in a period of one or two months/days. Nonmoving items should be reviewed periodically to prevent date expiry, obsolescence, and damage in storage. It may remain in the stock for several months/days.

Inventory control register

Name of the Material	Code No.	Max Level	Min. level	Reorder Level	EOQ	Units

7. **Issue/distribution:** Items held in inventory by the stores may be issued through indents to the user department on a periodical basis or as and when necessary. Systems of stocks replenishment towards are of following types:

- **Requisition or drug basket system:** At definite intervals when the departmental stock level gets low, a requisition is prepared for replenishing the stock and sent to stores. The stores then issue items in compliance with the request.

- **Par level or topping up systems:** The maximum stock level for each ward is predetermined based on usage range and frequency of replenishment. This departmental stock is stored in an assigned location.
- **Exchange cart systems:** This system is similar to the par level system in that there are predetermined maximum stock levels and predetermined intervals for stock replenishment. At predetermined intervals, the full cart from the stores is taken to the user area and exchanged for the depleted cart.

8. **Usage:** Every effort must be made at all levels in the organization to utilize supplies to avoid any form of wastage. Monitoring of consumption should be effected through monthly supply usage reports to work which summarize items consumed department wise. The material cost can also be decreased by appropriate selection of materials, cheaper substitutes, and standardization of supplies.

9. **Maintenance:** Proper maintenance of equipment, furniture, and fixtures not only ensure their almost continuous availability for use but also an extended life and productivity for the items, thus resulting in lower material costs. Time and costs of maintenance can be reduced by consideration of the following factors during the purchase of the capital assets.

- **Durability:** Since the equipment will be handled by multiple users the item should be more sturdy than that available for single person use in the home environment.
- **Periodical disinfections:** The external surface of the items should be washable, and it should provide for sterilization by moist heat, formalin vapor, spirit, or other disinfectants.
- **Repairability:** Go for items that are more easily repairable.
- **Spare parts availability:** Standardization of items and opting for those readily available in the market ensures easy availability of spare parts required for repair and maintenance.
- **Operation and service manuals:** When purchasing sophisticated equipment, it is essential to obtain the operating and service manuals so that repairs can be attended to by the hospital maintenance department without relying perpetually on the supplier.
- **Service contracts:** Better terms for service are possible by negotiating service contracts for maintenance before the purchase of the equipment. Such agreements should specify a minimum number of preventive maintenance over hard schedules, service charges, etc.
- **Stand by units:** In the hospital, work must carry on even when the equipment is down, wherever possible. It is necessary to provide for replacements to tide throughout the repair.

10. **Disposal/Condemnation:** Indents are often improperly scrutinized, and unofficial inventory builds up inwards/departments because of the hoarding of supplies. Thus the nursing supervisors should periodically inspect the stocks attached to each ward and arrange for the return of excess stock/equipment. Each hospital should also have a condemnation to review used materials that are to be disposed of. At times it is possible to recycle or reuse materials or find some other use for the item. If no further use can be found for disposables, used consumables and damaged equipment, it may still have value as scrap.

Criteria for condemnation: The equipment has become:
- Non-functional and beyond economical repair
- Non-functional and obsolete
- Functional but obsolete
- Functional but hazardous
- Functional, but no longer required

Procedure for Condemnation
- Verify records
- Preparation of history sheet of equipment
- Logbook of maintenance and repairs
- The performance record of equipment
- Put up in proper form and to the appropriate authority

Disposal
- Circulate to other units, where it is needed
- Return to the vendor, if willing to accept
- Sell to agencies, scrap dealers, etc.
- Auction
- Local destruction

11. **Collusion:** Frauds involving buyer-vendor collusion can account for a significant percentage of avoidable material costs. For the sake of commission either in the form of cash or any other kind, purchase personnel may compromise the interests of the hospital. The vendor finances such payment by infiltrating the price, overstating the quantity or through fraudulent payments. Such fraud can be prevented by intensive internal audit and by involving two or more departments or persons in purchase transactions. It is for this purchase that many hospitals set up separate departments for purchase and stores.

- **Pilferage:** Theft is not common. Items may be pilfered or stolen by the transporters, receivers, store personnel, or the users. Control of hospital theft is possible with intensive vigilance.

Material Management for Nursing Care Unit and Hospital

This department manages the materials and supplies required for a hospital to function. Supplies indicate the consumables in the hospital. A hospital requires the supplies such as medicines, surgical items, which may include glass as well as disposable items, IV fluids and other materials used for perfusion, biomedical machines, other life-supporting machine, bandages and dressing materials, antiseptics, chemicals, food and beverages, office stationery, linen, equipment maintenance materials and so on. Usually, the term equipment is referred to those items which are moreover fixed such as machinery, furniture, oxygen plants, marketing and advertising articles, public use facilities, other fixed devices, etc. The above said articles and equipment are also broadly classified as Medical and Non-Medical supplies for easy categorization. The process of purchasing the said supplies and equipment is processed through mainly three departments such as:

- General store
- Dietary division
- Pharmacy division

When getting ready for the purchase of articles, planning is done at the substantial cost of materials as well as for the extra fees that are included, for example, Transport charges, Incidental costs, Operating expenses such as hiring a technician and so on. While purchasing articles make sure to satisfy the standards such as Indian Standards Institution (ISI), which is a national body in India whose function is to monitor the quality and standard of the articles that are used by different organizations. Acquiring the said articles should be carried out remembering the accompanying viewpoints;

- The material utilized for any gear should be sturdy and safe to use. It should not be toxic or corroding.
- Should have standard shapes and measurements to fit into different circumstances.
- The article should be repairable and make sure that the spare parts are readily available.
- The article should be exchangeable.
- The surgical instruments and other supplies should pass all the mentioned quality tests and also should be sterilizable.
- Should have precision in estimations.
- It should be simple to use.

The majority of the hospital has a focal office where gear and supplies are put away and from which they are circulated to the units. The sort of materials that are kept in the focal supply room differs according to hospital policy.

Material Management during Emergencies and Disaster

The planning of crisis or emergency requires a wide assortment of provisions, gear, and assets, including personal protective equipment (PPE), cleaning equipment, and trained human resources. The process of planning ought to incorporate working together with neighborhood crisis committees and teams of state and local government bodies for deciding what all provisions, equipment, and supply should be kept by a health care organization to handle a catastrophe.

Numerous items that are readily accessible and routinely utilized in hospitals may likewise be used in a crisis. Each health care organization keeps a separate inventory to meet the emergency needs arisen due to a disaster. The following list is intended to exhibit an example of the said inventory.

General Considerations in Material Management during a Disaster

- **Supplies and Equipment:**
  - Obtain extra supplies from runners through the purchasing department.
  - Outside supplies will be requested by the Purchasing Director and conveyed to the clinic.
  - Be in charge of setting up additional beds in the hospital if necessary, and also transporting storeroom supplies and acquiring other provisions from different zones.
  - Be willing to help affected people from rescue vehicles to Triage.
- **Material Management – Purchasing.**
  - Department Head will bring in their very own workforce as required after answering to Command Center.
  - Be arranged to supply all offices with the required supplies.
  - Director will assign a deputy for the supply of additional supplies.
  - Have a state-of-the-art rundown of providers who can rapidly supply additional materials.
- **Valuables and Clothing:** Large paper or plastic packs are accessible in the treatment areas and the storeroom for patient's apparel and assets.
- **Housekeeping and Laundry:** Additional human resources may be allocated for carrying out the added burden of cleaning and maintenance of the hospital. Make sure to keep the corridors and passageways free of cleaning materials and equipment.
- **Operating Room and CSSD:** Should be equipped completely. Keep a base rundown of provisions close by and be set up to process extra sterile supplies rapidly. The anesthetists should keep up a satisfactory amount of anesthesia and other medical supplies.
- **Hospital Unit** - Supervisor will:
  - Prepare for an extension by informing the support staff of many additional beds required and where to set them up.
  - Send for additional provisions required for Purchasing, CSSD, Laundry, and Dietary.
  - Make sure the availability of supportive devices such as wheelchairs, stretchers, etc.
- **Laboratory:** There should be availability of extra blood, blood components, and if not, the necessary arrangments should be made.
- **Pharmacy:** The pharmacy department has to prepare a list prior in the hand of vendors who can provide medicines in an emergency. The pharmacy has to be opened all the time

with sufficient human resources to meet the emergency needs of the situation. The inventory and supply chain has to be monitored.

Nurses' Role in Material Management

A ward is frequently alluded to as a nursing unit. This infers a ward is in reality under the control of the nurse or in charge nurse for its support and for running its usual patient care. The nursing duties in connection to material management are recorded underneath.

Roles of Head Nurse or Nurse-in-Charge

- Responsible for keeping an adequate amount of equipment and supplies in the ward
- Make sure that equipment and supplies are in good conditions
- Put in a requisition for necessary equipment for repair and maintenance when needed.
- Make sure that equipment and supplies are conveniently located
- Make sure that all the personnel in the ward should know who may use ward articles and equipment and who assumes responsibility for it.
- The head nurse must be vigilant and prevent waste or misuse by educating the staff in the economical and appropriate use of all equipment and materials.
- She may sometimes arrange a ward class to enable the staff to know the cost of the equipment and materials.
- She should take three steps to ensure an adequate stock of available supplies in the ward or unit.
- Set a standard for the quantity of each item to be maintained in the ward all the time.
- Have a satisfactory system for the replacement of broken or worn-out equipment.
- Make regular inventories of all the items.

Responsibilities of the Ward Sister

- Materials should be in good condition.
- Indenting, accepting, storage, checking of articles, and supplies.
- Keeping up the stocks, both emergency and buffer.
- Giving responsibilities to handle supply and equipment.
- Checking for misuse and how to minimize it.
- Educating the ward staff and other health care workers in the economical use of materials.

NURSING AUDIT AND MAINTENANCE

Nursing audit refers to the assessment of the quality of clinical nursing. The nursing audit is an exercise to find out whether good nursing practices are followed. The audit is a means by which nurses can define standards from their point of view and describe the actual practice of nursing.

Clinical Audit is a quality improvement process that seeks to improve care and outcomes through a systematic review of care against criteria and the implementation of change.

Purposes of Nursing Audit

- Evaluating the nursing care given.
- Achieves deserved and available quality of nursing care.
- Stimulant to better records.
- Focuses on care provided and not on the care provider
- It contributes to research.
- To orient nurses with the quality control program for nursing.
- To justify the proposal for additional staffing or resources to the management.

Types of Audit

- **Internal auditing:** Internal auditing is a method of control carried out by an auditor who is an organization's employee. He makes an independent policy assessment, plans, and notes the deficits in policies or procedures and gives a proposal to eliminate deficiencies.
- **External auditing:** It is an independent assessment of the financial account and statements of the organization. An external auditor is a qualified person who is required to certify the annual profit and loss account and prepare a balance sheet after a thorough review of the appropriate report and document books.

Methods of Nursing Audit

There are two methods:
1. **Retrospective view:** This relates to an in-depth quality assessment after discharging the patient, having the reference of the patient's record as a source of information. The retrospective audit is a technique for assessing the quality of nursing care by examining nursing care, as reflected in the discharged patient's care documents. Specific behaviors are described in this sort of audit, then they are transformed into issues, and the auditor looks in the record for responses.
2. **The concurrent review:** This relates to assessments carried out on behalf of patients still undergoing care. It involves evaluating the patient at the bedside concerning predetermined criteria; interviewing the employees accountable for this care and assess the record and care plan of the patient.

Audit Committee

Before carrying out an audit, an audit committee should be formed, comprising of a minimum of five members who are interested in quality assurance and are clinically competent and able to work together in a group. It is recommended that each member should review not more than ten patients each month and that the auditor should have the ability to carry out an audit in about 15 minutes. If there are less than fifty discharges per month, then all the records may be audited, if there are a large number of documents to be reviewed, then an auditor may select 10% of discharges.

Process for Nursing Audit

- Formulation of nursing audit committee consists of a chairman (e.g., senior nurse) and 3-4 members (supervisors /head nurse).
- The committee should meet once a month to audit records of patients discharged during that time.
- The chairman should assign the number of charts to each member to be audited. Steps should be outlined for evaluation/auditing care.
  - Visit the unit to complete the evaluation form.
  - Compile the score for each patient.
  - Meet the committee to discuss the findings.
- Members should be sincere and impartial in their judgment. A confidential note should be sent to the individual if something very outstanding has been recorded.
- A review of the audit is done by the members of the committee, compiled and submitted to the authorities with recommendations for future action.

Nursing Audit Cycle

Below are the phases of a nursing audit cycle (Fig. 6).

- **Identify a problem or issue.** This may come from personal experience. A problem may be identified from everyday practice or a feeling that something could or should have been done better. Problems can be identified in three essential areas of practice work:
  - Structure - This refers to the resources required, for example, the number of staff and the skills they need, space, and equipment.
  - Process - This refers to the actions and decisions taken by practitioners, such as communication, assessment, education, investigations, prescribing, interventions, evaluation, and documentation.

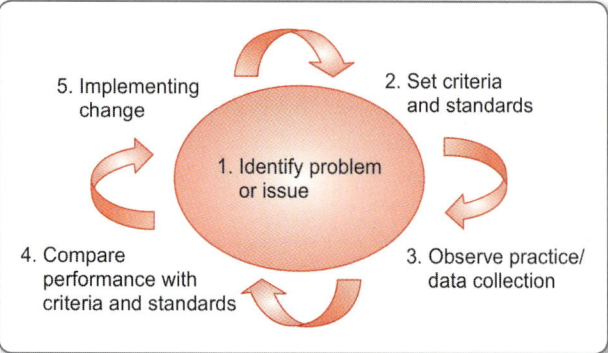

Fig. 6: Nursing audit cycle

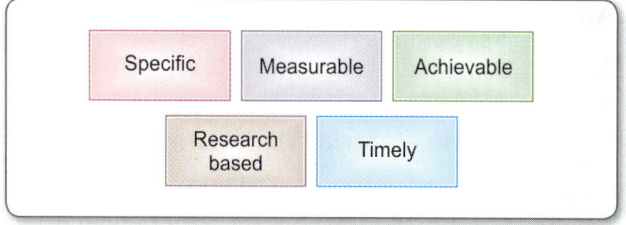

Fig. 7: SMART

- Outcome - This refers to the result of interventions such as healthy levels, patient knowledge, or satisfaction and problem priorities.
- **Set criteria and standards.** This is where you can say what should be happening. A criterion is an item of care or an aspect of practice that can be used to assess quality. The criterion is written as a statement defining what you want to measure. The criteria and standards should follow the line of **"SMART."** (Fig. 7)
  - **S: Specific**: Standards should relate to a specific area of care and should give appropriate boundaries. They should be unambiguous.
  - **M: Measurable**: If standards are vague and woolly, how can you compare your practice against them. The physically measurable aspect of a standard will facilitate comparison.
  - **A: Achievable**: There are no point writing standards that are not achievable either due to the resource or clinical limitations.
  - **R: Research-based**: Peer-reviewed research evidence will have shown the best available treatment/method for your topic area.
  - **T: Timely**: Standards should reflect current practice, not what you thought you did two years ago.
- **Collecting data on performance.** Recognize what information requires to be gathered, how it needs to be obtained and in what type, and who will retrieve it. Remember only to collect vital data.
- **Assess performance against criteria and standards.** Once the required data or information is obtained, then the analysis is carried out for the identification of problems and areas of the issues. It also helps in recognizing the field of nursing care that is below the level of established standards. This understanding of the difficulties and area below the predetermined organization standards will help in the formation of the action plan so that the identified deficiencies may be rectified. Additionally, it is also determined that how, when, and who is going to rectify the same.
- **Identify the need for change/Implementing change.** The audit cycle does not complete until the re-evaluation of the care provided is done. It is carried out to evaluate the extent of efficiency of care and practice provided. It helps in adopting the recommendations to improve the level of care.

Audit as a Tool for Quality Control

An audit is a comprehensive and formal review of the quality, and it is formally done by reviewing the records, observing the process, and evaluating the output. Healthcare auditing provides executives with a tool to apply monitoring processes to determine the value of the service provided. The nursing audit is the method of evaluating the information on the outcome of the patient, based on the nursing process. It evaluates the efficiency of nursing interventions that are provided to solve the problems identified at the stage of assessment. Structure audit, Process audit, and Outcome audit are the audits most frequently used in quality control.

- **Structure audit:** The structural review supervises the framework or the location in which patient treatment takes place, such as financial expenses of the procedure, nursing care quality, the physical facilities of the health care organization and records that are maintained including the workplace environment. This audit implies that there is a connection between the qualities of the care provided and the context in which it is provided. These can take place retrospectively, simultaneously and prospectively.
- **Process audit:** It is the assessment of the process of care or the way how the nursing care was delivered to the patient. It is mainly based on the established criteria or standards that are governing the administration of different nursing procedures. It is based on the concept that a relationship exists between the quality of the care and the quality of the nurse. The quality of the nurse is explained as the ability to follow the standards and norms.
- **Outcome audit:** These are the 'end' results or output of nursing care. This is based on patient health status. The improvement in the patient's health status can be attributed to the quality delivery of nursing care. It assumes the relationship between quality care and progressive outcome. The assessment of the rate of mortality, morbidity, duration of hospital stay is based on this outcome audit. It is a traditional method of quality assurance.

Advantages of Nursing Audit

- It can be used as a method of measurement in all areas of nursing.
- It is a scoring system, relatively simple, and its results are easily understood.
- It assesses the work of all those involved in recording care.
- It may be a useful tool as part of a quality assurance program in areas where accurate records of care are kept.

Disadvantages of the Nursing Audit

- It appraises the outcomes of the nursing process, so it is not so useful in areas where the nursing process has not been implemented.
- It is time-consuming since it requires a team of trained auditors.

 REVIEW QUESTIONS

1. Define staffing. Enlist the objectives of staffing and explain its methods in detail.
2. Explain staff scheduling and scheduling policies.
3. Define recruitment and explain the purpose and its types.
4. Explain the sources of recruitment.
5. Explain training and development.
6. Explain the selection and various steps in the selection process.
7. Define placement. Explain its process and significance.
8. What are the methods of Projecting Staffing Requirements?
9. Explain credentialing.
10. Explain the concept of transfer.
11. Explain human resource management in the hospital and community.
12. What is staff welfare? Explain the methods of staff welfare.
13. Define job description and elaborate on the job description of nursing personnel in a hospital.
14. Define SIU. Explain its recommendation.
15. Brief the staffing requirement according to IPHs norms.
16. Explain the PCS.
17. Brief absenteeism and employee turnover.
18. Define In-service education. Explain the objectives and approaches in detail.
19. Discuss the components of in-service education. Explain the scope of in-service education.
20. Enumerate problems of in-service education.

Contd…

21. Discuss the types of in-service education and its evaluation.
22. Explain the concept of Adult Education; discuss its objectives.
23. Discuss the principles of adult learning.
24. Enumerate the types and importance of adult learning.
25. Explain material management and its process.
26. Explain material management during the disaster and the role of a nurse manager in material management.
27. Define nursing audit. Brief the types and methods of the nursing audit. Explain Nursing Audit Cycle.

Further Readings

1. Banerjee, Shyamal. Principles and Practice of Management. Oxford and IBM Publishing, New Delhi; 2000.
2. Basavanthappa BT. Nursing Administration. 2nd Edition: Jaypee Brothers Medical Publishers (P) Ltd., New Delhi; 2009.
3. Barrett, Jean. Ward Management and Teaching. Konark Publishers, Delhi; 1992.
4. Warren, Stevens, F. Management and Leadership in Nursing. McGraw – Hill Inc, New York; 1978.
5. Alexander et al. Nursing Service Administration. Mosby Publishers, US; 1962.
6. Park K. Preventive and Social Medicine, 19th Edition: M/s. Banarasidas Bhanot Publishers, Jabalpur; 2007.
7. Basavanthappa BT. Nursing Administration, 1st Edition: Jaypee Brothers Medical Publishers (P) Ltd., New Delhi; 2002.
8. Goel SL, Kumar R. Management of Hospitals – Hospital Administration in the 21st century, Vol. 4, Deep and Deep Publication, New Delhi; 2002.
9. Ranga Rao SP. Administration of Primary Health Centers in India, 1st Edition: Mittal Publications, New Delhi; 1993.
10. Lucita M. Nursing: Practice and Public Health Administration. Current Concepts and Trends. B. I. Churchill Living Stone Pvt. Ltd., New Delhi; 2002.
11. Sakharkar BM. Principles of Hospital Administration and Planning, 2nd Edition: Jaypee Brothers Medical Publishers (P) Ltd., New Delhi; 2009.
12. Patricia S Yoder-Wise. Leading and Managing in Nursing. 2nd Edition: Mosby Publication, US; 1999.
13. Bessie L Marquis, Carol J Huston. Leadership Roles and Management Functions in Nursing: Theory and Application. 5th Edition: Lippincott Williams and Wilkins, New York; 2006.
14. Linda Roussel. Management and Leadership for Nurse Administrators. 4th Edition: Jones and Bartlett Publication, USA; 2006.
15. Wehrich H, Koontz H. Management A Global Perspective. 11th Edition: Tata McGraw-Hill Publishing Company, Ltd., New Delhi; 2005.
16. Marquis BL, Huston CJ. Leadership and Management Functions in Nursing- Theory, and Application. 5th Edition: Lippincott Williams and Wilkins, Philadelphia; 2006.
17. Douglass LM. The Effective Nurse: Leader and Manager. 5th Edition: Mosby Publication, US; 1996.
18. Trained Nurses Association of India, Nursing Administration, and Management.
19. Samson Rebecca. Leadership and Management in Nursing Practice and Education 1st Edition: Jaypee Brothers Medical Publishers (P) Ltd., New Delhi; 2009.
20. Kunders GD. Designing for Total Quality in Health Care, Prism Book Pvt. Ltd., Bangalore; 2002.
21. Chandorkar AG. Hospital Administration and Planning. 2nd Edition: Paras Medical Publisher, New Delhi; 2009.
22. Joshi DC, Joshi Mamta. Hospital Administration. 1st Edition: Jaypee Brothers Medical Publishers (P) Ltd., New Delhi; 2009.
23. Eleanor J Sullivan, Philip J Decker. Effective Leadership and Management in Nursing. 4th Edition: Published by Addison Wesely; 2011.
24. Kulkarni GR. Financial Management for Hospital Administration, Jaypee Brothers Medical Publishers (P) Ltd., New Delhi; 2009.

Unit

6

Directing and Leading

 Unit Outline

BASIC CONCEPTS OF DIRECTING

In the ordinary sense, directing means giving instructions and guiding people in doing work. In our daily life, we come across many situations like a hotel owner directing his employees to complete certain activities for organizing a function, a teacher directing his student to complete an assignment, a film director directing the artists about how they should act in the film, etc. In all these situations, we can observe that directing is done to achieve some predetermined objective. In the context of management of an organization, directing refers to the process of instructing, guiding, counseling, motivating and leading people in the organization to achieve its objectives. You can observe here that directing is not a mere issue of communication but encompasses many elements like supervision, motivation, and leadership. It is one of the key managerial functions performed by every manager.

Direction means giving orders to start the operation for the implementation of a policy or a plan. The direction is the issuance of orders, assignments, and instructions that permit the subordinate to understand what is expected of him, and the guidance and overseeing of the subordinate so that he can contribute effectively and efficiently to the attainment of organizational objectives. Directing is a managerial process that takes place throughout the life of an organization. The main characteristics of directing are discussed below:

- Directing initiates action: Directing is a key managerial function. A manager has to perform this function along with planning, organizing, staffing and controlling while discharging his duties in the organization.
- Directing takes place at every level of management: Every manager, from the top executive to supervisor performs the function of directing. The directing takes place wherever superior-subordinate relations exist.
- Directing is a continuous process: It takes place throughout the life of the organization irrespective of people occupying managerial positions.
- Directing flows from top to bottom: Directing is first initiated at the top level and flows to the bottom through the organizational hierarchy.

Definitions

The direction is a complex function that includes all those activities that are designed to encourage subordinates to work effectively and efficiently in both the short and long run.

—**Koonts and O'Donnell**

Direction consists of process and technique utilized in issuing the instructions and making certain that operations are carried on as originally planned, Directing is the process around which all the performances revolve.

—**Theo Haimann**

Importance of Directing

The importance of directing can be understood by the fact that every action in the organization is initiated through directing only. Directing guides towards the achievement of common objectives.

- Directing helps to initiate action by people in the organization towards the attainment of desired objectives.
- Directing integrates employees' efforts in the organization in such a way that every individual effort contributes to organizational performance. Thus, it ensures that individuals work for organizational goals.
- Directing guides employees to fully realize their potential and capabilities by motivating and providing effective leadership. A good leader can always identify the potential of his employees and motivate them to extract work up to their full potential.
- Directing facilitates the introduction of needed changes in the organization. Generally, people tend to resist changes in the organization. Effective directing through motivation, communication, and leadership helps to reduce such resistance and develop required cooperation in introducing changes in the organization.
- Effective directing help to bring stability and balance in the organization since it fosters cooperation and commitment among the people and helps to achieve balance among various groups, activities, and departments.

Elements of direction: Directing includes the following activities:

- **Giving orders:** The central task of directing is giving orders. The order is the technical means through which a subordinate understands what is to be done. An order or instruction initiates, modifies, guides, and terminates activities in the organization. A good order consists of the following characteristics:
  - Clear and complete
  - Easily understandable
  - Reasonable and attainable
  - Avoid offensive communication
  - Specification of time to be followed to carry out the order.
- **Supervision:** Supervision is the activity of the management that is concerned with the training and discipline of the workforce. It includes follow up to assure the prompt and proper execution of orders. Supervision is the act of overseeing, watching, and directing with authority, the work and behavior of others. The term supervision can be understood in two ways. Firstly, it can be understood as an element of directing and secondly, as a function performed by supervisors in the organizational hierarchy. Supervision being an element of directing, every manager in the organization supervises his/her subordinates. In this sense, supervision can be understood as the process of guiding

the efforts of employees and other resources to accomplish the desired objectives.

Importance of Supervision

- The supervisor maintains day-to-day contact and maintains friendly relations with workers.
- The supervisor acts as a link between workers and management.
- The supervisor plays a key role in maintaining group unity among workers placed under his control.
- The supervisor ensures the performance of work according to the targets set.

- **Leading:** Leadership is the ability to inspire and influence others to contribute to the attainment of the objectives. Successful leadership is the result of the interaction between the leader and his subordinates in a particular organizational situation. Whenever we hear the success stories of any organization, we are immediately reminded of their leaders. Can you imagine Microsoft without Bill Gates, Reliance Industries without Ambanis, Infosys without Narayana Murthy, Tata without J.R.D. Tata or Wipro without Azim Premji. You would say it is not possible to achieve success without such great leaders. The leaders always play a key role in the success and excellence of any organization.

  - Leadership indicates the ability of an individual to influence others.
  - Leadership tries to bring change in the behavior of others.
  - Leadership indicates interpersonal relations between leaders and followers.
  - Leadership is exercised to achieve the common goals of the organization.
  - Leadership is a continuous process.

- **Motivating:** Motivation refers to how the needs (urges, aspirations, and desires) control and direct to explain the behavior of human beings. The manager must motivate or cause the employee to follow directives. While discussing motivation, we need to understand three interrelated terms motive, motivation, and motivators.

  - **Motive:** A motive is an inner state that energizes, activates or moves and directs behavior towards goals. Motives arise out of the needs of individuals. The realization of a motive causes restlessness in the individual, which prompts some action to reduce such restlessness.
  - **Motivation:** Motivation is the process of stimulating people to action to accomplish the desired goals. Motivation depends on satisfying the needs of people.
  - **Motivators:** Motivator is the technique used to motivate people in an organization. Managers use diverse motivators like pay, bonus, promotion, recognition, praise, responsibility, etc., in the organization to influence people to contribute their best.

- **Communicating:** Communication is the passing of information and understanding from a sender to the receiver. Communication is vital to the directing function of the management; one way to visualize this importance is to view the manager on one side of a barrier and the workgroup on the other. Communication is how the manager can reach through the fence to attain workgroup activity. Communication plays a key role in the success of a manager. How much professional knowledge and intelligence a manager possesses becomes immaterial if he is not able to communicate effectively with his subordinates and create an understanding in them. The abilities of a manager mainly depends upon his communication skills. That is why the organization always emphasize on improving communication skills of managers as well as employees.

- **Coordination:** It is the synchronization of people and activities so that they can function smoothly in the attainment of organizational objectives. For example, in a hospital, the actions of doctors, nurses, ward attendants, and lab technicians must be appropriately coordinated if we desire to provide the best care to the patient.

Principles of Direction

The principles to be observed by management in the direction of its subordinates are as follows:

- **Leadership:** It is necessary for the boss to possess the qualities of a good leader. The subordinates feel happy to work when they get useful commands from their boss. It includes solutions for professional as well as personal problems.

- **Motivation:** Motivated workers always work hard to achieve the objectives of the organization. The authority of direction should always be motivating to the workers/subordinates.

- **Harmony of objectives:** The balance of individual objectives and organizational objectives is a must in any organization. The direction should be in such a way that the individual feels that they can integrate their targets with the purposes of the organization.

- **Maximum individual contribution:** The progress of the organization always relies on the maximum participation of its employees.

- **Unity of command:** This principle requires that the employees should receive orders from one superior only. The violation of this principle may lead to confusion and indiscipline.

- **Direct supervision:** Personal contact and face to face interaction always foster the organization's climate. It also ensures a successful direction.

- **Comprehension:** The accuracy of the direction largely depends on how instruction is given to a subordinate and what the education is.

- **Appropriateness of direction technique:** The technique used by the management for direction should be appropriate to ensure effective instruction. The different methods of direction briefed below.

Approaches/ Techniques of Direction

- **Consultative direction:** Here, the Boss decides after consulting the subordinates regarding the feasibility and workability of the task and issues a direction to the assistants.
- **Autocratic direction:** Here, the Boss takes a decision and issues a direction to the subordinates, but no consultation or suggestion is expected from the subordinates regarding the feasibility and workability of the task.
- **Free-rein direction:** Under this method, the subordinates are encouraged and enabled to show his/her initiative and give independent thought to the solution of the problem. This technique is used only if the assistants are highly educated, efficient, and sincere.

Importance of Direction

- Direction initiates action. It acts as the driving force of all execution.
- It integrates the efforts of the actions of the members in the group towards the achievement of the desired goals.
- It brings about healthy changes in the organization.
- It helps in bringing out the maximum potential of the individual.
- It is referred to as the heart of the organization as it helps in the achievement of the mission and vision of the organization.

SUPERVISION

Supervision and guidance are some of the essential functions of any organization. Every organization has a provision for supervision. In common man's language supervision means overseeing the employees at work. Here let us discuss in detail the role of a supervisor and supervision in managing people.

Definition

It has been defined as the authoritative direction of the work of one's subordinates.
Supervision is defined as guiding and directing efforts of the employees and other resources to accomplish stated work outputs.   —**Terry and Franklin**
It is the act of watching a person or activity and making certain that everything is done correctly and safely.

—**Cambridge Dictionary**

Objectives of Supervision

- To help the staff to carry out their responsibility skillfully and adequately to give the most extreme yield with the least assets cost viability.
- Improves the autonomy and productivity of the individual.
- To guide and help with meeting foreordained works.
- To help to persuade subordinates to keep up high confidence, i.e., the advancement of inspiration and trust among all the nursing staff.
- To help the individuals from the group to perceive issues, recognize an answer, and to make a move.
- To help to create camaraderie and advance cooperation for successful working.
- To help to enhance the mentalities of the individuals towards the work or program, i.e., crossing over any barrier between individual and group/organizational objectives by giving direction the correct way.

Principles of Supervision

- Supervision must be practiced without giving the subordinate a feeling that they are being administered.
- Supervision endeavors to make the unit a decent learning circumstance. It should be a learning process.
- Supervision should cultivate the capacity of each staff to think and represent himself/herself.
- Supervision ought to energize the participatory approach in planning and decision making through effective communication.
- Supervision ought to have the solidarity to impact downwards based on their ability to influence upwards.
- Supervision ought to make a reasonable atmosphere for profitable work.
- Supervision should offer self-governance to laborers contingent upon identity, competence, and attributes and continue to aim at staff development and improvement.

Types of Supervision

Generally, there are two types of supervision:
1. **Direct supervision:** This is done through face to face talk with the workers. This can be exercised at the educational institutions, ward/unit level in the hospital or PHC or sub-center of the community setting.
2. **Indirect supervision:** It is done in reference to records and reports of the workers and through written instructions or some agency between the supervisor and supervisee.

Methods/Approaches to Supervision

Supervision is an effective procedure with a goal for the enhancement of nursing administration. To accomplish this goal, there are diverse techniques or ways to deal with supervision, which include:

- **Creative versus technical supervision:** Creative supervision gives the most significant adjustment to the circumstance. E.g. Rather than an introduction time of about fourteen days for each new staff, a variable arrangement should be designed according to the needs of the individual in both the content and duration. Technical strategies are a portion of the fundamental supervisory aptitudes that should be prepared. Gathering meetings, conducting discussions in a group, etc.
- **Cooperative versus authoritarian supervision:** In the first type, there is a full interest of every individual in arranging and decision making while in the second type, it is dictator supervision that fixates entirely on the chief, with the staff following his/her requests. Both are required by circumstances and conditions.
- **Scientific versus intuitive supervision:** The Scientific Supervision is based on facts, rules, and regulations derived scientifically. The second type is based on the law of marinating relationships. This supervision needs a delicate and automatic response to accomplish the ideal objective.

Supervisory Styles

Each manager has an alternate style of directing. This might be depicted as following;

- **Task-centered:** Here, the boss concentrates on the work and output rather than the human resources required for it. The attention is focused on the productivity of higher outcomes, but the human element is not regarded.
- **Employee centered manager:** Here, the administrator focuses on fellow workers more than the task or output. It is more human but lacks the focus on the task assigned.
- **Autocratic or critical supervisor:** A dictator who cannot endure any deviation from standards and nature of work. The choices are made independent from anyone else.
- **Benevolent supervisor:** The leader is very protective of his/her subordinates, keep telling them what they should do and what they should not, thus providing constant direction, such supervisor is usually liked by the workers but is valid as long as they are physically present as they tend to develop the subordinates as dependent followers.
- **Democratic supervisor:** A leader who believes in a style of—let us agree on what we are to do in dealing with the subordinates. Such a supervisor provides guidance only when requested by the assistants.

Functions of Supervisor

- **The orientation of newly posted staff:** Transfers and postings, or new postings of personnel are shared in all organization. All newcomers should be informed about their functions, the method that they should adopt, the staff with whom they will work and the community wherein they will work, through an orientation.

- **Check the workload of employees:** It must be ensured that the workload is within the physical and mental competence of a worker. Otherwise, the job should not be assigned to them. A supervisor should not expect workers a level of effort that is beyond them.
- **Arranging for the flow of materials:** A supervisor must find out the needs for supplies and equipment and arrange for their supply in a good time.
- **Coordination of the efforts:** A supervisor coordinates the work of his/her workers and agencies and promotes teamwork.
- **Promotion of effectiveness of workers:** This may be done through performance evaluation and introducing concepts of staff development.
- **Promotion of social contact and flow of communication:** Social connections help to bring the staff together and increase group cohesiveness. A free flow of communication among members is necessary for teamwork. A good supervisor should provide equal opportunity to all the workers.
- **Assist the individuals in managing their issues:** Personal problems are likely to come up while dealing with workers. Those may not be the supervisors' duties, but a sympathetic understanding of his part improves individual morale.
- **Raising the level of motivation:** All good work should be given due credit through recognition. The supervisor must provide opportunities for growth and achievements.
- **Establishment of control:** Supervision is a control measure as well as a leadership technique. The supervisor must know what is being done and with what effectiveness. Several technologies, such as observation and record review, can be used for this purpose.
- **Development of confidence:** Supervisors must know the background of workers and try to develop trust. There is a need to combine understanding with firmness and to take a personal interest without sacrificing impracticality or discipline.
- **Emphasis on achievement:** It has been proved that the development of a monotonous work routine and the improvement of human relations without a corresponding focus on goal achievement are not likely to increase productivity.
- **Record keeping:** The supervisor should maintain a proper record system.

GUIDANCE

A unique feature of guidance is the presentation of knowledge, information, or advice to individuals or groups in a structured way that provides sufficient material upon which choices or decisions are made.

Definitions

Guidance involves giving personal help, which is designed to assist a person in deciding where he wants to go, what he wants to do, or how he can best accomplish his goals.

—**Jones (1951)**

The fundamentals of all guidance include the assistance given by a competent person to an individual so that the latter may make his own decisions and carry them out.

—**Crow and Crow**

Elements of Guidance

- The guidance focuses on the individual rather than the problem.
- It helps to the discovery of one's abilities and potential.
- It is based on interests, abilities, assets, needs, and limitations of the individual.
- It gives rise to self-direction and self-development.
- It makes the individual plan wisely for the present and future.
- It helps the individual adapt to the new environments.
- It helps in achieving success and happiness.

Purposes of Guidance

- **Understanding the individual:** The primary purpose of the guidance is to discover and understand capacities, potentials, abilities, aptitudes, interests, weak and strong points of the individual and to evaluate the self concerning personal and social experiences to use the person more efficiently in everyday living.
- **Helping the individual to make adjustments:** Guidance assists an individual to make satisfactory and maximum adjustments at home, school or society by giving him informational services such as individual inventory and occupational information services, counseling services, placement and follow up services.
- **Developing personal abilities and potentials:** Guidance helps individuals improve their talents and potentialities. It helps them utilize their efforts and make their own decisions and choices. It also helps them to direct their lives.
- **Improving school activities:** A guidance program helps the school staff to solve various problems and promote all operations of the school.
- **Coordinating home, school, and society:** Erickson has correctly said that one of the essential purposes of guidance has been to organize the home, school, and community influences on the child.

  According to Erickson, the purposes of guidance can be as below:
  - Coordination
  - A careful study of individual

- Assisting the school staff
- Counseling
- Informational services
- Placement and follow up

Types of Guidance

- **Educational guidance:** Guidance services are meant to help students make proper adjustments with the environment in which they are living and also make the best possible contributions commensurate with one's strengths and limitations. Educational guidance refers to the guidance that the students get in all aspects of education such as how to study, using the standard tools of learning, adjusting the school life and other activities, regularly attending the school tasks, learning to speak, interview, compose in writing, take examinations, use libraries, make critical educational decisions at each stage.
- **Vocational guidance:** Vocational guidance is functionally an effort that reinforces the priceless native capacities of youth and the costly training provided in schools. It helps the individual to invest and use his capabilities where they will bring the highest satisfaction and success to him and benefit to society. It helps the individual develop his or her potentials to an optimum level. It is a process that allows an individual to choose and occupation in life, prepare for it and find a suitable job.
- **Personal guidance:** Personal guidance is the assistance offered to an individual to solve his emotional, social, ethical, moral, and health problems. It deals with all of the issues of life. It is concerned with social and civic activities, health and physical activities, proper use of leisure time and character-building activities. It is majorly concerned with the individual and social problems. It also helps the individual in his moral and spiritual development.
- **Recreational guidance:** An individual needs assistance in choosing recreational activities that are suited to his characteristics.
- **Group guidance:** It improves students' attitudes and behavior. It helps in assisting an individual in the group in solving his problems and making necessary adjustments.

PARTICIPATORY MANAGEMENT

Participative Management alludes to an open type of administration where workers have effectively collaborated with the association's essential leadership and decision-making process. This idea is used by the directors who comprehend the significance of human judgment and look for a robust association with their workers. They understand that the workers are the facilitators who bargain straightforwardly with the clients and fulfill their requirements. To beat the opposition in the market and to remain in front of the debate, this type of board has been used by numerous associations. They welcome the inventive thoughts, ideas, and considerations from the workers and include them in the necessary leadership, planning, and decision-making process.

Participative Management can likewise be named as 'Mechanical Democracy,' 'Co-assurance,' 'Representative Involvement,' and additionally 'Participative Decision Making.' The idea of worker interest in the association's essential leadership is not new. Even though the hypothesis of participative administration is as old as the establishment of workers' businesses, still, it is not connected by a large extent of associations. Usage of the rationality of participatory decision making by high-level administration sets the phase for including more individuals and maybe even the whole staff in settling on choices at the dimension at which activity happens. The participatory approach in administration is beneficial for an result orientated functioning. Here the allotted target is achieved with great zeal and commitment and the workers acknowledges their role, functions and performance.

In nursing, as like any other profession participatory decision making in assignment and delegation of responsibilities improves responsibility, cooperation and collaboration. The first line supervisor with assigned power and authority maintain the liaison with other departments that are involved in care giving process.

Advantages

- It relieves high-level administrators from the weight of overseeing.
- Motivates subordinates to embrace duty, and it gives more freedom to the higher officials.
- Create provisions for competitions among departments and promotes growth.
- The manager will be prepared for rapid modifications in the company/department.

Limitations

- Maintenance of uniform arrangement all through association may be troublesome.
- It increases the multifaceted nature of coordination and increases the risk of loss of control.
- Require extensive training for employees.
- An insufficient number of trained staff at a lower level.
- It might be constrained by outside elements like government directions, and so on.

Decision making lies deeply embedded in the management process and is the only vehicle for carrying the managerial workload. Nurses should be actively involved in decision making at all levels rather than merely obeying the decisions. It is valid only when it is timely done. It needs courage as well as creative thinking on the part of the nurse administrator.

INTERPROFESSIONAL COLLABORATION

We have all participated in teams, but the culture of health care has long emphasized solo acts. The nurse acts apart from the physician, who is unaware of the physical therapist's role. Meanwhile, the pharmacist fails to communicate with members of the medical office staff. This series will emphasize why interprofessional collaboration (IPC) is important, and it will provide concrete examples of how to make IPC work across multiple settings.

Interprofessional collaboration is defined as "when multiple health workers from different professional backgrounds work together with patients, families, carers (caregivers), and communities to deliver the highest quality of care." It is based on the concept that when providers consider each other's perspective, including that of the patient, they can deliver better care. Interprofessional education occurs "when two or more professionals learn with, about, and from each other to enable effective collaboration and improve health outcomes."

To provide proper care and improve patient outcomes, today's nurses must collaborate effectively with members of the healthcare team from other disciplines. That means working together as team members and team leaders. To do that, they must understand each member's education, the scope of practice, and areas of expertise. Learning the language, norms, and special foci of other disciplines foster a more effective use of resources and knowledge.

Benefits of Interprofessional Collaboration

- Reduced error in the provision of care
- Decreased length of stays for every patient as a healthy outcome is easily obtained
- Improved health of patients of caregivers
- Better pain management through easy communication and collaboration
- Improved quality of life
- Higher patient satisfaction
- Cost savings
- Healthy work environments and Job satisfaction

However, currently, IPC is the exception, not the rule. Each of the health professions must shift its focus toward collaboration, partnerships, and sharing, rather than operate in silos. The quality and safety of care, and the need to contain costs, require all professions to work together in an environment of respect. With a projected shortage of healthcare providers, including physicians and nurses, it is imperative to rely on interprofessional practice to work collaboratively and more efficiently. If the team's professionals do not communicate and collaborate, their performance suffers. In the healthcare field, poor communication is often cited as a root cause of medical errors. Effective teamwork and good working relationships can reduce errors and improve outcomes. Besides, patients are "handed off" with each transition in care, increasing the risk for error to the patient with each handoff. With the efficient transfer of essential information, IPC can mitigate some of the risks associated with these transitions. IPC optimizes patient outcomes by improving communication and teamwork.

Another reason IPC is important is that it promotes coordination of care across the continuum of health care in all settings. Working as a team, the patient's care is coordinated throughout the healthcare continuum. This promotes the sharing of knowledge and working toward a common goal where each professional learns about each other's roles and responsibilities from each other.

Furthermore, IPC is critical for the success of patient-centered care. Patient-centered care is "providing care that is respectful of and responsive to individual patient preferences, needs, and values and ensuring that patient values guide all clinical decisions." This replaces the traditional physician-centered system with one that revolves around the patient. Such a system works well with the team-based approach of IPC.

Barriers to Interprofessional Collaboration

Despite these benefits, it is clear that creating IPC is not easy. Many influential factors affect the relationship with one another. Although data are starting to emerge showing the value of team-based care, there are many obstacles to its implementation. Some of these include:

- Gender, power, socialization, education, status, cultural differences between professions. The traditional culture of healthcare training and practice has been to work in silos. Professionals are not used to working collaboratively across disciplines. There is little exposure to each other's roles and perspectives. This fosters miscommunication, mistrust, conflict, and a lack of coordinated care.
- Lack of a payment system and structures that reward interprofessional collaboration.
- The misunderstanding of the scope and contribution of each profession.
- Turf protection: Physicians historically have been autonomous and dominant of other health professions, rather than collaborative. Hence, the decision on the boundary of the care, rights and decision-making influence the spirit of IPC.

There are many benefits to IPC. It can improve safety and healthcare delivery, as well as reduce costs. It puts the patient at the center of the healthcare team's focus and allows all health professionals, with the patient, to collaboratively provide input, be part of the decision making, and improve outcomes. Although there are several obstacles to IPC, adopting this team-based culture of mutual respect and understanding is possible and, in fact, necessary.

MANAGEMENT BY OBJECTIVES

It is also known as management by results (MBR). It was popularized by Peter Drucker in 1954 through his book *The Practice of Management*. It is the process where the manager defines some specific objectives and conveys to the members of the organization. The members decide the methods to achieve each target in a sequence. It helps the manager to organize the work and maintain a productive environment.

Definitions

The MBO is a management system in which the objectives of an organization are agreed upon so that the management and employees understand a common way forward.

—**Business Dictionary**

A process whereby the superior and subordinate managers of an enterprise jointly identify its common goals, define each individual's area of responsibility in terms of the results expected of him and use these measures as guides for operating the units and assessing the contribution of each of its members. —**George S Odiorne**

Purposes

- MBO helps to identify the goals, aims, and objectives of the organization.
- It attempts to achieve the defined goals by giving individual managers, supervisors, and other sub-goals or targets related to significant purposes.
- It also gives a provision to make an assessment of the degree of achievement of goals or targets set.

In **MBO** the goals are expected to be **SMART** (Fig. 1)

Features of MBO

- An attempt is made by the management to integrate the goals of an organization and individuals. This will lead to effective management.
- MBO tries to combine the long-range goals of the organization with short-range goals.
- Management tries to relate to the organization's goals with social goals.

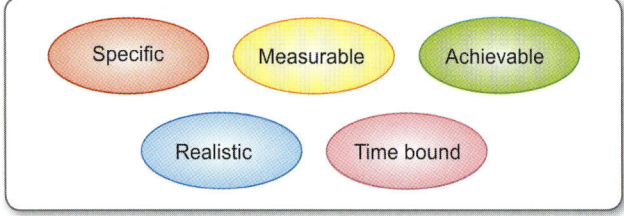

Fig. 1: SMART

- It pays consistent attention to refining, modifying, and improving the goals and changing the approaches to achieve the objectives based on experience.
- It increases the organizational capability of achieving the goals at all levels.
- MBO's emphasis is not only on goals but also on productive performance.
- A high degree of motivation and satisfaction is available to employees through MBO. (Recognizes the participation of employees in the goal-setting process).
- Encourages a climate of trust, goodwill, and a will to perform.

Process of MBO

The MBO process is characterized by the balance of objectives of the organization and individual. The method of MBO is given below:

- **Defining organizational goals:** Initially, corporate goals are framed by the top-level employees of an organization which then moves downwards. The definition of organizational goals states why the business is started and exists. First, long-term goals are framed then short-term goals are framed, taking into account the feasibility of achieving long-term goals.
- **Goals of each section:** Objectives of each chapter, department, or division are framed based on the overall objectives of the organization. The period within which these objectives should be achieved is also fixed. (Goals or objectives are expressed in a meaningful manner).
- **Fixing key result areas:** Profitability, Market standing, Innovation, etc., are set based on organizational objectives and arranged on a priority basis. It indicates the strength of the organization.
- **Setting subordinate/sub-objectives or targets:** The objectives of each subordinate or individual are fixed. There should be a free and frank discussion between the superior and his subordinates. Subordinates are induced to set standards themselves by giving an opportunity.
- **Matching resources with objectives:** The objectives are framed based on the availability of resources. If specific resources (technical personnel or raw material) are not adequately available, the purposes of an organization are changed accordingly. So there is a need for matching resources with goals. Next, the available resources should be appropriately allocated and utilized.
- **Periodic review meetings:** The superior and the subordinates should hold meetings periodically in which they discuss the progress in the accomplishment of objectives. The fixed standards may be changed in light of growth and development. But the underlying conditions do not change.
- **Appraising of activities:**
  - At the end of the fixed period for achieving the objectives, there should be a discussion between the superior and subordinates. (The discussion is related to subordinates' performance against the specific standards).
  - The superior should take corrective action. The superior should identify the reasons for the failure of achieving the objectives.
  - The problems faced by the subordinates should be identified, and steps should be taken to tackle such issues.
- **Reappraisal of objectives:** An organization is living in a dynamic world. (There are a lot of changes within a short period). The survival and growth of a modern business organization largely depend on putting up with the changing conditions. So the top-level executive should review the organization's objective to frame the goals according to the changing situation.

Advantages

- MBO is a well-known approach to plan and evaluate the work done in organizations, and it can be used by any individual in the organization.
- It can be used as a total system of management throughout the organization, including financial management.
- They serve as a planning guide and encourage goal-directed behavior rather than random activity.
- It helps the managers to understand their role in the entire organization.

Disadvantages

- MBO can be a meaningless exercise if the objectives are not used after they are written.
- The objectives will become an overly demanding and rigid standard if it is used in an authoritarian manner, and it appears to staff as a punishment/control system rather than as a guide.
- The objectives may become a source of unrealistic demands, especially if goals are set higher and higher each year.

Implications of MBO in Nursing

- Measures and judge the performance of the staff.
- Correlates individual performance to organizational goals.
- Clarifies job responsibilities expected from staff.
- Increase the competency and growth of subordinates.

TEAM MANAGEMENT

A team is an association or group of individuals working together to achieve a goal. In other words, when one person cannot accomplish a job alone and several individuals cooperate to fulfill a mission, then a team is required. The better the cooperation, communication, and coordination among team members, the more efficient the team is.

Structuring an organization into teams should be seen as a strategic initiative to achieve operational effectiveness. Strategic positioning is essential to long term performance. However, the formation of teams without effective position and focus will not lead to successful sustained performance. It is designed to improve the bottom line of the organization's performance. Teams are not an end in themselves but a means to involve people in managing their piece of business more effectively.

Characteristics of High Performing Teams

- Clearly-defined goals matching with reasonable outcomes
- Accurate effective two-way communication
- Leadership is shared and participation encouraged
- Effective decision making and problem-solving
- Team identity and cohesiveness
- Diverse backgrounds and experience
- Cooperation and collaboration

Team Development

As per Tuckman's theory/hypothesis, there are five phases in development of team.

1. **Forming:** This stage is typically described by some perplexity and vulnerability. The real objectives of the team have not been set up. The idea of the errand or authority of the team has not been resolved. Accordingly, forming is an introductory period when individuals become acquainted with each other and offer assumptions regarding the team. These sentiments fortify in later phases of improvement. People are regularly confounded amid this stage since jobs are not clear, and there may not be a solid head.

2. **Storming:** Here, the team is probably going to see the largest amount of difference and struggle. Individuals frequently challenge aggregate objectives and the battle for power. People often compete for the initial position amid this phase of advancement.

3. **Norming:** This stage is portrayed by the acknowledgment of individual contrasts and shared desires. Ideally, at this stage, the team individuals will start to build up a sentiment of team union and character.

4. **Performing:** Performing happens when the team has developed and achieved a sentiment of cohesiveness. Amid this phase of advancement, people acknowledge each other, and strife is settled through group talk. Individuals from the team decide on choices through a sound procedure that is centered around significant objectives as opposed to severe subject matters.

5. **Adjourning:** All the teams do not undergo this stage since it is described by the disbandment of the group. Reasons may vary, but the common cause is the accomplishment of the objectives. Members may express fear of closure and sadness as the termination phase begins.

Process of Team Management

While each team will respond to their work process and priorities, at some point in the process each team should do the following:

- **Define team principles:** Define your team's principles around your organization's vision and how you want to work as a team. Principles may include things such as the agreement to conduct discussions with absolute frankness and honesty; to agree to adhere to the decision in unity as if they were your own; to listen to all input with respect, and to maintain a constant focus on the requirements of customers.

- **Clarify roles and responsibilities:** One of the most common misunderstandings of team management is that teams reduce responsibility and result in the chaos of unclear roles. Roles may include facilitation, data collection and presentation, customer and supplier communication, training, and responsibility for specific process steps.

- **Define key customers and requirements:** Without a doubt, one of the most useful concepts to come out of the quality movement is the focus on customers and their requirements. The team management process institutionalizes this focus as a routine responsibility of every employee in every team. Each team will decide how to define their customers best and how to gather data on requirements.

- **Develop a balanced scorecard:** The purpose of the team management process is to improve business performance. Every team should know their data. They should define measures that reflect the output of their work process as well as measures of customer satisfaction. Measures typically include productivity, quality, costs and cycle time.

- **Analyze the work processes:** Teams are formed around responsibility for specific work processes. The processes may be assembling a certain product in a manufacturing environment, servicing a group of customers, selling to a defined market group. Each team should be an expert in those processes for which it is responsible.

- **Prioritize problems:** Problems are a normal part of all work environments. It is the purpose of teams to assume ownership of all problems related to their work process and to solve those problems most effectively and rapidly. Teams are trained in data analysis and problem-solving techniques.

- **Recognize contributions:** In past years, managers were encouraged to "catch someone-doing-something-good-today" on the assumption that it was they who were responsible for the performance of their people. While that is still true, it is also true in a high performing organization that all employees share in the responsibility to celebrate success, to recognize the accomplishments of their peers and teams.

- **Evaluation:** Evaluation of the entire process, from customer requirements, to work process, and results, the functioning of the group as a team is an ongoing responsibility of the team. By periodic evaluation, the team develops the sensitivity and flexibility to make adjustments as they develop greater skill as circumstances change.

Leadership's Role in Team

In creating a team-based organization, there are some critical change agents. These change agents all have a role in the success of the process. They are the leadership team who steer the process; the team consultants or coaches who assist the teams in their assimilation of the new skills; and the customers and suppliers to the organization and the teams. The leadership team has the following role:

- **Define the mission, vision, and values:** What is our purpose as an organization? Whom do we want to become in relation to our market place? The vision includes the questions, "What it will be like to work here?" and, "What performance results do we expect to be achieving?"
- **Plan the change process:** The senior team should be heavily involved in planning the improvement effort with their change agents. If the senior team does not understand all the implications of the change effort, it often leaves the consultants or coaches without the credibility to move the process forward.
- **Learn and practice:** The senior team should undergo all the same training and implementation steps expected of the rest of the organization. It is the experience that teamwork at the top is often no better than the subordinates and more critical in arriving at effective and unifying decisions.
- **Model the desired behavior:** One of the keys to effective leadership is to become the model of the desired behavior. Every individual in the organization watch the senior team member that if his/her behavior changes during the implementation process.
- **Reinforce improvement:** The only way organizations survive the agonies of rearranging themselves is through experiencing success along the way. The senior team needs to play an active role in giving recognition to those who are even attempting to change.
- **Evaluate results:** This makes the organization continuously healthier and more competitive.

Barriers to Team Building

- The credibility of the project leader
- Unclear project objectives
- Changing goals and priorities
- Lack of team definition and structure
- Confusion about roles and responsibilities
- Performance appraisals that fail to recognize teamwork
- Excessive team size (Optimum size 7–25)

ASSIGNMENTS IN NURSING

Assignment in general means to divide the work among persons on the unit depending upon the workload, the number of skilled workers, type of work, etc. to get the job done smoothly and efficiently.

Types of Assignments in Nursing

- Patient assignment: According to the condition of the patient.
- Work assignment: According to the entire work of the ward.
- Student assignment: Students are assigned to patients for fulfilling their clinical tasks under the supervision of staff.
- Individual assignment: Such as taking inventory.
- Functional assignment: Depends on the functions to be carried out by each health professionals and others.
- Team assignment.

Objectives of Assignment

- To give the best possible care to the patient
- To consider the learning needs of the staff
- To develop excellent managerial skills

PATIENT ASSIGNMENT

Planning of patient assignment is not a matter merely of dividing up the patients among the available members of the staff but also of assigning an individual patient or group of patients to nurses according to the needs of the patient and nurse's ability to handle them.

Principles of Patient Assignment

- There should be a regular caseload on each staff nurse depending upon the ability of the nurse and the needs of the patient.
- In a training hospital, the patient assignments should include student nurses too.
- Assignments help in improving professional competency.
- Assignments of patients and duties should not be changed more frequently until it is necessary.
- Assignment planning should be in accordance with the timing available for providing the service.

Types of Patient Assignment

- **The patient method:** A nurse is expected to give complete nursing care to one or more patients. The responsibility includes general nursing measures, treatment, medications, taking vitals, serving nourishments, and providing health instructions.
- **The functional method:** It is a task-oriented method in which distinct duties are assigned to specific personnel.

One nurse does all the vital signs, and another person makes all the beds.

- **The team method:** Two or more members of the nursing staff are assigned, along with a leader to work together. The team leader is always a professional nurse.

CONCEPT OF ROTATION PLAN IN NURSING

Planning is the function of a managing authority which decides in advance what has to be done. It is an intellectual process in which creative thinking and imagination are essential. Planning is the first function of an executive. Planning plays an important role in everybody's life. Every moment every individual has to plan for future action.

A master plan is the overall plan of all students in a particular educational institution, showing the placement of the students belonging to the total program, including both theory and practice denotes the study block, practical block, placement of student of the clinical block, team nursing, examinations, vacation, and co-curricular activities, etc.

The clinical rotation plan is the complete planning of clinical experience for a student. Clinical experience is an integral part of learning where the student will be actively participating to obtain skills in clinical practice by applying the principles of learning by doing. The time the student spends and learns in the clinical fields is an important and integral part of the total study program. In nursing education, rotation refers to the regular, successive and recurrent posting of various groups of nursing students belonging to different classes in specific nursing fields i.e., OPDs, specialty wards, OT, delivery room, clinics, community health fields, clinics, outreach centers, sub-centers, health centers, schools, etc.

Definitions

The rotation plan is more than a tool that schedules the student period of experiences in various clinical departments.
—**Seckler Hudson**

It is a device that helps to ensure a well-organized plan of educational experiences. —**Fiffner**

Types of Rotation Plan

- **Master plan:** Master rotation plan is an overall plan of rotation of all students in a particular educational institution showing the entire teaching-learning activities and related events during an academic year like details of theoretical instruction, duration and areas of clinical instruction, particulars of community health nursing, posting, the period of vacation, study leave for university examinations, examination week, etc. Usually, master rotation plans of all batches are prepared as a combined

chart for getting a unified view regarding the placement of students on various occasions. This will help to avoid duplication and the resulting confusion.

- **Individual rotation plan:** It is made to make sure that each student in a particular block posting undergoes experience in each area. For example, in four weeks of operation theater posting where the student needs to gain experience from different theaters like gastroenterology, orthopedics, etc. an individual rotation plan can be made for each student by indicating different areas of posting during this period to ensure adequate experience.

- **Clinical rotation plan:** Clinical rotation plan refers to the regular successive and recurrent posting of various groups of nursing students belonging to different classes in specific nursing areas, i.e. OPDs, specialty wards, OT, delivery, clinics, community health fields, clinics, outreach centers, sub-centers, schools and so on.

MASTER ROTATION PLAN

The overall plan of rotation of all students in a particular educational institution, showing the placement of the students belonging to total program (4 years in BSc Nursing and 3 years in GNM) includes both theory and practice denoting the study block, practical block, placement of a student in clinical blocks, team nursing, examinations, vacation, co-curricular activities, etc.

The master rotation plan (MRP) is an overall plan which shows the rotation of all the students in a particular educational institution. —**Nurses of India-Journal**

The master rotation plan shows the placement of the students belonging to various groups/classes in clinical nursing as well as the community. —**Nurses of India-Journal**

Purposes of Master Rotation Plan

- Availability of an advance plan before the implementation of curricular activity during an academic year, for the entire program.
- All concerned are aware of the placement of students in clinical fields.
- Co-ordination becomes more effective when theory and practice correlates and integrity exist.
- It helps the students and teachers to prepare themselves for working in the areas.
- Effective coordination can be made for the smooth running of organizational activities between the faculty and service staff.
- Evaluation of the program is more effective.
- It helps to make tentative advance plans for leave or vacation.

Principles of Master Rotation Plan

- The plan should be as per the curriculum for the entire course/program.
- Plan in advance for each student in the class for all years.
- Plan the activities by following the maxims of teaching.
- Post the students based on their background preparation and the extent of guidance available.
- Select areas that can provide the expected learning experience.
- Plan to build on previous experiences.
- Acquaint the clinical staff/clinical supervisor with clinical objectives and rotation plan.
- Provide each clinical experience of the same duration to all the students.
- Rotate each student through each learning experience or block.
- Plan for all students to enter and leave on the same schedule.

Features of Master Rotation Plan

- It shows the relationship between classroom teaching and experience.
- Each area of clinical experience is indicated by a code to which a guide is attached.
- The period of clinical experience varies in length each year but the total duration of such experience is the same for all students.
- Students of one class are divided into groups and rotated through some clinical areas.
- It is prepared in advance for the whole year.
- It gives a complete and clear picture of the students.
- It must include the period of vacation, teaching block, preparation time and examination.
- The teacher should be aware of the student's placement.
- Overlapping a particular area or shortage in a particular area can be noted.
- The teacher should follow the Indian nursing council and university syllabus.
- The teacher should consider all three domains.

Factors to be Considered while Preparing Master Rotation Plan

- Objectives of the courses
- Number of students in the class
- Number of departments or areas
- Size of the department e.g.: Surgical Ward, Medical Ward, Critical Care Units, Post-operative Wards and so on.
- Duration of experiences
- Number of persons available for supervision
- Indian Nursing Council University requirements

Responsibility of Teaching Staff in Preparing Master Rotation Plan

- Correlate theory and practice.
- Participate in teaching, supervision, and evaluation.

- Prepare the students in theory block before they enter the clinical block.
- Maintain adequate and regular attendance at both the classroom and clinical areas.
- Report to the principal or concerned person for any change or modification.
- Plan for a regular meeting to evaluate the effectiveness of a plan.

CLINICAL ROTATION PLAN

Clinical rotation plan refers to regular successive and current postings of various groups of nursing students belonging to different classes in specific nursing fields. i.e. OPDS, especially, wards, OT, delivery room, clinical, community health fields, clinics outreach center, sub-center, health center, schools.

Clinical rotation plan is a statement that explains the order of the clinical postings of various groups of nursing students belonging to different classes in relevant clinical areas and community health settings as per the requirements laid down by the statutory bodies.

Factors to be Considered in Planning Rotation

- The objectives of the course have to be clearly stated.
- The number of students in each class.
- The number and size of the departments, agencies, areas, technical units or wards where students will be given an opportunity for gaining clinical experience.
- Presence of students of other programs in the same field.
- The agency and authority's concern should be considered.
- The duration of clinical experience in each area.
- The number of people available for clinical supervision.
- Indian Nursing Council requirements, i.e., the individual schools have the freedom to organize the clinical experience the way they choose but all must meet the minimum prescribed by the council.
- The number of staff nurses employed to provide nursing services in the hospital/field.
- Sectors that are solely dependent on student services during day and night.
- The sequence of experience required.
- Select wards depending on learning experiences to be provided.
- Adhere to the rotation plan.

Basic Principles in Planning Clinical Rotation

- The clinical rotation plan must be in accordance with the total curriculum.
- It must be made in advance.
- Theoretical instructions should precede closely as possible with clinical experience simultaneously the ward teachings. case presentations, bedside clinics, etc can be conducted.

- The teacher and student ratio will be 1:4 or as prescribed by INC or according to the types of patients nursed e.g, in critical care unit 1: 1.
- Select the type of learning experience from simple to complex.
- Clinical supervisors must be familiar with the rotation plan; a copy of the rotation plan should be available in each area.
- The students should be posted where they will get maximum supervision from clinical supervisors and qualified nursing staff.
- Each student should get all the experience on rotation wise.
- Overcrowding in any clinical area should be avoided.
- Avoid overlapping of work.
- All students should enter and leave the particular clinical area at the same time and should complete the assignments on time.
- Continuity in the clinical area is needed.

Criteria for Organizing Clinical Experience

- **Continuity:** Refers to the vertical organization of major curriculum events.
- **Sequence:** Each successive experience builds upon the proceeding one, but go more broadly and deeply in the matters involved. It is a logical order, based on psychology and educational needs and standards of the curriculum. The student experiences have to be planned.
- **Integration:** Refers to the horizontal relationship of the curriculum, to get a unified view and unified behavior concerning the elements dealt with. The courses are going so organized that they reinforce one another and point toward general objectives. E.g. integration of medical–surgical nursing to nutrition and psychology.
- **Coordination:** Coordination promotes improved efficiency, quality and safety of nursing care. The training has to consistent with the clinical outcome. It is necessary to understand that the optimum health is always the outcome of a multidisciplinary approach. To ensure this the teachers and students must have good understanding of other disciplines/courses of health care.

Role of Teachers in Rotation Plan

- The teacher has to prepare the master plan and clinical rotation plan based on the curriculum program and INC guidelines.
- Based on objectives clinical experience has to be planned to provide a specific planned learning experience.
- If necessary, some of the topics provide spot clinical teaching and such teaching has to be repeated to each group of students as they rotate.
- Plan the course outline and so that theory can be correlated to practice.

- Get permission from clinical authorities: place the necessary material for clinical care, plan the assignments and evaluation tools.
- Participate in teaching, supervision, and evaluation of students on the wards. Arranging of ward teachings, ward discussions, and case presentation.
- Criticize constructively the students' activities, which improves their performance.
- Help the students for the effective charting of records and reports. Depending upon the ward postings, the evaluation tools have to be prepared.
- Along with theory and practice provide the chances and opportunities for the student, to develop personality also. Overcrowding should be avoided.

Advantages of Preparing Rotations

- Every student should be exposed to all experiences.
- Supervision will be easy.
- Overcrowding can be avoided.
- Reduce confusion among teachers and students.
- Easy for evaluation
- Students can fulfill all the objectives.

It is prepared well in advance for the whole year so that it gives a complete and clear picture of student's placement either in theory or field during an academic session. For each year, it can be prepared either separately or for the total program. It also makes sure that every faculty/staff is aware of students' placements. It promotes the availability of ambient time for mutual preparation to work in their respective areas.

MAINTENANCE OF DISCIPLINE

Discipline can act as a natural control by which a worker brings his or her conduct into a concurrence with the organization's legitimate conduct code, or it tends to be an administrative action to implement worker consistency with office principles and directions. It alludes to working as per certain perceived principles, instructions and traditions, regardless of whether they are composed or understood in character.

Discipline is defined as training or molding of the mind and character to bring about desired behaviors.

Discipline is the practice of making people to obey rules or standards of behavior, and punishing them when they do not.
—**Collins Dictionary**

Aims and Objectives of the Discipline

- To get an acknowledgment of the principles, directions, and strategies of an association with the goal that authoritative objectives can be accomplished.
- To bestow a component of assurance, despite a few contrasts in casual personal conduct and other related change in an association.

- To build up tolerance and adjustment among employees.
- To make a climate of regard for human identity and human relations.
- To increment the working effectiveness and confidence of the workers/representatives with the goal that their efficiency is ventured up, the expense of generation is cut down, and quality is increased.

Types of Discipline

- **Self-controlled discipline:** For the situation of Self-controlled discipline, the worker brings her or his conduct into a concurrence with the associations authentic conduct code, i.e. the worker controls his/her very own exercises for the benefit of all of the association. Therefore, individuals are acquainting with work for a pinnacle execution under controlled discipline.
- **Enforced discipline/control:** Here, an administrative activity authorizes worker consistency with the association's tenets and directions, i.e., it is a typical control forced from the higher level. Here, the supervisor practices his power to urge the workers to carry on with a specific goal in mind.

Approaches to Discipline

- **Traditional methodology:** It accentuates correction/punishment for unfortunate conduct. The reasons for conventional order are punishment for wrongdoing, implement an adjustment to custom, and fortify the power of the old over the youth.
- **Developmental methodology:** It accentuates discipline as a shaper of attractive conduct. The reason for formative discipline is to shape behavior by giving excellent results to the correct functioning and severe modifications for the wrong conduct; and shirking of physical punishments, defend the privileges of the blamed and swap for individual discretionary decisions of the blame.
- **Positive approach:** It depends on the presumption that a good worker with a sense of pride, regard for power, and enthusiasm for the activity will stick to brilliant work benchmarks; and when an intrigued, conscious and self-regarding employee briefly strays from his/her typically exclusive expectations, an amicable reminder/update is sufficient to divert their endeavors in the ideal bearing.

Principles of Disciplinary Action

- **Have an inspirational frame of mind:** The supervisor's demeanor is imperative in averting or amending unwanted conduct. Individuals will, in general, do what is anticipated from them. Subsequently, the administrator must keep up an uplifting frame of mind by anticipating the best from the staff.
- **Investigate cautiously:** If staff nurse is restrained unreasonably or superfluously, the consequences for the whole staff members might be severe and hence the administrators must continue with an alert. They should gather certainties, check charges, and even approach the blamed representatives for their side of the story.
- **Be prompt:** If the disciplinary action is postponed, the connection between the corrective measure and the mistakes turns out to be less precise.
- **Protect privacy:** Disciplinary activities influence the sense of self of the staff nurse. Talking about the circumstance in private causes less hatred and a more possibility for future co-activity.
- Focus on the mistake or act but not the employee as the action was not acceptable, not the worker.
- **The consistency of rules:** It diminishes the likelihood of bias, advances uniformity, and cultivates acknowledgment of punishments.
- **Be adaptable:** Individuals and conditions are never the equivalents. Punishment ought to be resolved merely after the whole record is looked into.
- **Take remedial, reliable action:** The administrator ought to make sure that the staff nurse comprehends that the conduct was in opposition to the association's prerequisites.
- **Follow up:** The supervisor ought to unobtrusively explore to decide if the staff nurse's conduct has changed. If not, the administrator ought to determine the explanation behind that mentality.

Punishments/Penalties

- **Oral reprimands:** It is recommended in case of minor faults due to any reason. An oral warning will be given by the Nurse Manager but add the same in the anecdotal record with nature of the event, time, and place.
- **Written reprimands:** It is advised in times of serious faults. A notice may be issued by the supervisor to prevent and the same in the future. It should include the name of the worker and the supervisor, the idea of the issue, the punishment, and the outcomes of future redundancy. The worker needs to sign it, to demonstrate that the worker has perused it. A duplicate should be given to the person who is getting punished and one held for the staff record. On the off chance that again, the terms are not met, different punishments will most likely be vital.
- **Other punishments:**
  - Financial punishments may be initiated, such as deducting salary, etc.
  - Loss of benefits may incorporate exchange to a less attractive position and loss of inclination for nursing assignments.
  - Demotion is a sketchy arrangement. It makes hard emotions which might be infectious and more probable spots for wrongdoers in a situation of low grade.
  - Suspension from the employment for a timeframe, withholding an appraisal/salary hike.

■ **Termination (rejection):** Perpetual end of employment in the organization.

Advantages of Discipline

- Discipline establishes a pattern for acceptable conduct and performance. It provides a code of conduct for all the students and employees.
- It promotes individual growth, develops human efficiency, and enhances the will power to perform higher.
- It creates an environment under which individual excellence gets a boost, group performance is improved, and harmonious working evolves.

LEADERSHIP IN MANAGEMENT

Leadership has most likely been expounded on, formally examined, and casually talked about more than some other single subject. It is still understood as an unexplainable wonder. It is known to exist since time immemorial and impacts the execution of all human activities, yet its inward activities and precise measurements cannot be accurately illuminated.

Significance of Leadership

Leadership is an essential factor for making any associations fruitful. The following are the significance of better leadership.

- **Motivating employees:** Motivation is fundamental for work execution, higher the inspiration, better the implementation. A decent pioneer, practicing his leadership/authority, spurs the workers for better performance.
- **Creating confidence/certainty:** A great leader may make trust in his adherents by guiding them, giving them counseling and increases productivity and meet organizational objectives through them.
- **Building morale:** Morale is communicated as the demeanor of workers towards the association, the leaders of the association, and voluntary cooperation to offer their capacity to the association. High morale prompts high efficiency and the association's strength.

Note: The concepts of leadership are detailed in the upcoming Units.

REVIEW QUESTIONS

1. Define direction. Explain the principles of direction.
2. What are the elements of direction?
3. Define supervision. Explain the objectives and principles of supervision.
4. Explain the significance of supervision and guidance in nursing.
5. What are the approaches to supervision and explain the role of Nurse Manager in supervising?
6. Define guidance. Explain the purpose and types of guidance.
7. Explain participatory management. What are its merits and demerits?
8. Explain interprofessional collaboration.
9. What is MBO? Explain its process and uses in nursing.
10. What is patient assignment? Explain its principles and types.
11. What are rotations? Explain the type of rotations.
12. Define discipline. Explain the types and approaches to disciplines.
13. What are the principles of disciplinary action and enlist the type of punishments in an organization?

Further Readings

1. Banerjee, Shyamal. Principles and Practice of Management. Oxford and IBM Publishing, New Delhi; 2000.
2. Basavanthappa BT. Nursing Administration. 2nd Edition: Jaypee Brothers Medical Publishers (P) Ltd., New Delhi; 2009.
3. Barrett, Jean. Ward Management and Teaching. Konark Publishers, Delhi; 1992.
4. Warren, Stevens, F. Management and Leadership in Nursing. McGraw – Hill Inc, New York; 1978.
5. Alexander et al. Nursing Service Administration. Mosby Publishers, US; 1962.
6. Park K. Preventive and Social Medicine, 19th Edition: M/s. Banarasidas Bhanot Publishers, Jabalpur; 2007.
7. Basavanthappa BT. Nursing Administration, 1st Edition: Jaypee Brothers Medical Publishers (P) Ltd., New Delhi; 2002.
8. Goel SL, Kumar R. Management of Hospitals – Hospital Administration in the 21st century, Vol. 4, Deep and Deep Publication, New Delhi; 2002.
9. Ranga Rao SP. Administration of Primary Health Centers in India, 1st Edition: Mittal Publications, New Delhi; 1993.
10. Lucita M. Nursing: Practice and Public Health Administration. Current Concepts and Trends. B. I. Churchill Living Stone Pvt. Ltd., New Delhi; 2002.
11. Sakharkar BM. Principles of Hospital Administration and Planning, 2nd Edition: Jaypee Brothers Medical Publishers (P) Ltd., New Delhi; 2009.
12. Patricia S Yoder-Wise. Leading and Managing in Nursing. 2nd Edition: Mosby Publication, US; 1999.
13. Bessie L Marquis, Carol J Huston. Leadership Roles and Management Functions in Nursing: Theory and Application. 5th Edition: Lippincott Williams and Wilkins, New York; 2006.
14. Linda Roussel. Management and Leadership for Nurse Administrators. 4th Edition: Jones and Bartlett Publication, USA; 2006.
15. Wehrich H, Koontz H. Management A Global Perspective. 11th Edition: Tata McGraw-Hill Publishing Company, Ltd., New Delhi; 2005.
16. Marquis BL, Huston CJ. Leadership and Management Functions in Nursing- Theory, and Application. 5th Edition: Lippincott Williams and Wilkins, Philadelphia; 2006.
17. Douglass LM. The Effective Nurse: Leader and Manager. 5th Edition: Mosby Publication, US; 1996.
18. Trained Nurses Association of India, Nursing Administration, and Management.
19. Samson Rebecca. Leadership and Management in Nursing Practice and Education 1st Edition: Jaypee Brothers Medical Publishers (P) Ltd., New Delhi; 2009.
20. Kunders GD. Designing for Total Quality in Health Care, Prism Book Pvt. Ltd., Bangalore; 2002.
21. Chandorkar AG. Hospital Administration and Planning. 2nd Edition: Paras Medical Publisher, New Delhi; 2009.
22. Joshi DC, Joshi Mamta. Hospital Administration. 1st Edition: Jaypee Brothers Medical Publishers (P) Ltd., New Delhi; 2009.
23. Eleanor J Sullivan, Philip J Decker. Effective Leadership and Management in Nursing. 4th Edition: Published by Addison Wesely; 2011.
24. Kulkarni GR. Financial Management for Hospital Administration, Jaypee Brothers Medical Publishers (P) Ltd., New Delhi; 2009.

Unit
7

Leadership

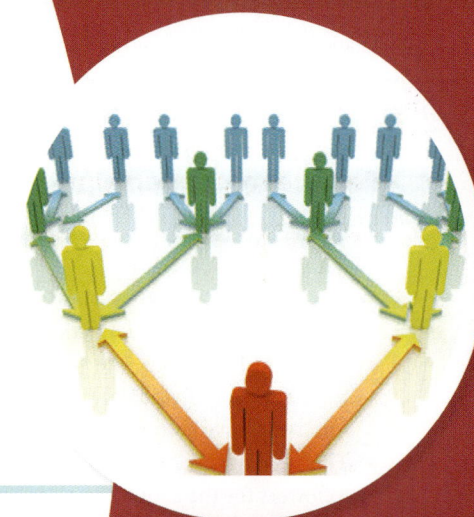

 Unit Outline

BASIC CONCEPTS OF LEADERSHIP IN NURSING

Leadership has most likely been expounded on, formally examined, and casually talked about more than some other single subject. It is still understood as an unexplainable wonder. It is known to exist since time immemorial and impacts the execution of all human activities, yet its inward activities and precise measurements cannot be accurately illuminated.

Leadership is interpersonal influence exercised in a situation and directed through the communication process, towards the attainment of a specific goal or goals. —**LM Prasad, 2006**

Leadership is the process of influencing and supporting others to work enthusiastically towards achieving objectives.

—**Barnard Keys, 1990**

Features of Leadership

- Leadership is a continuous process of behaviors, and it is not a one-shot activity.
- Leadership is the relation between a leader and his followers, and it arises from their functioning for common goals.
- Through leadership the leader tries to influence the behavior of individuals or groups of individuals around him to achieve common goals.
- The willingness and enthusiasm are observed among followers for the achievement of common goals.

Types of Leadership

According to the personal research board of Ohio University, there are five types of leadership; these are:

1. **Bureaucrat leadership:** A leader who sticks to the routine, appeases his superiors, and avoids his subordinates. The priority of concern is pleasing higher authority than taking care of the assistants.

2. **Diplomat leadership:** The leader is highly opportunistic. He/She tries to exploit the people or his/her assistant and fellow workers. He/She generally raises distrust.

3. **Autocrat leadership:** A leader who is directive in nature and expects the obedience of subordinates. Generally, his/her subordinates are antagonistic to him/her as less interaction exists in the relationship.

4. **Expert:** Expert leader is concerned only with his field of specialization. The job or targets are given higher priority. He treats his subordinates as fellow-workers.

5. **Quarterback:** The leader, who identifies himself with his subordinates even at risk of displeasing his superiors.

The Significance of Leadership

Leadership is an essential factor for making any association fruitful. The following are the significance of better leadership.

- **Motivating employees:** Motivation is fundamental for work execution; higher the inspiration, better the implementation. A decent pioneer, by practicing his leadership/authority, spurs the workers for better performance.

- **Creating confidence/certainty:** A great leader may make trust in his adherents by guiding them and giving them counseling thus increasing productivity and meet in organizational objectives through them.

- **Building morale:** Morale is communicated as the demeanor of workers towards the association, the leaders of the association, and voluntary co-operation to offer their capacity to the association. High morale prompts high efficiency and the association's strength.

Functions of Leaders

According to **Krech and Crutchfield,** there are 14 functions performed by leaders in general (Fig. 1). They are:

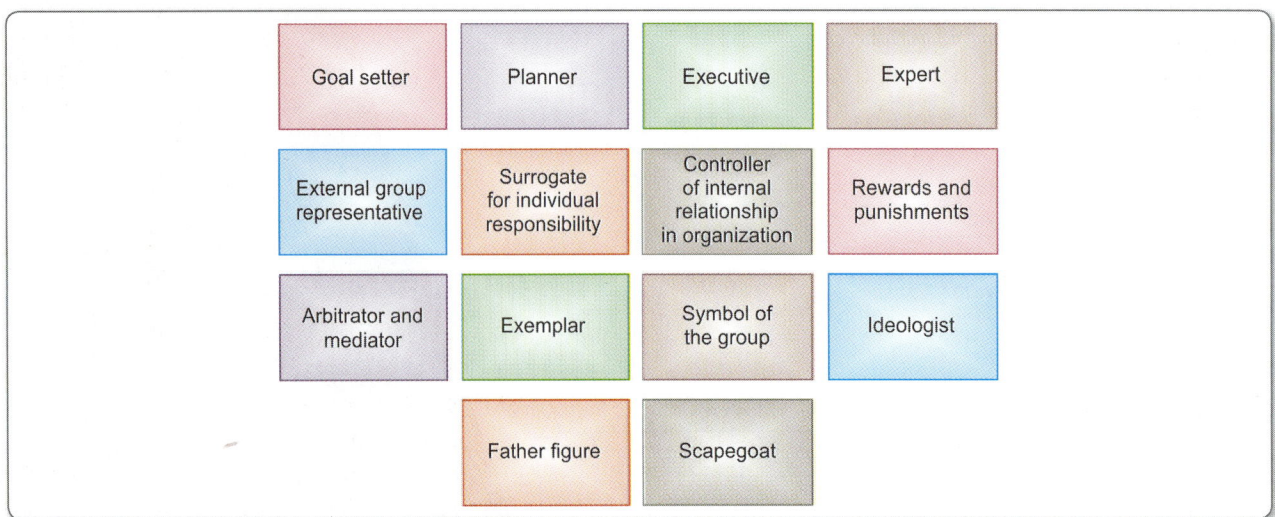

Fig. 1: Functions of leaders

THEORIES OF LEADERSHIP

Great Man Theory or Charismatic Theory

A leader possesses an extraordinary ability referred to as "charisma," which act as an influencer. It is a Greek word signifying "Gift/Blessing." It is a personal attribute present in every leader commonly believed as the gift of God, which makes him a pioneer independent of the circumstances in which he works. The leader motivates his employees through his vision and vitality.

Characteristics of Charismatic Leaders

- Charismatic leaders have substantial power of influencing others.
- They have incredibly high levels of self-confidence, dominance, and the ability to convince followers.
- Leaders possess some exceptional inborn qualities of leadership, which are sufficient to make a leader successful.
- As these qualities are inborn, the enhancement of these qualities is not possible through education and training.
- It cannot be transferred or shared with others as these qualities are personal.
- The effectiveness of a leader relies on these qualities and not on situational factors.

Limitations

- It suggests that there is no hope to create leaders in the associations.
- A charismatic leader may not be successful in the changed circumstance, and hence, the situational variables influence the effectiveness of leadership.

Trait Theory

Ralph M Stogdill (1974) suggested the trait theory after the evaluation of various traits indicated by the researchers. According to the behavioral psychologist and related researches, the attributes for an effective leader are not purely inborn as many of the traits are acquired through learning and experience. Different characteristics needed for leadership can be categorized as inborn traits and acquired traits.

- **Innate qualities:** It corresponds to those qualities that are possessed by an individual since birth. These characteristics are often referred to as God-gifted. Based on these characteristics, the statement is made "leaders are conceived and not created." Individuals can not acquire these characteristics. The main components are the following:

  Physical features: Heredity variables determine the physical characteristics of a person. Heredity is the distribution of attributes by a process mainly in the chromosomes of the germ cells from the parent to the offspring. To some point, leadership needs physique, wellness, and personality.

  Intelligence: Intelligence is mandatory for effective leadership. Intelligence is usually conveyed in cognitive capacity. Intelligence is a natural value in people to a functional part, as it is connected straight with the nervous system.

- **Acquired qualities:** These are leadership characteristics that can be gained and enhanced through different procedures. Many of these characteristics can be improved by practice. The main components of leadership are provided below:

  Emotional Stability: A leader should possess emotional stability at a high standard. He should be safe of prejudice, act consistently, and abstain from wrath. He should be comfortable in himself and should think that he can cope effectively with most circumstances.

  Human relations: A good leader must know adequately how natural relationships are to be handled by people. A leader's role is to develop individuals and learn about individuals and their relationships with each other through mutual collaboration.

  Empathy: Empathy is the concept of observing things and situations from a different perspective. A significant element of effective leadership is the capacity to see things objectively and understand them from others perspective.

  Objectivity: It explains that the leader's action should be based on facts and figures. The leader should assess the things and situations in an organization without any bias. The impartial approach of a leader is termed as objectivity.

  Motivating skill: The leader should be self-motivated so that he can motivate his followers. Although many external pressures encourage an individual to perform better, individuals have an internal urge to function as well.

  Technical skills: People's leadership needs to be consistent in defining values to be grasped and applied to higher achievement. It involves the application of significant capabilities, which represent a technical management competency to schedule, arrange, assign, evaluate, pursue consultation, decide, monitor, and gain the collaboration.

  Communicative skills: A good leader can interact efficiently. Communication has excellent strength to obtain recognition from contact recipients. For convincing, informative, and engaging purposes, the leader utilizes communication expertly. In contrast to an introvert, a good leader usually is an extrovert.

  Social skills: A good leader must have sufficient social skills. He recognizes individuals and identifies their shortcomings and strengths. He can function with all and leads to become trustworthy and loyal. He collaborates with all voluntarily.

Limitations

- **Generalization of traits:** There are issues in applying the traits of a particular leader in all similar situations. Some traits may be viable, and some may not be.
- **The relevance of qualities:** The impediments that obstruct the full use of trait theory, is that authority as a procedure of impact reflects in pioneer's conduct and not his characteristics.

Behavioral Theory

The behavioral theory of leadership given by Lewin K Lippitt (1953) emphasizes that stable leadership is the aftereffect of viable role behavior. The leadership is exhibited more by an individual's actions than his qualities. For a leader to work viably, two significant functions need to be performed by the group:

- **Task-related functions:** They are problem-solving functions related to providing a solution to the problems faced by the group, in performing jobs and activities.
- **Group related functions:** These are social functions of a leader, referred to as actions of mediating and solving the disputes in the group and ensuring that individuals feel valued by the group. An individual who performs both roles successfully would be an effective leader. Leadership behavior may be viewed in two ways: functional and dysfunctional. Functional behavior influences followers positively and includes setting clear goals, motivating, building team spirit, etc. Dysfunctional behavior may be an inability to accept employees ideas, so it is unfavorable to the followers and denotes ineffective leadership.

The implication of the behavioral theory of leadership for managers is that they can shape or modify the behavior that makes the group functional and avoid or discard the behavior that hinders the functioning of the group.

Limitations

- Specific conduct might be useful at a point of time, yet it might be useless at another point of time. Hence, the time components will decide the adequacy of the conduct and not the manner alone.
- The adequacy of leader's behavior relies upon different external elements such as the nature of the group of the leader, and the circumstance under which the leader behavior happens. Here these factors are not given sufficient attention.

Situational Theory

Situational leadership theory is also known as contingency theory, and it was given by Paul Hersey and Ken Blanchard. It was applied for the first time in 1920 among the armed forces of Germany. It was aimed to get good Generals under different situations. Here the primary focus is on the circumstance/

situation where the leadership is exercised. There are various factors affecting the effectiveness of leadership. It may be broadly classified as:

- **Leader's behavior**
- **Situational factors**

The effectiveness of leadership is determined by the combination of these factors.

- **Leader's behavior:** Leader's behavior is affected by two variables. Leader's characteristics and his hierarchical position in the organization.

  Leader's characteristics: The intelligence and ability of an individual are highly regarded as a leader. Additionally, the attributes like his personality, attitudes, interest, motivation, and physical features such as age, sex, and physical characteristics also contribute to the effectiveness of leadership. All these factors are internal to the leader.

  Leader's hierarchical position: Leader's hierarchical position in the organization is vital because persons at different levels face different kinds of problems. That affects the degree of participation between the superior and his subordinates in arriving at decisions to solve the issues. Managers at higher levels are more concerned with the right issues, which require more involvement in decision making. Managers at lower levels are more concerned with short-run issues involving the daily operations, which may not require a high level of engagement. The degree of involvement affects the leader's behavior.

- **Situational factors:** It includes subordinates characteristics, leader's situation, group factors, and organizational factors:

  Subordinates characteristics: The effectiveness of leadership is based on the characteristics of subordinates such as attitude, motivation, personality, and interest, including physical features such as age, sex, and so on.

  Leader's situation: The condition of the leader concerning his fellow officers affects the efficiency of management. The position of the leader is determined by two primary factors. The power of the position and the relationship with subordinates. The leader's power of designation enables influence others, while the small strength of position makes it harder for the leader. The classic exchange theory indicates that two-way influence exists between the leader and subordinates, which is another factor for leaders' situation. Therefore, with the assistance of the leader, healthy supporters must perform in their employment their responsibilities keeping in view of the interest of the leader. Thus, the effectiveness of a leader is likely to be influenced by competent subordinates and the relationship with them.

  Group factors: Different group variables such as job layout, team structure, team norms, team cohesion, and peer group connection influence the efficiency of leadership. The leader will be efficient if these variables are favorable.

Organizational factors: The efficacy of management is affected by organizational variables such as organizational climate and corporate culture. If these are conductive, efficiency will be the ruler.

Implications of the Theory

- It provides hints as to why a manager who succeeds in one scenario loses when the scene changes.
- A manager can do faster by embracing management methods that suit situational factors, including leadership.

Limitations

- Although this theory tends to be appropriate and useful, owing to various internal variables, it is quite complicated in reality.
- This concept lacks management understanding and the conditions overwhelm the manager.

New Theory of Leadership

Bennis and Manus (1995) proposed a new management theory centered on comprehensive research of 90 members who took part in an experiment to find out what is prevalent in management and governance. This study's results found that leaders share four kinds of human management abilities. The writers worked out the specifics of these abilities in excellent depth and referred to them as policies. Those policies are:

- **Vision**
- **Communication**
- **Trust and positioning**
- **Positive self-regard**

Vision: It is a vision-based awareness leadership that relates to the capacity of the leader to generate a concentrate or a positive result image or planned outcome. All the research participants/leaders were result-oriented. The concepts they retained in their minds were apparent, making it simple for people to see where they were going.

Communication: Communication's significance implies the ability of leaders to transform their vision into pictures that others could comprehend. These leaders were able to convert their thoughts with real significance into symbols. Through this skill of communication, leaders can influence and capture the imagination of others too.

Trust and positioning: It refers to the capacity of the leader to promote confidence in others by adding to the stability of the organization. This implies that the leader never loses sight of the existence of the organization. The second element of the commitment of a leader is to facilitate constancy or to stay the course. The leader brings the organization on the correct path like a pilot and an airplane. A leader thus maintains the harmony and purpose of the organization through positioning, but also acknowledges the need for change and inconsistencies and promotes creativity.

Positive self-regard: It implies that a leader is self-developing and is leading in a very personal manner. A favorable self-image and particularly self-respect is displayed by the leader. The leader acknowledges his or her abilities and compensates for failure while fostering the talents and skills he or she possesses.

Implications of the Theory

- It is possible to learn and cultivate leadership.
- The charismatic trait is not mandatory for leaders. Indeed, management is more than a feature and charisma, and it can only be the consequence of efficient management.
- Leadership is not restricted to the top officers of the organization. Instead, possibilities for management occur at all stages of the organization. It is not exercising power or authority instead, it is all about empowering others.

PRINCIPLES OF LEADERSHIP

- **Self-understanding and self-improvement:** One leader must understand the attributes of oneself clearly. Seeking self-improvement means to continually strengthen one's attributes. This can be accomplished through self-study, formal classes, reflection, and interacting with others.
- **Technical proficiency:** As a leader, one must know the job and have a solid familiarity with one's employees' tasks.
- **Seek responsibility and take responsibility:** As a leader one must strive to guide the organization to new heights. When things go wrong; instead of blaming the employees, analyze the situation and take corrective action and move to the next challenge.
- **Make sound and timely decisions:** Use good problem solving, decision making, and planning tools.
- **Set the example:** Be a good role model for the employees. They must not only hear what they are expected to do, but also see the actions to be taken.
- **Understand the employees and look after their well being:** Know human nature and the importance of sincerely caring for the workers.
- **Sharing information:** There should be a proper communication channel established between the leaders and workers.
- **Develop a sense of responsibility among workers:** The development of good character traits will help the employees to carry out their professional responsibilities.

LEADERSHIP STYLES

Autocratic Style of Leadership

It is portrayed as an authoritarian or imperious approach to leadership. It is a directive approach, and the leader is considered as an extraordinary type of "Dictator/Tyrant" who uses his total power to make behavior. The said powers are not distributed or delegated to any other person irrespective of the levels or positions of employees. It is a centralized approach.

Personality of the Leader

- Corporate personality, persistent, self-assured, extremely dominant, with or without purpose.
- Has an intense preoccupation with the job than with the individuals who do the job.
- Using the workers' attempts to the finest of their ability and demonstrates no consideration for the employees concerns.
- Sets strict efficiency norms and techniques and requires subordinates to follow and obey the guidelines.
- Makes all choices about the job and transfers instructions to the employees on his own and force them to obey the orders.
- The concept of group participation is not present, or it is very less.
- Thinks that his intentions and actions are the best. May listen to others without any influence.
- In short, he/has no trust or trust in the subordinates.
- Maintains the center of attention by exercising power and manipulating the subordinates.

Advantages and disadvantages of autocratic leadership are given in Table 1.

Democratic Leadership Style

- Democratic leadership is portrayed as a cooperative and associated style of authority. It is consultative and participative. This style is described by a feeling of correspondence among leaders and supporters.
  - This style is characterized by a sense of equality among leaders and followers. The leader is people-oriented, focuses on the human aspects, builds productive workgroup, and togetherness is emphasized.
  - An open system of communication prevails. The group participates in work-related decisions (sharing the thoughts in problem-solving).
  - The interaction between the leader and the group is friendly and trusting.
  - The leader works not by domination but by suggestions and persuasions of the fellow workers. The workers are motivated by the leader to set their own goals, make their work plans, and evaluate their performance. Informs the overall purpose and the progress of the organization.
  - Performance standards exist to provide guidelines and permit appraisal of workers, thus results in high productivity.

Advantages and disadvantages of a democratic leadership style are given in Table 2.

TABLE 1: Advantages and disadvantages of autocratic leadership

Sr. no.	Advantages	Disadvantages
1	Proficient during an emergency, easy to settle on a choice by one individual than by group. Also, less tedious.	It does not empower a person's development and does not understand the capacity and initiative of employees and makes less collaboration among individuals.
2	It is valuable when the main person/leader is experienced having new and necessary data while subordinates are fresh and newly recruited without much experience.	Though the decisions are wise and correct, the leader is not supported by the group.
3	It is helpful when the employees are uncertain of making a choice and anticipate that the leader should guide them.	Hinders group support, which results in the absence of development, less employment fulfillment, and it can prompt less pledge to the objectives of the association.

TABLE 2: Advantages and disadvantages of democratic leadership

Sr. no.	Advantages	Disadvantages
1	The employees are allowed and urged to practice essential leadership aptitudes such as decision making.	It requires more significant investment for settling on the choices by the group than by a leader. In any case, favorable circumstances overweigh the negative results.
2	It advances individual association; recommendations are respected; this outcome is based on commitment and improved occupation fulfillment.	
3	Choices made by the group are more compelling than by the leader alone. Individuals may have more information/data than the leader.	

Laissez-Faire leadership style

Otherwise called permissive, ultra-liberal, anarchic, or free - rein type of authority. The leader surrenders all capacity to the subordinates/group. This supports free movement and functioning by a group of employees. An external member will not be able to differentiate the leader and other members of the group. There is absence of focal course, supervision, coordination, and control.

Characteristic Features

- This promotes the autonomy of group members. An external person may not be able to recognize the leader of the organization. The manager has little or no impact on the employees of the group. Centralized orientation, supervision, alignment, and monitoring are lacking.
- Group participants are entitled to define their objectives, decide their tasks, and do almost what they want to do. Each person can put a range of targets, and it becomes difficult for the group to fulfill them.
- The leader may choose this style if he or she is too poor to influence and command the group members, or it can be an attempt to make everyone comfortable. And as a result, it does not work out efficiently as a leader.
- It is found useful in case of a highly motivated professional employee who shares mutual responsibilities. E.g. The research work of the scholar and its guidance by the supervisor.
- In an exceptionally organized health care delivery system or organization, this mode is not helpful.
- The group where there is no appointed leader will fall into this category.

Advantages and disadvantages of Laissez-faire leadership style are given in Table 3.

Bureaucratic Style of Leadership

In this sort of leadership initiative, the leader performs his roles and responsibilities just on lines with the standard norms. The leader is adaptable and dislikes to alter to the criteria. He is not able to take any risk action or decision beyond the said norms. Example: Defense leaders. They are strictly adhering to the rules and maintain the discipline of the group.

TABLE 3: Advantages and disadvantages of Laissez-faire leadership

Sr. no.	Advantages	Disadvantages
1	In constrained circumstances, innovativeness might be empowered for explicit purposes. Eg. Exceedingly qualified individuals plan another way to deal with an issue that needs the free opportunity of action.	May prompt unsteadiness, confusion, wastefulness, no solidarity of activities.
2	To attempt new strategies for activities.	Neither the gathering nor anybody in the forum will feel to be dependable to take care of the issues that may emerge
		The individual will lose intrigue activity and want for accomplishment.

Transactional versus Transformational Leadership

This classification is based on the leader's approach to influence the followers. In Transactional Leadership, the leader views the leader-follower relationship as a process of exchange. He tends to gain compliance by offering rewards for performance and threatening punishment for non performance. In contrast, Transformational Leadership, leaders are more visionary and inspirational in approach. They tend to communicate a clear and acceptable vision and goals, with which employees can identify and tend to engender intense emotions in their followers. Rather than giving rewards and punishments, here leaders attempt to build ownership on the part of group members, by involving the group in the decision process.

Situational Leadership

It is a leadership style proposed by Paul Hersey and Ken Blanchard based on the situational theory of leadership. Situational Leadership emerged as one of a related group of two-factor theories of leadership, many of which originated in research done at Ohio State University in the 1960s. These two-factor theories hold that possibilities in leadership style and are composed of combinations of two main variables: task behavior and relationship behavior. Various terms are used to describe these two concepts, such as initiating structure or direction for task behavior and consideration or socioemotional support for relationship behavior. The fundamental principle of the situational leadership model is that there is no single "best" style of leadership. Effective leadership is task-relevant, and the most successful leaders are those who adapt their leadership style to the performance readiness (ability and willingness) of the individual or group they are attempting to lead or influence. Effective leadership varies, not only with the person or group that is being influenced, but it also depends on the task, job, or function that needs to be accomplished. The Situational Leadership Model has two fundamental concepts: leadership style and the individual or group's performance readiness level, also referred to as maturity level or development level. The leadership style is composed of four behavior styles such as Telling, Selling, Participating and Delegating. These behavior styles explain the leader part of leadership. The second part of situational leadership is the maturity level of the person or group who is lead. The group based on maturity is classified into four types such as very capable and confident, capable and but unwilling, unable but confident and unable and insecure.

COMPETENCIES/QUALITIES OF A GOOD LEADER

- **Managerial abilities:**
  - Plans, organizes and makes decisions effectively, encourages cooperation and participation.

- Assists nurse/subordinates in solving the problems and provides consistent feedback.
- Provides a rationale for difficult decisions.
- Assesses the abilities of the workers, guides them to develop new skills.
- Provides the workers with adequate facilities.
- **Interpersonal relationships:**
  - Shows supportive and caring behavior towards subordinates.
  - A good listener and sensitive to others' needs.
  - Guides and motivates them to act and work together.

Temperament

- (Nature or character)
  - Reliable, open, honest, and sincere.
  - Shows a sense of humor courteous, friendly, and loyal.
  - Calm and charismatic, modest, neat, and patient.
  - Positive, energetic, hard worker, happy, and enthusiastic.
  - Shows a balance between work life and personal life.
- **Credibility and forward-thinking:**
  - Acts as an activist, challenger, creative thinker, change agent, innovator, risk-taker, and courageous.
  - Acts as a facilitator and solution seeker.
- **Professionalism:**
  - Committed to the profession and maintains confidentiality.
  - Instills hope and pride in the profession.
- **Advocacy:**
  - Acts as an advocate for others, especially for the nursing profession and for nursing staff.
  - Acts as an advocate with a physician.
  - Acts as an advocate for nursing education and students for the rights and standards.

Implications for Nursing

Regardless of the style selected, the nurse managers should be aware of the effect of the method adopted in the hospital, unit, or educational institution, staff, and on the level of work performance. Effective leadership improves job performance and quality on the whole.

LEADER AND LEADERSHIP DEVELOPMENT

Leader development is typically focused on individual-based knowledge and the skills and abilities associated with the formal leadership roles.

Leadership development is "expanding the collective capacity of organizational members to engage effectively in leadership roles and processes."   —**McCauley et al. 1998**
Leadership processes are those that enable groups of people to work together in meaningful ways, whereas management processes tend to be position and organizational skills.

—**Keys and Wolfe, 1988**

Methods of Leadership Development

To develop the leadership talents and induce a positive attitude towards certain leadership qualities among nurse managers, and also keeping in mind the other factors, the following methods can be adopted to improve leadership effectiveness among the nurse leaders.

- **Leadership training programs:** These are mostly found to be effective not just in bringing about short term change, but also in the long term. These trainings are successful if the individual is committed to change, the organizational environment is supportive and the behavioral change required is reasonable.
- **Competency training:** The competencies that can be taught during leadership training programs are relationship skills, effective communication, and approachability, characteristics of relationally focused leadership.
- **Educational activities:** The given educational activities for modeling and practicing leadership can be followed. It includes Classroom-based learning and Sensitivity Training or T-group learning. The T-group training is a small group interaction process in the unstructured form, which requires people to become sensitive to other's feelings to develop reasonable group activity. The objective of these types of training is to create awareness of the emotional reaction to others and self, to increase the ability of perception, to develop personal values and to inculcate the sense of achievement.
- **360-degree feedback:** It is multi-source feedback that is systematic collection of the individuals' perceptions from peers. This is not proved to be effective in leadership development, rather may be useful when combined with executive coaching.
- **Coaching:** This is for improving individual performance and enhancing organizational effectiveness and is an ongoing process. There is little empirical evidence on the impact of coaching on leadership development.
- **Mentoring:** Mentorship facilitates learning opportunities, helping to supervise and assess staff in the practice setting.
- **On-site programs:** It includes the training program provided at the real setting of leadership execution such as contact with caregivers, empowerment, transformational leadership practices and so on.

MENTORING AND PRECEPTORSHIP IN NURSING

Mentoring

Mentoring empowers faculties through encouraging senior academics to share their unique talents and skills to young or new academics promoting their professional growth. The essential characteristics of mentoring identified in literature concludes that mentoring strengthens intellectual growth, research, professional career development and from an academic view, assists new faculty members with academic guidance, and skill development. The value of mentoring is unequivocal and when conducted successfully, new academics can meet expectations vital to their professional growth.

In higher education, the primary goal is to professionally encourage the new faculty members to succeed in teaching, research and service activities. From a teaching perspective a mentor can enhance new academics instructional abilities. This is valuable as the new staff has limited experience in course development and design, and teaching within the professional standards of the university. Mentors additionally assist the faculty member to adjust to the day-to-day activities of university organization and structure. A mentor provides the junior faculty member with guidance thereby increasing confidence so that they become productive scholars and researchers (Table 4).

Preceptorship

The role of preceptorship within the context of nursing education, shows considerable interest in the socialisation of the learners (the undergraduate nurse student) into the professional nurse role. This involves the student developing attitudes, competence, interpersonal communication skills, clinical problem-solving abilities and perhaps most importantly, their critical thinking skills. Preceptorship believes that it is incumbent on nurse educators to create a teaching-learning environment conducive to developing and promoting these skills within nursing students. Preceptorship within academia is seen to arise from this perspective, where the preceptor is the academic and the preceptee is the undergraduate student nurse. Although the literature on the usefulness of preceptorship for new academics is scarce there are several attributes evident, such as orientation and socialisation to the work environment, which can be beneficial to newly fledged academics (Table 5).

TABLE 4: Mentoring According to American Psychiatric Nurses Association

Definition	Mentoring implies a knowledge or competence gradient, in which the teaching-learning process contributes to a sharing of advice or expertise, role development, and formal and informal support to influence the career of the protégé.
Role/ Relationship	Mentoring is a reciprocal and collaborative learning relationship between two individuals with mutual goals and shared accountability for the success of the relationship. The mentor is the guide, expert, and role model who helps develop a new or less experienced mentee.
Initiation:	Negotiation between parties
Duration:	Longer-term/Ongoing. It ends via mutual and negotiated consent.

TABLE 5: Preceptor-ship according to American Psychiatric Nurses Association

Definition:	A preceptor is typically a nurse assigned based on her/his knowledge, skills, and experience in the specialty to assist an entry-level nurse or Advanced practice registered nurse (APRN) student with competency in the skill and knowledge of philosophies, goals, policies and procedures, expectations, physical environment, and services in learning the practice of nursing.
Role/ Relationship	An experienced nurse who serves as a short-term clinical teacher, role model, supporter, supervisor, and evaluator to a nurse orientee who is acclimating to the complexities of patient care and the role of professional nurse in a given clinical setting and during work hours.
Initiation:	Ascribed or appointed by educational institution, employer, or individual
Duration:	Defined period of time determined by established standards and institutional requirements.

DELEGATION

Delegating roles is an essential component of the coordinating capacity of nursing administration. It is a productive efficiency of the nurse managers by which they complete the work through their representatives. It is to make others work or direct and control the work of someone to achieve common objectives. It is to assign authority and responsibility to someone and make sure of his actions and accountability.

Dimensions of Delegation

- **Assignment of obligations:** One cannot perform all the tasks; hence, it should be distributed.
- **Grant of power:** It is the distribution of power and obligations. This is essential for their empowerment and to meet the goals of the organization.
- **Creation of responsibility**: The subordinates are made accountable. They should be directed and controlled.

Principles of Delegation

- It should be based on anticipated outcomes.
- Parity of power and responsibility. Keep a balance of power and responsibility.
- **Clarification of boundary of authority/power:** The subordinates should be aware of the extent of the authority.
- **Unity of command:** There shall be a single controlling/reporting authority for employees. It encourages uniform direction, control, and supervision, and one director who will set up work needs and will mastermind collaboration.

Types of Delegation

- **Formal delegation:** This is found in the exercise of authority defined by an organization's role.
- **Fimak delegation:** This is a downward delegation. It is useful to the extent of the acceptance and respect for formal authority.
- **Informal delegation:** It occurs because people want to do something apart from what they are told to do. It is something that is not formally required to be done. When there is a problem in the exercise of formal authority, informal delegation is accepted.

List of Ways or Steps for Nurse Managers to Successfully Delegate

- Train and develop subordinates: It is an investment. Give them reasons for the task, authority, details, opportunity for growth, and written instructions if needed.
- Plan ahead. It prevents problems.
- Control and coordinate the work of subordinates. Develop ways of measuring the accomplishment of objectives with communication, standards, measurements, and feedback to prevent errors.
- Visit subordinates frequently. Spot potential problems of morale, disagreement, and grievance.
- Coordination to prevent duplication of effort.
- Solve problems and think about new ideas. Emphasize employees to solve their problems.
- Know subordinate's capabilities and match tasks or duties to the employee. Be sure the employee considers it essential.
- Assess results. The nurse manager should accept the fact that employees will perform delegated tasks in their style.
- Give appropriate tasks.
- Do not take back delegated tasks.

Reasons for Delegation

- Assigning routine tasks.
- Assigning tasks for which the nurse manager does not have time.
- Problem-solving.
- Changes in the nurse manager's job emphasis.
- Capability building.

The nurse manager should be careful not to misuse the clinical nurse by delegating tasks that can be done by non-nurses or non-licensed personnel.

Barriers to Delegation

- **Barriers in the delegator**
  - Preference for working independently.
  - No participation in delegating.
  - Refusal to permit botches, fear of being disdained, and less trust in subordinates.
  - Perfectionism, prompting over the top control.
  - Lack of authoritative ability in adjusting outstanding burdens.
  - Failure to appoint specialist comparable with an obligation.
- **Barriers in the delegate**
  - Lack of experience and skill.
  - Avoidance of duty and disorganization.
  - Overdependence on the manager.
  - Overload of work.
- **Barriers to the situation**
  - Confusion in duties.
  - No toleration of oversights and criticality of choices.
  - Understaffing.
  - Urgency, leaving no opportunity to clarify.

Advantages of Delegation

- Delegation promotes co-appointment, and hence, all dimensions of the association are utilized fittingly.
- It lessens the burden of workers. Delegation helps the senior officials to be free from less critical tasks, and he will be able to concentrate on tasks of more importance.
- A sound arrangement of designation will result in general, build-up, an expanded awareness of other's expectations and upgraded potential work limits of an individual worker.
- It helps in improving the business by enhancing the personal abilities of the supervisor.
- Delegation allows the subordinates to amplify their work, expand their comprehension and build up their ability.

CONCEPT OF POWER IN NURSING

Nursing is a fast-developing professional field. One of the characteristics of a profession is that professionals have power over the practice of their discipline, which is often referred to as professional autonomy. In an earlier period, nurses were unaware of the term "power". Autonomy represents one kind of power that nurses need, and has been defined as "the freedom to act on what one knows". Therefore, power is a key element of empowerment which is the nurse's control over their practice.

Historical Perspectives

Power was considered as a taboo in nursing. Anyone (nurse) who excised power was not appreciated; it was looked upon as inappropriate, and out of the nursing profession. Major decisions about nursing education and practice were taken by persons not related to nursing. Slowly and gradually nurses began to exercise their collective power, as there was a rise of nursing leaders like Lillian Wald, Isabel Stewart, Auvie Goodrish, Lavinia Dock, M. A Delaide Nutting and Isabel Hamptal Robb. Also, there was the development of organizations and associations at the national level for nurses. Over the last century, many social, technological, scientific, and economic trends have shaped nursing and nurses, and their ability to exercise power towards the development of the profession. However, even these days the nurses behave like oppressed groups and get involved in intra and intergroup conflicts and do not feel the need to join professional organizations/associations.

Definitions

Power is the force of energy to accomplish a task, meet a goal, promote changes or influence others. Power is the capacity to control behaviors surrounding life events, the freedom to make choices and decisions, the capacity to create order and sustain influence.

Power can be defined as the capacity to produce or prevent changes. —**Sullivan and Decker, 1997**

Power is a means of protecting ourselves against the cruelty, indifference or ruthlessness of other people. —**Korda, 1975**

Power implies the ability to change the attitude and behaviors of individual people and groups. —**Henin, 1998**

Characteristics of Power

- Power is fleeting, never permanent.
- Power is a neutral concept, neither good nor bad in itself.
- Power can be constructive and useful/it can be destructive and harmful.
- Power controls, corrects and corrupts.
- Power is reciprocal i.e., when one person answers control other person gives it up.

Types of Power

Power is to influence, and the most important ingredient of a leader or manager in an organization. Types and usage of power is given in Table 6.

- **Reward power:** Reward Power is obtained by the ability to grant favors or reward others with whatever they value. The arsenal of reward that a manager can dispense to get employees to work toward meeting organization goals is very broad and a great deal of loyalty towards the leader.
- **Punishment power:** The Punishment Power is the opposite of Reward power and is based on fear of punishment if the expectation is not met. The manager may obtain compliance through the Threat of Transfer, demotion, or dismissal.
- **Legitimate power:** It is the position of power. Authority also is called legitimate power. It is the power gained by a title or official position within an organization. The socialization and culture of subordinate employees will influence to some degree how much power a manager has due to his or her position.

TABLE 6: Types and usage of power

Types of power	Basis	How to use the power
Legitimate power	Given by an organization according to the position e.g. principal.	• Make polite requests • Use clear and simple language • Explain the reason • A follow-up to check compliance.
Reward power	The leader can provide for the subordinates and value by the group.	• Do not over emphasize • Reinforce good behavior • Size of the reward should reflect the total performance • Money is not only the reward e.g, awards, certificates.
Punishment power	Found in fear e.g: oral or written warnings, suspension, and termination	• Avoid it except when needed. • Determine genuine fault. • Discipline promptly without favoritism. • State warnings without hostility. • Fit the punishment to the seriousness of the fault • Warn before punishing.
Expert power	Special ability, skill and knowledge by virtue of education and experience.	• Avoid careless decisions, rash statements. • Remain calm in crisis and act confidently. • Respect staff ideas and include them • Keep abreast with current development • Do not threaten self esteem of the staff
Referent power	The fating of admiration and respect the staff feels towards a leader.	• Treat them fairly • Avoid hostility and indifference • Make requests reasonable. • Be a good role model.

- **Expert power:** It is gained through knowledge, expertise or experience having critical knowledge that allows a manager to gain power over others who needs that knowledge. This type of power is limited to a specialized area. For e.g. Someone with vast expertise in music would only be powerful in that area, not in another specialization.
- **Referent power:** Referent power is the power that a person has because others identify with that leader. Referent power is given to others through association with the powerful. People also may develop referent power because others perceive them as powerful and it is based on respect.

Other Types of Power

- **Personal power**: It is the drive within a person to overcome both internal and external resistance to reaching one's goal; not to exercise control over others, but to have control within oneself.
- **Shared power:** It is the inter-dependence in relationships and human interaction as a source of power. Research indicates that women tend to prefer shared power more than personal power.
- **Political power:** It is associated with governmental control of people, using the prestige of office and the coercive power of the state.
- **Collective power/associative power**: It is the power of a group of members that raises from the sheer weight of numbers of people, uniting their collective energy to achieve a goal. When a professional group exercises such power, it is called Professional Power. For example, nurses Professional Power.
- **Position power**: It is the power of being a Dean, Principal or Chief Executive.
- **Knowledge-based power**: It is the power used by an expert in any field to affect an outcome.
- **Latent power**: Power hidden within an individual. Recently more nurses are using their expertise to participate in the development of health policy, and knowledge with legislature and serve in community organization to develop health services.
- **Charismatic power**: It arises from a personal sense of self-care and ability to communicate personal attributes so that others admire, identify and get motivated to follow the person, e.g., natural leaders, respected teachers.

Individual Skills and Attributes as Sources of Power

Pfeffer's (1992) research and observations emphasize the following characteristics as being especially important for acquiring and maintaining strategic power bases:

- *High energy and physical endurance* is the ability and motivation to work long. Without this attribute other skills and characteristics may not be of much value.
- *Directing energy* is the ability and skill to focus on a clear objective and to subordinate other interests to that objective. *Attention to small details* embedded in the objective is critical for getting things done.
- *Successfully reading the behavior of others* is the ability and skill to understand who are the key players, their positions and what strategy to follow in communicating with and influencing them. Equally essential in using this skill is correctly assessing their willingness or resistance to follow the Strategic Leader's direction.
- *Adaptability and flexibility* is the ability and skill to modify one's behavior. This skill requires the capacity to re-direct

energy, abandon a course of action that is not working, and manage emotional or ego concerns in the situation.

- *Motivation to engage and confront conflict* is the ability and skill to deal with conflict in order to get done what you want to accomplish. The willingness to take on the tough issues and challenges and execute a successful strategic decision is a source of power in any organization.
- *Subordinating one's ego* is the ability and skill to submerge one's ego for the collective good of the team or organization. Possessing this attribute is related to the characteristics of adaptability and flexibility. Depending on the situation and players, and by exercising discipline and restraint an opportunity may be present to generate greater power and resources in a future scenario.

The skills and attributes are relevant not only to the work of strategic leaders but may contribute to the overall capacity to acquire and use power effectively. These skills and attributes are grouped as conceptual skills attributes and positive attributes.

Conceptual Skills

- Professional competence is one of the many ways leaders "add value" by grasping the essential nature of work to be done and providing the organizing guidance so it can be done quickly, efficiently, and well.
- Conceptual flexibility is the capacity to see problems from multiple perspectives. It includes a rapid grasp of complex and difficult situations as they unfold, and the ability to understand complex and perhaps unstructured problems quickly.
- Future vision reflects strategic vision, appreciation of long-range planning, and a good sense of the broad span of time over which strategic cause and effect play out.
- Political sensitivity is being skilled in assessing political issues and interests beyond narrow organizational interests. It means possessing the ability to compete in an arena immersed in the political frame to ensure that your organization is adequately resourced to support your stated organization's interests and those of the nation.

Positive Attributes

- Interpersonal competence is essential for effectiveness in influencing others outside your chain of command, or negotiating across agency lines. It suggests high confidence in the worth of other people, which is reflected in openness and trust in others.
- Empowering subordinates goes beyond simple delegation of tasks and is crucial for creating and leading high performing organizations. It involves the personal capacity to develop meaningful roles for subordinates and then to encourage initiative in the execution of these roles.
- Team performance facilitation includes selecting good people in assembling a team, getting team members

the resources to do a job, providing coordination to get tasks done and moving quickly to confront problem of individuals.

- Objectivity is the ability to "keep one's cool" and maintain composure under conditions that might otherwise be personally threatening.
- Initiative/Commitment is the ability to stay involved and committed to one's work, get things done, be part of a team effort and take charge in situations as required.

Strategies for Developing Power/Powerful Image

- Self-image
- Grooming and well dressed, grounded hair and face, good clothing and neat appearance.
- Good manners – treating people with courtesy and respect.
- Good body language – good postures, good eye contact, confident movement.
- Speech - firm, confident voice, good grammar, appropriate vocabulary, good communication skills.
- Own values, attitude and beliefs.
- Career commitment.
- Networking political skill
- Mentoring mentors are competent, experienced professionals who develop a relationship with a trainee for the purpose of providing advice and support.

Power in Nursing

There are at least three types of power that nurses need to be able to include in their optimum contribution. The various types of power can all be categorized as stemming from nurses' control in three domains:

- Control over the content of practice,
- Control over the context of practice, and
- Control over competence.

The continued lack of control over both the content and context of nursing work suggests that power remains an elusive attribute for many nurses. Now power will be discussed as it is manifested by nurses' control over the content, context, and competence of nursing practice.

Power and Roles of Nurses

Nurses historically had limited power in the health care system. But now nursing organizations are working to provide nurses with a voice at a higher decision-making level in health care.

- **Working together:** By understanding the political realities and the way in which decisions are made by working together to speak with a unified voice, nurses can increase their power in the system.
- **Nursing education programs:** Increasingly try to educate nurses to act as client advocates and agents of change. The higher educations like MSc (N), M Phil (N), and PhD in

nursing and specialized courses will help the nurses to gain team or group power in the health system.

- **Collective bargaining and shared governance:** It helps the nurses with the mechanism for demanding recognition of the importance of their role for being participants in the decision-making process.
- **Power as a tool for leadership:** Power is an increasingly important form of influence for nursing leaders. Leaders are found throughout the organization and have formal and informal leadership, responsibility, respect and regard for the knowledge and good judgment of individuals.

POLITICS IN NURSING

Politics can be science or art. It is the business of conducting the affairs of state or organization, exploring public policy and implementing laws that affect the lives of the public. Nurses are even still uncomfortable about politics, treating "politics" as if it is a dirty word.

History of Politics in Nursing

Nurses' involvement in politics is limited. Florence Nightingale used her contacts with powerful men in the government to obtain supplies and the personnel she needed to care for wounded soldiers. Hannah Ropes was able to fight incompetence and obtain decent care for wound civil war soldiers because she understood who the influential people in Washington are. Lillian and Margaret Sangar have influenced decision making in areas such as sanitation, nutrition, and birth control. In 1974, the American Nurses Association (ANA) formed the nurse's coalition in politics (N-CAP), which was the first political action committee (PAC) for nurses.

Definitions

Politics is the art of influencing the allocation of scarce resources. —**Mason and Abbott, 1985**

Politics means influencing the allocation of scarce resources. —**Talbott and Vance, 1981**

Politics is a means to an end, a means for influencing events and the decisions of others. —**Stevens, 1980**

Purposes

- Protection of the interests of the whole group or a particular part of a group against subordinates' groups.
- The preservation of order in the interest of the group of power or of the whole population.
- It is important for analysis and planning.

What nurses do in their everyday practice is influenced by, and in turn influences. What governments do; what professional organization does. These are overall political power.

- **Politics in the workplace:** Politics in the workplace is often regarded with disdain, as reflected in the Remark, she plays politics. This statement is used to imply that the individual got what he or she wanted because of personal connections rather than on merit.
- **Politics in government:** Politics in government can influence who gets what kind of health care, where, and why. Despite many efforts to limit health care costs, they continue to rise much faster than inflation in general.
- **Politics in financing:** Which individual qualifying to be cared for by a nurse in an organization is, to a certain extent, determined by the politics of health care financing. In metropolitan regions, one can find at least two tiers of health care. One for the poor (Public Hospital) and one for the middle and upper classes (Private Institution and Private Physician).

Political Action

Political action means getting involved in the process of changes, such involvement is most effective when nurses use what Vance (1985) calls the 3 C's of political action.

- Communication is assertive, clear and concise.
- Collectivists, a source of power and the foundation for neat networking coalition- building and collaboration.
- Collegiality, a sense of community, birthhood and foundation for building esteem.

Framework for Political Action

Although most people associate the word politics with government, it pertains to every aspect of life that involves competition for allocating scarce resources or influencing decision making. As such, it is relevant to what nurse do in their daily practice, whether as a nurse in a home health agency, a nurse practitioner in a clinic, or a nurse manager in a hospital.

- **Politics in organization:** Once a patient gets into a hospital bed, the kind and quality of nursing care he or she receives also can be influenced by politics. Politics decides policies of government; they also determine the shape and focus of nursing organizations. These organizations are an important forum for nurses to learn, develop, and apply their political skills.
- **Politics in the community:** The workplace, government and organization all interact with the community, whether local, regional, national or international. One nurse found that her leadership as a community effort to eliminate improper garbage dumping in her town enabled her to develop an important connection to government officials on both the state and local levels.

Applying Power and Politics to Managing Nursing Care

The delivery of nursing services occurs at many levels in health care organizations. The effectiveness of care depends or linked to the application of power and politics and marketing. For the staff nurse, the politics beside care involve influencing the allocation of scarce resources (e.g.- equipment, supplies, time) for the delivery of nursing care. To maintain access to the resources needed for patient care nurses must connect to the whole organization and beyond and not just their nursing unit. Staff nurse can use their power when the limitation interferes with and place restrictions on patient care whether the restriction come in the form of limited supply, money or time. Nurse can use their power and the political skills of artful collaboration and networking to obtain the necessary resources to provide care. Politics of nursing care calls for an action plan, not just a care plan. It is time to force those who seek to establish policy without nursing's input to listen to what nurses have to say.

Political Focus

- In the community—nurses can become politically active in the community e.g., school lunch committee, health facilities and prisons, infant and aged care, highway safety, air quality, self-help groups, food distribution centers.
- In the professional organizations—for the advancement of profession, influencing health care, advisory capacity to governmental agencies, support public and private initiative.
- In the workplace—political action at the workplace of nurses is limited because of the enormous workload.

Impact of Power and Politics on Nursing's Future

Health care is in a state of constant change. Acute care hospitals are downsizing and reorganizing, while, at the same time, community sites to deliver nursing care are expanding. Nurses know the problems and have many of the solutions. Making a case for nursing input into health care policy is no longer an option for the nurse. Nurses can have a tremendous impact on health care policy. The best impact is often made with a bit of luck and timing, but never without knowledge of the whole system. This includes knowledge of the policy agenda, the policymakers, and the politics that are involved. Once you gain this knowledge; you are ready to move forward with a political base to promote Nursing. To convert your policy ideas into political realities, consider the following power points:

- **Use Persuasion over coercion:** Persuasion is the ability to share reasons and rational when making strong care for your position.
- **Use patience over impatience:** Despite the inconveniences and failing caused by health care restructuring, impatience in the nursing community can be detrimental. Patience, along with a long-term perspective on health care reform, is needed.
- **Be open-minded rather than closed-minded:** Acquiring accurate information is essential if you want to influence others effectively.

- **Use compassion over confrontation:** In times of change, error and mistakes are easy to pinpoint.
- **Use integrity over dishonesty:** Honest discourse must be matched with kind thoughts and actions. To manage nursing care in the future, nurses must come to realize that nursing expertise and clinical judgment are the best combination to effectively influence nursing practice and policy changes. By applying power and politics to the workplace, nurse increases their professional influence.

So far, we have discussed in this seminar about the introduction of power and politics, definitions, types, sources, use in the organization, power as a tool for leadership, the framework of political action, applying power to manage nursing care, the impact of power and politics on nursing future.

EMPOWERMENT IN NURSING

The concept of empowering the members of your team is talked about a lot these days and with good reason. Good leaders are characterized by their ability to empower their teams to achieve maximum success. It is important to think through what empowerment means and how best to employ it so the organization can harness its strength. The US Army's definition of leadership contains implied references to empowerment: "influencing people by providing purpose, direction, and motivation while operating to accomplish the mission and improve the organization." Empowerment does all of those things.

Empowerment is a means to include the team in decision making, to give them a participatory role that capitalizes on their expertise and judgment, and that increases their sense of both individual worth and commitment to the organization. Empowerment also demonstrates that the leader has good listening skills and that the leader cares about the input of everyone in the team. Empowerment sounds great, but leadership is principally about the human dimension so nothing is always simple. Embracing empowerment may run counter to the personality of some leaders.

Empowering Team Members

No leader can lead organization to success on his own. It is the collective excellence of the that builds success. A leader leads based on the considerable work of everyone in the team who contributes and commits to the same commonly stated goals. Techniques for successful empowerment includes:

- **Share the vision with the future leaders:** Once you have a compelling vision, share it in a simple and straightforward message.
- **Provide ways to contribute to the vision:** Offer ways for the future leaders to pour into the vision. Better yet, offer incentives for them to come up with their ways of contributing.

- **Respect the employees, their opinions and their input:** Nothing can disempower workers faster than feeling disrespected. Second to that is when employees feel that a supervisor doesn't respect an idea or suggestion they've put forward.
- **Communicate well and often:** To empower future leaders, the leader must cultivate an environment that encourages open dialogue.
- **Reward effort and success:** Genuine effort and success should never go unnoticed. An empowering leader recognizes and rewards effort and success.
- **Use failures and mistakes as learning opportunities:** One strategy for empowering leaders is to build them up, not tear them down. It sounds easy but the implementation can be tough and requires honest, objective analysis.
- **Reward in public; correct in private:** Strive to reward your employees in public and not correct them in front of others. Nothing can disempower a worker faster than public correction, which is humiliating and makes an adult feel like a child. Such correction is likely to create disempowered, disengaged employees.
- **Avoid being a "Helicopter-Supervisor":** The "helicopter-supervisor," like the helicopter-parent, hovers, corrects, and squelches independence and creativity. Such helicoptering breeds resentment because no one likes being monitored and evaluated all the time. Another word for this is micromanager.

COACHING LEADERSHIP STYLE

The Coaching Leadership Style is a relatively new and guiding leadership style. Instead of making all decisions and delegating tasks by oneself, as is the case in the autocratic leadership style, the coaching leader takes the lead to get the best out of his employees or team. A coaching leader must not be confused with a coach, but does have coaching skills. The leader has these skills when he is able to develop and improve the performance and competences of his employees.

The basis of the Coaching Leadership Style is the dynamic interaction between the leader and the employee. This gives rise to valuable insights and the achieved results are discussed and analyzed. This is done by means of providing and receiving feedback, asking questions and conducting motivating conversations. A good coach encourages the learning process of the coached person and promotes the responsibility and independence of the employees. A coaching attitude of the leader ensures that the employees continue to work autonomously and independently without removing the initiative from them. A good coaching leader has his employees perform their work independently, but still makes them feel supported and involved in their work. The independent aspect of coaching makes this style excellently suitable for independent teams.

Conditions for Effective Coaching Leadership

Because coaching and leading are certainly two different matters, the leader must have a number of additional competences. The coaching leader is closer to his employees than the authoritarian leader and will probably know his employees better. The coaching leader looks where opportunities exist for employees to improve themselves, but also takes their preferences into account. By taking this into account, everyone will be working in the right place, which will advance productivity. A requirement is that the leader knows exactly what is happening on the work floor and what the role of the coached person is. It includes:

- Good Social skills and tactics
- Good Communication skills
- Periodical and regular feedback
- Ask questions from the employees

Merits of Coaching Leadership Style

- **Positive organizational culture:** A coaching style encourages a sense of responsibility and commitment in employees.
- **Advanced self-development:** The coaching leader offers his employees sufficient space and freedom to brainstorm about the tasks that must be carried out.
- **Knowledge:** The leader is closer to the activities on the work floor than an external coach and therefore has a better idea of the jobs/project in the organization.

Demerits of Coaching Leadership Style

- **Coaching leadership is pointless with unmotivated employees:** Coaching means developing qualities, but when the employees do not feel motivated, they will not invest any effort in self-development.
- **Coaching is not always the key to the better functioning of an employee:** Often, coaching is used as an instrument to solve the dysfunction of an employee.

DECISION MAKING

Effective decision-making is an art. It involves finding and selecting the best alternative and having the most appropriate person to make and implement the decision at the right time. To function successfully the nurse must constantly demonstrate the ability to solve problems in rapidly changing and uncertain situations in which indecisive man and poor decisions are costly. The ability to foster organized decision making and problem-solving is an essential skill for nurses.

Definitions

Decision-making is a necessary component of leadership, power, influence, authority, and delegations. —**John, 1993**

Decision-making calls for a systematic process in which a manager chooses among the alternatives to come to a conclusion and select an action. —**Rebecca Samson**

Decision making is a systematic process of choosing among alternatives and putting the choice into action.

—**Lancaster and Lancaster**

Decision making is the heart of all managerial and administrative functions. It is true that decision making is a part of everyday life. Decision making is at the core of all planned activities. It is the last step of the process by which an individual chooses one alternative from several to achieve the desired objective.

Types of Decision Making

There are four managerial decisions:
1. **Mechanistic decision making**
   - It is routine and repetitive in nature.
   - It usually occurs in a situation involving a limited number of decision variables where the outcome of each alternative is known.
   - Tools used for these kinds of decisions are charts, lists, decision trees, etc.
2. **Analytical decision making**
   - This decision helps to solve complex problems.
   - It involves a problem with a large number of decision variables where the outcome of each decision alternatives can be computed.
   - Computational techniques involve linear programming and statistical analysis.
3. **Judgmental decision making**
   - The decision involves a problem with a limited number of decision variables.
   - These types of decisions are useful in marketing investment and to solve personal problems.
4. **Adaptive decision making**
   - Decisions involving a problem with a large number of decision variables where outcomes are not predictable.
   - Such ill-structured problems require the contribution of many people with a diverse technical background. E.g. research finding.

Steps in Decision Making

The decision-making task can be divided into six steps which are stated in the order of their sequence as:
1. **Making the diagnosis:** The first step is to determine what the real problem is. The diagnosis should not be merely based on one or two visible symptoms. But it should be diagnosed after the analysis of the whole situation.
2. **Analyzing the problem:** The problem should be thoroughly analyzed to find out adequate background information and data relating to the situation. This analysis will provide

the manager with an insight into the problem. From the information gathered the facts should be identified and separated to provide a solid foundation for making a sound decision.

3. **Searching an alternative solution:** After analyzing, the problem attempts are made to find alternative solutions to the problem. In the absence of alternatives, the decision-making process will become mechanical.

4. **Selecting the best possible solution:** Selection of one best course of action among the several alternatives developed; requires an ability to draw distinctions between tangible and intangible factors as well as facts and guesses. The four criteria have been suggested by Mr. Dracker in selecting the best solution.

   - The proportion of risk to the expected gain
   - Relevance between the economy of effort and the possibility of results
   - The time considerations that meet the needs of the situation
   - The limitation of recourses

   Instead of picking the best solution managers need to focus really on a course of action that is satisfactory enough under the existing circumstances and limitations.

5. **Putting the decision into effort:** The decisions can be made effective through the action of other people. To overcome the opposition on the part of employee's managers can make three important preparations.

   - Communication of decisions
   - Securing employee acceptance
   - The timing of decisions.

6. **Follow up the decision:** As a safeguard against the incorrect decisions, managers are required to a system of follow-up care of the decisions to modify them at the earliest.

Decision-making Authorities

- **Individual:** The autocratic managers' fears that decisions made by others may be more costly, less effective and represents a threat to his/her position. There are mainly three behavioral characteristics that influence decision making such as Perception of the problem, Personal value system and the Role theory that predicts how actions will be performed in certain roles.
- **Group:** Group comprises two or more people who share a common interest and come together to accomplish an activity through face to face interaction. Commitment to the decision and the implementation is important and may be increased by participation in the decision-making process.
- **Committees:** A committee is a group of people chosen to deal with a particular topic or problem. It can be a formal or informal committee. A committee is appointed to collect data, analyze findings, and make recommendations. It is an ad-hoc committee.

Factors Affecting Decision Making

Internal Factors

- Physical and emotional status of decision makers
- Personal characteristics and values
- Past experiences and interests
- Knowledge and Attitude
- Self-awareness and courage
- Energy and creativity
- Resistance to change
- Sensitivity and flexibility

External Factors

- Cultural environment
- Philosophical environment
- Social background
- Time
- Poor communication
- Cooperation
- Coordination

Tools of Decision Making

- **Judgmental technique:** This is the oldest technique and subjective in decision making. It is based on past experiences and intuition about the future. It is useful in making routine decisions and cheap and less time-consuming. There is a risk of taking the wrong decision.
- **Operational research technique:** It can be defined as the analysis of problems and using the scientific method to provide the needed quantitative information to manager in making the decision. Operational research makes the decisions analytic, objective and quantitative-based. It includes linear programming, Program Evaluation and Review Technique (PERT), Critical Path Method (CPM) and so on.
- **Delphi technique:** It allows members who are dispersed over a geographic area to participate in decision making without meeting face to face. This is possible through the use of a questionnaire. The members will return the questionnaires anonymously; the results of the first questionnaire are centrally compiled and sent to each member. Again, the members are asked for suggestions. This process continues until the consensus is reached. Little changes usually occur after the second round. The Delphi technique is free from others' influence.
- **Decision trees:** A decision tree is a graphic method that can help the supervisor in visualizing the alternatives available, outcomes, risk and information needs for a specific problem over a while. It helps to see the possible directions that actions may take from each decision point and evaluate the consequences of a series of decisions. The process begins with a primary decision having at least two alternatives. Then the predicted outcome of each

decision considered and the need for further decision is contemplated.

Advantages of Decision Making

- It is characterized by order and direction that enables managers to determine where they are.
- Provide a framework data gathering which is relevant to the decision.
- It allows the application of previous knowledge and experience that minimizes errors and improves the quality of patient care and work of an organization.
- Increase the manager's confidence and ability in making the decision.

CONCEPT OF PROBLEM SOLVING

It is a part of decision making. A systematic process that focuses on analyzing a difficult situation, problem-solving always includes a decision-making step.

Problem-solving Process

Different decision-making procedures are required in different situations depending on the nature of the problem, environment, internal and external, time and cost. Each decision-making process involves the following steps, known as the elements of problem solving.

Elements of the Problem-solving Process

- **Identification of problem:** The process of problem solving starts with the discovering of the problem for which internal and external situations are analyzed. The problem may relate to an area of operation or may be related to the external environment. Along with the location of the problem, its basic nature is ascertained as to whether it calls for a strategic operational, major or minor, and long and short-term decision.
- **Definition of the problem:** Once the problem has been perceived, the manager proceeds to analyze it to determine its nature. Here, the manager has to clearly define the problem. A well-defined problem is half-solved. The efficiency of the decision-making process and its quality depends on the clear definition of the problem, which is a difficult task because the real problem may be quite different from what it appears. The problem of the situation has to be defined and described in terms of its origin, scope, symptom causes, importance, gravity, intensity, and ramifications. Defining a problem is a time-consuming job and the manager may prefer to define its strategic and critical components.
- **Specification of objectives:** The decision-making process does not work in isolation. It has certain objectives. Decisions are directed towards the achievement of objectives. The managers are expected to prepare a statement of the objectives, which may be quantitative and qualitative and serve as a yardstick for measuring and evaluating the efficiency and effectiveness of the various alternative course of action, particularly, the one, chosen or solving the problem. For example, the company facing the problem of cut-throat competition may achieve the objectives of survival or maintenance of market share by solving the problem.

- **Collection of data:** Required, relevant and reliable information has a very important role in decision making. Information is required not only for uncovering and defining the problem but is equally useful for others involved in the process. The required information is gathered from internal and external sources to provide a factual framework to managers. Availability and reliability of information is a critical input for decision making.

- **Developing an alternative course of action:** After defining a problem and collecting information, a manager has to develop an alternative solution. The process of decision making becomes relevant, meaningful and challenging exercise for managers, only if they have more alternatives to be examined for making a final decision. Alternative solutions may not be obvious and apparent. It is the duty of managers by reference to experience and expertise and generate alternatives through research and analysis, creative thinking and innovativeness.

- **Evaluation of alternative course of action:** The objectives of decision making is to choose an alternative that will provide the greatest amount of wanted and the smallest amount of unwanted consequences. Each alternative is evaluated to satisfy the objectives of the managers. The probable consequence of alternatives can be estimated through forecasting and other devices. An alternative should be thoroughly evaluated in terms of risk, time consumed, efficiency and resource position. While choosing an alternative, both quantitative and qualitative factors should be taken into account.

- **Selection of appropriate alternatives:** Here, the final choice is made by screening and conducting a critical evaluation to eliminate a large number of alternatives. But, for the final choice, the managers have to rely on experience, skill and judgment and feasibility, acceptability, practicability, and simplicity of the choice. Various organizational plans, policies, rules, basic philosophy of management and other human factors are given due weightage.

- **Implementation of the decision:** Implementation of decision implies a series of actions and utilization of resources. To implement the decision, necessary structural administrative and logistic arrangements are made such as delegation of authority, allocation of resources, assignment of activities and installation of controlling mechanism. To secure maximum co-operation, commitment and acceptance for implementing the decision, the concerned employees are taken into confidence or involved in the process.

CONFLICT MANAGEMENT

Conflict is generally defined as the internal or external discord that results from differences in ideas, values, or feelings between two or more people. Because managers have interpersonal relationships with people having a variety of different values, beliefs, backgrounds, and goals, conflict is an expected outcome. Conflict is also created when there are differences in economic and professional values and when there is competition among professionals.

Meaning and Definition of Conflict

Conflict can be defined as an expressed struggle between at least two interdependent parties, who perceive that incompatible goals, scarce resources, or interference from others are preventing them from achieving their goals.

—Wilmot and Hocker, 2001

Conflict is related to feelings, including feelings of neglect, of being viewed as taken for granted, of being treated like a servant, of not being appreciated, of being ignored, of being overloaded, and other instances of perceived unfairness.

Conflict management is the process of planning to avoid conflict where possible and organizing to resolve conflict where it does happen, as rapidly and smoothly as possible.

Types of Conflicts

The conflict has been described and studied from the standpoint of its context, or where it occurs. Three types of conflicts are:

1. **Intrapersonal conflict:** An intrapersonal conflict occurs within an individual in situations in which he or she must choose between two alternatives. Choosing one alternative means that he or she cannot have the other; they are mutually exclusive. E.g. we might internally debate whether to complete an assignment that is due the next day or watch a favorite television program.
2. **Interpersonal conflict:** It is the conflict between two or more individuals. It occurs because of differing values, goals, actions, or perceptions. E.g. when you want to go to a science fiction movie, but your partner may prefer to attend an opera. Interpersonal conflict becomes more difficult when we are involved in issues relating to racial, ethnic and lifestyle values and norms.
3. **Organizational conflicts:** Conflict also occurs in an organization because of differing perceptions or goals. Organizational conflicts may be intrapersonal or interpersonal, but they originate in the structure and function of the organization. Typically, aspects of the organizations' style of management, rules, policies, and procedures give rise to conflict. When a conflict occurs within an organization, it is important that the conflict is resolved constructively to maintain the team's motivation. The leader's role takes on special significance. Two areas responsible for the conflict in organizations are role ambiguity and role conflict.

Conflict Process

Before managers can or should attempt to intervene in the conflict, they must be able to assess its five stages accurately:

1. **Latent conflict:** The first stage in the conflict process, latent conflict, implies the existence of antecedent conditions such as short staffing and rapid change. In this stage, conditions are ripe for conflict, although no conflict has actually occurred and none may ever occur. Many unnecessary conflicts could be prevented or reduced if managers examined the organization more closely for antecedent conditions.
2. **Perceived conflict:** If the conflict progresses, it may develop into the second stage: perceived conflict. Perceived or substantive conflict is intellectualized and often involves issues and roles. The person recognizes it logically and impersonally as occurring. Sometimes, conflict can be resolved at this stage before it is internalized or felt.
3. **Felt conflict:** The third stage, felt conflict, occurs when the conflict is emotionalized. Felt emotions include hostility, fear, mistrust, and anger. It is also referred to as affective conflict. It is possible to perceive conflict and not feel it. A person also can feel the conflict but not perceive the problem.
4. **Manifest conflict:** It is also called an overt conflict, the action is taken. The action may be to withdraw, compete, debate, or seek conflict resolution. People often learn the pattern of dealing with manifest conflict early in their lives, and family background and experiences often directly affect how conflict is dealt with in adulthood. Gender also may play a role in how we respond to conflict. Men are socialized to respond more aggressively to conflict, while women are more apt to try to avoid conflicts or to pacify them.
5. **Conflict aftermath:** The final stage in the conflict process is conflict aftermath. There is always conflict aftermath-positive or negative. If the conflict is managed well, people involved in the conflict will believe that their position was given a fair hearing. If the conflict is managed poorly the conflict issues frequently remain and may return later to cause more conflict.

Outcomes of Conflict

We often hear people hear about conflict situations resulting in win-win, win-lose and lose-lose. Filley (1975) identified these three different positions or outcomes of conflict.

- **Win-lose outcome:** Occurs when one person obtains his or her desired ends in the situation and the other individual fails to obtain what is desired. Often winning occurs because of power and authority within the organization or situation.
- **Lose-lose outcome:** In a lose-lose situation, there is no winner. The resolution of the conflict is unsatisfactory to both parties.
- **Win-win outcomes:** Are of course the most desirable. In these situations, both parties walk away from the conflict and have achieved all or most of their goals or desires.

Effects of Conflict in Organizations

- Stress
- Absenteeism
- Staff turnover
- De-motivation
- Non-productivity

Signs of Conflict between Individuals

- Colleagues not speaking to each other or ignoring each other
- Contradicting and bad-mouthing one another
- Deliberately undermining or not co-operating with each other, to the downfall of the team

Conflict Management

The optimal goal in resolving conflict is creating a win-win solution for all involved. This outcome is not possible in every situation, and often the manager's goal is to manage the conflict in a way that lessens the perceptual differences that exist between the involved parties. A leader recognizes the most appropriate conflict management strategy for each situation. The choice of most appropriate strategy depends on many variables, such as the situation itself, the urgency of the decision, the power and status of the players, the importance of the issue, and the maturity of the people involved in the conflict.

- **Discipline:** In using discipline to manage or prevent conflict, the nurse manager must know and understand the organization's rules and regulations on discipline. If they are not clear, the nurse manager should seek help to clarify them.
- **Consider life stages:** Most organizations will have nurses at all life stages in their employ. Conflict can be managed by supporting individual nurses in attaining goals that pertain to their life stages. Three developmental stages are young adult nurses, middle age, and age after 50 years. Each age group has its vision and the conflict may be accordingly managed.
- **Communication:** Communication is an art that is essential to maintain a therapeutic environment. It is necessary for accomplishing work and resolving emotional and social issues. Supervisors prevent conflict with effective communication and should make it a way of life.
- **Active listening:** Active or assertive listening is essential for managing conflict. To be sure that their perceptions are correct, nurse managers can paraphrase what the angry or defiant employee is saying. Paraphrasing clarifies the message for both. Paraphrasing can help cool off the situation because it gives the employee time and the opportunity to hear the supervisor's perceptions of the emotions expressed.
- **Assertiveness training:** Assertive nurses, including managers, will stand up for their rights while recognizing the rights of others. They are straightforward and know that they are responsible for their thoughts, feelings, and actions. Assertive nurses also know their strengths and limitations. Rather than attack or defend, assertive nurses assess, collaborate, support, and remain neutral and non-threatening. They can accept challenges and prevent conflict by helping others deal with their anger. Assertiveness can be taught through staff development programs. Greenhalgh has developed a system for assessing the dimensions of the conflict. His view is that conflict may be considered to be managed when it does not interfere with ongoing functional relationships. Participants in conflict have to be persuaded to rethink their views. A third party must understand the situation empathetically from the participants' viewpoints. The conflict may be the result of a deeply rooted antagonistic relationship.

Greenhalgh's Conflict Diagnostic Model of Conflict has seven dimensions, each with a continuum from "difficult to resolve" to "easy to resolve." Once the dimensions of the conflict have been assessed, those should be shifted to the easy-to-resolve domain.

- **The issue in question:** It has already been stated that values, beliefs, and goals are difficult issues to bring to a reasonable compromise. Principles fall into the same category since they involve integrity and ethical imperatives. The third-party must persuade the conflicting parties to acknowledge each other's legitimate point of view.
- **The size of the stakes:** The size of the stakes can make conflict hard to manage. If change threatens somebody's job or income, the stakes are high. The third-party must try to keep egos from being hunt, postponing action if necessary.
- **The interdependence of the parties:** People must view resources in terms of interdependence. If one group sees no benefits from the distribution of resources, it will be antagonistic. A positive-sum interdependence of mutual gain is needed.
- **Continuity of interaction:** Long-term relationships reduce conflict. Managers should opt for continuous, not episodic, interaction.

- **Structure of the parties:** Strong leaders who unify constituents to accept and implement agreements reduce conflict. When informal coalitions occur, involve their representatives to find and implement agreements.
- **Involvement of third parties:** Conflicts are difficult to resolve when participants are highly emotional and resort to distorting nonrational arguments, unreasonable stances, impaired communication, or personal attacks. Such conflicts can be solved with a prestigious, powerful, trusted, and neutral third mediator, or arbitrator.

Manage and Resolve Conflict Situations

- **Collective bargaining:** Especially in workplace situations, it is necessary to have agreed with mechanisms in place for groups of people who may be antagonistic (e.g. management and workers) to collectively discuss and resolve issues. This process is often called "collective bargaining" because representatives of each group come together with a mandate to work out a solution collectively.
- **Conciliation:** The dictionary defines conciliation as "the act of procuring goodwill or inducing a friendly feeling." It refers to the activity of a third party to help disputants reach an agreement.
- **Negotiation:** This is the process where mandated representatives of groups in a conflict situation meet together to resolve their differences and to reach an agreement. It is a deliberate process, conducted by representatives of groups, designed to reconcile differences and to reach agreements by consensus. The outcome is often dependent on the power relationship between the groups.
- **Mediation:** When negotiations fail or get stuck, parties often call in an independent mediator. This person or group will try to facilitate the settlement of the conflict. The mediator plays an active part in the process, advises both or all groups, acts as an intermediary and suggests a possible solution.
- **Arbitration:** Means the appointment of an independent person to act as an adjudicator (or judge) in a dispute, to decide on the terms of a settlement. Both parties in a conflict have to agree about who the arbitrator should be, and that the decision of the arbitrator will be binding on them all.

NEGOTIATION

Negotiation is a dialogue between two or more people or parties intended to reach a beneficial outcome over one or more issues where a conflict exists concerning at least one of these issues. Negotiation is an interaction and process between entities who compromise to agree on matters of mutual interest while optimizing their utilities. This beneficial outcome can be for all of the parties involved, or just for one or some of them. Negotiators need to understand the negotiation process and other negotiators to increase their chances to close deals, avoid conflicts, establishing a relationship with other parties and gain profit.

It is aimed to resolve points of difference, to gain an advantage for an individual or collective, or to craft outcomes to satisfy various interests. It is often conducted by putting forward a position and making concessions to achieve an agreement. The degree to which the negotiating parties trust each other to implement the negotiated solution is a major factor in determining whether negotiations are successful.

Types of Negotiation

- **Distributive negotiation** is also sometimes called positional or hard-bargaining negotiation and attempts to distribute a "fixed pie" of benefits. Distributive negotiation operates under zero-sum conditions and implies that any gain one party makes is at the expense of the other and vice versa. For this reason, distributive negotiation is also sometimes called *win-lose* because of the assumption that one person's gain is another person's loss.
- **Integrative negotiation** is also called interest-based, merit-based, or principled negotiation. It is a set of techniques that attempts to improve the quality and likelihood of negotiated agreement by taking advantage of the fact that different parties often value various outcomes differently. While distributive negotiation assumes there is a fixed amount of value to be divided between the parties, integrative negotiation attempts to create value in the course of negotiation by either "compensating" loss of one item with gains from another or by constructing or reframing the issues of the conflict in such a way that both parties benefit. Integrative negotiation often involves a higher degree of trust and the formation of a relationship. It can also involve creative problem-solving that aims to achieve mutual gains. Productive negotiation focuses on the underlying interests of the parties rather than their starting positions, approaches negotiation as a shared problem-solving rather than a personalized battle, and insists upon adherence to objective, principled criteria as the basis for agreement.
- **Integrated negotiation:** An integrated negotiation is a strategic approach to influence that maximizes value in any single negotiation through the astute linking and sequencing of other negotiations and decisions related to one's operating activities. This approach in complex settings is best executed by mapping out all potentially relevant negotiations, conflicts, and operating decisions to integrate helpful connections among them while minimizing any potentially harmful connections. In sports, athletes in the final year of their contracts will ideally hit peak performance so they can negotiate robust, long-term contracts in their favor.

Stages in the Negotiation Process

However, negotiators need not sacrifice effective negotiation in favor of a positive relationship between parties. Rather than conceding, each side can appreciate that the other has emotions and motivations of their own and use this to their advantage in discussing the issue. Perspective-taking can help move parties toward a more integrative solution. Fisher et al. illustrate a few techniques that effectively improve perspective-taking through the following, negotiators can separate people from the problem itself.

- **Put yourself in their shoes:** People tend to search for information that confirms his or her own beliefs and often ignore information that contradicts prior beliefs. To negotiate effectively, it is important to empathize with the other party's point of view. One should be open to other views and attempt to approach an issue from the perspective of the other.
- **Discuss each other's perceptions:** A more direct approach to understanding the other party is to explicitly discuss each other's perceptions. Each individual should openly and honestly share his or her perceptions without assigning blame or judgment to the other.
- **Find opportunities to act inconsistently with his/her views:** The other party may have prior perceptions and expectations about the other side. The other side can act in a way that directly contradicts those preconceptions, which can effectively send a message that the party is interested in an integrative negotiation.
- **Face-saving:** This approach refers to justifying a stance based on one's previously expressed principles and values in a negotiation. This approach to an issue is less arbitrary, and thus, it is more understandable from the opposing party's perspective.
- **Active listening:** Listening is more than just hearing what the other side is saying. Active listening involves paying close attention to what is being said verbally and nonverbally.
- **Speak for a purpose:** Too much information can be as harmful as too little. Before starting an important point, determine exactly what you wish to communicate with the other party. Determine the exact purpose that this shared information will serve.

Results of Negotiation

- **Accommodating:** Individuals who enjoy solving the other party's problems and preserving personal relationships. Accommodators are sensitive to the emotional states, body language, and verbal signals of the other parties. They can, however, feel taken advantage of in situations when the other party places little emphasis on the relationship. Accommodation is a passive but prosocial approach to conflict. People solve both large and small conflicts by giving in to the demands of others.

- **Avoiding:** Individuals who do not like to negotiate and don't do it unless warranted. When negotiating, avoiders tend to defer and dodge the confrontational aspects of negotiating; however, they may be perceived as tactful and diplomatic. Inaction is a passive means of dealing with disputes. Those who avoid conflicts adopt a "wait and see" attitude, hoping that problems will solve themselves. Avoiders often tolerate conflicts, allowing them to simmer without doing anything to minimize them.
- **Collaborating:** Individuals who enjoy negotiations that involve solving tough problems in creative ways. Collaborators are good at using negotiations to understand the concerns and interests of the other parties. Collaborating is an active, pro-social, and pro-self-approach to conflict resolution. Collaborating people identify the issues underlying the dispute and then work together to identify a solution that is satisfying to both sides.
- **Competing:** Individuals who enjoy negotiations because they present an opportunity to win something. Competitive negotiators have strong instincts for all aspects of negotiating and are often strategic. Because their style can dominate the bargaining process, competitive negotiators often neglect the importance of relationships. Competing is an active, pro-self means of dealing with conflict that involves forcing others to accept one's view.
- **Compromising:** Individuals who are eager to close the deal by doing what is fair and equal for all parties involved in the negotiation. Compromisers can be useful when there is limited time to complete the deal; however, compromisers often unnecessarily rush the negotiation process and make concessions too quickly.

PLANNED CHANGE

Bringing change in a planned manner is the prime responsibility of all forward-looking managers. The planned change aims to prepare the total organization to adapt to the significant changes in the organization's goal and direction.

"Planned change is the deliberate design and implementation of a structural innovation, a new policy or goal, or a change in operating philosophy, climate or style."

The pace of global, economic, and technological development makes change an inevitable feature of organizational life. However, the change that happens to an organization can be distinguished from the change that is planned by its members. Organization development is directed at bringing about planned change to increase an organization's effectiveness and capability to change itself. It is generally initiated and implemented by managers, often with the help of an Organization Development (OD) practitioner from either inside or outside of the organization.

Organizations can use planned change to solve problems, to learn from experience, to reframe shared perceptions, to adapt to external environmental changes, to improve performance, and to influence future changes. All approaches to organization development (OD) rely on some theory about planned change. The theories describe the different stages through which planned change may be affected in organizations and explain the temporal process of applying OD methods to help organization members manage change. There are three major theories of organizational change that have received considerable attention in the field: Lewin's change model, the action research model, and the positive model.

- **Lewin's change model:** One of the earliest models of planned change was provided by Kurt Lewin. He conceived change as a modification of those forces keeping a system's behavior stable. Lewin viewed this change process as consisting of the following three steps: **(1) Unfreezing:** This step usually involves reducing those forces maintaining the organization's behavior at its present level. Unfreezing is sometimes accomplished through the process of "psychological disconfirmation." By introducing information that shows discrepancies between behaviors desired by organization members and those behaviors currently exhibited, members can be motivated to engage in change activities. **(2) Moving:** This step shifts the behavior of the organization, department, or individual to a new level. It involves intervening in the system to develop new behaviors, values, and attitudes through changes in organizational structures and processes. **(3) Refreezing:** This step stabilizes the organization at a new state of equilibrium. It is frequently accomplished through the use of supporting mechanisms that reinforce the new organizational state, such as organizational culture, rewards, and structures.

- **The action research model:** The classic action research model focuses on the planned change as a cyclical process in which initial research about the organization provides information to guide subsequent action. Then the results of the action are assessed to provide further information to guide further action, and so on. This iterative cycle of research and action involves considerable collaboration among organization members and OD practitioners. It places heavy emphasis on data gathering and diagnosis before action planning and implementation, as well as careful evaluation of results after an action, is taken. The cyclical process includes the following steps: (Fig. 2)

- **The positive model:** The third model of change, the positive model, represents an important departure from Lewin's model and the action research process. The positive model focuses on what the organization is doing right. It helps members understand their organization when it is working at its best and builds off those capabilities to achieve even better results. This positive approach to change is consistent with a growing movement in the social sciences called "positive organizational scholarship,"

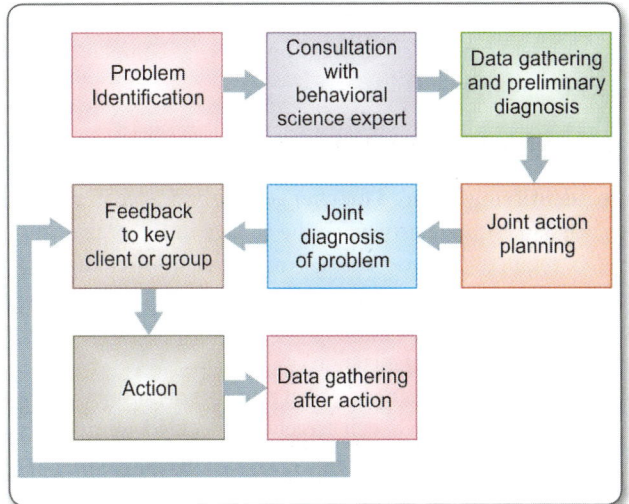

Fig. 2: Action research model

which focuses on positive dynamics in organizations that give rise to extraordinary outcomes. Considerable research on expectation effects also supports this model of planned change. It shows that people tend to act in ways that make their expectations occur. Thus, positive expectations about the organization can create anticipation that energizes and directs behavior toward making those beliefs happen. The positive model includes five stages such as **(1)** Initiate the enquiry, **(2)** Enquire into best practices, **(3)** Discover the themes. **(4)** Envision a preferred future and **(5)** Design and deliver ways to create the future.

Planned change attempts at all aspects of the closely interrelated organization; technology, task, structure, people.

- **Technology related change:** Technology refers to the total of knowledge providing ways to do things. It may include invention and techniques, which affect the way of doing things, i.e., designing, producing, distributing products. Technology related changes may include the changes in problem solving, decision-making procedures and introduction of automated data processing devices.

- **Task-related changes:** Technology related changes determine the types of tasks that may be the number of ways ranging from job simplification to job enrichment. Task-related changes must focus on high internal work motivation and quality work performance.

- **Structure related changes:** Structural changes redefined nature of relationships among various organizational positions and may include changing the number of hierarchical levels, changing one form of organization to another form, changing span of management and changing line staff and functional authority.

- **People related changes:** Changes of any type such as technology, task and structural require changes in people in an organization. These changes may be of two types; i.e., skills and behavior. For example, if there is a change in technology from manual to automated, it requires different types of skills in the operators as compared to the previously used skills.

Process of Planned Change

- **Identifying the need for change:** The basic step in planned change is to identify when the change in the organization is required because change for the sake of change may produce much stronger resistance while useful and necessary. Though various external forces are necessitating a change in an organization.
- **Elements to be changed:** What elements of the organization should be changed will largely be decided by need and objectives of change. While the process of the identification of change will provide the clue why change should take place, this stage takes the analysis further by diagnosing the problems caused because of which the change is necessary. For example, declining profit may require change but does not specify what elements are to be changed. Therefore, it is necessary to diagnose the factors, which are responsible for declining.
- **Planning for change:** At this stage, managers should plan about how the change can be brought in the light. Planning for change includes who will bring change when to bring change and how to bring change.
- **Assessing change forces:** In a group process, there are some forces favoring change and some opposing it to maintain equilibrium. In a situation, there are both driving and restraining forces that influence any change that may occur. Driving forces are those which affect a situation by pushing it in a particular direction; they tend to initiate a change and keep it go. Restraining forces act to restrain change or to decrease the driving forces. Equilibrium is reached when the sum of driving forces equals the sum of restraining forces.
- **Action for change:** Actions for change comprise three stages such as unfreezing, changing and refreezing.

 REVIEW QUESTIONS

1. Define leadership. Explain the types and significance of leadership.
2. Explain the theories of leadership.
3. What are the types of leadership styles? Enlist the qualities of a good leader.
4. Explain mentorship and preceptorship.
5. What is transformational leadership?
6. Define delegation and explain its principles and types.
7. What are the barriers to delegate? What are the advantages of delegation?
8. What is power in management? What are the types of power? Brief the skills and attributes that act as the source of power.
9. Explain application of politics in the nursing management.
10. What is decision making? Explain its types and processes.
11. What is conflict? Explain the types and conflict resolution.
12. What is negotiation? Explain its types. What is the possible outcome of a negotiation?
13. What is planned change? Explain the models of planned change.

Further Readings

1. Banerjee, Shyamal. Principles and Practice of Management. Oxford and IBM Publishing, New Delhi; 2000.
2. Basavanthappa BT. Nursing Administration. 2nd Edition: Jaypee Brothers Medical Publishers (P) Ltd., New Delhi; 2009.
3. Barrett, Jean. Ward Management and Teaching. Konark Publishers, Delhi; 1992.
4. Warren, Stevens, F. Management and Leadership in Nursing. McGraw – Hill Inc, New York; 1978.
5. Alexander et al. Nursing Service Administration. Mosby Publishers, US; 1962.
6. Park K. Preventive and Social Medicine, 19th Edition: M/s. Banarasidas Bhanot Publishers, Jabalpur; 2007.
7. Basavanthappa BT. Nursing Administration, 1st Edition: Jaypee Brothers Medical Publishers (P) Ltd., New Delhi; 2002.
8. Goel SL, Kumar R. Management of Hospitals – Hospital Administration in the 21st century, Vol. 4, Deep and Deep Publication, New Delhi; 2002.
9. Ranga Rao SP. Administration of Primary Health Centers in India, 1st Edition: Mittal Publications, New Delhi; 1993.
10. Lucita M. Nursing: Practice and Public Health Administration. Current Concepts and Trends. B. I. Churchill Living Stone Pvt. Ltd., New Delhi; 2002.
11. Sakharkar BM. Principles of Hospital Administration and Planning, 2nd Edition: Jaypee Brothers Medical Publishers (P) Ltd., New Delhi; 2009.
12. Patricia S Yoder-Wise. Leading and Managing in Nursing. 2nd Edition: Mosby Publication, US; 1999.
13. Bessie L Marquis, Carol J Huston. Leadership Roles and Management Functions in Nursing: Theory and Application. 5th Edition: Lippincott Williams and Wilkins, New York; 2006.
14. Linda Roussel. Management and Leadership for Nurse Administrators. 4th Edition: Jones and Bartlett Publication, USA; 2006.
15. Wehrich H, Koontz H. Management A Global Perspective. 11th Edition: Tata McGraw-Hill Publishing Company, Ltd., New Delhi; 2005.
16. Marquis BL, Huston CJ. Leadership and Management Functions in Nursing- Theory, and Application. 5th Edition: Lippincott Williams and Wilkins, Philadelphia; 2006.
17. Douglass LM. The Effective Nurse: Leader and Manager. 5th Edition: Mosby Publication, US; 1996.
18. Trained Nurses Association of India, Nursing Administration, and Management.
19. Samson Rebecca. Leadership and Management in Nursing Practice and Education 1st Edition: Jaypee Brothers Medical Publishers (P) Ltd., New Delhi; 2009.
20. Kunders GD. Designing for Total Quality in Health Care, Prism Book Pvt. Ltd., Bangalore; 2002.
21. Chandorkar AG. Hospital Administration and Planning. 2nd Edition: Paras Medical Publisher, New Delhi; 2009.
22. Joshi DC, Joshi Mamta. Hospital Administration. 1st Edition: Jaypee Brothers Medical Publishers (P) Ltd., New Delhi; 2009.
23. Eleanor J Sullivan, Philip J Decker. Effective Leadership and Management in Nursing. 4th Edition: Published by Addison Wesely; 2011.
24. Kulkarni GR. Financial Management for Hospital Administration, Jaypee Brothers Medical Publishers (P) Ltd., New Delhi; 2009.

Unit

8

Controlling

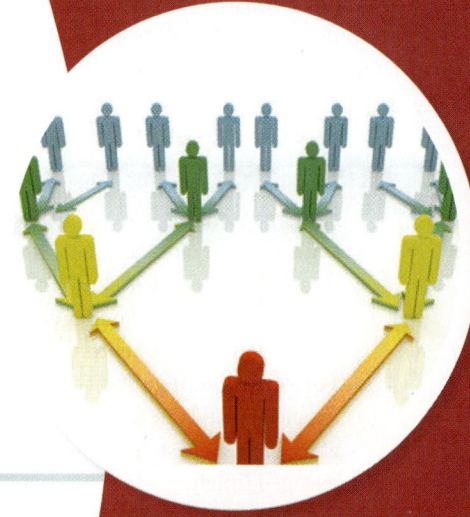

Unit Outline

- Basics of Controlling
- Nursing Standards
- Policy: Nursing View
- Nursing Rounds/Visits
- Nursing Protocols
- Nursing Manuals
- Nursing Procedures
- Records in Nursing
- Nursing Reports
- Quality Management
- Quality and Quality Assurance
- Performance Appraisal
- Program Evaluation and Review Technique
- Gantt Charts (Activity Plan)
- Benchmarking
- Critical Path Method/Analysis

BASICS OF CONTROLLING

Controlling is a crucial element of the management process. It is the process of comparing and verifying the actions against the desired outcome.

Definitions

Control is checking current performances against predetermined standards contained in the plans to ensure adequate progress and satisfactory accomplishments.

—EFL Brech

Control consists of verifying whether everything occurs in conformity of the plans adopted, the instructions issued, and the principles established. —Henry Fayol

Components of an Effective Control System

- **Reflect organization needs:** The control system of an organization should be by the objectives of the organization. For instance, the control system of the financial department and human resource department should be different. Similar criteria should not be used for two various departments.
- **Forward-Looking:** The control system of an organization should be efficient to detect the shortcoming of execution at its early stage so that the necessary modifications can be engaged timely.
- **Flexible Control:** The control system should fit the needs of the organization to a particular extent though it has to be based on the predetermined policies of the organization.
- **Acceptability:** The system should be satisfactory to the organization members. When upper-level managers set one-sided standards, there is a probability that employees will consider those standards as unreasonable or impossible.
- **Corrective System:** The control system should not only detect deviations from the predetermined standards but should also provide solutions to the problems that are responsible for variations.

Characteristics of Control

- Control is a continuous process
- Control is forward-looking
- Control process is universal
- Control involves measurement
- Control is an influence process

Types of Control System

- **Budgeting:** Budget is the heart of administrative management. It serves as a powerful tool of coordination and a capable device for eliminating duplication and wastage.
- **Auditing:** Auditing is a control technique performed by an auditor. It can be an internal auditing or external auditing.

Usually, the internal auditor is a person from within the organization, whereas the external auditor is a technically qualified external person.

- **Reports:** The report prepared from each unit is also a control mechanism. It provides the information required by the management for planning and devising control mechanisms.
- **Standing orders and limitations:** They help in defining the role performance area of an individual in the absence of reporting authority.
- **Job description:** This provides and serves as an excellent tool for defining one's role in an organization. It helps in removing the unnecessary transfer of responsibility among the workforce.
- **Personal observation/Supervision:** A manager can also exercise fruitful control over his/her subordinates by observing them while they are engaged in work.
- **Program evaluation and review technique (PERT):** It is a useful management tool for planning, coordinating, and controlling large, complex projects such as the formulation of the master budget.
- **Human resource accounting:** The concept of human resource accounting is recent. It can be understood as a process by which we identify the investments made in the human resources of an organization.

Role of Nurse/Nurse Manager in Ward Control

- Maintain a clean and cheerful environment for the patients.
- Carry out the orders of medical officers, observe and record the progress of the treatment.
- Maintenance of ward furniture, inventory, and other gadgets and carry out a periodical audit.
- Patient and duty allocation to fellow workers.
- Overall monitoring of the work of the staff and ensure timely completion of all assigned tasks.
- Maintain drug inventory.
- Timely updating of treatment aspects in the patient management system.

Importance of Controlling

- **Facilitates decision making:** The process of control involves correct actions to bring actual performances and standards together. The corrective measure includes the right decisions as to what and how deviations can be rectified.
- **Facilitates decentralization:** Executives wish to decentralize and delegate when there is an efficient system of control. They can ascertain through the monitoring that the decisions taken by subordinates are coherent with the policies of the organization and whether the delegated authority is being correctly used.
- **Stimulates action:** Control provides the basis for further action by spotting and correcting mistakes.

- **Enhances employee morale:** A sound control system is vital to the motivation and confidence of employees.
- **Promotes efficiency of operation:** Control contributes to organization efficiency by focusing on the achievement of the objectives.
- **Promote coordination:** It provides a sense of direction as to which line the employees should perform to achieve the objective.
- **Psychological pressure:** The control system creates a mental influence on the employees regarding what to do and what not to do. The employees become cautious while performing their duties.

NURSING STANDARDS

Standard is a recognized proportion of examination for any value, norm, or criterion, either quantitative or qualitative. A standard is an approach that appreciates general acknowledgment and similarity among experts or a definitive proclamation of the judgment of practice and education. A nursing care standard is a reference for the evaluation of expected quality.

A standard is a powerful statement that frames the legal and professional base for nursing practice.

A standard is a regulation that guides to provide complete care with good quality and established standards.

Purposes of Standards

- Standards provide guidance and give rules to the functioning of nurses.
- It suggests the basics against which the nursing care quality can be compared and thus, it helps in the up-gradation of nursing care efficiency.
- Standards assist managers in guiding nursing staff to enhance execution and enhancing the essential leadership capacity.
- Standards may help legitimize requests for supply and its association.
- It helps in defining the nurses' area of functioning and the extent of responsibility.

Sources of Nursing Standards

- Established health care institutions, such as NIMHANS, PGIMER, JIPMER, and other nursing universities.
- Specific patient care units where research is done after providing evidence-based care such as ICU, CCU, NICU.
- Ministry of Health and Family Welfare and other government bodies.
- Professional Nursing bodies such as TNAI, ANA.
- Nursing licensing organizations such as State Nursing Council, Indian Nursing Council, International Council of Nurses.

Classification of Standards

- **Normative and empirical standards:** Normative standards portray some practices as 'great' or 'perfect' based on the reference or considerations of some legitimate groups. Empirical Standards portray the same that is seen in multiple settings of patient care. Normative standards are easily and commonly followed. For the most part, proficient associations (ANA/TNAI) proclaim standardizing measures (Normative standards) while law authorization and administrative bodies (INC/MCI) declare experimental guidelines(Empirical Standards).
- **Ends and means standards:** This categorization is based on what is significant or expected in patient care. The first one (End Standard) mainly focuses on the outcome of the patient after the patient care, such as physical/mental/emotional changes or modifications. Mean standards are nursing oriented, and it explains the approaches and activities/models applied by nurses to achieve the end standard. Moreover, these are the sides of the same coin since one is the target, and another one is the mode of attaining the objective.
- **Structure, process and outcome standards:** It can be arranged and figured by edges of references identifying with nursing structure, process, and outcome because the standard is an enlightening articulation of the ideal dimension of execution against which to assess the nature of the administration.
  - **Structure standard:** It includes the 'set-up' of the organization. It consists of the aims and objectives of the organization, its physical amenities, the scope of facilities, eligibility and qualification of the human resources, types of equipment and types of machinery, supplies, financial capacity, feedback system and, other factors associated with the organization in obtaining the goals. The structure directly influences the standard of care.
  - **Process standard:** It highlights the ideal execution of the nursing practice. The criteria that indicate the perfect strategy for the explicit nursing profession is the process guidelines. A process/procedure standard includes the exercises linked with providing patient care. In this manner, the process standards help with estimating the level of aptitude, with which strategy or system was completed, the level of customer support or the idea of the cooperation among health professionals and customers/patients. It incorporates nursing care strategies, methods, regimens, and procedures.
  - **Outcome standards:** The result of patient care sets the framework and guidelines for setting the benchmarks for defining the standards. It estimates modification/improvement/change in the patient wellbeing status.

Legal Significance of Standards

They are the rules by which health professionals are governed in their practice. On the off chance that nurses or other professionals do not perform obligations according to acknowledged principles of standards, they may put themselves in the risk of the lawful activity. The negligence and malpractice suit will be filed against health workers if the patient gets offended due to the nurse's inability to maintain the standards.

Quality affirmation is highly significant; nurses must create guidelines for patient service and suitable assessment instruments with the goal that proficient parts of nursing can be accomplished, including scholarly and relational exercises. The patients will be assured of the quality. The organization needs to set benchmarks and should define the milestones. The parameters act as a reference on which care and concern are rated. It should be based on standard practice norms. The principles must be composed, routinely checked on, and understood by the nursing staff.

POLICY: NURSING VIEW

A policy is an announcement or general understanding which gives rules in making decisions to individuals of an association regarding any strategy. It is a human-made principle of a foreordained policy that is cultivated to the execution of work towards obtaining the aims of the organization. According to Joint Commission Accreditation (JCA, USA), the hospital policy should contain the essential elements:

- **Hospital philosophy:** The strategy/policy/guidelines should have a short articulation that talks about the philosophy of the hospital.
- **Policy statement:** Write and depict what the strategy is, the point at which it applies and what it is expected to achieve.
- **Definitions of terms:** Define the relevant terms that are important and utilized inside the hospital such as pharmacists, direct caregivers, key staff members, etc. to avoid unexpected results.
- **Patient contact algorithm:** Set forward rules for patient contacts:
  - **Initial patient contact:** The employees designated for initial communications such as receptionists, front office employees, call centre employees should be set up for this experience whether it is reasonable or unforeseen and whether it is by phone, face to face or through an agent. Managing troublesome discussions and feelings is a communication and correspondence ability for which all staff individuals should get training.
  - **Directing the patient to the appropriate individual(s):** Based on the initial patient contact data and considering the need and situation, the staff should settle on the choice of the patient and their attendants

whom to coordinate for further care and direction. A well thoroughly considered choice tree that is a piece of a policy/strategy rule will be advantageous to diminish staff wavering and perplexity amid critical situations.
- Investigate unanticipated outcomes in detail if any, and convey subtleties of the assessment to the concerned staff individuals.

NURSING ROUNDS/VISITS

In nursing rounds/visits, a subgroup of nurses out of the staff/employees, not more than five to six with a leader take rounds of the hospital wards to know about the patients in the department and their problems. The group typically consists of the department in charge, and the nursing superintendent and supervisor.

Purposes of Nursing Rounds

- To observe clients' conditions and to check the recovery status.
- To illustrate the nursing care procedures.
- The instructional purpose for student nurses.
- To learn more about the disease and its method of care and treatment.
- Improving patient care and ward management.
- To rectify the deficiencies with the ward and caring personnel.
- To give information to others about patient status.

Procedure for Conducting Nursing Rounds

- Constitution of the group for nursing rounds.
- Planning the schedule for the rounds.
- Information should be given to the pertaining wards.
- The concerned student nurses/staff nurses should briefly explain about each patient, the care given, and the treatment status.
- The case presentation should be brief and should be related to the immediate needs of the patients.

Limitations of Nursing Rounds

- It requires careful planning.
- It is time-consuming.
- The number of members is less on the team.

NURSING PROTOCOLS

These are detailed plans that describe particular patient care. It is essential to follow specific protocols when practicing patient care so that uniformity of care can be maintained. Nursing Protocol helps in quality control elements. Nursing tasks are always initiated by nurses. The nurses have a responsibility to make sure that the sick or ill people are given comprehensive and qualitative nursing care. Keeping all these elements in mind, the nursing protocols shall be developed. The nursing protocol is mainly divided into three parts:

1. Definitions and details such as etiology, objectives, and assessment of the condition.
2. The actual nursing care plan, including diagnostic studies, therapeutic methods, client education, counseling, follow up, and referral.
3. Scientific reasons to justify the nursing care plan, such as a proper reference to support the protocol.

Nurse Protocol is the written statement mutually agreed by a registered nurse and a licensed physician, by which a registered nurse is permitted to perform specific procedures, administration of certain medications, and other services. This may also be interpreted as a standing instruction.

NURSING MANUALS

The nursing manuals or procedure manuals provide guidelines to ensure adherence to consistently recognized standards of nursing practice. All the nursing procedures should be developed and performed based on current scientific knowledge and the upcoming technology.

Functions of Nursing Manuals

- It provides a tool for a training program to enable new nursing service personnel to become acquainted with the standards of care to be followed.
- It works as a ready reference for the staff members who are already working.
- It helps in the standardization of procedures and equipment.
- It is a reference to evaluation.

NURSING PROCEDURES

Nursing procedures are standardized procedures used by nurses to achieve a high level of patient care. By creating routine responses to medical situations, nursing procedures keep nurses on task and allow them to ensure that patients are getting the care they need. Many hospitals have specific nursing guidelines, which they expect their staff to follow, while other procedures are taught in nursing school. In both cases, the guidelines reflect years of experience and collaboration between doctors, nurses, and other medical personnel.

Benefits

- Having standard procedures is a critical part of medical care.
- Nursing procedures establish priorities of care so that nurses can work quickly to stabilize a patient, focusing on critical issues first and moving to less serious medical problems.
- They also act as a checklist, which can be used to confirm that every step necessary for the patient's wellbeing has been taken and that these steps have been followed in the right order.
- These procedures also dictate the number of patients a nurse can care for at once, the maximum hours in a day a nurse can work and how the nurse handles administrative duties like charting.

In a simple example of a nursing procedure, many hospitals require nurses to double-check the labels used on bags of intravenous medication, to confirm that the medication is correct before administering it to a patient. Dangerous medications may have brightly colored labels so that nurses are reminded that the contents of the bag could be dangerous to some patients.

While procedures for nursing are designed to standardize responses to situations to increase patient safety and make nursing more effective, nurses may at times be required to go outside procedural guidelines to deal with unique situations. A good nurse has sound judgment which helps the nurse identify situations in which standard procedures do not apply, and he or she is not afraid to question actions and medical orders which could endanger a patient. When nurses start work at a hospital, they are typically given a nursing policy handbook, which provides information about working in that hospital. The handbook includes information about uniforms, hospital procedures, and expected standards of behavior, and it also includes a discussion of standard nursing procedures in that medical facility.

Note: The concept of "Nursing Audit" is mentioned in detail in Unit 5; Page 121 to 123; under Nursing Audit and Maintenance.

RECORDS IN NURSING

Every individual should be responsible for the execution of their obligations to general society, especially the professionals. Since nursing has been considered as a calling, nurses need to record their work on consummation. Records are the indispensable and unavoidable guide to the professional practitioner in giving the ideal support and service to their care recipients.

A record is defined as a permanent written communication that documents information relevant to a client's health care management.

A record is a scientific, clinical, administrative as well as legal document about the medical and nursing care given to the individual family or community.

Purposes of Records

- It provides vital information for planning and evaluation, and this data is also crucial in improving individual and family health.

- It is used as the correspondence material between health professionals and the family.
- A well-maintained record demonstrates the medical issue in the family and different variables that influence their wellbeing.
- It is vital in future planning and helpful in the research development of nursing services.

Principles of Writing the Record

- Nurses should build up their technique for articulation and frame in record composing.
- It is written plainly, properly and enough.
- Contain realities dependent on perception, discussion, and activity.
- Since records are legally significant, it should be dealt cautiously, and represented.
- Records should be composed on the same day about action/incident.
- Maintain confidentiality.
- Do not include any awkward phrases, double meaning words, etc.
- The record has to be signed by the person who prepares it with proper date and time.

Advantages of Records

For the individual and family:
- It contains the complete history of the patient and hence helps in continued care and follow up.
- Records fill in as proof to help or to oversee or confront the legal inquiries that emerge.
- As it contains health information, it can be used as an educative and research tool.

For the doctor:
- It is a guide to health care services from diagnosis to follow up, including evaluation.
- Indicates advancement and congruity of care.
- It help in self-assessment and provides legal protection.
- Useful in education and research.

For the nurse:
- It is the evidence of services provided to the patient since it exhibits the health status of the patient.
- It is the resource for further planning and advancements.
- Helps in self-growth/self-assessment and judgment of the services provided in terms of quality and quantity.
- Serves as a communicative tool among colleagues and helps in future planning.

For authorities:
- Provide the administration with measurable data essential for choice as to use of assets, making arrangements for authoritative control and future references.
- Help the manager assess the administrations rendered, teaching done, and an individual's activity and responses.

Types of Records

- **Cumulative records:** It is otherwise called as continuous records. It is economical and time-saving. It contains the complete information of the individual and helpful in the long term evaluation.
- **Family records:** It contains all the documents of the whole family members, such as their health issues. It will give a picture of total family health status, and mostly, it is applied in community health care settings.
- **Anecdotal record:** An anecdotal record is a simple statement of an incident prepared by the observer, which seems to be significant with the pertaining incident. In elaboration, it is the recording of all incidents in an organization concerning a particular event or person.

Common Records

- Admission register
- Lab investigations register
- MRD register
- Discharge register
- Medicine inventory checking register
- General inventory checking register
- Biomedical equipment register
- Record of lost/condemned articles
- Billing register

Community Health Center

- Forms, case cards, and registers
- Family record
- The eligible couple and child register
- Sterilization and IUD register
- MCH Card/register
- Child Card/register
- Birth and death register
- Stock and Issue register
- Malaria parasite positive case register and others

Educational Institution

- Admission register
- Attendance register
- Clinical experience records
- Common health record
- Internal assessment register
- External marks register
- Reports of various committee
- Other regulatory and affiliating bodies correspondence

Tips to Improve Record Keeping

- Get into the propensity for utilizing real, predictable, precise, objective, and unambiguous patient data.
- Ensure there is a contemplated method of reasoning (proof) for any information recorded.

- Ensure notes are precisely attested with time and date, along with the credentials of the person.
- Write the notes, where conceivable, with the inclusion and comprehension of the patient/bystanders.
- Errors should be remedied by putting a separate line through the inaccurate explanation and attest it with time and date. Do not use corrective fluids as it lacks transparency.
- Follow the SMART model (Specific, Measurable, Achievable, Realistic, and Time-based).
- Write up notes within 24 hours of the occasion. Subsequent modifications are not allowed.

NURSING REPORTS

Reports are oral or composed data traded between the health professionals in a hospital or similar place. A report is an outline of the activities of the individual or staff and the organization. Reports can be assembled every day, week after week, month to month, once in four months or annually.

Importance/Significance of Reports

- Useful reports spare duplication of exertion and take out the requirement for an examination to learn the certainties of a circumstance.
- Patients get better consideration when reports are intensive and give every single appropriate information.
- Complete reports help in getting all facts, and it provides a sense of security.
- It aides in proficient administration of the ward.

Criteria for Good/Decent Report

- Reports should be made instantly to serve its purpose.
- An excellent report is definite, total, and compact.
- It is to be composed of all appropriate, distinguishing information, incorporate the date and time, the general population concerned, the circumstance, with proper credentials and attestations of the author of the report.
- Do not add self-perceptions and extra materials.
- Useful oral reports are communicated and shared intriguingly.

Types of Reports

- **Oral reports:** It is essential when the data is for quick use and not for the long term. E.g. The nurse makes it to another nurse during the shift of allocation of patients.
- **Written reports:** Reports are to be composed when the data is to be utilized by numerous faculty, which is pretty much of lasting worth, e.g., daily reports, patient census, interdepartmental reports, required by the circumstance, occasions, and conditions.

- **Change of shift reports or 24 hours report:** Provide just primary foundation data about the client such as name, age, sex, medical and surgical history, and treatment. Other details are omitted.
- **Transfer reports:** It is the correspondence of data about the patient in detail from one nurse to another nurse during the process of transfer of the patient from one area to another area.
- **Incident reports:** The health professional who saw the episode or who found the patient during the event should document the report. The health professional portrays in brief what happened explicitly. The health professional does not translate or endeavor to clarify the reason for the occurrence. The health professional portrays impartially the patients and conditions when the event was found. Any actions taken by the health professional or some other nurses are also reported.
- **Census report:** This is to count the number of patients daily and is usually carried out at midnight by the supervisor. The report will demonstrate the aggregate number of patients, the number of admission and discharges, birth and death, shifts if any.
- **Birth and death report:** The compilation of birth and death data and its forwarding to the concerned government department is the responsibility of the nurse.

Attributes of a Good Report

- Before anything can be composed plainly, it must be clear as far as one could tell.
- Reports, lacking actualities, might be one-sided or useless.
- Conciseness, exactness, and fulfillment are fundamental to great reports.
- It is smarter to compose a few reports than single when there is more than one fundamental subject at which point to report.
- Terminology should be short, straightforward, commonly utilized words for nontechnical reports. Logical terms can be used when issuing statements to professionals.
- Observes mechanics of suitable composition. Use better language and sentences.
- If the report is composed of another person, check/proofread it before signing/marking it.

Role of Nurse in Records and Reports

The patient has a privilege to review and duplicate the record in the wake of being discharged. The inability to record critical patient data on case file makes the nurse liable for legal actions and carelessness. The medical record must be precise to give a sound premise to the care provided. Mistakes in charting must be adjusted quickly in a way that leaves no questions about the certainties. In detailing data about criminal acts got amid patient consideration, the nurse must uncover such data just to the police since it is viewed as a favored correspondence. The obligations of Nurse Manager in Records and Reports can be summed as pursues:

- **Fact:** Information about patients and their treatment and care must be practical. A record should contain precise, targeted data about what a nurse has perceived about the patient with her senses.
- **Accuracy:** The record should be trustworthy. Precise data will make certainty among the colleagues.
- **Completeness:** Unfinished data in the record to be avoided. Make sure the entry of complete and thorough data of all the events is related to the patient.
- **Currentness:** Do not delay the recording/reporting as it creates suspicion of legal complications. A late entry in a register or any other record/report is negligence.
- **Organization:** The supervisor imparts data in a consistent and logical manner so that it is better to comprehend the data by the second person.
- **Confidentiality:** It is the legal, ethical, and moral responsibility of the health professionals to keep the privacy of the patient information.

Maintaining good quality records and reports has both immediate and long-term benefits for staff. In the long term, it protects individuals and teams from accusations of poor record-keeping and the resulting drop in morale. It also ensures that the professional and legal standing of nurses is not undermined by absent or incomplete records if they are called to account at a hearing.

QUALITY MANAGEMENT

Quality management and quality improvement are the basic concepts derived from the philosophy of total quality management. Now it is preferred to use the term continuous quality improvement, and the method of monitoring of healthcare for CQI is done with quality assurance.

Quality assurance is a judgment concerning the process of care based on the extent to which that care contributes to valued outcomes. **—Donabedian 1982**

Quality assurance is the measurement of provision against expectations with declared intention and ability to correct any demonstrated weakness. **—Shaw**

Purposes of Continuous Quality Improvement

- Rising expectations of the consumer of services.
- Increasing pressure from national, international, government, and other professional bodies to demonstrate that the allocation of funds produces satisfactory results in terms of patient care.
- The increasing complexity of healthcare organizations.
- Improvement of job satisfaction.
- Highly informed consumer.
- To prevent rising medical errors.

- The rise in the health insurance industry.
- Accreditation bodies.
- Reducing global boundaries.

Elements/Components of Quality Assurance

According to Donabedian

- **Structure element:** The physical, financial, and organizational resources provided for health care.
- **Process element:** The activities of a health system or healthcare personnel in the provision of care.
- **Outcome element:** A change in the patients current or future health that results from nursing interventions.

According to Manwell, Shaw, and Beurri, there are 3A's and 3E's

- Access to healthcare
- Acceptability
- Appropriateness and relevance to need
- Effectiveness
- Efficiency
- Equity

Principles of Continuous Quality Improvement

- It operates most effectively within a flat, democratic, and organizational structure.
- Managers and workers must be committed to quality improvement.
- The goal of QM is to improve systems and processes and not to assign blame.
- Customers define quality.
- Quality improvement focuses on the outcome.
- Decisions must be based on data.

Principles of Quality Improvement According to W Edward Deming; (Deming's 14 Points)

1. Create consistency of purpose for improvement of product and service.
2. Adopt the new philosophy.
3. Cease dependence on inspection to achieve quality.
4. End the practice of awarding business based on the price tag.
5. Improve continually and forever the systems of production and service.
6. Institute training on the job.
7. Institute leadership.
8. Drive out fear.
9. Break down barriers between departments.
10. Eliminate slogans, exhortations, and targets for the workforce.
11. Eliminate various quotas for the workforce and numerical goals of management.
12. Remove barriers that rob people of pride and quality.

13. Institute a vigorous program of education and self-improvement for everyone.
14. Put everyone in the company to work to accomplish the transformation.

Approaches

- **General approach:** It involves large governing or official bodies evaluating a person or agencies' ability to meet established criteria or standard during a given time.
  - **Credentialing:** It is the formal recognition of professional or technical competence and attainment of minimum standards by a person and agency.
  - **Licensure:** It is a contract between the profession and the state in which the profession is granted control over entry into an exit from the profession and over the quality of professional practice.
  - **Accreditation:** It is a process in which certification of competency, authority, or credibility is presented to an organization with necessary standards.
  - **Recognition:** It is defined as a process whereby one agency accepts the credentialing states and the credential confined by another.
- **Specific approach:** These are methods used to evaluate identified instances of provider and client interactions.
  - **Audit:** It is an independent review conducted to compare some aspects of quality performance, with a standard for that performance.
  - **Direct observation:** Structured or unstructured based on the presence of set criteria.
  - **Peer review:** Comparison of individual provider's practice either with practice by the provider's peer or with an acceptable standard of care.
  - **Benchmarking:** A process used in performance improvement to compare oneself with best practice.
  - **Staging:** It is the measurement of adverse outcomes and the investigation of its antecedence.

QUALITY AND QUALITY ASSURANCE

"Quality is defined as the degree to which health services for the individuals and populations increase the likelihood of the desired health outcomes and are consistent with current professional knowledge."

—**JCA of Healthcare Organizations, 2002**

"Quality of a service is defined as the totality of features and characteristics of a service that bear on its ability to satisfy the stated and implied needs of the patients."

—**International Organization for Standardization (ISO 8402)**

Quality assurance is a judgment concerning the process of care based on the extent to which that care contributes to valued outcomes. — **Donabedian, 1982**

"Quality Assurance is an on-going, systematic, comprehensive evaluation of health care services and the impact of those services on health care services." —**Kozier**

Goals of Quality Assurance

- It accomplishes continued enhancement in medical services and to the configuration of procedures to address the issues of patients.
- To screen, dissect, and enhance execution to inspire better outcomes of patients.
- To structure a framework dependent on traditional, unsurprising procedures and best practices.
- Set incremental objectives as required.
- **Public responsibility:** It gives proof that the money is being spent successfully bringing about ideal usage of the resources and thus bring out operational effectiveness and productivity of the offered services.
- **Improvement of administration:** This is to give a quality confirmation program as an instrument for critical administrative thinking.
- **Adopt innovations:** It incorporates the assessment of the services given, and there is an arrangement of proper criteria for appraisal.

Principles

- The effective functioning of quality assurance occurs in an organization when it is democratic, flat, and with proper structure.
- Quality improvement is the responsibility of workers as well as managers.
- The objective of quality assurance is to enhance frameworks, forms, and services and not to find fault with anyone.
- Quality is defined by customers/recipients.
- Quality enhancement centers around the result.
- Decisions must be founded on the information.

Approaches/Methodologies

- **General methodology:** It includes huge overseeing or authority bodies assessing an individual or organizations' capacity to meet the built-up criteria or standard amid a given time.
  - **Credentialing:** A formal acknowledgment or certifying a person's essential and least ability/standards to perform and act by an organization.
  - **Licensure:** It is an agreement amid profession and the state in which it is practiced within the set limits and controls.
  - **Accreditation:** A procedure in which the certification and affirmation of competence, credibility, and power are given to an association with standards that are required.

- **Charter:** It is a component by which a state government stipends corporate status to institutions/foundations with or without the privilege to grant degrees.
- **Recognition:** A procedure of approving or accepting the standards of an organization by a competent authority.
- **Academic degree:** Basic educational imperatives for a higher education/practice granted by the concerned authority.

- **Specific methodology:** These are strategies used to assess recognized examples of supplier and customer communications.
  - **Audit:** It is an independent survey directed to look at some part of quality execution, with a set standard for that execution.
  - **Direct observation:** It may be organized or disorganized, dependent on the set criteria.
  - **Appropriateness assessment:** The degree to which the association gives vital and in-time care at the right dimensions of service.
  - **Peer review/audit:** Comparison of two or more individuals caregiving or with some established norms and standards.
  - **Benchmarking:** A procedure utilized in execution enhancement to contrast oneself and best practice.
  - Self-assessment.

Models of Quality Assurance

- **Donabedian Model (1985):** It is based on the three pillars of the basic understanding of the quality, i.e, structure, process, and outcome. Many significant models in quality assurance (QA) is based on it. The model is frequently spoken to by a chain of three boxes containing structure, process, and result/outcome associated with unidirectional bolts in a specific order. These crates speak to three sorts of data that might be gathered to draw surmisings about the nature of care in a given framework (Fig. 1).
  - The structure incorporates every one of the components that influence the setting in which care is conveyed. This combines the physical office, machinery, and HR, and besides, authoritative attributes, for example, employee training and their compensation structure. These variables control how suppliers and patients in a medical services framework act, and are the evaluation of the quality of services provided in the said framework. The structure is frequently simple to watch and evaluate, and it might be the upstream reason for issues distinguished all the while.
  - The process is the aggregate of all activities that make up human services. These generally incorporate finding the disease, treatment, preventive consideration, and patient training; however, it might be extended to the activities of patients and their families. The process can be additionally named technical/specialized process,

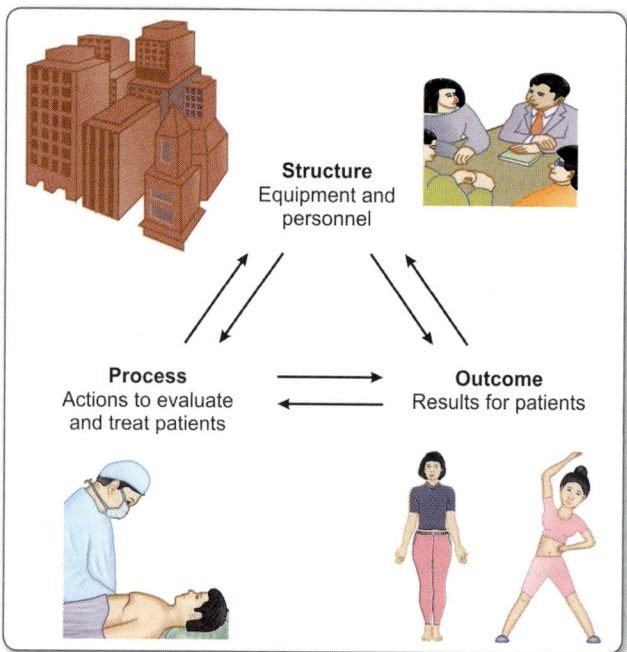

Fig. 1: Donabedian model

how care is conveyed, or Inter-Personal Relationship (IPR)/relational process, which all envelop how care is given. As per Donabedian, the estimation of the process is about proportionate to the evaluation of quality since the process contains the significant actions of the health care system. Data about the process can be acquired from the Medical Records Department (MRD), interviews with patients and professionals, or direct observation.

- The outcome contains every impact of health services on patients, including changes to wellbeing status, conduct, or learning and also persistent fulfillment and wellbeing related personal satisfaction. The outcome is in some cases seen as the most critical markers of quality because enhancing persistent wellbeing status is the essential objective of health services. Be that as it may, precisely estimating results that can be credited only to health care is exceptionally troublesome. Drawing associations among process and outcome regularly require expansive populaces, alterations of the case, and follow up for a longer duration as the outcome may set aside extensive opportunity to end up as a recognizable one.

- **ANA Model:** It was proposed by Long and Black in 1975. It explains the concept of self-assurance of the patient, his/her family, their preference for health, the expectation of quality, and the role of nurses. As per the Donabedian Model, structure, process, and outcome criteria are altogether fundamental for a precise evaluation of the quality of health care. Even though consistency with structure and process criteria was sufficient, the result may have been unexpected. According to the updated ANA model, the below-mentioned parameters may be taken into consideration to assure the quality (Fig. 2).

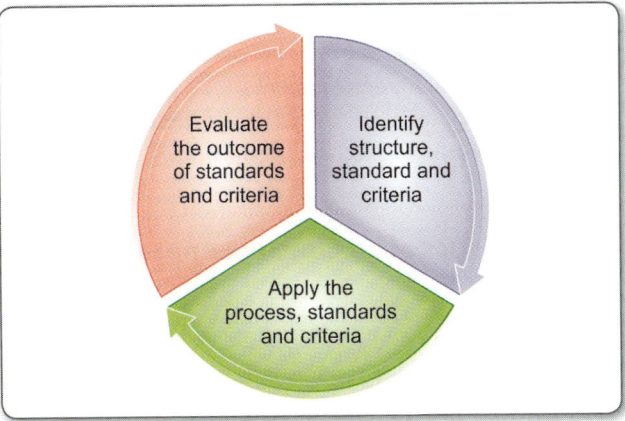

Fig. 2: ANA model

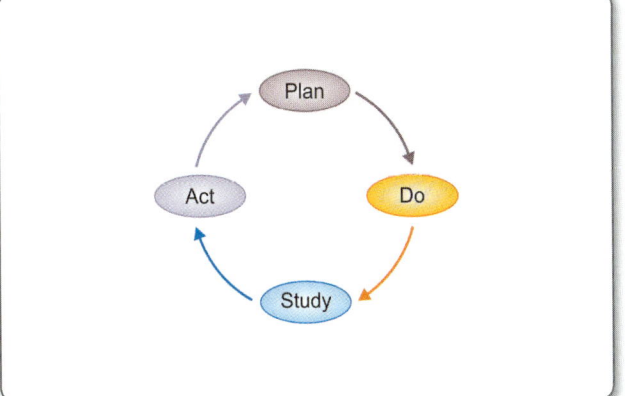

Fig. 4: Plan, do, study, and act cycle

- Identify the structure, standard, and criteria for estimations to decide the quality. We should likewise translate the merits and shortcomings of estimation strategies.
- Enact the process or activity with legal measures and criteria. The action should be considered distinctive techniques to enhance the nature of nursing care, for example, proceeding with different modes of staff development programs, new approaches, advanced policies, research, and reward or correctional activity.
- Evaluate the aftereffects of the move/actions made: It is pivotal in portraying quality assurance/affirmation. It is an effective procedure that helps to bring out innovations and newer trends in any sector.

- **Quality health outcome model:** It is put forward by Mitchell and Co. It is based on the fact that the indicators of quality are directly and reciprocally connected showing the evidence of the existence of dynamic relationships among the said components (Fig. 3). According to this model, there are four factors which are interconnected in quality health outcome such as:
1. Care environment or system
2. The outcome of the care
3. Patient characteristics
4. Interventions

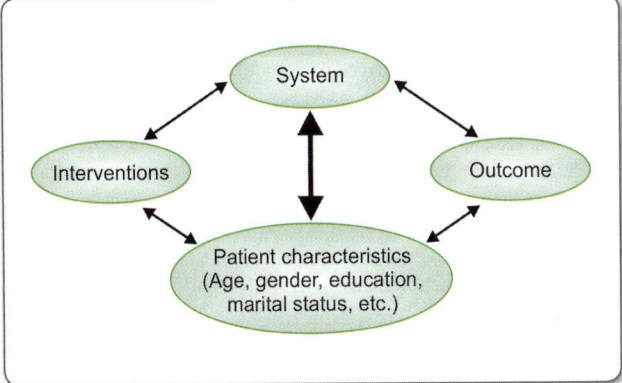

Fig. 3: Quality health outcome model

Donabedian's point of view was direct, expecting that structures influence processes/actions, which thus influence the outcome/results. Patient qualities are at times considered as interceding results, and clinical mediations are viewed as prepared. It expands past models by setting dynamic associations with markers that follow up on as well as proportionally influence the different segments.

- **Plan, do, study, and act cycle:** Suggested by Dr. Deming, which is generally applied, and it contains a particular enhancement stage. The PDSA concept expects that an issue has been recognized and examined for it doubtlessly reasons and change is suggested for wiping out the probable causes. Once the initial analysis of the problem is finished: (Fig. 4).
  - A Plan is created to test one of the enhancement changes. It depends on the appraisal of requirements.
  - During the Do stage, the execution or change is made.
  - During the Study stage, information is gathered to assess the outcomes. The examination includes the investigation of the information collected. Data is evaluated for proof that enhancement has been made.
  - The act step includes taking activities that will design the change, so the additions made by the enhancement are supported after some time. There are three kinds of events, for example, agree, adjust or desert.
- **Six sigma:** It is a statistically based quality assurance model. It alludes to six standard deviations from the mean and is commonly utilized in quality enhancement to characterize the number of agreeable imperfections or mistakes created by a process. A fault in the yield of the care delivery system is not expected by the recipient. We are supposed to ensure the best output of care by reducing the defects. The term Six Sigma is used to show zero defects in nursing care since; statistically, six sigma produces the least error (near to zero) when compared to another sigma. (four sigmas and five sigmas). In a preview of the principles of six sigma, the organizations list out five functions abbreviated as DMAIC (Fig. 5).

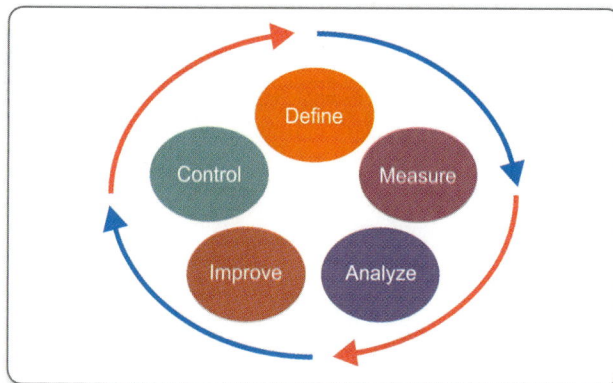

Fig. 5: DMAIC

- Define the critical client prerequisites and essential procedures to help those necessities.
- Measure the essential procedures and gather the information.
- Analyze the information collected to find the reason for the variations identified.
- Improve this stage that creates arrangements and makes and measures process changes.
- Control the processes so that it functions as preplanned in the acceptable limits of operation.

Quality assurance is the responsibility of hospital management and (workers) health personnel to assure a higher quality of care. The administrators generally have to face the consequences in terms of the poor reputation of the hospital, legal expenses, and higher hospital costs.

PERFORMANCE APPRAISAL

It implies the orderly assessment of the execution of an employee by his reporting authority. It helps in the evaluation of the quality and quantity of work in a given setting. Performance is understood as a measurement of one's activity in a particular field, and the appraisal reveals the demand satisfaction of the job. It acts as a record for apprentices and regular employees and helpful in deciding promotions, transfer or demotions, increments, and bonuses.

Irancerich, Donnelly, and Gibson identified five possible parties who could evaluate or rate another person. They are:

- Supervisor
- Peers
- Raters inside the organizational environment
- Subordinates
- Raters outside the organizational environment

Definitions

Performance appraisal is the systematic, periodic and an impartial rating of an employee's excellence in the matters pertaining to his present job and his potential for a better job.

—**Flippo**

It is the method of evaluating the behavior of employees of the individual concerning his or her performance on the job and his or her potential for development. —**Beach DS**

Performance appraisal is a systematic description of an employee's job-relevant strengths and weaknesses.

—**Cascio Wayne**

Characteristics of an Effective Appraisal System

A performance appraisal system should be effective as several crucial decisions are made on the basis score or rating given by the appraiser, which in turn, is heavily based on the appraisal system. So an appraisal to be effective should possess the following essential characteristics:

- **Reliability and validity:** The appraisal system should provide consistent, reliable and valid information and data, which can be used to defend the organization-even in legal challenges.
- **Job relatedness:** The appraisal system should measure the performance and provide information in job-related activities/areas.
- **Standardization:** Appraisal forms, procedures, administration of techniques, ratings, should be standardized as appraisal decisions' affect all employees of the group.
- **Practical viability:** The techniques should be practically viable to administer, possible to implement and economical to undertake continuously.
- **Legal sanction:** Appraisals must meet the laws of the land. They must comply with provisions of various statutes relating to labor.
- **Training to appraisers:** Because the appraisal is important and sometimes difficult, it would be useful to provide training appraisers. Some ideas on documenting, rating, conducting appraisal interviews should be provided.
- **Open communication:** A good appraisal system provides the needed feedback continuously. The appraisal interviews should permit both parties to learn about the gaps and prepare themselves for the future.
- **Employee access to results:** Employees should know the rules of the game. They should receive adequate feedback on their performance. If performance appraisals are meant for improving employee performance, then withholding appraisal result would not serve any purpose. Permitting employees to review the results of their appraisal allows them to detect any errors that may have been made.

Purposes/Importance

- It gives reinforcement information to administrative plans concerning pay norms, promotions, transfers, or selection/termination of service.
- It acts as an eligibility platform for recruitment and other HR services.

- It helps with employee motivation by providing the correct feedback.
- It helps in recognizing employee objectives and desires to acquaint them with organizational policies and objectives.
- To accept and reward the workers for their doings.
- To enhance correspondence among different levels of management, which fosters the collective achievement of organizational objectives.
- To reserve/select persons for the supervisory and higher management, designations to meet the organizational objectives.

Further, the purpose of performance appraisal may be categorized as follows:

- For Employees
  - It is one of the criteria for promotion
  - It is a measurement of job performance
  - It helps in improving the job of the employees
  - It helps to identify training needs and planning for training programs.
  - It is helpful in the planning and administration of compensation for employees.
  - It facilitates feedback, self-examination, and maintains control in the organization.
- For Organization
  - Measurement of organizational objectives.
  - Measurement of work standards.
  - It generates information regarding the employees and their personal planning.
  - It reduces the grievances of the employee.
  - It helps in manpower management.
- Specific Uses
  - It facilitates promotion decisions.
  - It is helpful to plan and analyze the training and development programs.
  - Evaluation of supervisors and managers.
  - It helps in performance feedback and personal development.

Principles

- A single worker is evaluated by two persons, and both reports are analyzed for a precise result.
- It should be done by the immediate superiors.
- Useful performance appraisal is obtained by an ongoing and individual observation of a worker.
- The development of an independent department for performance appraisal is appreciable.
- The result of the appraisal should be shared with the concerned worker. The person can comprehend the position where he stands and where he should go.
- The benefits of a worker should be perceived, and less focus is given to the shortcomings but mentioned.
- The administration must be credible in terms of appraisal of its workers.

Approaches to Performance Appraisal

- **Traditional approach:** The traditional approach is based on past performance. The main purpose is to determine and justify the salary and perks of the employees and not considered for development purposes. This is to judge the organizational performance as a whole by the past performance of its employees.
- **Modern approach:** The purpose of performance appraisal ha snow been taken for development purposes, for taking the corrective actions timely so that the organizational goals can be achieved within the time frame and also help in re-planning. It is more formal and structured so that training needs can be identified and accordingly the training programs can be planned. Hence the modern approach is future-oriented.

Process of Performance Appraisal

Performance appraisal is planned, developed and implemented through a series of steps. They are as

- **Establish performance standards:** Appraisal systems require performance standards that serve as a benchmark against which performance is measured. To be useful, standards should be related to the desired results of each job. The performance standard should be clear to both appraiser and the appraise. Performance standards should be written down after a thorough analysis of the job. They must be measurable within a short period.
- **Communicating the standard:** Performance appraisal involves at least two parties, the appraiser and the appraise. The appraiser should prepare job descriptions clearly, help appraise to set his goals and targets, analyze results objectively. Performance standards must be communicated to appraises clearly.
- **Measure actual performance:** After the performance standard is set and accepted, the next step is to measure actual performance. This requires the use of dependable performance measures to be helpful and must be easy to use, reliable, and report on the critical behaviors that determine performance. Four common sources of information, which are generally used by managers regarding how to measure actual performance are personal observation, statistical reports, an oral report, and written report.
- **Compare actual performance with standards and discuss the appraisal:** Actual performance may be better than expected and sometimes it may go off the track. Whatever the consequences, there is a way to communicate and discuss the outcome. The assessment of another person's contribution and ability is not an easy task. It has serious emotional overtones as it may affect the self-esteem of the employee.
- **Taking corrective action, if necessary:** Corrective action is of two types: One puts out the fires immediately, while

the other destroys the root of the problem permanently. Immediate action sets things right and get things back on track whereas the basic corrective action gets to the source of deviation and seeks to adjust the difference permanently.

Methods of Performance Appraisal

There are numerous sorts of performance appraisal accessible, and they can use any methods. Generally, there are two approaches to assessment; one is trait-oriented, and the other one is result-oriented. The traits approach evaluates the conduct and attitudes of the worker, while the other one focuses only on the results of the tasks assigned to the worker. The methods of performance appraisal are categorized as:

- **Individual evaluation methods:** This method is mostly used in government organizations. This is one of the old and traditional methods of evaluating the employees. The mechanisms are

  - **Essay appraisal method:** Under this, the rater expresses in detail, the employee's strong and weak points. The suggestions for improvement are also mentioned.
  - **Critical incidence technique:** Under this method, the rater rates the employee based on the critical events that have taken place in the past and brief about positive and negative points of the employee. It is a rating method wherein rating is done for all the incidents about a particular employee that has happened during a specific period. The incidences might have occurred due to the ability/disability of the employee based on the nature of incidents.
  - **Checklists and weighted checklists:** A checklist is a set of descriptive statements about the employee and the rater has marked it accordingly. The assessment of the capacity of a worker through finding solutions to various inquiries is known as a checklist. These inquiries/ questions are identified with the conduct of a worker.
  - **Graphic rating scales:** The appraisee marks the quantity and quality of the employee based on a particular trait. The trait may be predefined. The rater has the option to rate the employee on a scale-like Likert's scale.
  - **Behaviorally anchored rating scales:** BARS are systematically developed checklist using critical incidents in combination with graphic rating scales. It consists of predetermined statements of job performance and behavior based on critical incidents. They are time-consuming and costly to construct.
  - **Management by objectives:** As already discussed in one of the previous units, here the employee and employer sit together to set the objectives of the organization. The evaluation of the employee is based on the attainment of mutually set objectives.

- **Multiple person evaluation methods:**
  - **Ranking strategy:** It is the simplest and oldest type of performance appraisal. Here a worker is ranked/ positioned against the other in the same group. In a group of 10 workers, the best performer is placed under the first rank, and the least performer is placed under the tenth rank.
  - **Paired comparison method:** This method is impractical in a large organization. Here the evaluator compares an employee against all his colleagues, and marking is done for favorable parameters upon which the appraisal is done. The evaluator repeats this exercise with each employee individually, and this is followed by the final tabulation and summary. At long last, a worker who gets the most extreme ticks is the best.
  - **Forced distribution strategy:** The evaluation is done on a group, and it is suitable for large organizations. Here the traits are not assessed; rather, the results are focused. A group of workers is selected by the supervisor/evaluator, and they are categorized into few subgroups based on outcomes such as very good, good, average, and below average. The number of subsets may be increased or decreased as per the requirement.
  - **Grading:** It also follows the moreover similar criteria of forced distribution method. Here the traits and results are assessed. A group of workers is selected by the supervisor/evaluator, and they are categorized into few subgroups based on attributes as well as consequences such as very good, good, Average, and below average. The number of subsets may be increased or decreased as per the requirement.

- **Other methods:**
  - **Assessment centers:** This is a system or organization, where the assessment of many employees is done by various experts using the various techniques. The methods include simulation exercises, role play and so on.
  - **Group appraisal method:** Here the appraisal is done by many appraisers including the immediate superior. The group may use different techniques for appraisal. This method helps in the elimination of personal bias.
  - **Field review method:** Here the employee is evaluated by a different person than the superior. The appraiser interacts with the supervisor and employee and makes the report.
  - **360-degree appraisal:** This system is also known as multi-rater feedback. A 360-degree appraisal is a type of employee performance review in which subordinates, co-workers, and managers all anonymously rate the employee. This information is then incorporated into that person's performance review. The 360-degree performance appraisal system is an advanced kind of appraisal that is used by many organizations where the performance of the employee is judged using the review of around 7–12 people. These people are working with the employee and they share some of

their work environment. The feedback is gathered in the form of reviews in terms of the competencies of the employee. The employee himself or herself also takes part in this appraisal with the help of self-assessment. The 360-degree performance appraisal system is a way to improve the understanding of the strength and weaknesses of the employee with the help of creative feedback forms.

Essentials of Good Appraisal System

- **Ease of understanding:** If an appraisal system is too complicated or too time-consuming, it may be grounded by its dead weight of complications, which nobody but only the experts understand.
- **Support of line workers:** If the line workers think that the system is too ambitious or unrealistic or that has been imposed on them by ivory-towered, staff or consultants who have no comprehension of the actual demands on the time of line workers, they will resent it.
- **Suitability to the operations and structure:** A system may function exceptionally well at an organization whose activities are compact.
- **Validity and reliability:** The efficacy of rating is the degree to which the system indeed indicates the intrinsic merit of the employees. Reliability refers to the consistency of the ratings.

Guidelines for Nurse Manager for Conducting Appraisal

The objective of a personal interview is to evaluate the past, present, and future potential of an individual. The following points are general guidelines for the nurse manager:

- Establish a friendly atmosphere by selecting the right time and place for the interview. Be sure the interview will be free of interruptions.
- Ensure freedom from a work assignment. Arrange for coverage during the time of the meeting. Begin and end the session on time.
- Establish rapport. A few brief chit-chats before the actual interview.
- Let the individual talk first. Include all the important issues in the discussion. Be alert and present criticism carefully. Never combine positive and negative comments and use the guidance approach. Use a concerned tone of voice. Discuss the work never the worker.
- Make a final overall judgment about the individual progress, as well as any recommendations on the evaluations form.
- Let the individual sign the report and explain that the signatures do not necessarily signify that he/she agrees with the content, but it indicates that she/he has read the report.

Limitations of Performance Appraisal

- The performance appraisal will be influenced by the familiarity of the employee with the employer.
- If the supervisor is not capable of the appraisal, then the employee cannot be evaluated.
- Some characteristics of a worker cannot be effortlessly evaluated through any assessment strategy.
- A manager may assess a worker to be great to make the employee happy.
- The individual difference among managers influences performance appraisal.

Potential Problems in Performance Appraisal

- **Leniency error:** The inclination of an administrator to overrate staff work.
- **Recency error:** The inclination of an administrator to rate a worker dependent on ongoing occasions as opposed to over the whole assessment time frame.
- **Halo error:** The inability to separate among different parameters of performance appraisal during its execution.
- **Horn Effect:** A tendency to rate another under a negative attitude or drive.
- **Ambiguous evaluation:** The propensity of evaluators to put vague remarks on the rating scale.

Performance Evaluation Report

Employee reviews and appraisals are some of the hardest meetings to have, and writing the report can create conflict or fear. Rather than being a manager who instills negative feelings in his employees, it can be written in such a way that the employee feels prepared to meet new challenges or fix current issues.

- **Step 1:** Decide on the criteria for review. Any manager that goes into a review completely subjective will be respected less, and all business notes that many employees already find written reviews to be "artificial and unfair." A good idea is to think about the role of the employee under review, create categories regarding that role (punctuality, work ethic, ability to meet deadlines, etc.) and use a numeric scale to rate the employee's effectiveness.
- **Step 2:** Prepare a report based on current conditions. In other words, how the employee is currently performing. Rehashing the first few weeks of the employee's work history, often the most difficult and awkward will make the employee feel despondent and unmotivated. Compliment the ways the employee is contributing, note where she can perform better, and recommend ways that the employee can contribute further in the future.
- **Step 3:** Evaluate based on your observations, not hearsay. Office gossip is not an accurate indicator of an employee's performance. For instance, saying, "I hear that many of the employees see you with personal email sites open," would

cause the employee to feel upset and vulnerable. Only bring up a point if you have witnessed it yourself.

- **Step 4:** Use specific examples for your employee review. In any observation whether positive or negative, be sure to have an example to back it up. For instance, if you want the employee to note his punctuality, say, "I appreciate the days you make it into the office by 8:30. Perhaps if you are going to be later, you could give a phone call." Employees will not grow unless they can understand what they did right or wrong in a specific scenario.
- **Step 5:** Encourage the employee under review to indicate her goals for the next year. This type of positive reinforcement makes the manager-worker relationship feel more reciprocal and motivates the employee to achieve more than she already has. Ask, "What do you feel you are capable of adding on to your duties?" or recommend a new task yourself, "I think that you are ready to move into increased client invoicing responsibility."

PROGRAM EVALUATION AND REVIEW TECHNIQUE

The program evaluation and review technique (PERT) was developed by the Special Projects Office of the U.S. Navy and applied to the planning and control of the Polaris Weapon system in 1958. It worked then, it still works, and it has been widely used as a controlling process in the business and industry.

Definition

"PERT is a network system model for planning and control under uncertain conditions. It involves identifying the key activities in a project, sequencing the activities in a flow diagram (critical pathways), and assigning the duration of each phase of the work."

The activities that cause the progress from one event to another are indicated by arrows, with the direction of the arrow showing the course of the workflow.

Steps for Accomplishing the Project

PERT also deals with the problem of uncertainty concerning time by estimating the time variances associated with the expected time of completion of the subtasks. It is a statistical method of time planning for a project/work. Three projected times are generally determined.

- **The optimistic time (O):** This occasionally happens when everything goes right. Optimistic time(t_o), which estimates the completion time without complication.
- **The most likely time (M):** It represents the most accurate forecast based on standard developments. The most likely time(t_m), which estimated the completion time with routine problems.

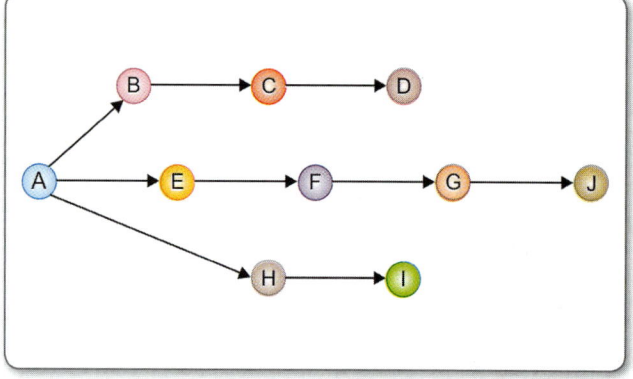

Fig. 6: Critical path method

- **The pessimistic time (P):** This is estimated at maximum potential difficulties. Pessimistic time(t_p), which determines the completion time given numerous problems.

The expected time of completion of a particular project by using beta probability distribution using the formula:

$$\frac{(t_e) = t_o + 4(t_m) + t_p}{6}$$

Example: A nurse administrator is planning to set up a new ICU in a particular hospital. The Critical Path Method (CPM) is used to plan, coordinate, and control the activities of this project (Fig. 6). The following subtasks are listed:

A: Meeting to finalize the idea of setting up an ICU.
B: Planning the infrastructure. (1 week)
C: Prepare the list of articles needed for the unit and put tender. (1 week)
D: Finalize the bid. (1 week)
E: Prepare the budget, both capital and operating. (1 week)
F: Draw the plan of ICU, and estimate the cost. (1 week)
G: Order for the articles. (1 week)
H: Give the work to the contractors to start the work. (1 week)
I: Get the materials like cement gravel tiles, electric and plumbing materials. (1 week)
J: Start the project.

PERT model indicates that subtask A should be done at first. Task C and D can be done only after the completion of task B. Task E is the predecessor of task F. Task A, B, C, D, E, and F must be completed before Task G. Finally Task J can be achieved after the completion of task G and I. If the optimistic time is 8 weeks, the most likely time 10 weeks, and the pessimistic time 12 weeks, the expected time is,

$$t_e = \frac{8 \text{ weeks} + 4\,(10 \text{ weeks}) + 12 \text{ weeks}}{6} = \frac{60 \text{ weeks}}{6} = 10 \text{ weeks}$$

Using the critical pathways, one can also plan the time duration for completing each subtask, the sum of which can be the total expected time.

Advantages of PERT

- It encourages logical discipline in planning, scheduling, and control of the project.
- It encourages more long-range and detailed project planning.
- It provides a standard method of documenting and communicating project plans, schedules, and time and cost-performance.
- It identifies the most critical elements in the plan, thus focusing management attention, i.e., most constraining on the schedule.
- It illustrates the effects of technical procedural changes on overall schedules.
- It is used for complicated and extensive projects.
- It is forward-looking.

GANTT CHARTS (ACTIVITY PLAN)

Early in this century, **Henry L. Gantt** developed the Gantt Chart as a means of controlling production/projects. It depicted a series of events essential to the completion of a project or program. It is usually used for production activities. It is typically a bar chart that explains a project schedule. It illustrates the start and finishes dates of the critical elements in a project. It is commonly used in combination with PERT as a medium to plot and represent the figures of PERT. PERT and GANTT CHARTS can be easily understood with the help of the same example as mentioned before.

Example: A nurse administrator is planning to set up a new ICU in a particular hospital. The Critical Path Method (CPM) is used to plan, coordinate, and control the activities of this project. The following subtasks are listed:

Sub task	Predecessor	Expected time
A: Meeting to finalize the idea of setting up an ICU.	Nil	0 days
B: Planning the infrastructure.	A (Start)	Seven days
C: Prepare the list of articles needed for the unit and put tender.	B	Seven days
D: Finalize the tender.	C	Seven days
E: Prepare the budget, both capital and operating.	A	Seven days
F: Draw the plan of ICU, and estimate the cost.	E	Seven days
G: Order for the articles.	D, F	Seven days
H: Give the work to the contractors to start the work.	A	Seven days
I: Get the materials like cement gravel tiles, electric and plumbing materials.	H	Seven days
J: Start the project.	G, I (Finish)	0 days

PERT model indicates that subtask A should be done at first. Task C and D can be done only after the completion of task B. Task E is the predecessor of task F. Task A, B, C, D, E, and F must be completed before Task G. Finally Task J can be achieved after the completion of task G and I.

In the above table, there are ten tasks labeled from A to J. Some jobs can be done concurrently while others cannot be done until their predecessor task is complete. Additionally, each job has three-time estimates: the optimistic time estimate (O), the most likely time estimate (M), and the pessimistic time estimate (P). (Only the expected time is mentioned in the table which is calculated using PERT formula.)

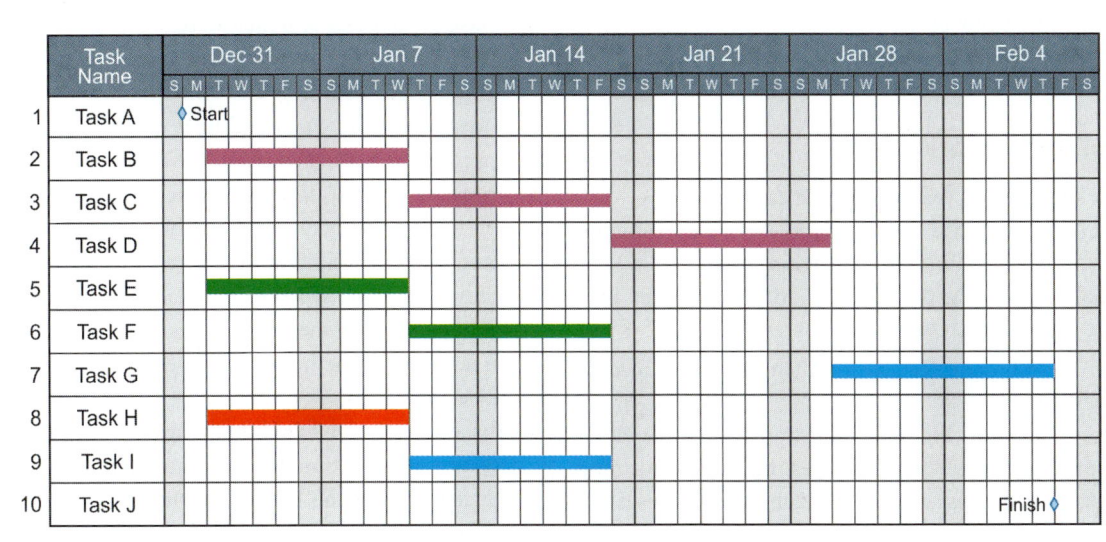

Advantages of Gantt Charts

- It forces planning and shows how pieces fit together.
- It does this for all the nursing line managers involved.
- It establishes a system for periodic evaluation and control at critical points in the program.
- It reveals problems and is forward-looking.

BENCHMARKING

Benchmarking is the process of evaluating our services by comparison with an established standard. In the context of nursing management, it is the comparison of a healthcare organization against other reputed ones of the same type. It gives an insight to the managers as for where we stand and provide a chance to observe the best practices such as evidence-based practices of other healthcare organizations. It can easily be applied to specific areas of nursing practice, such as Hospitals and Educational Institutes. The benchmarking in clinical practice improves customer satisfaction; maintain quality and helps in continuous improvement.

Definition

Benchmarking is defined as a continuous process to identify and implement the best practices that lead to superior or excellent performance.

It is a practice of identifying, understanding and adapting successful business practices and processes used by other companies, which help to improve chances in one's own company.

Purposes

- To improve the competitive position of a company.
- To recognize the strength and weaknesses of an organization.
- To gain a better understanding of efficiency, the effectiveness of organizational activities.
- To create a positive driving force in the organization and thus promotes profit gain.
- To incorporate the best practices.
- To widen the organization's experience.

Types of Benchmarking

Benchmarking can be broadly classified as (Fig. 7):
- Internal (comparing performance between different groups or teams within an organization) or
- External (comparing performance with companies in a specific industry or across industries).

Within these broader categories, there are three specific types of benchmarking:
- **Process benchmarking:** It demonstrates the methods of accomplishing particular processes by top-performing organizations. This is achieved through means of research, interviews, and visits. This supports and affirms the decision-making process.

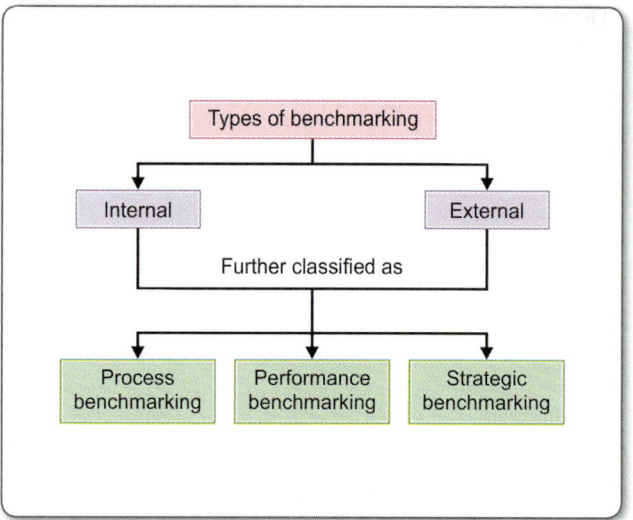

Fig. 7: Classification of benchmarking

- **Performance benchmarking:** Allows the initiator firm to assess their competitive position by comparing products and services with those of target firms. This can be done through a detailed survey.
- **Strategic benchmarking:** It is the identification of fundamental lessons and winning strategies of successful organizations. It includes all dimensions of the particular organization, which is ideal for growth with a long-term perspective. E.g. Benchmarking against the accredited/awarded organization.

Benchmarking Process

- **Phase 1: Planning:** It includes what is to be benchmarked, who are the members and partners, and what data collection method should be employed. Through this, one will come to know-how to understand the business strategy in a better way.
- **Phase 2: Analysis of benchmarking:** It involves analyzing the performance of the partners and comparing their work to figure out how and why they are better. What we understood from them and how we can use and apply to improve our performances in the organization.
- **Phase 3: Integration of benchmarking:** It involves developing the goals and combining them to perform standard benchmarking to improve the performance. The main focus is on whether the management agrees on the findings whether there is any need to modify goals based on results and whether all purposes are clearly explained to all partners involved or not.
- **Phase 4: Action in benchmarking:** This phase involves the creation of an action phase on modified goals. There is a recalibration of the benchmark in this phase. It includes new plans to achieve the goals, plans to evaluate the progress and work schedule for recalibration of the benchmarks.

The process of benchmarking follows the following stages:

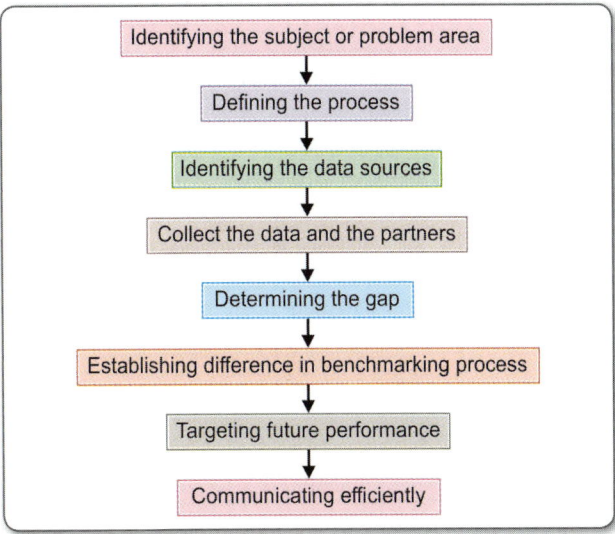

Advantages of Benchmarking

- It estimates the strength and weaknesses of the firm.
- Improve communication.
- Professionalization and growth of the organization and its services.
- Budgetary reasons.
- Self-improvement.
- Creates yardstick comparison within the industry.

CRITICAL PATH METHOD/ANALYSIS

CPM is the most versatile planning and control technique used in business. It was first employed by the E.I. Nemours Company. Unlike PERT, it is applied in those projects where activity timings are relatively well known. It is used for planning and controlling the most logical sequences of activities for accomplishing a project. The critical path method is a technique to reduce the time required to implement a project. By breaking the project into activities that must be undertaken for its implementation and by determining their time sequence, it is possible to isolate the most critical path schedule in their implementation. Under CPM, the project is analyzed into different operations or activities and their relationships are determined and show on the network diagram. The network or flow plan is then used for optimizing the use of resources and time. It is based on the assumption that the expected time is the time taken to complete the project. CPM is suitable for the construction of projects and plant maintenance. CPM requires greater planning than required otherwise it increases the planning cost, but this increase in cost is justified by concentrating on critical paths and avoiding expenses on the strict supervision and control of the whole project. Besides asserting the schedule, CPM provides a standard method of communication project plans, schedules, and costs.

Advantages

- It provides an analytical approach to the achievement of project objectives which are defined clearly.
- It identifies the most critical demands and paths more attention on these activities.
- It helps in ascertaining the time schedules.
- It makes use of better and detailed planning.
- It assists in avoiding the waste time, energy and money on unimportant activities.
- It provides a standard method for communication project plan schedules and costs.

Steps in CPM: The Steps in CPM is similar to that of PERT. The application of network techniques in project management involves the following steps. E.g. a construction company having a project for the construction of a multi-storied hospital complex.

- **Identification of component:** The first step in the application of CPM is the identification of all key activities and phases or events necessary for the completion of the project. It is denoted by a circle in a network diagram. The construction can be identified as the broad activities from 1 to 10.

Sr. no.	Activity	Expected time in weeks
1	Procurement of materials	5
2	Foundation of work	10
3	Construction of 1st floor	20
4	Construction of 2nd floor	22
5	Plumbing	6
6	Electrical fittings	10
7	Installation of doors and windows	8
8	Plastering	15
9	Flooring	8
10	Painting	8

- **Sequencing of activities and events:** A network diagram is prepared to show the sequence of activities and events. It has a beginning point and a termination point of the project. It also depicts the number of paths or activities from beginning to completion of the project. Each event is given a serial number for the sake of convenience. It may be noted that some activities have to be undertaken sequentially while others are to be carried out concurrently.
- **Determination of estimated time:** It is essential to determine the expected time required to complete each activity.
- **The determinant of critical path:** Under this stage, it is required to identify the sequence of those activities in the completion of the project. The line in the network diagram

connecting the critical activities from start to finish of the project is the critical path.

- **Modification of initial plan:** Once the critical path has been framed, an analysis shall made to check the deviation from the initial plan if any. The time (both early starting/ending and late starting/ending) shall be estimated to finalize the CPM. The potential exits for a substantial gain may alter the initial plan.

- **Controlling the project:** The project managing has to be in constant touch with the persons engaged in the critical activities. If there have been any difficulties or obstacles, they have to be removed.

- **Planning, programming and budgeting system (PPBS):** PPBS is a system to help decision-makers to allocate resources of an organization and most effectively in achieving its objectives. Another approach is known as zero budget approach, i.e., the budget starts a zero or fresh without considering the previous budget prepared. Usually Zero budget is prepared for a specified period of time such an year only.

- **Job analysis:** Job analysis is the process of gathering information on all aspects of a specific job. Job analysis is a scientific study and statement of all the facts about the job.

 REVIEW QUESTIONS

1. Define controlling. Explain the types and significance of controlling in the hospital. Brief the role of a nurse in controlling the ward.
2. Define nursing standards. Explain the types and legal significance of standards.
3. Define nursing audit. What are the methods of auditing? Explain nursing audit cycle.
4. Explain the significance of records. What are the principles of record writing? Enlist the types of records.
5. Define reports. Explain the types, significance, and role of a nurse in report making.
6. Define quality and quality assurance. Explain the principles and approaches.
7. Define continuous quality improvement. Explain in detail the quality assurance model.
8. Define performance appraisal. Explain its principles and types. Enlist the problems in performance appraisal.
9. What is performance appraisal? What are the methods of performance appraisal?
10. Explain the types of evaluation. Explain employee evaluation reports.
11. Define benchmarking and explain the purpose and process of benchmarking.

Further Readings

1. Banerjee, Shyamal. Principles and Practice of Management. Oxford and IBM Publishing, New Delhi; 2000.
2. Basavanthappa BT. Nursing Administration. 2nd Edition: Jaypee Brothers Medical Publishers (P) Ltd., New Delhi; 2009.
3. Barrett, Jean. Ward Management and Teaching. Konark Publishers, Delhi; 1992.
4. Warren, Stevens, F. Management and Leadership in Nursing. McGraw – Hill Inc, New York; 1978.
5. Alexander et al. Nursing Service Administration. Mosby Publishers, US; 1962.
6. Park K. Preventive and Social Medicine, 19th Edition: M/s. Banarasidas Bhanot Publishers, Jabalpur; 2007.
7. Basavanthappa BT. Nursing Administration, 1st Edition: Jaypee Brothers Medical Publishers (P) Ltd., New Delhi; 2002.
8. Goel SL, Kumar R. Management of Hospitals – Hospital Administration in the 21st century, Vol. 4, Deep and Deep Publication, New Delhi; 2002.
9. Ranga Rao SP. Administration of Primary Health Centers in India, 1st Edition: Mittal Publications, New Delhi; 1993.
10. Lucita M. Nursing: Practice and Public Health Administration. Current Concepts and Trends. B. I. Churchill Living Stone Pvt. Ltd., New Delhi; 2002.
11. Sakharkar BM. Principles of Hospital Administration and Planning, 2nd Edition: Jaypee Brothers Medical Publishers (P) Ltd., New Delhi; 2009.
12. Patricia S Yoder-Wise. Leading and Managing in Nursing. 2nd Edition: Mosby Publication, US; 1999.
13. Bessie L Marquis, Carol J Huston. Leadership Roles and Management Functions in Nursing: Theory and Application. 5th Edition: Lippincott Williams and Wilkins, New York; 2006.
14. Linda Roussel. Management and Leadership for Nurse Administrators. 4th Edition: Jones and Bartlett Publication, USA; 2006.
15. Wehrich H, Koontz H. Management A Global Perspective. 11th Edition: Tata McGraw-Hill Publishing Company, Ltd., New Delhi; 2005.
16. Marquis BL, Huston CJ. Leadership and Management Functions in Nursing- Theory, and Application. 5th Edition: Lippincott Williams and Wilkins, Philadelphia; 2006.
17. Douglass LM. The Effective Nurse: Leader and Manager. 5th Edition: Mosby Publication, US; 1996.
18. Trained Nurses Association of India, Nursing Administration, and Management.
19. Samson Rebecca. Leadership and Management in Nursing Practice and Education 1st Edition: Jaypee Brothers Medical Publishers (P) Ltd., New Delhi; 2009.
20. Kunders GD. Designing for Total Quality in Health Care, Prism Book Pvt. Ltd., Bangalore; 2002.
21. Chandorkar AG. Hospital Administration and Planning. 2nd Edition: Paras Medical Publisher, New Delhi; 2009.
22. Joshi DC, Joshi Mamta. Hospital Administration. 1st Edition: Jaypee Brothers Medical Publishers (P) Ltd., New Delhi; 2009.
23. Eleanor J Sullivan, Philip J Decker. Effective Leadership and Management in Nursing. 4th Edition: Published by Addison Wesely; 2011.
24. Kulkarni GR. Financial Management for Hospital Administration, Jaypee Brothers Medical Publishers (P) Ltd., New Delhi; 2009.

Unit

9

Organizational Behavior and Human Relations

 Unit Outline

- Concept and Theories of Organization
- Organizational Behavior
- Group Dynamics
- Interpersonal Relationship
- Human Relations
- Public Relations
- Relations with Professional Organizations
- Collective Bargaining
- Motivation
- Motive
- Concept of Employee Morale
- Communication
- Assertive Communication in the Workplace
- Committees

CONCEPT AND THEORIES OF ORGANIZATION

The organization is "a group of people working together and with each other towards the achievement of the common goals."

Characteristics of an Organization

- Group of people with common goals or objectives.
- There is a division of work.
- Vertical and horizontal relationship is the relationship between supervisor and subordinates or the relationship between different departments and divisions.
- Chain of command with laid down channels of communication. (flow of authority from the higher to the lower levels of management in the hierarchy).
- Group dynamics is the interactions that take place between the individuals and groups within the organization, based on their values, needs, sentiments, attitudes, beliefs, and interests. It is a social, self-generating, and dynamic interactive process that gives rise to an informal group.

Principles of Organization

- **The principle of a chain of command:** The flow of communication is through the chain of command. The channel of communication tends to be one way downward.
- **The principle of unity of command:** It is the concept of responsibility/guideline of duty. The authoritative set up should be masterminded so that a subordinate should get the guidance or heading from one manager.
- **The principle of the span of control:** It alludes to the most significant number of individuals adequately directed by a solitary person. The count of individuals might be expanded or diminished by the type of work done by the subordinates or the capacity of the chief. It empowers the smooth working of the association.
- **The principle of specialization or division of work:** Every worker must perform one's respective function with full authority and accountability. The labor must be scientifically divided. Division of labor is differentiation among kinds of duties. Specialization helps in the control of actions among individuals and groups. It will aid in keeping the correct man for the right activity and save resources and time.
- **Hierarchy/Scalar chain:** It is the order of rank from top to bottom in an organization. It is the line through which authority is passed on, or the command is exercised.
- **Centrality:** It is the position or distance the person has on the organizational chart from other workers.
- **Unity of objectives:** Every establishment functions to achieve specific predetermined objectives. The organization requires employees who are being geared towards the fulfillment of these objectives.

- **Definition of jobs/principle of definition:** It is essential to characterize and settle the obligations, duties, and power of every laborer. Notwithstanding that, the authoritative relationship of every laborer with others should be unmistakably described in the hierarchical setup.
- **The principle of balance:** Many units are working independently under an authoritative setup. The duty of one group may have been initiated after the fulfillment of the work by another group. So, the grouping of work should be masterminded logically.
- **The principle of equilibrium balance:** In specific periods, a few segments are over-burdened. Amid this period, due importance may be given to a department based on the new remaining task at hand. The over-burden areas or offices can be additionally separated into subsections or sub-divisions. It would involve in the compelling command over all the actions of the association.
- **The principle of continuity:** The process of administration is a continuing or ongoing process, recycling the structure of the organization based on the economic, environmental, and socio-political changes.
- **The principle of exception:** It implies to the fact that the routine decision making should rest with lower levels of management within the policy framework. The unusual or exceptional matters should be referred to as the higher levels of management for taking decisions.
- **The principle of unity of direction:** It is the rule of coordination. Many subdivisions are made on the original plan. Each sub-plan is assigned to a specific section/ department. Every section is asked to collaborate to achieve the principle targets or in executing the main aims of the association.
- **The principle of communication:** A two-way communication flow from upward to downward and vice versa is a prerequisite to obtaining an active organizational setup.
- **The principle of flexibility:** To meet the challenges of the increasing and changing demands of the environment, an organization structure is subjected to change. As such rigidity has to be avoided and flexibility is essential in the organization structure so that changes can be brought about without disrupting the basic design of the structure.

ORGANIZATIONAL BEHAVIOR

An organization needs to achieve effectiveness in its activities. It refers to the behavior of individuals and groups within organizations and the interaction between its members and their external environment.

Definitions

Organizational behavior is a field of study that investigates the impact that individuals, groups, and structure have on behavior within an organization to apply such knowledge towards improving an organization's effectiveness.

—Stephen P Robbins

Organizational behavior is directly concerned with the understanding of prediction and control of human behavior.

—**Fred Luthans**

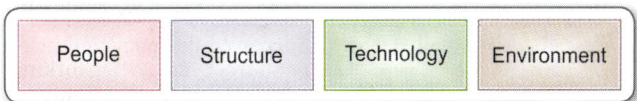

- **People:** People are the central resource of any organization. It is the individuals who constitute the organization.
- **Structure:** Organization is a social system. Any social system has its structure, and that could be either formal or informal.
- **Technology:** The company purchases technological tools for purposes of production and service, and this is an essential element of an organization's behavioral system.
- **Environment:** There are two types of environment in which an organization operate: internal and external.

Theories of Organization/Organizational Behavior

- **Classical theory:** It was found by Frederick W. Taylor, the father of scientific management. He proposed this theory based on four principles. They are:
  - The principle of division of labor
  - Principle of scalar and functional processes
  - Principle of structure
  - The principle of span of control

Classic organizational theorists believe that the size, structure, division of labor, number of supervisory levels, and span of control are critical variables in determining the success or efficiency of an organization. It is based on the belief that breaking down the operation into specialized components is necessary for the assignment and completion of responsibilities. Creating these specialized segments demands coordination that is best handled by a delegation of authority to supervisory personnel, such as the nursing administrator or a head nurse.

Classic organization theory tries to differentiate staff and line relationships. According to the line roles a head nurse is directly responsible for employees and their services. Traditionally lines authority is designated to hire and fire the employees. In contrast, the clinical specialist has traditionally held a staff position, indirectly responsible for the same services through employee education, consulting, and role modeling.

Criticism

Lack of decision-making opportunities for employees is a result of the structure itself. Often the individual who makes the decisions and the individual who implements them occupy different positions on the organizational chart. This criticism has led to a study of the psychology of work behavior and research into employee participation as a means of increasing motivation and commitment. This theory is based on an authoritarian approach.

- It does not care about the human element in an organization.
- It does not give two-way communication.
- The motivational assumptions underlying the theories are incomplete and consequently inaccurate.
- The outside factors on individual behavior are ignored.
- The generalizations of classical theories have not been tested by strictly scientific methods.

- **Neo-classical theory:** This theory is produced to fill the holes and inadequacies in the classical approach. It focuses on the movement of human relationships. Investigation of the association depends on human conduct, for example, how individuals carry on and why they do as such in a specific circumstance. It calls attention to the reasonable troubles of the working of scalar and functional aspects. The primary commitment of this theory features the significance of the advisory groups and better communication/correspondence. This theory also underscores that laborers should be urged and persuaded to display active involvement in the production. The emotions and suppositions of the employees should be considered and regarded before any change is presented in the association. In a nutshell, if the classical theory is production-oriented, then the neoclassical approach is employee-oriented.
  - The person should be the basis of an organization.
  - The organization should be viewed as a total unity.
  - Individual goals and organization goals must be integrated.
  - There should be a flow of communication from bottom to top and from top to bottom.
  - The employee should be given more power, responsibility, authority, and control.
  - Preparation of working standards and decision making should be participative.
  - Members usually belong to formal and informal groups and interact with others within each group or subgroup.

- **Modern organizational theory: (Flatter organization):** It was organized in the early 1950s. Modern or Contemporary organizational theorists suggest that an essential element in understanding and predicting organizational behavior is the ability to predict the functioning of the persons within an organization. These theorists contend that the following aspects are keys to organizational harmony and success.
  - Motivation
  - Satisfaction
  - Leadership
  - How conflicts are resolved

Unlike the classic approach, which focuses on structure and function, this approach maximizes the value of the individual. It recognizes that each employee has a set of unique processes, feelings, and thoughts that may not fit with those of the organization and may create tension among employers and employees. The supervisor's role becomes one of initiating activities that help the employee and supervisor to succeed together.

Criticism of Modern Theory

- This theory puts old wine into a new bottle.
- It does not represent a unified body of knowledge. There is nothing new in this theory because it is based on past empirical studies.
- This theory forms only the questions and not the answers. It is based on behavioral, social, and mathematical methods. These are management theories in themselves.

- **Motivation theory:** It is related to the work inspiration of workers of the association. The works are performed viably if appropriate inspiration is given to the representatives. The motivation might be financial incentives or non-financial incentives. The internal gifts of any individual can be recognized in the wake of providing sufficient inspiration to him or her. Maslow's hierarchy of needs theory and Herzberg's two-factor theory are some of the examples of motivation theory.

- **Decision theory:** It was proposed by Herbert. A. Simon, and he won the Nobel Prize for it in the year 1978. He viewed the association as a structure of decision makers/leaders. The decisions/choices were taken at all areas of the association, but the decisions related to policy matters are entrusted with higher levels. Simon has recommended that the hierarchical structure is planned through an examination that focuses on what decisions/plans/choices are made and the people from whom data is required if decisions/plans/choices should be acceptable.

GROUP DYNAMICS

It is defined as a force or actions of a group within. The group dynamic is concerned with the dynamic interaction of individuals in a face to face relationship. The task goal of the group originating from the fundamental organization objectives provides for their continued cooperation. As a leader, understanding the group dynamics is essential to both compose and guide individuals within a group for successfully and efficiently completing an assignment.

Group dynamics might be characterized as the standard procedure by which individuals associate up close and personal in groups. It is a part of social psychology which ponders issues, including the structure of a group/gathering.

Type of Groups

- **Formal and informal groups:** Formal type alludes to those which are built up under the lawful or formal specialist with the view to accomplishing specific results. E.g., trade unions. The casual or informal type alludes to the total of individual contact and connection and a system of the relationship among the person. E.g., group of friends.

- **Primary and secondary gatherings:** Primary ones are described by small size, with increased intimacy and face to face relationships. E.g., family, neighbors, etc. The latter ones are characterized by expansive size, and individual identity features more than the usual and natural interactions. E.g., professional associations.

- **Social groups** Allude to a coordinated arrangement of the people with similar mentality and objectives. E.g., political parties, public clubs, etc.

- **Reference group:** It is a kind of group that individuals use to assess themselves.

- **Functional groups:** The people who cooperate and perform similar tasks every day.

Principles of Group Dynamics

- The individuals/members must have a solid feeling of belongingness in the group.
- Any single change in a group can create tension for others too, and hence it can be overcome by wiping out the replacement or rearrangement of the group.
- The group functioning is controlled by common motives.
- Groups make due by setting the individuals into the useful chain of designation/importance and encouraging the activity towards the objectives.
- The organization of the group, participation of members, and their internal relations makes the group productive.
- Information identifying with a requirement for change, plan for change, and the result of changes must be shared by group members.

Elements of Group Dynamics

- **Communication:** One of the most straight forward parts of group formation is their communication pattern. The sorts of perceptions we make give us pieces of information to other essential things which might go on in the group, for example, who drives whom or who impacts whom.

- **Content versus process:** When we see what the group is discussing, we are concentrating on the content. When we attempt to see how the group is taking care of its correspondence, i.e., who talks how much or who converses with whom, we are discussing the process. The content of the discussion in a group explains its plan of process/function.

- **Decision:** Many sorts of choices are made in groups without considering the impacts these choices have on different individuals. Some endeavor to force their own decisions on the group, while others need all individuals to take an interest or offer in the decisions that are made. A few choices are made intentionally after much discussion and casting a ballot. Others are made quietly when nobody gives a recommendation.

- **Influence:** Some individuals may talk practically nothing, yet they may catch the consideration of the group. Others may be talkative, but members may not listen to him/her.

Group Development

Group dynamics is also concerned with the development of new groups and why and how they develop. As per Tuckman's theory/hypothesis, there are five phases in the development of groups.

1. **Forming:** This stage is typically described by some perplexity and vulnerability. The real objectives of the group have not been set up. The idea of the errand or authority of the group has not been resolved. Accordingly, forming is an introductory period when individuals become acquainted with each other and offer assumptions regarding the group. These sentiments fortify in later phases of improvement. People are regularly confounded amid this stage since jobs are not clear, and there may not be a solid head.

2. **Storming:** Here, the group is probably going to see the largest amount of difference and struggle. Individuals frequently challenge aggregate objectives and the battle for power. People often compete for the initial position amid this phase of advancement.

3. **Norming:** This stage is portrayed by the acknowledgment of individual contrasts and shared desires. Ideally, at this stage, the group individuals will start to build up a sentiment of group union and character.

4. **Performing:** Performing happens when the group has developed and achieves a sentiment of cohesiveness. Amid this phase of advancement, people acknowledge each other, and strife is settled through group talk. Individuals from the group decide on choices through a sound procedure that is centered around significant objectives as opposed to severe subject matters.

5. **Adjourning:** All the groups do not undergo this stage since it is described by the disbandment of the group. Reasons may vary, but the common cause is the accomplishment of the objectives. Members may express fear of closure and sadness as the termination phase begins.

Roles of Nurse Manager in Group Dynamics

- Supervise and deal with the general working of staff in the division.
- Analyzing, detailing, giving suggestions, and creating techniques on the most proficient method to enhance the quality of nursing care.
- Accomplish the objectives and vision of the organization.
- Involve in human resource management, in-service education, working out pay and rewards, and other staff development activities.

- Identifying issues, making decisions, and giving alternative courses of action.

INTERPERSONAL RELATIONSHIP

One of the most distinctive aspects of human beings is that we are social beings. Interpersonal relationships are and have been the core of our social system since the dawn of civilization. Nursing is a therapeutic process and demands an association between the nurse and the patient. The interpersonal relationship between an employee and his/her supervisor is critical to the employee's motivation level. We often forget that the only way to achieve our goals is through the people who work with us. Therefore, although managers cannot directly motivate, they can create a climate that demonstrates positive rewards for their employees, encourages open communication as well as growth and productivity and recognizes achievement.

Interpersonal relationships refer to reciprocal social and emotional interactions between two or more individuals in an environment.

An interpersonal relationship is defined as a close association between individuals who share common interests and goals.

Dynamics of Interpersonal Relationship

The dynamics of interpersonal relationship consists of three kinds: Dyad, Triad and Group (Fig. 1).

- **Dyad:** A dyad consists of two interacting people. It is the simplest of the three interpersonal dynamics. One person relays a message and the other listens. It is one of the most unstable interpersonal dynamics. The interaction ends when one constituent of the dyad refuses to listen or share his or her message. It is also one of the most intimate interpersonal dynamics as the focus of listening and communication is centered on only one person.

- **Triad:** A triad consists of three interacting people. The members engage in the relay and reception of thoughts and ideas. It is more stable than the dyad as the third member may act as a mediator when there is a conflict between the other two.

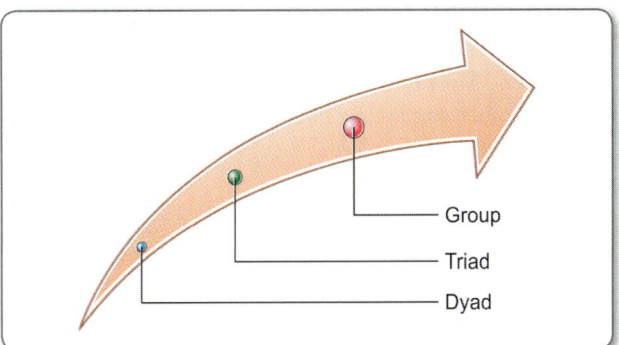

Fig. 1: Dynamics of interpersonal relationship

- **Group:** A group consists of more than three members and is a collection of triads and dyads. It is the most stable form of interpersonal relationships.

Purposes of Interpersonal Relationship

- The interpersonal relationship for an individual are:
  - Personal growth and development
  - Source of enjoyment
  - Sense of security
  - Context of understanding
  - Interpersonal needs
  - Establishing personal identity
- The interpersonal relationship for nurses are:
  - Building a positive functional multidisciplinary team
  - Improving intra and/or inter-team communication, coordination and cooperation
  - Building mutual understanding and cooperation
  - Understanding self
  - Improved decision making and problem-solving
- The interpersonal relationship for patients are:
  - Developing a sense of security and comfort
  - Fostering trust and cooperation
  - Facilitating communication
  - Improving socialization
  - Developing and maintaining positive feelings

Types of Interpersonal Relationship

Interpersonal relationships are classified based on relational contexts of interaction and the types of mutual expectations between communicators. Some common types of interpersonal relationships are:

- **Friendship:** Theories of friendship emphasize the concept as a freely chosen association where individuals develop a common ground of thinking and behaving when they enter into the relationship by including mutual love, trust, respect and unconditional acceptance for each other. Friendship is a relationship with no formalities and the individuals enjoy each other's presence.
- **Family and kinship:** Family communication patterns establish roles and identify and enable personal and social growth of individuals. Family relationships can get distorted if there is an unresolved conflict between members. Most of the time, a significant family member senses other family member has significant emotional difficulties but fails to bring them out unless the physician or nurse enquires.
- **Professional relationship:** Individuals working for the same organization are said to share a professional relationship and are called colleagues. Colleagues may or may not like each other.
- **Love:** A informalized intimate relationship characterized by passion, intimacy, trust and respect is called love.

Individuals in a romantic relationship are deeply attached and share a special bond.

- **Marriage:** Marriage is a formalize intimate relationship or a long-term relationship where two individuals decide to enter into wedlock and stay together life-long after knowing each other well.
- **Platonic relationship:** A relationship between two individuals without feelings of sexual desire for each other is called a platonic relationship. In such a relationship, a man and a woman are just friends and do not mix love with friendship. Platonic relationships might end in a romantic relationship with partners developing feelings of love for each other.
- **Casual relationships:** In these relationships, the individuals usually develop a relationship that exclusively lacks mutual love and consists of sexual behavior only that does not extend beyond one night. These individuals may be known as sexual partners in a wider sense of friends with benefits who consider sexual intercourse only in their relationship.
- **Brotherhood and sisterhood:** Individuals united for a common cause or a common interest (may involve formal membership in clubs, organizations, associations, societies, etc.) may be termed as a brotherhood or a sisterhood. In this relationship, individuals are committed to doing good deeds for fellow members and people.
- **Acquaintances:** An acquaintance is a relationship where someone is simply known to someone by introduction or by a few interactions. The close relationship is absent and the individuals lack in-depth personal information about others. This could also be the beginning of a future close relationship.

Phases of Interpersonal Relationship

Hildegard Peplau (1952) gave the interpersonal relationship model which explains the four phases of the interpersonal relationship (Fig. 2).

1. **Orientation phase:** The orientation phase defines the problem. It starts when the nurse meets the patient, and the two are strangers. After defining the problem, the orientation phase identifies the type of service needed by the patient. The patient seeks assistance, tells the nurse what he or she needs, asks questions, and shares preconceptions and expectations based on past experiences. Essentially, the orientation phase is the nurse's assessment of the patient's health and situation.

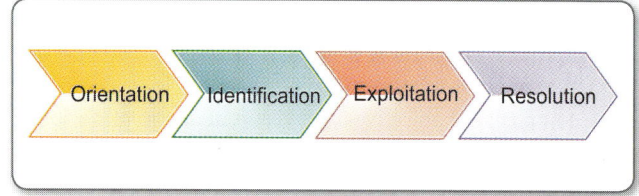

Fig. 2: Phases of interpersonal relationship

2. **Identification phase:** The identification phase includes the selection of the appropriate assistance by a professional. In this phase, the patient begins to feel as if he or she belongs, and feels capable of dealing with the problem which decreases the feeling of helplessness and hopelessness. The identification phase is the development of a nursing care plan based on the patient's situation and goals.

3. **Exploitation phase:** The exploitation phase uses professional assistance for problem-solving alternatives. The advantages of the professional services used are based on the needs and interests of the patients. In the exploitation phase, the patient feels like an integral part of the helping environment and may make minor requests or use attention-getting techniques. When communicating with the patient, the nurse should use interview techniques to explore, understand, and adequately deal with the underlying problem. The nurse must also be aware of the various phases of communication since the patient's independence is likely to fluctuate. The nurse should help the patient exploit all avenues of help as progress is made toward the final phase. This phase is the implementation of the nursing plan, taking actions toward meeting the goals set in the identification phase.

4. **Resolution phase:** It is the termination of the professional relationship since the patient's needs have been met through the collaboration of the patient and nurse. They must sever their relationship and dissolve any ties between them. This can be difficult for both if psychological dependence still exists. The patient drifts away from the nurse and breaks the bond between them. A healthier emotional balance is achieved and both become mature individuals. This is the evaluation of the nursing process. The nurse and patient evaluate the situation based on the goals set and whether or not they were met.

The goal of psychobdynamic nursing is to help understand one's behavior, help others identify felt difficulties, and apply principles of human relations to the problems that come up at all experience levels. Peplau explains that nursing is therapeutic because it is a healing art, assisting a patient who is sick or in need of health care. It is also an interpersonal process because of the interaction between two or more individuals who have a common goal. The nurse and patient work together so both become mature and knowledgeable in the care process.

The nurse has a variety of roles in Hildegard Peplau's nursing theory. The six main roles are stranger, teacher, resource person, counselor, surrogate, and leader. As a stranger, the nurse receives the patient in the same way the patient meets a stranger in other life situations. The nurse should create an environment that builds trust. As a teacher,

the nurse imparts knowledge about the needs or interests of the patient. In this way, a nurse is also a resource person, providing specific information needed by the patient that helps the patient understand a problem or situation. The nurse's role as a counselor helps the patient understand and integrate the meaning of current life situations, as well as provide guidance and encouragement to make changes. As a surrogate, the nurse helps the patient clarify the domains of dependence, interdependence, and independence, and acts as an advocate for the patient. As a leader, the nurse helps the patient take on maximum responsibility for meeting his or her treatment goals. Additional roles of a nurse include technical expert, consultant, tutor, socializing and safety agent, environment manager, mediator, administrator, record observer, and researcher.

Barriers of Interpersonal Relationship

There are three barriers of interpersonal relationship (Fig. 3).
1. **Personal barriers:** Personal barriers may include fear of rejection, Gender, Psychiatric problems, Lack of honesty and trust, lack of compatibility, feeling of insecurity, ineffective communication, distorted self-concept, lack of flexibility, lack of respect for the rights of others, and so on.
2. **Situational factors:** Situational factors include complex interaction setting, Adverse environmental situations, Lack of territoriality, High density of individuals, large distance and lack of time.
3. **Sociocultural barriers:** It includes cultural diversity, ethnic diversity, social diversity, and language diversity.

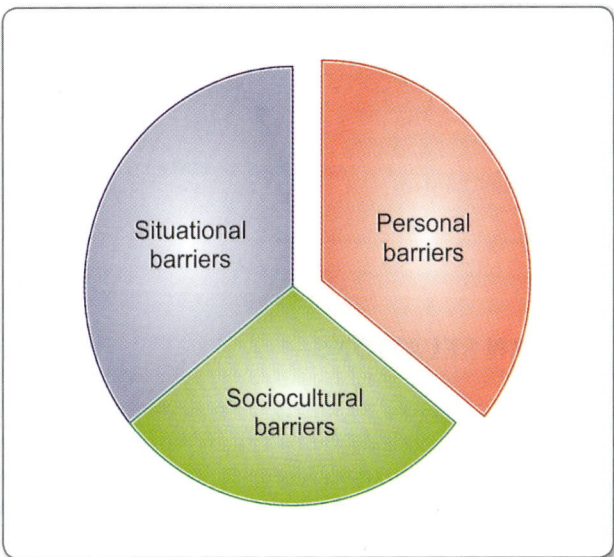

Fig. 3: Barriers of interpersonal relationship

Methods to Overcome the Barriers

The methods of overcome the barriers of interpersonal relationship are given in Table 1.

TABLE 1: Methods to overcome the barriers of interpersonal relationship

Categories of barriers	Description of barriers	Methods to overcome
Personal barriers	Gender variation	In IPR, gender must be given due consideration
	Lack of honesty and trust	Honesty and trust must be maintained while establishing and building IPRs
	Lack of compatibility	Compatibility between the individual involved in IPR must be ensured.
	Feeling of insecurity	A sense of security must be ensured between the people involved in an IPR
	Ineffective communication	Effective communication is a key aspect of efficient IPRs; therefore, effective communication must be ensured.
	Distorted self-concept	Individuals involved in IPRs must have a sound self-concept and +ve self-esteem
	Lack of flexibility	There must be flexibility in ideology and philosophy of the individuals in a relationship for an effective adaptation and success of the IPR
	Lack of respect for others' rights	A mutual sense of respect must be ensured by the people involved in personal and professional relationships
	Fear of rejection	Fear of rejection must be eliminated between the individual involved in a relationship
	Pre-existing psychiatric problem	Skilled therapeutic communication is required to interact with individuals who suffers from psychiatric or personality problems.
Situational barriers	Complex interaction setting	The individuals must try to make the interaction setting simple and familiar and must make the other person feel important.
	Adverse environmental situations Lack of territoriality A high density of individuals	Special care must be taken while developing a relationship between individuals of diversified territories and high density or interaction in adverse environmental situations.
	Lack of distance Lack of time	Even in an organization, individuals must spend quality time with their co-workers to strengthen the bond between them
Sociocultural barriers	Cultural diversity Ethnic diversity Social diversity	An individual can try to overcome cultural diversity in trying to enhance the four primary factors that decide interaction patterns (such as openness, trust, owing and risk to experiment)
	Language diversity	Individuals must try to enhance interpersonal communication skills (such as maintaining good eye contact, appropriate body language, listening with patience, etc.)

HUMAN RELATIONS

Human relations and organizational behaviors are two vital aspects to any organization especially in the present scenario of technical and modern advancement. It helps to bring about productivity, a work culture, the essence of responsibility and accountability.

Human relations is the skill or ability to work effectively through and with other people.

Human relations is defined as a phenomenon of organized human activity directed towards the promotion of cooperative and happy work relationships. It is getting the work done by people with their hearts in the job.

Goals of Human Relation

- **Self-esteem:** Self-esteem is at the core of most issues in human relations. Self-esteem is a feeling of confidence and worth as a person. Psychological research has shown that low self-esteem is related to a variety of mental health problems including alcoholism, anxiety, depression; all of which cause problems on the job. High self-esteem on the other hand, healthy self-esteem is the key to top performance and high-quality work, especially when the work directly affects other staff.

- **Mutual respect:** Mutual respect is the positive consideration or regard that two persons have for each other, can exist only when self-esteem is stable. Without trust, mutual trust is meaningless. Nurses at all levels of an organization need trust and mutual respect to performing at their best.

- **Self-awareness and self-disclosure:** Self-awareness is the knowledge of how you are being perceived by others. Self-disclosure is the process of letting other nurses know what you are thinking and feeling. Self-awareness allows one to know what is one's behavior and is being perceived as real by other nurses; self-disclosure involves 'being real' with others and reflects the positive side of human relationships.

Elements of Human Relation

- **Human need satisfaction:** According to Maslow's theory, there is a hierarchy of needs: physiological, safety, social, esteem and self-actualization needs. These needs are prepotent for motivating factors.
- **Motivation:** Motivation is the act of stimulating an individual or oneself to contribute the utmost to achieve the desired objectives. It can be induced through monetary sources, positive reinforcement, participation, and job enrichment.
- **Distribution of status and roles:** The employees should be inspired and encouraged in updating the knowledge for staff and professional development.
- **Informal social groups:** It is important to have a social gathering to exchange views and to share their feelings.
- **Spontaneity of group formation:** These are a form of associations through which they can work together and can take decisions for the betterment of staff.

Principles of Human Relation

- Recognition and appreciation should be given
- Fair treatment with an understanding of emotions and feelings
- Informal relations should be encouraged along with a formal relationship.
- Job security and job satisfaction
- Effective communication
- Decentralization of work and give autonomy to staff and functional departments
- Participatory decision making
- Concern for developing self motivated nurses

Advantages of Human Relation

- It has a great impact on the efficiency, productivity, and profitability of the nursing organization
- Reduces the incidence of absenteeism, strikes, and acts of indiscipline.
- It is more preventive in nature than curative.
- It can provide a nurse manager with an overall picture of the individual and group needs of the behavioral pattern of staff.

Roles of Nurse Manager in Developing Human Relations

- Recognize the importance of the individual and humanly deal with them.
- There must be a mutual understanding of their position.
- The nurse employees and administrators should have a common interest.
- Mutual discussion, exchange of views and good communication must be inculcated among nurses.
- Set a good example.
- Be fair and impartial
- Develop a promotion ladder for nurses
- Give clear, concise and complete instructions.
- Evaluate the effectiveness of work performed by nurses and of her own.

PUBLIC RELATIONS

Public relation is knowing what the public expects and explaining how the administration is meeting these desires.

—**John Millet**

Public relations in the government is the composite of all the primary and secondary contacts between the bureaucracy and citizens and all the interactions of influences and attitudes established in these contracts.

—**J L McCamy**

Need for Public Relation

Four increasing necessities signify public relations such as the updated norm of the government, increased population and associated communication issues, highly educated customers, and advancements in communication techniques.

Functions of Public Relations

- Public Relations is establishing the relationship between the two groups (organization and public).
- Art or Science of developing mutual understanding and goodwill.
- It analyzes the public perception and attitude, identifies the organization policy with the public interest, and then executes the programs for communication with the public.

Elements of Public Relation

- **Human relations:** Getting along with people. One should be aware of another person and interested in his/her progress.
- **Empathy:** Feeling with others.
- **Persuasion:** Causing somebody to do something by reasoning with him; compelling is against the principles of social contact.
- **Dialogue:** Conversation with a purpose. It is used for influencing behavior, selling goods, or inspiring ideas. Conciliation and compromise are involved in the dialogue.

Forms/Types of Public Relation

It is a general term that may incorporate numerous other "relations" with diverse crowds, methodologies, and strategies. For instance:

- **Employee relations:** It is an element of the public relations that incorporates reacting to the feelings and concerns of the employee and providing information and inspiration. A few strategies utilized for this relations may incorporate an excellent induction program for the new employee, an award for employee of the month, giving recognition through newsletters and media.
- **Community relations:** It is the capacity of effectively arranging and taking part in all the activities of the community that is in favor of the society and the health care organization. The typical strategies in the community are different events, sponsored programs, voluntarily initiated programs. This also helps in improving community relations along with their development both economically and socially.
- **Government relations:** It is a component of identifying with government authorities and organizations about issues that affect the hospital and its consumers.
- **Media relations:** It is regularly viewed as synonymous with the public relation, is the capacity of working with the media to impart the news. Media relations can be effectively looking for positive attention for a newsworthy subject at the hospital or receptive reacting to a news request about a positive or negative story remarkable to the media and its perusers or watchers.

Public Relation Plan for a Hospital

Each hospital should have an updated plan for public relations that aims/diagrams objectives and wanted results for a time of three to five years. When a general PR plan is set up, intermittent planning and modifications are necessary. The arrangements and its updates not only help the workers but also act as a tool that is effective in communicating with others of higher rank. Following are the critical components of a viable PR plan:

- **Goals/Objectives:** Public relations objectives help to coordinate the methodologies and strategies in future public relations. The purpose should bolster the mission of the hospital.
- **Target audiences:** Detail the group of individuals that are essential to advise or impact, and why, for example, patients, doctors, media, and so on.
- **Tactics:** It is simple for occupied hospital experts to consider strategies first; however, it is essential to have a substantial procedure set up. Seeking for the strategy will help to accomplish the objectives. Here are some "best uses" for explicit strategy, for example, brochure, letters, direct mail, and so forth.

- **Distribution methods:** How you disperse materials is frequently as imperative as what the association sends. It is a smart thshould know which strategies are best for the intended target groups, particularly the reporters.
- **Budgets:** Nothing is free—Consider cost both direct and indirect. Indeed, even an official press release has a price tag. It should be focused that it is carefully prepared, edited, printed, and published with minimum cost.

Method of Improving Public Relation in Hospital

As mentioned below the public relation in a hospital can further be improved by some tactics such as:

- **General:** High-quality patient care by the hospital is the theme of any public relations program. No amount of smiles, cheers, and propaganda will compensate for lousy administration and poor professional care in the hospital.
- **Physical facilities:** The hospital must be well-planned with sufficient waiting areas for the patient and accompanying people. There should be optimum floor space for each department of the hospital. It also must have the logical layout of the department and work areas. There should be adequate facilities like toilets, canteen, drinking water facility. All these factors help in improving the hospital image.
- **Staff:** In a hospital, the team consists of various individuals drawn from the different status of society with varying levels of education and background.
- **Name labels and uniform:** All functionaries should wear uniforms and name labels. This creates an initial good impression on patients and reflects proper administration.
- **Importance of color:** Color affects many of our moods and emotions. Proper choice of color can transform a depressing and monotonous atmosphere into a pleasing and exciting one. It stimulates an employee's productivity. Hospital is one area where color can be used with measured success not only in appearance but for the psychological uplifting which it brings to patients.
- **Waiting time:** The waiting time in the OPD is invariably the sore point of public grievances. Introduction of the appointment system, staggering of OPD timings for the registration, punctual attendance by doctors are some of the remedies which can be introduced to reduce waiting time and have successfully been implemented in many hospitals.
- **Delay in admission:** Anxiety and distress is the result of delays in admission due to the long waiting list.
- **Privacy:** The provision of screens around each bed would afford greater privacy.
- **Ward reception:** Patients are generally vulnerable to anxiety and fear on arrival in the ward. The way they are received in the department tends to leave a deep impression. Timely reception improves the confidence of the patients.

- **Cleanliness:** Clean environment is the signature of the hospital. It enhances the image of the hospital and also helps in preventing or controlling the infection. The cleaning should be done with an adequate amount of cleaning materials/solutions. Deodorants may be used to eliminate the stink, which is most dissatisfying.
- **Food:** Good food is well prepared, and attractively that served to patients, makes a very favorable impression. The presence of a dietitian or a nurse at the time of service creates a good impact on the patients.

RELATIONS WITH PROFESSIONAL ORGANIZATIONS

Professional associations in nursing are essential for creating the vitality, stream of thoughts, and proactive work expected to keep up a sound calling that advocates for the necessities of its customers and nurses, and the credibility by society.

Importance of Joining a Professional Organization

- **Broaden your knowledge:** Professional associations offer courses, workshops, classes as well as conferences and workshops to keep themselves and their individuals state-of-the-art on the most recent expert developments, research, and other patterns. Remaining trained and educated on the trends of one's profession will help one over the long haul and will put one on stage in front of the opposition.
- **Take charge of your career:** Take the preferred standpoint of vocation assets. Affiliations regularly have job vacancies on the web or in print accessible just to their individuals. This is an incredible method to discover focused on the occupation of one's taste.
- **Build a superior resume:** It gives more weight to the resume if our association and achievement with different professional organizations are mentioned in it. It creates an impression in the employer about one's relations with the profession and the updated knowledge that one possesses.
- **Enhancement of relationship and network:** We all realize that the relationship and networking are crucial for all the professional advancement. This can be obtained through initiating good relations with other members in the profession, and other professions (related) as well. It can be achieved by becoming a part of different Professional associations, and it gives the platform for making relations at the national and international levels.
- **Be a leader:** Professional affiliations offer you a chance to build up your aptitudes as a pioneer, and this is critical for your self-awareness as well as for your development in your firm.

- **Become a mentor:** Giving back can be the best reward and advantage. Taking part in panel discussions, conferences, workshops, and seminars is additionally an incredible method to develop your system. This enables you to make some extraordinary companions with indistinguishable interests from you.
- **Strength in numbers:** We indeed live in a time where it is mandated for any person to become proficient in the profession by a long time of hard work and less time for self-growth and self-development. Most of the time, the person may have bright ideas and concepts for professional advancement, but they may not be able to implement the same due to time constraints. The professional associations can help out the newcomers in this regard, and unity is the strength.

Various Professional Organizations in Nursing and their Functions

National Organizations

Indian Nursing Council (INC)

The Indian Nursing Council, which was approved by the Indian Nursing Council Act of 1947, was set up in 1949. It was set up as an independent statutory body for nursing training and practice under the Ministry of Health and Family Welfare, Government of India. It gave uniform gauges in Nursing training and correspondence in Nursing Registration all through the nation. The nurses enlisted in one state were not perceived for enrollment/practice in other states before the set up of INC. INC by setting up uniform standards in nursing education and training, brought the concept of mutual recognition all across the country, and it is termed as reciprocity in nursing practice recognition.

Functions of Indian Nursing Council

- Establish and monitor a uniform standard of nursing education for nurses, midwives, auxiliary nurse-midwives, and health visitors.
- Recognize the qualifications under section 10(2) (4) of the Indian Nursing Council Act, 1947 for registration and employment in India and abroad.
- Approve the registration of Indian and Foreign Nurses possessing foreign qualification under section 11(2) (a) of the Indian Nursing Council Act, 1947.
- To prescribe the syllabus and regulations for nursing programs to maintain uniform standards.
- Power to withdraw the recognition of qualification under section 14 of the Act in case the institution fails to maintain its standards under Section 14 (1)(b) that an institution recognized by a State Council for the training of nurses, midwives, auxiliary nurse-midwives or health visitors does not satisfy the requirements of the Council.

- To advise the State Nursing Councils, Examining Boards, State Governments, and Central Government in various essential aspects regarding Nursing Education in the Country.

State Nursing Council (SNC)

Like the Indian Nursing Council, every state/territory of India comprises an SNC/SNRC to direct the nursing exercises of the specific state and to give enrollment to student nurses and trained nurses. They also regulate the activities of the institution of training and nursing care and provide necessary required reports and suggestions to the government of the particular state as well as the organizations. Each State Nursing Council is governed by a Registrar and comes under the Indian Nursing Council, New Delhi. The State Nursing Council is formed by a legislative act in the particular state similar to the Indian Nursing Council. E.g. Punjab Nurses Registration Council (PNRC), Kerala Nursing Council (KNC), Karnataka State Nursing Council (KSNC), etc.

Functions of the State Nursing Council

- Regulation of training program for the diploma, graduate, and post graduate courses.
- Supervision of the practice of the profession by its member.
- Granting recognition to the training institutions and periodical inspection thereon, as the Council is governing authority of physical and clinical facilities in almost all the nursing courses conducted in the institution.
- Conducting examinations and other evaluations of different nursing training programs authorized by the respective government authority.
- Registration and granting a certificate to qualified persons to practice their profession and to watch and take action against the practice of the profession by quacks and check mal-practice as well and to take action.

Trained Nurses Association of India (TNAI)

It is the Autonomous National Association of the nursing profession in India. The present name and association were set up in 1922. In general, it points out the needs of the individual and issues in the nursing profession. It incorporates the development, upliftment, and streamlining of nursing training and education. It encourages you to be educated on recent developments in nursing and offers chances to distribute articles and opinions. The TNAI includes the following organization incorporated in it. **(1)** Health Visitors League **(2)** Auxiliary Nurse-Midwives Association, **(3)** Student Nurses Association. It is also affiliated to Commonwealth Nurses Federation. The membership in TNAI may be full, associate, or affiliate. The official organ of TNAI is The Nursing Journal of India.

Aims

- To develop, standardize, and upgrade nursing training and education.

- To enhance the employment conditions of the nurses in the country and foster their living.
- Provide membership in the organization for reciprocity of registration. A qualified nurse can get enrolled through the regular application process with the supporting evidence of the State Nursing Council registration certificate.

Benefits of TNAI Membership

- Allowed to attend and hold national level conferences.
- Provides professional development activities such as continuing education programs for knowledge enhancement.
- The registered members are also eligible for the election at the central, regional and state levels of TNAI for different professional positions.
- Support for Nursing Research.
- Scholarship for TNAI members and student nurses.

The Student Nurses Association (SNA)

The Student Nurses Association was set up in 1920, under the guidance of TNAI. It is a professional nurses association exclusively meant for nursing students. Once they become a member of SNA, they automatically become a member of TNAI after the completion of their nursing education/training.

Objectives of SNA

- It gives the student nurses an understanding of functioning in/of the professional organizations to maintain and improve the dignity and ideals of the profession.
- Develop and promote a corporate spirit among students.
- The SNA helps the student nurses bring out their talents, organizing ability, and it acts as a platform for student nurses to exchange their ideas and vision regionally and nationally.
- The SNA also provides the scholarship to the needy student nurses and organizes national conferences and meeting to improve and enhance the knowledge, networking, and relationships.

Activities of SNA

- Organization of meetings and conferences
- Maintenance of diary
- Project undertaking
- Propagation of the nursing profession
- Fundraising
- Sociocultural and recreational activities

International Organizations

International Council of Nurses (ICN)

It was framed in 1899 by Mrs Bedford Fenwick in collaboration with nurse leaders across the world. It is located in Geneva, Switzerland. Currently, around 128 countries are members of ICN. It is a federation of non-governmental and non-political nursing associations. It is a global relationship of all nurses on the planet. The ultimate destinations are to advance the improvement of national associations, help them to enhance the measures of nursing and the skill of nurses and fill in as the legitimate voice for nurses and nursing universally. All nurses who are registered with National associations are members of ICN by default. Individual membership in ICN is not permitted. Other International Professional Organizations such as the World Health Organization (WHO), UNESCO, UNICEF, Red Cross, etc. are also related to ICN.

Goals of ICN

- To influence nursing, health and social policy, professional, and socioeconomic standards worldwide.
- Advance the improvement of national associations, help them to enhance the measures of nursing and the skill of nurses and fill in as the legitimate voice for nurses and nursing universally.
- To establish, receive, and manage funds and trusts which contribute to the advancement of nursing and of ICN.

American Nurses Association (ANA)

It is a professional organization to improve quality, protect, and uplift nursing profession. Founded in 1911 and located in Maryland, United States, it encompasses the European regions.

Activities of ANA

- Establish and maintain the standards for nursing care.
- Develop and modify the educational standards governing nursing education and training.
- Promote nursing research.
- Establish a professional code of ethics.
- Monitor a credentialing system in nursing and regulate the legal aspects affecting professional practice.

The Commonwealth Nurses Federation

The Commonwealth Nurses Federation was formally sorted out in 1973 and works in six areas of the world which are East Africa, Atlantic, Australia, Pacific, South Asia, and Europe. The TNAI is additionally partnered with the Commonwealth Nurses Federation. It is comprised of nurses associations from federation member nations.

Cooperation in Professional Associations is of benefit to the nurses and nursing professions. It gives methods through which joined endeavors can be made to raise guidelines of nursing instruction and practice. It is also a platform for us to speak up our suggestions and getting updated with current trends and issues in nursing practice. Enrollment is essential for dynamic nursing practice either here or abroad. This is done through your State Nurses Registration Council. It gives legal protection to nurses and the recipients of nursing care.

COLLECTIVE BARGAINING

"Collective bargaining is an agreement between a single employer or an association of employers on one hand and a labor union on the other, which regulates the terms and conditions of employment." —**Ludwig Teller**

"Collective bargaining is a process of discussion and negotiation between two parties, one or both of whom is a group of persons acting in concert."

More specifically, it is the procedure by which an employer or employers and a group of employees agree upon the conditions of work". —**The Encyclopedia of Social Science**

Goals of Collective Bargaining

- To give a chance to the employees, to voice their issues that are identified with work.
- To encourage achieving an answer that is adequate for every one of the group/teams.
- To make solutions for all contentions and disagreements in a commonly pleasing way and prevent its occurrence in the future.
- To build up a conducive environment to cultivate great organizational relationships.
- To upgrade the profitability of the association by averting strikes and so on.

Characteristics of Collective Bargaining

- **It is a group process:** A group of people representing a considerable number of employees sits face to face with the leaders or employers or their representatives to bargain and negotiate the terms and demands of the work and work-related issues.
- **Negotiations:** It is a crucial part of collective bargaining with the scope of bargaining, discussions, and mutual understanding related to an issue.
- **Formalized:** It is a formalized procedure by employers and trade unions of employees to arrange terms and states of business and the manners by which specific work-related issues are to be directed within the organization and at the national/regional level.
- **Systematic:** It is systematic as it starts with the introduction of the sanction of requests and finishes with achieving an understanding, which would fill in as the law in the organization.
- **Continuous:** Collective bargaining is a persistent procedure. It empowers the existence of democracy in the industry. It utilizes collaboration and agreement for settling issues as opposed to strife and showdown.
- **Innovative:** Collective bargaining considers everyday changes, arrangements, possibilities, limits, and interests.

Collective Bargaining Process

It is the negotiations between two or more than two parties and mainly comprise of five steps.

1. **Prepare:** Before the process of the collective bargaining process, the negotiating teams have to be framed by both the team such as the employer and the trade unions of the employees. The representatives of the team should have excellent communication ability and should have a sound understanding of the issues to be discussed. It is also advisable to list down the most critical issues to be addressed rather than talking purposelessly.

2. **Discuss:** Here, the teams decide the general term of negotiations such as time and place of further actions. A procedure well started is half done, and this is no less valid if there should be an occurrence of collective bargaining. A location may be selected for mutual trust and acceptance.

3. **Propose:** It is a brainstorming stage, and the messages of both parties are exchanged, opinions are shared, possible options are suggested to resolve the problems by both parties.

4. **Bargain:** Negotiations are simple if a problem solving/critical thinking demeanor is embraced. This stage includes the ifs and buts of the issues, and desired agreements are made.

5. **Settlement:** Following the stage of bargaining, a consensual understanding is made by both parties, and they agree to the collective decisions of mutual agreement about the issues discussed.

Bargaining Form and Tactics

- **Distributive bargaining:** It is otherwise called conjunctive bargaining. It is mainly concerned with financial issues such as salaries, allowances, bonuses, etc. Mathematically it may be plotted with the help of a pie chart. In this type of bargaining, one group gains, and the other group loss. Disputants can try to make their part of the pie to make it larger. It is competitive.

- **Integrative bargaining:** It is a type of cooperative bargaining wherein both parties may gain, or at least neither of them loses anything. It discusses issues such as better in-service education programs, the introduction of new and enhanced evaluation systems, etc. Here both parties are demanding something more, and hence no one loses anything.

- **Attitudinal restructuring:** This includes forming and reshaping a few dispositions like trust or doubt, benevolence or threatening vibe among employees and employers. At the point when there is an accumulation of sharpness between both the groups, attitudinal rebuilding is required to keep up smooth and amicable relations.

- **Intraorganizational bargaining:** It is the method to resolve the internal conflicts in the organization. There may be more than two groups in the organization such as skilled and unskilled workers, men and women employees, etc. Every employee is unique and may have an interest in working. There are always chances for internal conflict in an organization. The trade unions, managers, and high-level employers/employees try to resolve these issues.

Significance/Advantages of Collective Bargaining

Significance to Workers

- It expands the quality of the workforce, in this manner, expanding their dealing limit as a group and enhances efficiency.
- It confines the employer's opportunity for subjective activity against the workers. Besides, unilateral actions by the employer are debilitated.
- Effective collective bargaining fortifies the trade unions' development, and the employees feel spurred to approach the administration for their issues.

Significance to Employers

- It is easy to resolve the issues at the bargaining level rather than at the individual level.
- Collective bargaining will result, in general, advance a feeling of professional stability among workers and in this way will, in general, lessen the expense of work turnover.
- Collective bargaining opens up the channel of correspondence between the workers and the administration, and it prevents disputes in the organization.

Significance to Society

- Harmonious organization climate bolsters the pace of a country's endeavors towards monetary and social improvement.
- The segregation and misuse of employees are always being checked.
- It helps in the formation of conditions and regulations of employment.

Conclusion

Collective bargaining has its particular manner between the work and association, yet at the same time, its fate is obscure to the nursing community. Collective bargaining is generally a relationship between the employee and employer/trade unions, which decides the working conditions and other aspects healthily.

MOTIVATION

It is an activity that stimulates a person to make a course of moves, which will result in the accomplishment of objectives, or fulfillment of specific material or mental needs of the person. Motivation/Inspiration is an integral asset in the hands of leaders. It can influence, persuade, and move individuals to act.

Definition

Motivation is "an inner impulse or an internal force that initiates and directs the individual to act in a certain manner to satisfy a need."

The motivating force is a need that comes from within an individual, e.g., to make a living, gain status and respect or to remove a source of frustration.

Types of Motivators

- **Intrinsic motivators: (Intrinsic factors)** Alludes to the motivation that originates from inside the individual, driving the person in question to be profitable. It is identified with an individual's dimension of motivation. The inspiration originates from the joy one gets from the errand itself or from the feeling of fulfillment in finishing or by enjoying the task itself without expecting any rewards. In any case, internal motivation does not imply that an individual will not look for remunerations. It just means that outer prizes are insufficient to keep an individual inspired.
- **Extrinsic motivators: (Extrinsic factors)** Alludes to the motivation that originates from outside an individual, i.e., improved by the workplace or outside remunerations, for example, cash or evaluations. The prizes give fulfillment and delight that the undertaking itself may not provide. An outwardly roused individual will take a shot at an errand even when they have little enthusiasm for it, because of the foreseen fulfillment they will get from the reward. e.g., a bonus for a student would obtain a good grade on an assignment or in the class.

MOTIVE

Motive is a force that determines the activity of an individual. It energizes and directs his behavior along with this or that channel. It initiates, sustains, and leads the movement of an organism in contrast to a stimulus. The physiological motives are temperature, pain, sleep, hunger, thirst, sex, maternal drive and so on.

General Motives

- **Activity:** Human beings and animals are powerful beings. They spend considerable time in moving around doing different things. It is a part of a healthy human life.
- **Exploratory drive:** Exploration of new environments, e.g., Mountaineers.

- **Curiosity:** This is similar to the previous one. All living beings are curious to know about the things around them.
- **Affection:** Love is an essential motive for life. We love our parents, siblings, friends, etc. We need the love and friendship of all to live on.
- **Fear:** Fear makes an individual to act against the will. It is instant and short-term and can get the job done quickly.

Social Motives

- **Affiliation:** It is a drive to identify with individuals on a social premise or social acceptance. People with this motivation perform work better when they are complimented for their positive disposition and co-task.
- **Social approval:** We seek social support for all the things we do, and we try our best to avoid doing anything that may evoke social disapproval.
- **Status:** All people are commonly motivated to achieve status among their fellow men.
- **Power:** It is the drive to impact individuals and change circumstances. Force propelled individuals wish to make an effect on their association and will take any risk for it.
- **Security:** It is a basic need. Insecurity is the haunting feeling that one may feel when he/she loses what one presently has.
- **Achievements:** It is the drive to scrutinize and achieve objectives. A person with motivation wishes to accomplish targets and advance up the stepping stool of success. Thus, the achievement is vital for the good of his/her own and not for the prizes that go with it.
- **Competence motivation:** It is an inclination to be great at something, enabling the person to perform fantastic work. Competence/aptitude persuaded people to look for mastery over their job and take pride in creating and in utilizing their critical thinking abilities and endeavor to be imaginative when gone up against with hindrances. They gain from their encounters.
- **Attitude motivation:** It is how individuals think and feel. It is their self-assurance, their faith in themselves and their demeanor to life. It is the way they feel about the future and how they respond to the past.
- **Incentive motivation;** Here the people are spurred by external rewards. Here, an individual or group receives a benefit from a movement. It is the sort of remunerations that drive individuals to work more earnestly.

Unconscious Motives

All the motives are not conscious. Many of them operate without being aware. In our behavior, we come across instances of acts that we cannot explain. The origin of unconscious behavior and motives can be found in the unconscious mind. Repression is an example of this act.

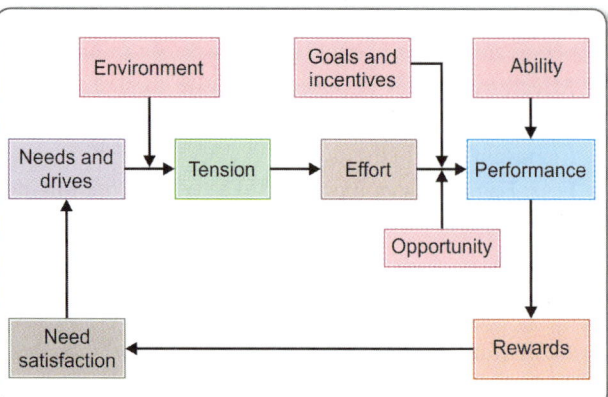

Fig. 4: Process of motivation

Process of Motivation

Initially, there is an excitement of need so critical, that the conveyor needs to wander in a hunt to fulfill it. This prompts the production of tension/pressure, which asks the individual to overlook everything else and oblige the stirred need first. This tension/pressure makes drives and mentalities concerning the sort of fulfillment that is wanted. This leads an individual to wander into the search of data. This, at last, prompts the assessment of choices where the best option is picked. After picking the alternative, a move is made. In light of the execution of the action, fulfillment is accomplished, which than assuages the tension/pressure in the person (Fig. 4).

Nature of Motivation

- A psychological concept deals with the human mind.
- The whole individual is motivated as it is based on the psychology of the individual.
- Motivation may be financial or non-financial. Financial includes increasing wages, allowance, bonus, etc.
- Motivation can be positive or negative: positive motivation means the use of incentives - financial or non-financial. E.g. of positive motivation: confirmation, pay rise, praise, etc. Negative motivation means emphasizing penalties. It is based on the force of fear. E.g., demotion, termination.
- Motivation is an internal feeling of an individual. It cannot be observed directly; we can see an individual's action and interpret his behavior in terms of underlying motives.
- Motivation is a continuous process that produces goal-directed behavior.

Sources of Motivation

- **Internal or push forces:**
  - Needs for security, self-esteem, achievement, and power.
  - Attitudes about self, job, supervisor, and organization.
  - Goals of task completion and performance level and career advancement.

- **External or pull forces:**
  - Characteristics of the job, such as feedback, timing, workload, tasks, variety, scope, discretion, and how the job is performed.
  - Characteristics of the work situation such as immediate social environment (supervisor, workgroup members and subordinates) and organizational actions such as rewards and compensation, availability of training and pressure for high levels of output.

Theories of Motivation

Content theories of motivation: It is also referred to as Need Theory. It centers around the inside variables that invigorate and coordinate human conduct. A few of them are:

- **Abraham Maslow Theory (1943) (Fig. 5):** It includes five fundamental needs such as physiological needs, safety, and security needs, love needs, self-esteem, and self-actualization.
  1. **Physiological needs:** Food, water, warmth, shelter, sleep, medicine, and education, etc. Once the physiological needs are met, the next level becomes predominant.
  2. **Safety and security need:** The necessity of freedom from danger and harm. It may arise from factors related to the loss of a job, property, food, or shelter. It also includes protection against any emotional injury.
  3. **Social needs:** Human beings are social beings. The necessity of belongingness and acceptance by the people is also a necessary need. People try to satisfy their need for affection, acceptance, and friendship. After the lower requirements are well met, affiliation or acceptance will emerge as dominant, and the person strives for meaningful social relationships.
  4. **Self-esteem needs:** The need for social needs is followed by the need to satisfy their self-esteem. The tendency of self-esteem is present in everyone, but it becomes a need after the achievement of lower requirements. This produces an inclination, and it is satisfied by the possession of power, status, and self-confidence. This can be either external or internal. The internal factors include self-respect and autonomy, and external factors are status, attention, and recognition.
  5. **Need for self-actualization:** Maslow regards this as the highest need in his hierarchy. It is the drive to become what one is capable of becoming; it includes growth, achieving one's potential, and self-fulfillment. It is to maximize one's potential and to accomplish something.

    Maslow proposed that human needs are requested in a chain of importance from easy to complex. More significant needs do not develop as sparks until the point that brings down requirements are fulfilled, and a met need never again rouses conduct.

- **Alderfer ERG theory:** ERG theory is like Maslow's chain of command of necessities.

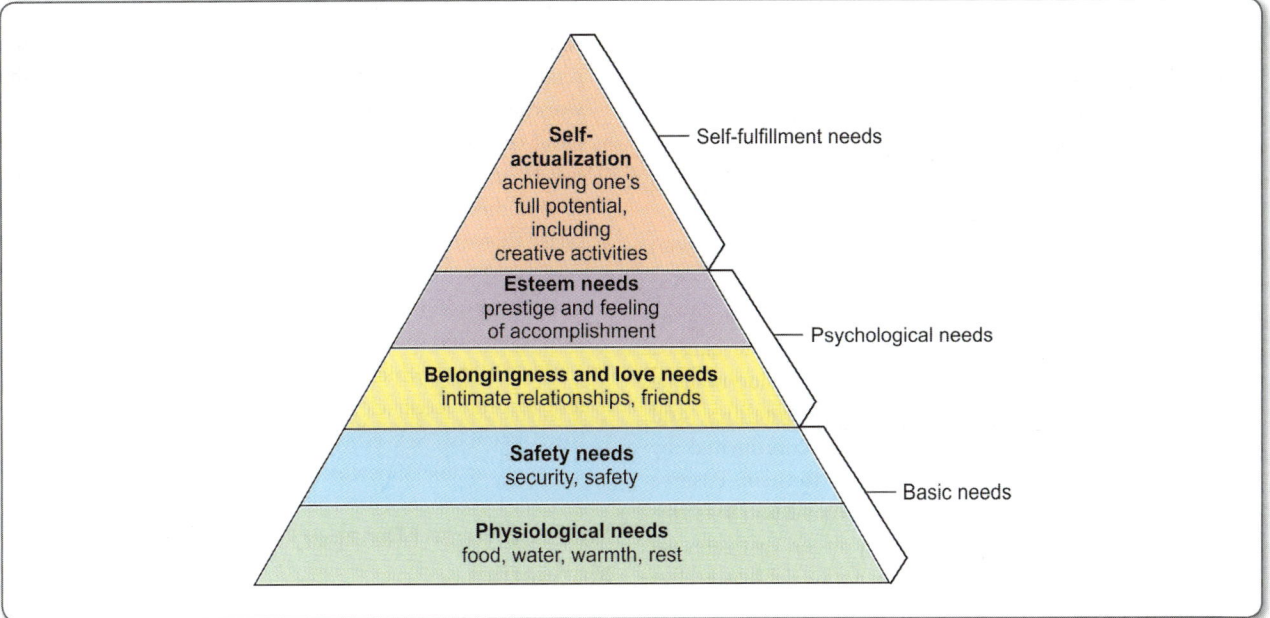

Fig. 5: Abraham Maslow theory

- The existence/presence (E) needs are proportionate to physiological and wellbeing needs.
- Relatedness (R) needs are related to belong, social, and love needs.
- The growth/development (G) needs are related to esteem/confidence and self-completion/actualization.

It concludes by the following: **(1)** People may have more than one need simultaneously. **(2)** On the off chance that a higher need goes unsatisfied, then the craving to fulfill a lower-level need increases. **(3)** Most of the time, the lower needs are met but not high-level requirements. **(4)** Regression of higher needs will cause a tendency to satisfy lower needs.

- **Frederick Herzberg two factor needs theory (1966):** Herzberg felt that activity fulfillment and disappointment exists on double scales. Laborers are spurred by two sorts of requirements/factors:
  - Needs identifying with the job/task/work itself are called essential/intrinsic/inspiration factors (satisfiers): challenging nature of work, accomplishment, included obligation, open doors for development and open doors for progression.
  - Needs identifying with working conditions are called outward/extrinsic/hygiene factors: Compensation, status, working conditions, nature of supervision, professional stability, and organizational arrangements.

As per Herzberg, the hygiene factors must be kept up sufficiently to avoid employee dislike. The dissatisfaction is mainly caused by unequal/partial administration and causes low execution and negative frames of mind. The inspiration factors make open doors for high fulfillment,

great inspiration, and elite. The absence of inspiration factors causes a deficiency of occupation fulfillment.

- **McGregor's Theory X and Theory Y:** Douglas McGregor proposed two diverse inspirational speculations hypothesis X and hypothesis Y. He expresses that individuals inside the association can be overseen in two different ways. The first is fundamentally contrary, which falls under the class X, and the other is optimistic, which falls under the classification Y.

As per hypothesis X, employees naturally, do not care for work and at whatever point conceivable, will endeavor to stay away from it. Since representatives hate the job, they must be constrained, forced, or compromised with the discipline to accomplish objectives. Representatives evade obligations and do not work until the point when formal bearings are issued.

As indicated by hypothesis Y, physical and mental exertion at work is as healthy as rest or play. Individuals do practice discretion and self-heading, and if they are focused on those objectives. Ordinary individuals will assume liability and exercise creative energy, inventiveness, and innovativeness in tackling the issues of the association.

On analysis of the assumptions, it can be detected that theory X assumes that lower-order needs dominate individuals, and theory Y understands that higher-order needs dominate individuals. An organization that is run on Theory X lines tend to be authoritarian—"power to enforce obedience" and the "right to command." In contrast, Theory Y organizations can be described as "participative," where the aims of the organization and the individuals in it are integrated; individuals can achieve their own goals best by directing their efforts towards the success of the organization.

Process theories of motivation: Process hypotheses of motivation give a chance to comprehend manners of thinking that impact conduct. The significant procedure hypotheses are—Vroom's expectancy theory, goal-setting theory, and reinforcement theory.

- **Reinforcement theory:** B.F. Skinner's hypothesis (1969) recommends that a worker's work inspiration is controlled by conditions of the outside environment, that is, by planning the background appropriately, people can be persuaded. Rather than considering inside/internal elements like impressions, sentiments, mentalities, and other intellectual conduct, people are coordinated by what occurs in the environment outside to them. Positive behavior should be strengthened or compensated as this expansion is the quality of a reaction or instigates its redundancy. Reinforcers will, in general, debilitate after some time and new ones must be produced. Negative rewards happen when the ideal conduct jumps out to maintain a strategic distance from adverse outcomes of punishment. Punishment makes a negative disposition and can expand costs.

- **Expectancy theory of Vroom:** It postulates that most practices are deliberately controlled by an individual and are subsequently propelled. It centers around individuals' exertion-execution-hope or an individual's conviction that an opportunity exists for a particular type and level of performance that is more acceptable. According to this theory, motivation relies on attractiveness, performance-remunerate linkage, and effort-performance.

  - **Attractiveness:** the person sees the outcome as desirable.
  - **Performance-reward linkage:** the person perceives that the desired outcome will result from a certain degree of performance.
  - **Effort-performance:** the person believes that a certain amount of effort will lead to performance.

- **Jeremy Bentham's "The Carrot and the Stick Approach":** Bentham's view was that all individuals are self-intrigued and are spurred by the longing to maintain a strategic distance from torment and pleasure/delight. Any laborer will work just if the reward is sufficiently massive, or the discipline adequately horrendous. With this view, the "carrot and stick" approach was incorporated. This metaphor relates to the use of rewards and penalties to induce the desired behavior. It came from the old story that to make a donkey move, one must put a carrot in front of him or dab him with a stick from behind. Despite all the research on the theories of motivation, reward and punishment are still considered strong motivators.

In almost all theories of motivation, the incitements or something to that effect of "carrot" is perceived. Frequently this is cash as pay or rewards and the "stick" is dread.

The dread of loss of occupation, loss of pay, decreased reward, downgrade, or some other punishment. It creates retaliation and results in the poor quality of work and working environment.

- **Goal-setting Theory of Edwin Locke:** This theory is based on goals as determinants of behavior. According to this theory, every organization sets the organizational goals that are high to achieve. The employees are then motivated to work hard to achieve the same. The specificity of the purpose brings out better results. The goals must be achievable, and their difficulty level must be increased only to the ceiling to which the person will commit. Goal clarity and accurate feedback increase security. It revolves around the concept of "Self-efficacy," i.e., individual's belief that he or she is capable of performing a hard task.

Roles of Nurse Manager to Facilitate Nurses Motivation

- Set self as an actual example with high standards, a positive attitude, and should possess skills and have the knowledge to perform different tasks.
- Initiate and keep up good personal relations by adopting two-way communication, non-critical, and friendly approach, with a sense of humor and abstain from getting furious.
- **Post each nurse where she can work best:** The nurse is bound to succeed and be persuaded if her/his advantages and abilities are considered in the task. Achievement is the best inspiration.
- **Use a participative style:** Participation and sharing data will propel nurses since they believe they are partaking in choices. Inspiration requires more than the physical contribution in an occupation. It likewise requests mental and passionate participation.
- **Guide, empower and bolster continuously:** Guidance implies helping the nurses in arranging, assessing their work, and in taking care of work and individual issues. Think about unique contrasts; be touchy to varieties in nurses.
- **Reward good work:** Offer acknowledgment to the fruitful accomplishment of the activity. It helps in making one prestigious in front of others. The reward incorporates pay increment, advancement, etc. and it increases self-reliance.
- Build cooperation (Teamwork).
- **Provide continuing education:** Nurses appreciate adapting new learning and abilities or refreshing the current information and aptitudes or taking new obligations through continuing education.

CONCEPT OF EMPLOYEE MORALE

Morale is a very widely used term. It generally refers to esprit de corps, a feeling of enthusiasm, zeal, confidence in individuals or groups that they will be able to cope with the tasks assigned to them. A person's enthusiasm for his job reflects his attitude of mind to work, environment and to his employer, and his willingness to strive for the goals set for him by the organization in which he is employed. Morale is a synthesis of superiors, his organization, his fellow-employees, his pay and so on. Feelings, emotions, sentiments, attitudes, and motives combine and lead to a particular type of behavior on the part of an individual or his group; and this is what is referred to as employee morale. It represents the attitudes of individuals and groups in an organization towards their work environment and towards voluntary cooperation to the full extent of their capabilities for the fulfillment of organizational goals.

Approaches to Morale

Morale is generally referred to as "willingness to work". Job satisfaction and dissatisfaction create the problem of low morale among the employees. Good motivation leads to high morale. It is a psychological concept, it is not easy to define it precisely. Different authorities have variously defined morale. Different definitions of morale can be classified into three major approaches:

1. **Classical approach:** According to this approach, the satisfaction of basic needs is the symbol of morale. If the basic needs of the employees are satisfied their morale will be high.
2. **Psychological approach:** According to this approach, morale is a psychological concept i.e., a state of mind. Emotions affect the willingness to work which in turn affects individual and organizational objectives. Accordingly, the attitudes and willingness to work is morale. Morale is a mental condition or attitude of individuals and groups which determine their willingness to cooperate.
3. **Social approach:** Morale is a social phenomenon that enables men to live in a society or group in pursuit of a common goal. Morale is the feeling of togetherness. There is a sense of identification with and interest in the elements of one's job, working conditions, fellow employees, supervisor, employer, and the company.

Characteristics of Morale

Morale is a feeling, somewhat related to esprit de corps, enthusiasm or zeal. For a group of employees' morale, according to the popular usage of the word, refers to the overall tone climate or atmosphere of work, perhaps vaguely sensed by the members. Morale is a group concept with five components:

1. A feeling of togetherness, i.e., of belonging to a group and not being isolated.
2. A clear goal which will be the target of production set before them.

3. There must be observed or perceived progress towards the attainment of the goal, i.e., the expectation of success.
4. Within the group, each member feels that he has a meaningful task to perform and.
5. Supportive or stimulating leadership.

Types of Morale

- **Individual morale:** An individual's morale is related to knowing one's expectations and living up to them. If one is clear of one's own needs and how to satisfy them, one's morale is high. An individual's morale is a single person's attitude toward life.
- **Group morale:** Group morale reflects the general esprit de corps of a collective group of personalities. Group morale is everyone's concern and it must be practiced continually, for it is never ultimately achieved and is constantly changing. Group morale and the morale of the individual are interrelated but not necessarily identical. They affect each other.
- **High morale/Good morale:** High morale exists when the employee's attitude is favorable to the total situation of a group and the attainment of its objectives. It is represented by the use of such terms as spirit, zest, enthusiasm, loyalty, honesty, dependability, resistance to frustration, etc. Possible effects of high morale are higher performance, better quality of work, job satisfaction, cheaper goods and services, lower cost, higher profits, employment stability, low absenteeism, and low labor turnover.
- **Low morale/Poor morale:** Low morale exists when attitudes inhibit the willingness and ability of an organization to attain its objectives. If employees seem to be dissatisfied, irritated, cranky, critical, restless, and pessimistic they are described as having poor or low morale. Effects of low morale are apathy and non-involvement, fatigue and monotony, high labor turnover, high rate of absenteeism, disciplinary problem and increased grievances.

Factors Influencing Employee Morale

Employee morale is a very complex phenomenon and is influenced by many factors on the shop floor. Factors influencing employee morale can well be divided into two groups namely organizational factors and personal factors.

Organizational Factors

- **The organization:** The goals of the organization influence the attitudes of employees greatly. If the goals set by the management are worthwhile, useful and acceptable, then employees develop a positive feeling towards the job and the organization.
- **Organizational design:** Organizational structure has an impact on the quality of labor relations, particularly on the level of morale. Large organizations tend to lengthen their

channels of vertical communication and to increase the difficulty of upward communication. Therefore, morale tends to be lower. Against this, a flat structure increases the level of morale.

- **The nature of work:** A meaningful and satisfying job helps to improve employee morale. In such a job each member of the group understands clearly how his specific task contributes to the attainment of group goals.
- **Work environment and conditions:** The building and its appearance, the condition of machine tools available at the workplace, provisions for safety, medical aid and repair to machinery, etc. have an impact on employee's morale. Physical work environment, job security, wages, and other allied factors exercise a significant influence on employee morale.
- **Leadership and supervision:** The actions of the management exercise a tremendous influence on the morale of employees. High rates of turn over, for example, indicate that the leadership is ineffective. Competent, dependable and fair-minded leadership can build and maintain high morale. The nature of supervision can better tell the attitudes of employees because a supervisor is in direct contact with the employees and can have a better influence on the activities of the employees.
- **Fellow employees:** Man, being a social animal, finds his work more satisfying if he feels that he has the acceptance and companionship of his fellows. If he has confidence in his fellow employees and faith in their loyalty, his morale will be high.
- **Future opportunities for rewards:** If the employee looks to the future and perceives opportunities for satisfaction and for attainment in the rewards and conditions that lie ahead, morale will tend to be high. If, on the other hand, the rewards and opportunities for the future appear to be bleak, morale will tend to be dampened.

Personal Factors

- **The employee's age:** The age and morale are directly related and that, other things being equal, older employees seem to have higher morale, because perhaps younger employees are more dissatisfied. They are a "new breed" with higher expectations than their elders. Studies have reported that employers, therefore, hire employees of a somewhat higher age.
- **Educational level:** An inverse relationship has been found between educational level and employee morale. In other words, the higher the educational level of an employee, the lower his morale because he compares his attainments with those of others.
- **Marital status:** The general impression is that married employees and employees who have more dependents tend to be more dissatisfied with greater responsibilities. But such employees may be more satisfied because they value their jobs more than unmarried employees.

- **Occupational level:** The occupational level of the employee also influences his level of morale. For example, executives are on the whole more satisfied than managers; managers are more satisfied than subordinates; and so forth.
- **Experience:** Morale tends to increase with increasing years of experience. But it may decrease after twenty years of experience particularly among people who have not realized their job expectations.

Effects of Morale

Since morale manifests itself in the attitudes of employees, it is important to find the results of high morale and low morale. The effects of morale are given below:

- **High morale–high productivity:** High morale reflects a predisposition to be more productive if proper leadership is provided. This situation is likely to occur when employees are motivated to achieve high-performance standards through financial and non-financial rewards.
- **High morale–low productivity:** The situation arises when employees spend their time and energy in satisfying their objectives unrelated to the company's goals. Faulty machinery, lack of training, ineffective supervision and restrictive norms of informal groups can also lead to low productivity on the part of employees with high morale.
- **Low morale–high productivity:** Low morale cannot result in high productivity for a long period. However, this situation can occur for a temporary period due to fear of loss of job, exceptionally good supervision and machine paced work in which only a part of employees' capabilities is used.
- **Low morale–low productivity:** This is a normal relationship. In the long run low morale is likely to result in low productivity. Thus, there is a complex relationship between morale and productivity. This is because morale is only one of the factors influencing productivity.

COMMUNICATION

Communication is a standout amongst the essential exercises in the nursing service and management. The obtaining of the organizational objectives is based on the communication pattern of the said organization. It is an active and purposeful process of change to achieve the expected results. Communication is a process in which a message is transferred from one person to another person through a suitable media, and the intended message is received and understood by the receiver.

Communication is defined as an exchange of ideas, facts, opinions, or emotions between two or more persons.

—Newman and Summer

Communication is the sum of all things a person does when he wants to create an understanding in the mind of another. It involves a systematic and continuous process of listening and understanding.

—Allen Louis

Elements of Communication

- **Source idea:** It is the formulation of a plan that needs to be conveyed to another person/group. This procedure can be affected by external variables such as books, television, internet, etc. or internal variables like own thinking, fantasies, etc. However, it is the core of communication.

- **Message:** The message is what is conveyed to another group/individual. It depends on the source idea, yet the message is made to address the issues of the receptor group. For instance, if the message is between two companions, the message will take an unexpected frame in comparison to if speaking the same with a senior person.

- **Encoding:** Encoding is the transformation of the message into a form capable of transmission to another group. The message is changed over into reasonable shape for transmission. The mechanism of transmission will decide the type of communication. For instance, the message will take another form if the mode of communication is via a talk or it to be composed.

- **Channel:** It is the route through which the message is conveyed. The channel must have the capacity to transmit the intact/unaltered message from the source to the other end. The circuit can be any medium such as a bit of paper, radio, or it tends to be an email. An email can utilize the internet as a channel.

- **Receiver:** It is the one who receives or accepts the message of communication. It may be an individual, group, instrument or mass public. The receiver is contingent upon the channel utilized for the communication.

- **Decoding:** It is the reverse form of encoding. The encoded message is decoded /translated to a meaningful interpretation. It is the internalization of the message by the receiver. It is influenced by past experiences of the receiver and external factors of the stimulus.

- **Feedback:** The feedback loop is essential part of all communication. It is the final stage of the communication whereby the receiver replies to the sender the acknowledgment of the message and its related matters.

Process of Communication

The six steps in the communication process are: (Fig. 6)

1. **Ideation/sender/source:** The initial step, ideation, starts when the sender chooses to impart his/her message to somebody, detects a need to convey, builds up an idea or chooses data to share.

2. **Encoding:** The second step, includes placing the idea of communication into a form of transmission such as representative symbols/structures, talking, composing, or nonverbal conduct. One's own, social, and educational inclinations influence the objectives and encoding process.

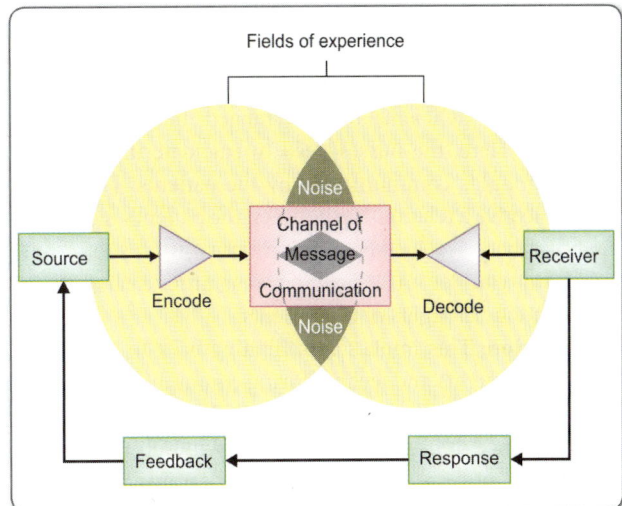

Fig. 6: Process of communication

3. **Transmission through channel:** The transfer of the message, through a channel, must conquer the problems of language, grammar, speaking/writing difficulties, the functionality of the devices used for transmission, and other factors associated with reading and writing.

4. **Decoding:** Decoding of the message by the beneficiary is critical. Composed messages consume more time for interpreting, as the receiver assesses for the explicit and implicit meaning of the words. The entire process of communication relies on the recipient's comprehension of the data.

5. **Receiving:** The process by which the beneficiary's sense organs are actuated as the transmitted message is got. Individuals will, in general, have particular consideration and the specific discernment that reasons inadequate and misshaped reception and understanding of the communication.

6. **Response or feedback:** The supervisor or sender needs to realize that the message has been got and precisely deciphered.

Techniques to Improve Communication

- **Listening:** It is a functioning procedure of getting data. The total consideration of the nurse is required, and there should be no distraction with oneself. Listening is an indication of regard for the individual who is talking and an amazing fortify of connections. It enables the patients to communicate more, without which the relationship cannot advance.

- **Broad openings:** These urge the patient to choose points for exchange, and show that health professional is focusing on him/her. E.g., what will we examine today? "Would you be able to reveal to me better about that?"

- **Restating:** The restatement of the communication reveals to the patient what the nurse is listening to or attending and considering as much important.

- **Clarification:** The individual's verbalization, mainly when he is exasperating or feeling profound, is not clear in communication. The patient's comments might be befuddled, deficient, or disarranged because of their disease. Here, the nurses need to elucidate the emotions and thoughts communicated by the patients. The nurses need to give a relationship between the patient's inclination and activity. For instance, "I don't know what you mean?" "Could you let me know once again?" clears up the ambiguous thoughts of the patients.

- **Reflection:** This implies coordinating back to the patient for his thoughts and feeling during communication.

- **Focusing:** It implies extending the dialogue on the point of significance. It causes the patient to wind up increasingly explicit, move from dubiousness to transparency, and spotlight on the correct aspects.

- **Sharing perceptions:** It is a process by which the nurse tries to comprehend the inner and hidden considerations or attitudes of the patient. For example, the nurse could ask the patient, as you are grinning. However, I sense that you are exceptionally irritated by me."

- **Theme identification:** This includes recognizing the fundamental issues or issues experienced by the patient that rises over and again throughout the interpersonal relationship (IPR). When we realize the underlying themes, it turns out to be easy to choose which of the patient's inclination and contemplations to react to and seek after.

- **Silence:** Here, the nurse uses silence to prompt the patient to speak. Nonverbal communication also signifies the interest of the therapist on the patient's discussion.

- **Humor:** This is the release of vitality through the comic delight. It is a socially adequate type of sublimation. It is a suitable type of coping, and by figuring out how to express humor, a patient figures out how to show feeling of others.

- **Informing:** It is the process by which the nurse shares straightforward realities and information with the patient.

- **Suggesting:** This is the introduction of elective thoughts identified with critical thinking. It is a necessary communication procedure when the patient has investigated his concern zone and is prepared to investigate elective ways of dealing with stress, and the suggestion helps understand the elective ways.

Types of Communication

- **Intrapersonal versus interpersonal communication:** In intrapersonal, the person communicates with oneself, such as thinking, imagining, meditation, problem-solving, etc. In interpersonal communication, the person interacts with others, such as two or more people.

- **Group versus mass communication:** In a group, the message is conveyed to a group of people who can be small or large. In the case of mass communication, it is delivered through mass media, and the message travels to a considerable number of people and cross over much distance.

- **One-way versus two-way communication:** In case of one way, it is the only sender to the receiver whereas the two-way process adds up the communication from receiver to sender too. The second one is dynamic, majority rule, and influential. The two-way communication is also referred to as cyclic or Socratic communication. It has the provision of feedback. For example, when a speaker presents the paper to a group, it is one-way communication, and when the audience is given the option of asking the question, it turns into two-way communication.

- **Formal/vertical communication:** It is commonly utilized for all practical purposes. This is definitive, explicit, exact, and available to everyone. The mechanism of official correspondence might be office meetings, gatherings, phone calls, interviews, rounds, and so on. It is also referred to as vertical communication considering the channel of communication.

- **Informal/horizontal/grapevine communication:** Gossip circles, for example, friends, WhatsApp groups, Facebook. Communication is quicker here. The casual channels might be progressively dynamic. It might be a reality, however, more in local gossip. It does not reach each one. It is swift and unconstrained. It is also referred to as horizontal or grapevine communication considering the route and channel of communication.

- **Physiological communication:** It explains the biological circuit of the process of perception where the sense organs pick up the stimuli, the brain interprets it, and the muscles create the action.

- **Psychic communication:** Extrasensory recognition happens, i.e., something which will occur in the future. The individual relates and predicts that ahead of time is called Psychic communication.

- **Visual communication:** The visual configuration of communication outlines charts, pictograms, tables, maps, and so forth.

- **Verbal communication:** The conventional method for communication has been by listening in on others' conversations. Dialect is the leading vehicle of communication. It fosters one to one interaction. It can easily be misinterpreted too.

- **Nonverbal communication:** Communication can happen even without a word. Non-verbal communication is message transmission through non-verbal communication without using words. It incorporates facial expressions and body movements. Quietness is also nonverbal communication. It can talk more intensely than words.

- **Oral communication:** Oral communication is transmitting a message orally through phone, internet, etc.

- **Written communication:** It is transmitting a message in composition. Composed communication can be pursued when a record of communication is vital.

- **Mechanical communication:** By utilizing mechanical gadgets, communication will be sent, e.g., web, radio, T.V., and so on.

Criteria for Good Communication

- Think clearly before communicating
- Ensure the purpose of communication
- Gain knowledge about the listeners thinking, expectations, feeling, etc.
- Be a democratic consultant
- Determine the medium of communication
- Manage the tone and content of the communication
- Be future-oriented
- Maintain trust and confidence
- Take feedback

Barriers to Communication

Communication obstructions make the issue of misconception and struggle between men who live respectively in a similar network, who cooperate on a related activity and even between men living in the particular parts of the world who have never observed each other. Following are the primary obstructions to survive:

- Structure of the organization.
- Status and position.
- Semantic barriers (the different meaning of words depends upon the situation).
- The tendency to evaluate.
- Heightened emotions: Lack of ability to communicate.
- Inattention.
- Un-clarified assumptions.
- Resistance to change.
- Closed minds.

ASSERTIVE COMMUNICATION IN THE WORKPLACE

Regardless of the level of communication skills, interacting with people can often be quite stressful. Learning to be assertive can help us to reduce and cope with this stress. Assertiveness is a communication style where we express our rights and feelings more openly. Everyone is assertive to some level, but the level of assertiveness could vary according to the social situation. For example, a man could be very assertive with his colleagues at work, but not with his wife and kids.

Definitions

Assertive behavior is "Behavior that enables a person to act in his own best interests, to stand up for himself without undue anxiety, to express his honest feeling comfortably, or to exercise his rights without denying the rights of others."

—**Calbert and Emmons, 1974**

Assertiveness is the expression of one's feelings, beliefs, opinions, and needs in a direct, honest and appropriate manner. Such assertive behavior will reflect a high regard for one's rights as well as the rights of others. Assertiveness training (AT) defines some basic concepts and skills to enhance our assertive behavior under varied social interactions. Assertiveness training defines three different communication styles used by us when we interact with someone:

- **Aggressive:** Examples of aggressive behavior are fighting, accusing, threatening, and a general disregard for the other person's feeling. Aggression is about dominance. A person is aggressive when he impose his will onto another person and tries to force him to submit.
- **Passive:** People behave passively when they let others push them around, when they do not stand up for themselves, and when they do what they are told regardless of how they feel about it. Passivity is about submission. Nobody likes being dominated, but it might seem like the smart thing to do at the time (perhaps to avoid disagreement or confrontation).
- **Assertive:** Assertiveness is about finding the middle path. We behave assertively when we stand up for ourselves (when required), express our true feelings, and do not let others take advantage of us while, at the same time, being considerate of others' feelings.

Assertiveness Training

Assertive nurses, including managers, will stand up for their rights while recognizing the rights of others. They are straightforward and know that they are responsible for their thoughts, feelings, and actions. Assertive nurses also know their strengths and limitations. Rather than attack or defend, assertive nurses assess, collaborate, support, and remain neutral and non-threatening. They can accept challenges and prevent conflict by helping others deal with their anger. Assertiveness can be taught through staff development programs. In these programs, nurses are taught to make learned, thoughtful responses and to know when to say no, even to the boss. They learn to hold people to a standard and to know when to accept responsibility rather than to blame others. When they are dissatisfied, they do something to increase their satisfaction. Most assertive behaviors can be learned with the use of case studies, role-playing, and group discussion. Assertive nurses focus on data and issues when offering constructive cretinism to the boss or constructive feedback to the staff, which encourages dialogue and produces solutions to problems rather than conflict. They ask for assistance or delay when needed. People generally respond positively to assertion and negatively to aggression; however, some people respond negatively to the assertion.

Assertive behavior: The behavioral characteristics of assertion include:

- **Openness** implies being clear and specific about what you want, think and feel. A lack of openness often leads to misunderstanding.
- **Directness** means addressing the person/situation directly. For example, if you are in a group and want to say something to someone, communicate directly with that person instead of addressing the whole group and hoping that the person gets the message.
- **Honesty** in communication implies that you should be truthful and not mislead the other person. Example: your friend says, "I don't like your body language" and you reply, "Yes, I don't like it too" when in fact you do. When we aren't honest, we deprive the other person of a chance to get to understand and know us better.
- **Appropriateness** implies taking the social and cultural context into consideration before communicating. The communication has to consider the context in which a person communicates with another person.

As we grow older and deal with more complex social interactions between friends, family, and co-workers, we also learn to be flexible. Here, flexibility implies learning to control emotions so that we can choose our communication style as per the situation, and not let our emotions dictate our approach. Nurse Leader's behavior includes expressing one's feelings, needs, ideas and standing up for one's right while considering the rights of others. An assertive person generally feels good about themselves and others.

Personal Boundaries/Rights in Communication Style

- **Assertive behavior is about a balanced approach:** It is not about simply choosing between an aggressive or passive style of communication. It's about respecting the rights (personal boundaries) and feelings of others and expecting others to respect your rights and feelings too. If someone doesn't respect your rights and feelings, you communicate it to them. It isn't about scoring points or getting even by lashing out at them (aggressive) or feeling hurt and not talking about it to not embarrass the other person (passive).
- **Assertiveness is about respect:** Assertiveness training emphasizes that to be assertive, one must be clear about their (and others) rights while communicating. The basic rights of every individual in this context are the right to do anything as long as it does not hurt someone, the right to maintain your dignity by being assertive, the right to request someone, as long as you recognize that the other person has the rights to say no.

Becoming Assertive

After understanding the basic concepts, the next step in assertiveness training is practicing it out. Assertiveness training deals with behaviors of various complexity.

- **Phase 1:** In the first phase, we need to practice our non-verbal cues. This means, while communicating stand straight, make eye contact and speak loud enough.
- **Phase 2:** In the second phase, we need to practice saying yes or no, when we want to ask favors and make requests to communicate our feelings and thoughts openly and directly and handle put-downs.
- **Phase 3:** In the third phase, we need to learn adaptive behaviors in job situations, the ability to form and maintain a social network and develop close and personal relationships.

COMMITTEES

Committees are found in every large organization since it is not always possible for the administrator to manage everything single-handed. A committee is a form of a formal group.

According to dictionary meaning, committee is "a group of people officially delegated to perform a function, such as investigating, considering, reporting, or acting on a matter". And also means, a group of people appointed or elected to administer, discuss, or make reports concerning a subject on which its members have authorities to perform a specified service or function.

A committee can be defined as a body of persons appointed to meet an organized basis for the discussion and dealing of matters brought before it. —**L M Prasad**

The committee is defined as a group of persons to whom, as a group, some matter is committed. It involves group decision making. —**Koontz**

Characteristics of Committee

- A committee is a group of persons.
- It has definite jurisdictions, i.e, it deliberates only on matters that are brought before it.
- It can be constituted at any level of organization
- The authority delegated to the committee depends on the nature of the committee.

Purposes of Committees

- **Decision making:** The committee has the responsibility to decide to establish organizational objectives, setting policies, and designing a strategy to guide the nursing activities.
- **Informational:** The committee is constituted to obtain and disseminate the information to implement organizational programs in different departments.
- **Coordination:** The main purpose of the committee is to facilitate the coordination of activities of different departments of the institution.
- **Advisory:** The committee is constituted to have continuous advice from the specialists by the top-level executive.

Types of Committees

- According to Authority:
  - **Line Committee:** If the authority involves the decision making or carry out managerial function affecting subordinate, it is called as a line committee.
  - **Staff Committee:** Authority relationship to a superior is advisory in nature.
- According to the delegation of authority:
  - **Formal:** The committees with specifically delegated duties and authorities are called formal committees.
  - **Informal:** The committees without a specific delegation of authority are called an informal committee.
- According to existence:
  - **Permanent:** Usually formal committees are permanent. These committees last until the organization stands.
  - **Temporary:** These committees are constituted for a short duration depending on the purpose of the committee. Once the task is over, the committees are abolished.

Advantages of Committee

- The pooling of knowledge and experience
- Promotes coordination and cooperation
- It encourages a comprehensiveness and democratic approach
- It brings an effective face to face two-way communication.
- It is a device or tool for management development
- Avoidance of a desired action or referral of a particular case from one person to other committees for decision making.

Disadvantages of Committee

- Delay in execution as it requires collective effort and contribution.
- Ineffective decision or wrong decision if the head is not competent.
- Increased economical expenditure in the constitution and maintenance of the committee.
- Divided responsibility of the group and less significance for the individual decision.

 REVIEW QUESTIONS

1. Define organization. Explain the principles of the organization.
2. What is organizational behavior and its elements? Explain the theories of organizational behavior.
3. Define group dynamics. Enlist the types of groups. Explain the principles of group dynamics.
4. Explain the stages of group development. Explain the role of the nurse manager in group dynamics.
5. Define the interpersonal relationship. What are the dynamics of IPR? Explain the types and phases of IPR building.
6. What are Human Relations? Brief the goals and principles of human relations. What is the role of a nurse in maintaining human relations?
7. Explain the concept of public relations. What are the functions and elements of public relations?
8. Explain the types/forms of public relations.
9. Elaborate public relation plan for a hospital and explain the methods to achieve it.
10. Explain various professional organizations in India and abroad, along with its functions.
11. Define collective bargaining. Explain its purpose and process.
12. What are the tactics of collective bargaining? Explain the significance of collective bargaining.
13. Define motivation and motive, types of motives and motivators. Explain the process of motivation.
14. Explain the theories of motivation. Explain the role of Nurse Manager to facilitate nurse's motivation.
15. Define communication. Explain the elements and processes of communication.
16. What are the types of communication? Explain the techniques of communication and its barriers.

Further Readings

1. Banerjee, Shyamal. Principles and Practice of Management. Oxford and IBM Publishing, New Delhi; 2000.
2. Basavanthappa BT. Nursing Administration. 2nd Edition: Jaypee Brothers Medical Publishers (P) Ltd., New Delhi; 2009.
3. Barrett, Jean. Ward Management and Teaching. Konark Publishers, Delhi; 1992.
4. Warren, Stevens, F. Management and Leadership in Nursing. McGraw – Hill Inc, New York; 1978.
5. Alexander et al. Nursing Service Administration. Mosby Publishers, US; 1962.
6. Park K. Preventive and Social Medicine, 19th Edition: M/s. Banarasidas Bhanot Publishers, Jabalpur; 2007.
7. Basavanthappa BT. Nursing Administration, 1st Edition: Jaypee Brothers Medical Publishers (P) Ltd., New Delhi; 2002.
8. Goel SL, Kumar R. Management of Hospitals – Hospital Administration in the 21st century, Vol. 4, Deep and Deep Publication, New Delhi; 2002.
9. Ranga Rao SP. Administration of Primary Health Centers in India, 1st Edition: Mittal Publications, New Delhi; 1993.
10. Lucita M. Nursing: Practice and Public Health Administration. Current Concepts and Trends. B. I. Churchill Living Stone Pvt. Ltd., New Delhi; 2002.
11. Sakharkar BM. Principles of Hospital Administration and Planning, 2nd Edition: Jaypee Brothers Medical Publishers (P) Ltd., New Delhi; 2009.
12. Patricia S Yoder-Wise. Leading and Managing in Nursing. 2nd Edition: Mosby Publication, US; 1999.
13. Bessie L Marquis, Carol J Huston. Leadership Roles and Management Functions in Nursing: Theory and Application. 5th Edition: Lippincott Williams and Wilkins, New York; 2006.
14. Linda Roussel. Management and Leadership for Nurse Administrators. 4th Edition: Jones and Bartlett Publication, USA; 2006.
15. Wehrich H, Koontz H. Management A Global Perspective. 11th Edition: Tata McGraw-Hill Publishing Company, Ltd., New Delhi; 2005.
16. Marquis BL, Huston CJ. Leadership and Management Functions in Nursing- Theory, and Application. 5th Edition: Lippincott Williams and Wilkins, Philadelphia; 2006.
17. Douglass LM. The Effective Nurse: Leader and Manager. 5th Edition: Mosby Publication, US; 1996.
18. Trained Nurses Association of India, Nursing Administration, and Management.
19. Samson Rebecca. Leadership and Management in Nursing Practice and Education 1st Edition: Jaypee Brothers Medical Publishers (P) Ltd., New Delhi; 2009.
20. Kunders GD. Designing for Total Quality in Health Care, Prism Book Pvt. Ltd., Bangalore; 2002.
21. Chandorkar AG. Hospital Administration and Planning. 2nd Edition: Paras Medical Publisher, New Delhi; 2009.
22. Joshi DC, Joshi Mamta. Hospital Administration. 1st Edition: Jaypee Brothers Medical Publishers (P) Ltd., New Delhi; 2009.
23. Eleanor J Sullivan, Philip J Decker. Effective Leadership and Management in Nursing. 4th Edition: Published by Addison Wesely; 2011.
24. Kulkarni GR. Financial Management for Hospital Administration, Jaypee Brothers Medical Publishers (P) Ltd., New Delhi; 2009.

Financial Management

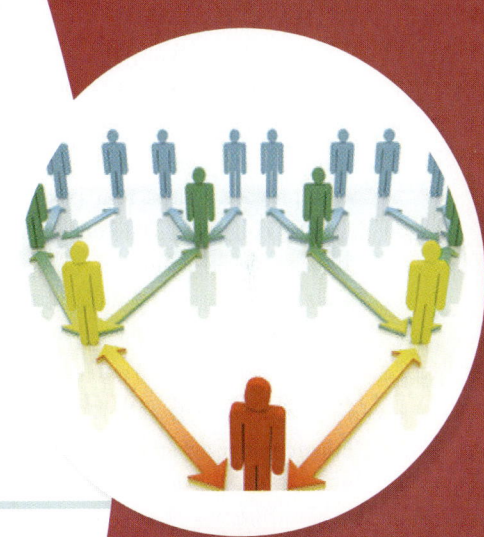

FINANCIAL MANAGEMENT

Introduction

The business concern needs finance to meet its requirements in the economic world. Any kind of business activity depends on finance. Hence, it is called the lifeblood of a business organization. Whether the business concerns are big or small, they need finance to fulfill their business activities. In the modern world, all the activities are concerned with economic activities and very particular for earning profit through any venture or activities. The entire business activities are directly related to making a profit.

Finance may be defined as the art and science of managing money. It includes financial services and financial instruments. Finance also is referred to as the provision of money at the time when it is needed. The finance function is the procurement of funds and their effective utilization in business concerns. The concept of finance includes capital, funds, money, and amount. But each word is having a unique meaning. Studying and understanding the concept of finance become an important part of the business concern.

Definitions of Finance

"Finance is the art and science of managing money".

—**Khan and Jain**

The word 'finance' connotes 'management of money'.

—**Oxford Dictionary**

Finance is defined as, "the Science or the study of the management of funds' as the system that includes the circulation of money, the granting of credit, the making of investments, and the provision of banking facilities.

—**Webster's Dictionary**

Definitions of Financial Management

Financial management is an integral part of overall management. It is concerned with the duties of the financial managers in the business firm. The term financial management has been defined as:

"It is concerned with the efficient use of an important economic resource namely, capital funds." —**Solomon**

"Financial Management deals with procurement of funds and their effective utilization in the business." —**SC Kuchal**

Financial management is defined as "an application of general managerial principles to the area of financial decision-making." —**Howard and Upton**

Thus, Financial Management is mainly concerned with effective funds management in the business. In simple words, Financial Management as practiced by business firms can be called as Corporation Finance or Business Finance.

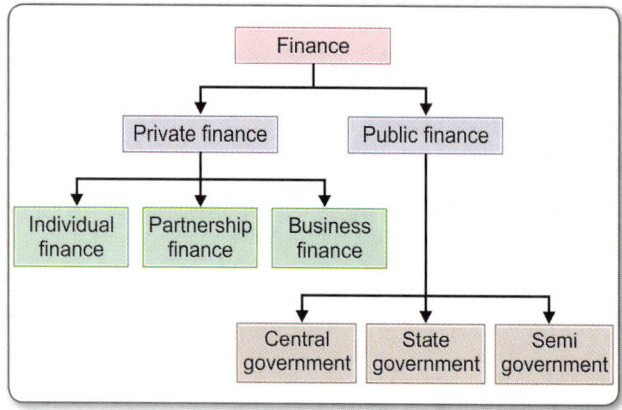

Fig. 1: Types of finance

Types of Finance

Finance is one of the important and integral parts of business concerns, hence, it plays a major role in every part of the business activities. It is used in all the areas of the activities under the different names. Finance can be classified into two major parts (Fig. 1).

Private Finance, which includes the Individual, Firms, Business or Corporate Financial activities to meet the requirements. Public Finance concerns with revenue and disbursement of Government such as Central Government, State Government, and Semi-Government financial matters.

Objectives of Financial Management

Effective procurement and efficient use of finance lead to proper utilization of finance by the business concern. It is an essential part of the financial manager. Hence, the financial manager must determine the basic objectives of financial management. Objectives of Financial Management may be broadly divided into two parts such as:

- **Profit maximization:** The main aim of any kind of economic activity is earning profit. A business concern is also functioning mainly to earn a profit. Profit is the measuring technique to understand the business efficiency of the concern. Profit maximization is also the traditional and narrow approach, which aims at, maximizing the profit of the concern. Profit maximization is also called as cash per share maximization. It leads to maximize the business operation for profit maximization. The ultimate aim of the business concern is earning a profit; hence, it considers all the possible ways to increase the profitability of the concern. Profit is the parameter of measuring the efficiency of the business concern. So, it shows the entire position of the business concern. Profit maximization objectives help to reduce the risk of the business.
- **Wealth maximization:** Wealth maximization is one of the modern approaches, which involves the latest innovations and improvements in the field of business concern.

The term wealth means shareholder wealth or the wealth of the persons who are involved in the business concern. Wealth maximization is also known as value maximization or net present worth maximization. This objective is a universally accepted concept in the field of business.

Elements of Financial Management

- **Investment decisions:** It includes investment in fixed assets called capital budgeting. Investment in current assets is also a part of investment decisions called working capital decisions.
- **Financial decisions:** They relate to the raising of finance from various resources that depends upon decision on the type of source, the period of financing, cost of financing and the returns thereby.
- **Dividend decision:** The finance manager has to decide with regards to the net profit distribution. Net profits are generally divided into two: dividends for shareholders and retained profits that is the amount of retained profits to be finalized that depends upon expansion and diversification plans of the organization.

Approaches to Financial Management

The financial management approach measures the scope of financial management in various fields, which include the essential part of finance. Financial management is not a revolutionary concept but an evolutionary. Theoretical points of view, and financial management approach may be broadly divided into two major parts:

1. **Traditional approach:** Traditional approach is the initial stage of financial management, which was followed in the early part of the years 1920 to 1950. This approach is based on past experience and the traditionally accepted methods. The main part of the traditional approach is the raising of funds for the business concern. The traditional approach consists of the following important area; Arrangement of funds from the lending body, Arrangement of funds through various financial instruments and Finding out the various sources of funds.

2. **Modern approach:** Modern approach views finance function in a broader sense. It includes both rising of funds as well as their effective utilization under the purview of finance. The finance function does not stop only by finding out sources of raising enough funds; their proper utilization is also to be considered. The cost of raising funds and the returns from their use should be compared. The funds raised should be able to give more returns than the costs involved in procuring them. The utilization of funds requires decision making. Finance has to be considered as an integral part of overall management. So, finance functions, according to this approach, cover financial planning, raising funds, allocation of funds, financial

control, etc. The modern approach considers the three basic management decisions, i.e., investment decisions, financing decisions and dividend decisions within the scope of the finance function.

The approaches to budgeting are further explained in the upcoming pages.

Principles of Financial Management

- **The principle of risk-return trade-off:** Risk and return are closely related to each other. More risk, more return is a common statement. Naturally, an investor expects more return for taking more risk.
- **The principle of net cash flows:** To implement any investment decision, it is important to determine the initial cash outflow to initiate the project and cash inflows received from the project.
- **The principle of internal financing:** It must be preferable to raise funds from the internal sources.
- **The principle of the time value of money:** The value of money changes due to change in time. One must refer today's ₹1/- than that of the future.
- **The principle of debt repayment:** It is important to repay the debt capital in time.
- **The principle of diversification:** It is not wise to invest all the funds in a single project. The fund must be diversified to diversify its risk.
- **Principle of liquidity and profitability:** There is a negative relationship between liquidity and profitability.
- **Principle of recovery:** An important principle of business finance is the principle of recovery. It is very crucial that whether the terms of recovery will be flexible or rigid.
- **The principle of minimum flotation costs:** Flotation costs are needed for external financing. The cost of capital increases due to the flotation cost. So, the matter of minimum flotation cost is to be kept in deep concern.
- **The principle of priority:** There may be several project profiles. Among them, which projects are to be given priority bears importance.

Functions of Financial Management

- **Estimation of capital requirements:** A finance manager has to estimate the capital requirements of the company. This will depend upon expected costs and profits and future programs and policies of a concern. Estimations have to be made in an adequate manner which increases the earning capacity of the enterprise.
- **Determination of capital composition:** Once the estimation has been made, the capital structure has to be decided. This involves short-term and long-term debt equity analysis. This depends upon the proportion of equity capital a company is possessing and additional funds that have to be raised from outside parties.

- **Choice of sources of funds:** For additional funds to be procured, the organization has many choices like the issue of shares and debentures, loans to be taken from banks and financial institutions and public deposits to be drawn like in form of bonds.
- **Investment of funds:** The finance manager has to decide to allocate funds into profitable ventures so that there is safety on investment and regular returns are possible.
- **Disposal of surplus:** The net profits decision has to be made by the finance manager. This can be done in two ways: Dividend declaration - It includes identifying the rate of dividends and other benefits like a bonus. Retained profits - The volume has to be decided which will depend upon expansion, innovative, diversification and plans of the company.
- **Management of cash:** The finance manager has to make decisions with regards to cash management. Cash is required for many purposes like payment of wages and salaries, payment of electricity and water bills, payment to creditors, meeting current liabilities, maintenance of enough stock, purchase of raw materials, etc.
- **Financial controls:** The finance manager has not only to plan, procure and utilize the funds but he also has to exercise control over finances. This can be done through many techniques like ratio analysis, financial forecasting, cost and profit control, etc.

Scope of Financial Management

Financial management is one of the important parts of overall management, which is directly related to various functional departments like personnel, marketing, and production. Financial management covers a wide area with multidimensional approaches. The following are the important scope of financial management.

- **Financial management and economics:** Economic concepts like micro- and macroeconomics are directly applied to financial management approaches. Investment decisions, micro- and macro-environmental factors are closely associated with the functions of the financial manager. Financial management also uses economic equations like money value discount factor, economic order quantity, etc. Financial economics is one of the emerging areas, which provides immense opportunities to finance and economical areas.
- **Financial management and accounting:** Accounting records include the financial information of the business concern. Hence, we can easily understand the relationship between financial management and accounting. In the olden periods, both financial management and accounting were treated as the same discipline and then it has been merged as Management Accounting because this part is very much helpful to finance managers to take decisions.

- **Financial management and mathematics:** Modern approaches to financial management applied a large number of mathematical and statistical tools and techniques. They are also called econometrics. Economic order quantity, discount factor, time value of money, the present value of money, cost of capital, capital structure theories, dividend theories, ratio analysis, and working capital analysis are used as mathematical and statistical tools and techniques in the field of financial management.
- **Financial management and production management:** Production management is the operational part of the business concern, which helps multiply the money into profit. The profit of the concern depends upon the production performance. Production performance needs finance because the production department requires raw material, machinery, wages, operating expenses, etc. These expenditures are decided and estimated by the financial department and the finance manager allocates the appropriate finance to the production department. The financial manager must be aware of the operational process and finance required for each process of production activities.
- **Financial management and marketing:** Produced goods are sold in the market with innovative and modern approaches. For this, the marketing department needs finance to meet their requirements. The financial manager or finance department is responsible to allocate adequate finance to the marketing department. Hence, marketing and financial management are interrelated and depend on each other.
- **Financial management and human resource:** Financial management is also related to the human resource department, which provides manpower to all the functional areas of the management. The financial manager should carefully evaluate the requirement of manpower to each department and allocate the finance to the human resource department as wages, salary, remuneration, commission, bonus, pension and other monetary benefits to the human resource department. Hence, financial management is directly related to human resource management.

FINANCIAL PLANNING

Budget planning is the estimated forecast of income and expenditure for a year or a few years. The budget is a yearly arrangement, planned to control the compelling utilization of human and material assets, items or benefits and dealing with it to enhance profitability. The concept of budgeting in nursing is an orderly arrangement by the nurse managers of income and expenses in nursing. The budget can be a solid help for creating composed goals for the nursing division and every one of its units.

Diverse sorts of methodologies are utilized in setting up the financial plan for a hospital. The essential purpose behind setting up a financial plan is to empower the hospital to successfully meet its money related prerequisites. A successful spending plan/budget is a rundown of the cautiously considered monetary policies. In this way, it should be evident to the organization regarding what the hospital's budgetary prerequisites will be. Funds will be used for the following purposes:

- **Capital funding:** For protection, redesigning, and substitution of physical offices and gear, innovation, development, etc.
- **Operating needs:** For working capital and working costs, employee compensations, materials, and supplies, upkeeping, utilities, and so on.
- **Reserves:** For crisis needs.

  Operating revenue is generated from:

  - **Direct patients who come for care:** IPD, OPD, Emergency, and other departments.
  - **Special services:** OT, labor, ICU, Physiotherapy, and so on.
  - **Supportive services:** All the diagnostic, imaging laboratory facilities.
  - **Hotel and catering benefit:** Room and Food.
  - Income from other services includes interest paid by bank, rents, grants from governments or any other organization and recuperation if any.

Steps in Making a Hospital Budget

Building a hospital expenses plan or budget is equally necessary for the routine functioning of the hospital. If a financial plan is not appropriately composed, the hospital might not able to deliver services by any stretch of the imagination. Such a large number of costs and wellsprings of income must be contemplated, so the process of preparing budget takes a specialist to overcome it effectively.

- **Determine the income of the organization:** Revenue and profit can emerge out of patient installments or payments, grants, and donations, insurance, etc. Consider the expense of unpaid bills, marketing works, social service, individual consideration for the poor and needy, etc.
- **Figure out costs or expenses:** It starts with stable structures such as building in terms of both setting up and maintenance. What is the upkeep cost of every office, building, cooling, warm water, different utilities? Recognize what gear or equipment costs, and what all things can be reused? Incorporate the non-restorative expense of each bed in the hospital, such as ads, publishing, etc.
- Know the expense of the workforce, all representatives, and auxiliary staff, including specialists, re-appropriated contracts, and all other human resources of the hospital from lower to an upper group, including the incidental advantages.
- Know the medicinal expenses of each bed. What number of hours are spent on each bed by the staff? Calculate this

figure to get an expense for every patient per year. Do not forget to add the nonmedical costs per bed, such as electricity, water, etc.

- Do not overlook parking structures and maintaining hospital premises, grounds, etc. Include hospital insurance and crisis fund also. Calamities happen, and the hospital must be well prepared for them when they arrive.

Mechanics of Budget Preparation

Income

- **Bed charges:** The beds are generally classified into four categories; A, B, C, and D. This classification is done more to segregate patients according to their ability to pay. The number of beds available under each category is predetermined. Facilities offered by each of these categories—such as space per bed, number of beds in a room, separate bed for patient's companion within the room, quality of linen and furniture, provision of TV and air conditioning, nurse or ward boy in attendance-are different. There may be little differentiation concerning the charges for doctors' rounds, laboratory analysis, nursing services, food supply, and so on.
- **Other hospital services:** Income from other hospital services such as OT, X-ray, and pathology tests for the budget year could be similarly computed. However, unlike in respect of beds, service offered by a department is identical to all patients. The fees charged for a service of that department, often, depends upon the class of bed occupied by them.
- **Other receipts:** The amount could be targeted at the previous year's level. Some hospital authorities leave their deficit from operations uncovered open-ended hoping to offset the same through donations. These are generally received from one or more business persons or collected by the leaders of the community with which the hospital is associated.
- **Donations:** Nonprofit healthcare institutions depend to a considerable extent on contributions from persons and organizations. These donations are not necessarily money always, rather it can be in the shape of assets like building, equipment, materials or land, etc.
- **Grants:** They are funds provided by a government body or department to an institution, for example, a hospital, to be used for a specific purpose, activity, or facility. Grants or permanent rights to grant are recognized as revenue in the period in which they are receiving.
- **Interest/dividend income:** Income from these sources is linked to investments provided in the balance sheet such as fluctuations (a) in exchange rates on capital funds and (b) rate of interest/dividend likely to prevail during the year.
- **Negative income/deductions from income:** To keep up with their images as a service organization and also to

secure tax concessions, hospitals offer concessions ranging from absolutely free service to marginal reduction in rates charged. Deductions should be shown separately grouped under indoor and outdoor patients and analyzed under (a) charities, the source of funding, community – if this is a relevant factor; (b) Staff, (c) Special schemes, and (d) Bad debts. Payment to Doctors: A percentage of fees charged on some hospital services or a fixed amount is paid to outside consultants and, sometimes, even to the medical staff on its payroll.

Expenses: Formats of costs could take the following forms: Major items of expenditures and their incidence in some hospitals are listed below. The figures indicate the percentage of the total cost. Payments should be accounted for on a mercantile basis.

- **General:** The pattern of expenses could vary by hospitals: Type, size, location, and other distinctive factors along with materials, employees expenses, dietary services, utilities—electricity and water, engineering and property maintenance, administration including consultancy fees, interest paid, depreciation and other hospital expenses. These factors influence the general liability of the hospitals.

   Materials budget expenses on medicines, injections, operation theatre material, X-ray plates, reagents used in the pathology laboratory, and such other material used while treating a patient in various departments, directly or indirectly, could be termed as direct material. The value of this type of material varies with the level of activity. Over a period, standards or norms are developed in terms of specifications and quantities for each material for different lines of treatment, operations, or procedures. If such norms are available, requirements of various categories of material could be computed by multiplying per unit requirements with activity level expressed in terms of numbers.

- **Fringe benefits:** Fringe benefits could be broadly categorized under:
  - **Retirement benefits:** These include Provident Fund, Gratuity, and Pension. These are predetermined by the corporate policy. These can be estimated as a percentage of regular pay.
  - **Cash benefits:** Such as Bonus, Leave-Travel Concession, House Rent, etc. These are related to the grade in which an employee is placed.
  - **Others:** Such as subsidized lunch, transportation, medical, training, uniforms, etc.

- **Overtime:** Overtime payments are necessary for emergency work and unplanned absenteeism. Some employees often create situations that need overtime payments artificially to generate additional income for themselves regularly each month and their colleagues. It creates terrible morale amongst other employees who are not similarly placed to take secure overtime payments.

Other operating expenses mainly include energy costs, maintenance, marketing, and administration.

Tips on Hospital Budget Planning

- **The paradigm of shift:** Plan the whole expenditure plan on the double. One reason for the planning of the budget to be double is a fragmented methodology. Building up a financial plan in storehouses will, without a doubt, make issues as every office is hollowed against the other in the battle for assets.
- **Be flexible:** Traditional planning can be insensitive and firm. Utilizing volume gauges to drive the monetary allowance gives a premise to both material and work accomplishment. Organizers should take a gander at the financial plan from a comprehensive viewpoint.
- **Benchmarking:** Use volume benchmarks to help decide the ideal income and cost levels. Benchmarks can emerge out of contending hospitals, earlier years' financial plans or best practice divisions.
- **Accountability:** Hold staff responsible for the financial plan. Build up an arrangement of fortification that incorporates both positive and negative criticism. One approach to fortify the financial plan while making the procedure less demanding is to spend more than once every year. Preferably, planning should be an all-year process, with multiyear checkpoints for responsibility.

NURSING BUDGET

The nursing budget is a plan for the allocation of resources based on preconceived needs for a proposed series of programs to deliver patient care during one fiscal year. A nursing budget is a systematic plan that is an informed best estimate by nurse managers of revenues and nursing expenses. The nursing budget projects how revenues will meet the expenses and it projects a return on equity that is profit.

Steps of Nursing Budget Preparation: There are main eight steps in nursing budget preparation:
1. **Determine the productivity goals:** The director of the nursing service and the nurse manager determine the unit's productivity goal for the coming fiscal year.
2. **Forecast the workload:** The number of patient days expected one each nursing unit for the coming fiscal year is calculated.
3. **Budget patient care hours:** The expected number of patient care hours devoted to the forecasted patient days is calculated.
4. **Budget patient care hours and the staffing schedule:** The budget patient care hours are reflected in the recommended staffing schedule by shift and day of the week.
5. Plan nonproductive hours and productive hours for the coming financial year.

6. To aid in the planning process a graph is used to show nurses and the level of forecasted patient days and therefore the staff requirement is expected to increase or decrease during the year, considering the educational activities.
7. Estimate costs for supplies and services. The supplies and services to be purchased for the year are budgeted.
8. Anticipate capital expenses. The expected capital investment for the coming year is included in the budget.

Advantages of Nursing Budgeting

- Budgeting can be strong support for developing written objectives for the nursing divisions and each of its units.
- It motivates effective planning and standard to evaluate the performance of nurse managers.
- Managing the financial end of nursing through an operational budget obviously can create a new sense of involvement for nurses.
- Effective planning provides for contingencies by indicating which progress or activities can be reduced or eliminated if budget goals are not met.
- The nursing budget plan ensures that clients receive nursing services from satisfied nursing staff.

Roles of Nurse Manager in Budgeting

Nurse managers set goals and design the budget (usually in collaboration with the finance department) for their responsibility center or nursing unit. After the budget has been developed and updated, it is submitted to administration and ultimately to the board of directors for approval. After the budget is approved and the fiscal year begins, the organization must deliver the planned services and programs. The budget-development workflow involves the following steps:

- **Collecting relevant data:** A critical task in creating a budget is collecting relevant data. The finance department ultimately collects the data, but this is done in collaboration with the nurse manager to create a functional budget. This includes the following information such as
  - Services offered/needed/demanded
  - Patient mix/case mix (This pertains to the complexity of care. Generally, the more complex the case, the higher the reimbursement)
  - Payer mix (This number reflects the patient demographics in terms of cash, TPA, Government support, charity and so on.)
  - Acuity index. The acuity index is a numeric calculation of the extent of care required by each patient, e.g. PCS.
  - Historical information of the prior years' operational performance.
  - Industry trends or a change in technology.
  - Organizational goals and objectives.
- **Planning services:** Nursing is aware of what types of services will be rendered in the next fiscal year. Finance may be aware if it is a large project with which the organization has been involved, but many times finance is not aware of every type of service that will be rendered. For example, a nurse manager in an emergency department may be planning on opening a fast-track part of the emergency department to accommodate the minor emergencies more efficiently. This type of new service will require additional staffing. This has to be planned in terms of additional revenue, expense and expected profit.
- **Planning activities:** An activity may be a particular treatment that is new to the department. This will also have to be planned accordingly in the budget. Based on the industry innovation the nurse manager must be aware of the newer caring technologies and its expenses.
- **Implementing the plan:** The budget plan is implemented by the nurse manager after approval by upper-level administration and ultimately the board of directors of the organization. Implementing the plan means providing the services. For many nursing managers, this process will be no different from previous years. For some nurse managers, this might entail the implementation of new services or treatments. Budgeted expenses and revenue will be compared to actual expenses and revenue.
- **Monitoring the budget:** The budget must be monitored, with accurate financial reporting on a routine basis. It is the responsibility of the nurse manager and the finance department to monitor the budget. Using reports, you must compare actual revenue and expenses to the budgeted revenue and expenses. Variances must be identified. A variance analysis must be completed, where appropriate, to analyze cost, efficiency, and volume variances.
- **Taking corrective measures when necessary:** Based on performance, the initial goals may need to be modified. A change in the types and levels of services and the resources used may also be required.

Divison of Role in Budget Preparation in a Health Care Setting

- **Department head:** Each department head or nurse manager is responsible for confirming the detailed operating expense budget for his or her department (cost center), consistent with organizational goals and objectives.
- **Director of the budget:** The director of the budget ensures that all budget forms are properly prepared and that data is accumulated within the specified timetable.
- **Vice presidents:** Vice presidents are responsible for the establishment of the basic annual budget formulation parameters. They assimilate departmental budgets into an organizational master budget consistent with organizational goals and objectives.
- **President/CEO:** The president or CEO has overall responsibility for the formulation and execution of the organization's budget. The president ensures consistency between the budget and divisional goals and objectives.

- **The finance committee and board of trustees:** These bodies are responsible for the review and approval of the completed operating budget.

In the Indian scenario, nurse administrators are not directly involved in the planning budget. Above mentioned steps are being exercised where they are involved in planning nursing services. The data also reveals that there is no separate budget for nursing services in Indian hospitals and most of the nurse administrators were unaware of the weightage given to the expenditure on nursing services in the hospital budget.

Approaches to Developing an Organization's Budget

Organizations adopt different approaches to preparing their budgets. One of the most common approaches is in the form of the traditional budget in which the current year's budget is taken as a base with the provisions of some additions and deductions in the next year's budget. The traditional approach of budgeting does not eliminate the drawback of the past. Therefore, newer approaches to budgeting have emerged. These have resulted in three types of budgeting.

- **Performance budgeting:** A performance budget is an input/output budget or cost and result budget. Performance budget emphasizes on non-financial measures of performance, which can be related to financial measures in explaining changes and deviations from planned performance. Performance measurements are useful for evaluating past performance and for planning future activities. Performance budgeting results in the following:
  - It correlates the financial and physical aspects of every program or activity.
  - It improves budget formulation, review and decision making at all levels of the organization.
  - It facilitates better appreciation and a review of organizational activities by the top management.
  - It makes possible more effective performance audits.
  - It measures progress towards long-term objectives.

  Advantages:
  - **Set accountability:** In the public sector organization and not for profit organizations, performance budget helps to increase accountability. The employees have to quantify a particular goal based on the priority and the tax payer's money.
  - **Clear purpose:** Performance budgeting indicates the objective on which the money is going to be spent. By making the purpose clear, it becomes easier to assess the performance and correct the deviations.
  - **Improvement in performance:** The performance budget improves the performance of the programs continuously. Besides, it leads to the overall operational efficiency of the organization. Also, it overcomes the limitations of traditional budgeting.

  - **Transparency:** Performance-based budgeting helps in bringing transparency in the budget preparation. The performance budget helps in taking better financial decisions for the allocation of resources.

  Disadvantages:
  - **Subjective:** Since the performance budget is subjective in nature, it creates disagreement amongst the management.
  - **A strong system of evaluation:** The performance budget requires a strong system of accounting. Therefore, the reporting system has to be strong for its successful implementation.
  - **Manipulation of data:** Staff may manipulate the data. Further, the calculation of the financial information is not reliable because of the errors in preparation.
  - **Difficult for long-term:** The period between the allocation of resources in the project and the achievement of the result might be more than a year. Undoubtedly, it makes difficult to measure the results of the projects in the long-term.

- **Zero base budgeting:** This was applied for the first time in preparing the divisional budgets of Texas instruments of the USA in 1971. Zero-based budgets are based on a system where each function, irrespective of the fact whether it is old or new, must be justified in its entirety each time a new budget is formed in detail from scratch that is zero bases. The process of zero bases involves four basic steps:
  - Identification of decision units, that is a cluster of activities or assignments within a manager's operations for which he is accountable.
  - Analysis of each decision unit in the context of the total decision package.
  - Evaluation and ranking of all decision units to develop the budget request.
  - Allocation of resources to each unit based.

  Advantages:
  - **Accuracy:** Against the regular methods of budgeting that involve just making some arbitrary changes to the previous year's budget, zero-based budgeting makes every department relook every item of the cash flow and compute their operation costs.
  - **Efficiency:** This helps in the efficient allocation of resources (department-wise) as it does not look at the historical numbers but looks at the actual numbers.
  - **Reduction in redundant activities:** It leads to the identification of opportunities and more cost-effective ways of doing things by removing all the unproductive or redundant activities.
  - **Budget inflation:** Since every line item is to be justified, the zero-based budget overcomes the weakness of incremental budgeting of budget inflation.
  - **Coordination and communication:** It also improves coordination and communication within the

department and motivates employees by involving them in decision-making.

Disadvantages:

- **Time-consuming:** Zero-based budgeting is a very time-intensive exercise for a company or government-funded entities to do every year as against incremental budgeting, which is a far easier method.
- **High manpower requirement:** Making an entire budget from scrap may require the involvement of a large number of employees. Many departments may not have adequate time and human resources for the same.
- **Lack of expertise:** Explaining every line item and every cost is a difficult task and requires training the managers.
- **Strategic budgeting:** It is used as a tool of resource allocation to various strategic business units and other units of an organization. Under strategic budgeting, the resource needs of various units are determined. It is usually long term in nature, more than one year. It supports the long-range vision of the organization. Strategic budgeting is the process of creating a long-range budget that spans a period of more than one year. The intent behind this type of budgeting is to develop a plan that supports a long-range vision for the future position of an entity. This may, for example, involve the development of new geographic markets, the research and development needed to introduce a new product line, converting to a new technology platform, and the restructuring of the organization. In these examples, it is not possible to complete the required activities within the period spanned by a single annual budget. Also, if only annual budgets are used, it is possible that the funding needed for a multi-year initiative will not be continued for the necessary full duration of the initiative, so that the project is never completed. Thus, only by engaging in strategic budgeting an organization can hope to achieve long-term improvements in its strategic position. A strategic budget is less concerned with the detailed revenue and expense line items typically found in an annual budget. Instead, these classifications are aggregated into a smaller number of line items. By doing so, there is less emphasis on the accuracy of specific items and a greater focus on the overall goals to be achieved.

PLANNING THE BUDGET

Planning yields forecasts for one year and several years. The budget is an annual plan, intended to guide the effective use of human and material resources, products or services and managing the environment to improve productivity. Budgetary planning ensures that the best methods are used to achieve financial objectives. In nursing, budgetary planning helps to ensure that clients or patients receive the nursing services they want and need from satisfied nursing workers.

A nursing budgeting is a systematic plan that is an informed best estimate by nurse administrators of revenue and nursing expenses. Managing the financial end of nursing through an operational budget obviously can create a new dimension for a nurse. The budget can be strong support for developing written objectives for the nursing division and each of its units.

Steps in the budgetary process: The nursing process provides a model for the steps in budget planning.

- **Assessment:** The first step is to assess what needs to be covered in the budget. Historically, top-level managers frequently developed the budget for the institution without input from the middle or first-level managers. Because unit managers who participated in fiscal planning were more up cost-conscious. A better understanding of the institutions' long and short term goals, budgeting today generally reflects input from all levels of the organizational hierarchy. Unit managers develop goals, objectives and budgetary estimates with input from colleagues and subordinates. Budgeting is most effective when all personnel using the resources are involved in the process. Managers, therefore, must be taught how to prepare a budget and must be supported by management throughout the budgeting process.
- **Develop a plan:** The second step is to develop a plan. The budget plan may be developed in many ways. A budgeting cycle that is set for 12 months is called a fiscal year budget. This fiscal year which may or may not coincide with the calendar year, is then usually broken down into quarters or subdivided into monthly, quarterly or semiannual periods. Most budgets are developed for one year, but a perpetual budget may be done continually each month. So that 12 months of future budget data are always available. Selecting the optimal time frame for budgeting is also important; a budget that is predicted too far in advance has a greater probability for error. If the budget is short-sighted, compensating for unexpected major expenses or purchasing capital equipment may be difficult.
- **Implementation:** The third step is implementation. In this step, ongoing monitoring and analysis occur to avoid inadequate or excess funds at the end of the fiscal year. In most health institutions, monthly-computerized statements outline each department's projected budget and any deviations from the budget. Each unit manager is accountable for budget deviations in their unit. Most units can expect some changes and remedial actions must be taken if necessary. Some managers artificially inflate their department's budgets as a cushion against budget cuts from a higher level of administration. If a major change in the budget is indicated, the entire budgeting process must be repeated. Top-level managers must watch for and correct unrealistic budget projection before they are implemented.
- **Evaluation:** This is the last step. The budget must be reviewed periodically and modified as needed throughout

the fiscal year. With each successive year of budgeting, managers can more accurately predict their unit as budgetary requirements.

Budget stages: The nursing budget follows three stages of development.

- **Formulation stage:** One of the first steps in writing a budget is gathering data for accurate prediction of expenses and revenues (income). Primary sources of data are the objectives for the division of nursing and each cost center. Other data include programs from other departments that will require use or expansion of nursing resources, expansion of nursing clinics and client teaching programs, incentive awards, library requirements, clinical and office supplies and equipment, etc.

- **Review and enactment stage:** Review and enactment stage are budget development processes that pull all the pieces together for approval of a final budget. Once the cost center managers present their budgets to the budget council, the chief nurse executive will consolidate the nursing budget. The chief executive officer of the organization and the governing board will then give their approval. Throughout this process, conferences will be held at which budget adjustments are made.

- **Execution stage:** Execution of the budget involves directing, executing, and evaluating activities. The nurse administrator and managers who planned the budget execute it. Revisions in the execution of the budgets are scheduled at stated intervals, frequently once or twice during the fiscal year. Certain procedures are followed for evaluating the budget at cost center levels.

Steps in the Preparation of an Operating Budget

- Collection of past data (historical data) as background material for the preparation of the budget in a cumulative form.

- Examining the expressed objectives of the previous years and to note in each instance the extent to which these objectives have been achieved or exceeded. Before setting programs for the future, it is necessary to assess the successes and failures of the past. Budget time is ideal for such reviews.

- Setting objectives for the forecast year. These objectives might include ways to increase the utilization of existing facilities and personnel.

- Stating the objectives in terms of units of production or services or activities. The indicated units are increased or decreased by the effect of expected achievements.

- Consideration of salary of wage adjustments. A complete schedule of cost of living increase and merit increase must be prepared of all cost centers, detailing the persons and months and the number of adjustments. However, these

increases should not exceed the ceiling salary/wages established under the job evaluation study.

- Preparation of report on the expenses related to insurance, taxes, supplies, services, maintenance and repair costs, etc. to be included in the budget schedule.

- Preparation of budget report: this report comprises of (a) narrative section summarizing the budget of explaining the budget plan for the year ahead, including the anticipated operating result and principal factors entering into increases and decreases in income and expenditure (b) budget statements and supporting schedules in a concrete manner (c) a comprehensive presentation of budget information by activities and cost centers.

- Review of the budget report by the administrator of the organization who ultimately presents it to the board of trustees.

- Evaluation of the budget as an operating plan, incorporating any changes and presenting it to the finance committee.

- The finance committee may further initiate any changes or modifications before finally presenting to the board for its consideration and decision.

- Final approval by the board.

Budget Manual: Since the budget is formulated at the instance of the top management, and its compliance ensured by the subordinates, there has to be a formal communication channel between the two. This could be in the form of oral or written instruction or directives. The Budget Officer initiates the work relating to the preparation of the Budget Manual. Heads of departments provide the details. The top management approves the first draft and subsequent changes. The policies and procedures are continuously updated and revalidated. A Budget Manual is tailored to fit the needs of each hospital or group of hospitals, where it is to be used.

Budget Committee: The Budget Committee generally consists of a representative cross-section of the major functional areas or divisions within the institution, with the designated budget director usually serving as the chairperson. Budget committees frequently include, those who hold the following positions:

- CEO/MD/Chairman, Director
- Director of Nursing
- Director of Human Resources
- Director of Material Management
- Chief Financial Officer
- Director of Engineering and Plant Operations
- Medical Superintendent

Budget Control: Budgets by themselves will achieve little unless they are supported by budgetary control procedures. Budgetary control mechanisms ensure that the actual results are in line with what was planned and agreed upon, and if there are deviations, identify the reasons and to the extent possible make individuals accountable for them. It can be achieved through:

- Continuous monitoring of the budget.
- Analyzing the changes in actual execution and making the required modification.
- Revising the financial plan if conditions change.

The definite fiscal summaries that come about because of planning from the activities of the hospital are the pay and consumption explanation and financial record, which mirror the money related execution of the clinic for the period and toward the finish of the period, separately.

Balance Sheet

The balance sheet speaks the money related position of an organization in a stipulated period. It reflects the loss and profit of the hospital. Just aggregate figures are given for every arrangement of the vital records. It principally contains:

- **Fixed resources:** These are physical resources for long-haul expected use. It includes the hospital building, different departments, and associated physical infrastructure. Further, it also contains the land, plants, various establishments to support the hospital, hospital furniture, machinery and equipment, vehicles, etc.
- **Current resources:** They comprise of cash balance, deposits, shares and insurances, pending payments to be received, stock materials, etc.
- **Other resources:** These comprise certain specific reason funds such as emergency fund, training and education fund, security funds, etc.
- **Liabilities:** It has current obligations such as payable compensations, other bills, taxes, etc. and long-term obligations, such as Mortgages and Long-term credits.

Problems in budgeting: Reasons why a budget may not deliver the desired benefits are:

- Lack of specific goals and objectives in the budgeting process may create issues.
- Lack of training and motivation. It is often perceived by the key personnel as a pressure technique imposed by the top management, and not as a planning device.
- Departmental goals may be at variance with the organizational/corporate goals. At the highest level, the management may like to deliver the best possible health care.
- Allocation of funds.
- Budgets are usually short term in nature that it is prepared annually, and hence for a long time, it may fail.

Sample Budget Proposal of Patient Care Units/ Hospital

Every budget proposal begins with an introduction to the organization, its philosophy, mission, and objectives. The expenditure is classified broadly into two categories before preparing the budget such as:

1. **Recurring:** Salary of employees and other employee benefits, Bus Maintenance, Electricity, Water, Telephone, Lab consumables, Stationery
2. **Non-recurring:** Building/Infrastructure set up, Furniture, Lab Equipments, Vehicles, Miscellaneous

Sr. no.	Particulars	Estimated cost in INR
1	**DIRECT COSTS**	
	Medical Supplies	
	Drugs	
	Nursing Service Expense	
	Diagnostic and Imaging expense including laboratory	
	Rehabilitation Services	
	Food Services	
	Laundry and other support services	
2	**INDIRECT COSTS**	
	Salaries and Wages	
	Fringe Benefits	
	Interest Expense	
	Facilities Service/Lease Agreements	
	Depreciation/Amortization	
	Credits and Adjustments	
	Material Maintenance	
	Other Expenses such as Electricity, Water, Telephone, Laundry, Dietary facility for indoor patients, Lab consumables, Stationary, Sanitary Maintenance, Engineering and maintenance, Transport, Security Services	
	Tax Payable	
	Others (Parking, Cafeteria, Stationery Shops and so on)	
	Total Expenditure (expected)	
3	**ANTICIPATED REVENUE (MONETARY)**	
	Income from Direct Patient Services	
	Interest from Banks/others	
	Dividend on current investments	
	Other Income (Charity Funds, Donations, Sponsors)	
	Others	
	Total Income (Expected)	

Sample Annual Balance Sheet of a Hospital

Revenue/Income	Amount	Expenditure	Amount
Revenue from Operations		Employee benefits expense	
Other Income (Charity Funds, Donations, Sponsors)		Cost of materials consumed	
Interest from Banks/others		Material Maintenance	
Dividend on current investments		Depreciation and amortization expense	
		Other Expenses such as Electricity, Water, Telephone, Laundry, Dietary facility for indoor patients, Lab consumables, Stationary Sanitary maintenance Engineering and maintenance, Pharmacy Transport	
		Tax Payable	
Any other gains		Others	
Total gain		**Total Expenditure**	

BUDGETING IN EMERGENCY AND DISASTER MANAGEMENT

Crisis management is a perplexing strategy subsystem that includes an intergovernmental, multiphased exertion to alleviate, plan for, react to, and recoup from catastrophe and comparative crisis circumstance.

Debacles or disaster are large scale natural or human-caused crisis occasions that all of a sudden outcome in broad negative monetary and social ramifications for the populaces they influence. While disaster/debacles change in scale, all undermine the general welfare of some people; accordingly, government mediation to limit the antagonistic outcomes of calamity and to reestablish the life of people is anticipated.

Emergency budgeting shows considerable difficulties for the government since there are unusual requests of the condition on various parameters.

Types of Budgeting During a Disaster

- **Pre-disaster budgeting:** It is the act of perceiving the expense of the relief of disaster or emergency before the misfortune occasion.

- **Post-disaster budgeting:** It is done after the misfortune or occasion. It is a financial detailing of the expenditure rather than a budget.

The types mentioned above of budgeting decide the preparation of the emergency and disaster management policy of a country.

Principles for Budgeting for Disasters

- The government policy should incorporate arrangements to build national funds/savings.
- It is difficult for the Government to give help straightforwardly to those enduring a misfortune.
- Lawmakers additionally should be aware of the monetary and political motivating forces confronting governments in the structure and execution of debacle approaches.
- If spending rules treat "crisis" spending as free (they do not need to be settled for with regulatory obligation increments or spending cuts), it will be hard to abstain from overspending for catastrophe alleviation.

Problems in Preparing a Budget for Disasters/Emergency

- Disasters are hard to foresee; putting a theoretical number in the monetary allowance may diminish the budget's efficiency and credibility.
- Since the disasters are unexpected, the policymakers may misuse the allocated funds/budget for some other purposes.
- A pre-planned budget diminishes the scope of external help, especially for underdeveloped and developing countries.

Nurse Administrator's Role in Budgeting

- The budget required for the nursing department should be a cooperative activity of the nursing superintendent and her associates, including the supervisors.
- He/she is a member of the budget planning team.
- Should seek an opinion from her/his fellow workers in determining the needs of the unit for ensuring the year based on information received.
- Submit a budget request with justification with proposed expenditure. The administrator defines her/ his budget so that the nursing unit will have enough money to conduct a program effectively. Money must be available to allow experimentation also.
- When the budget is allotted, the administrator should support the budget. He/she should interpret the subordinates, any changes that may affect instruction services for the adopted budget.
- Since the nurse administrator also is responsible for the budget, she/ he should cover the routine budget control.

Financial Audit

The audit is an independent appraisal activity within an organization for review of accounting, financial and other operations as a basis of services to the management. It is monitoring the budget process. Here, the budget reports are needed to monitor expenditure and keep the budget process focused on long-range objectives. The most common tools are:

- Capital inventory is an itemized list of a current capital asset that enumerates each piece of capital equipment, together with items serial number, current valuation, and physical location, e.g. checking stock register, and inventory.
- Supply inventory is an itemized list of available supplies. It is needed to implement the operating budget for each unit.
- The position control system is the status of each budgeted position. The serial number assigned to each budgeted position should indicate both the job classification and the budget unit and cost center in which the position is assigned it should be documented, dated and identified the nature of transactions and facilitates later retrieval information.
- Monthly account reports are reports of the amount spent and remaining per item, e.g., salary, T.A. etc.
- Cost accounting is a process of linking each expenditure to its purposes.
- **Variance analysis:** A variance is a discrepancy between the number of funds intended to be spent for a particular purpose and the number of funds used for that purpose. Variance analysis is a process that has the following four steps:
  1. Funds required for each budget item or expenditure are calculated for the expected level of activity.
  2. For each budget item, the difference between actual and planned expenditure is calculated.
  3. These differences or variances are examined and the cause of each variance is identified.
  4. Each positive variance (amount expended that exceeds the amount budgeted) is corrected either by increasing the funds allocated for the item or decreasing expenditure for it. The common causes of budget variance are:
     - Unanticipated increase in supply or equipment price.
     - Bills received in a different month when purchases were made.
     - Higher-than-expected inflation rate.
     - Failure to calculate the cost of disposable supplies needed for new equipment.
     - Professional practice charges that entail additional purchase.
     - Unforeseen technological improvement demanded by patients and doctors.
     - Reimbursement changes that alter the type and volume of service delivered.
     - New medical staff members who implement new treatments requiring new equipment and supplies.

- Changes in safety or injection –control standard.
- Excessive breakage of equipment by untrained staff.
- Opening or closing of nursing units.
- Improperly budgeting unproductive time.

The responsibility of nursing administration in the budget includes the following:

- Participation in planning budget.
- Consult and take the assistance of his /her subordinate in determining the needs of the unit for the ensuing year based on information received.
- Request sufficient funds to suggest a sound program such as provide for developing program provision, expansion of the program, to attract and hold qualified staff to provide for expansion of physical facilities, supplies, equipment, for improving instruction (school and college) and also to carry out adequate functions of the institution.
- Submit a budget request with justification with proposed expenditure. The administrators define his/her budget so that the nursing unit will have enough money to conduct the program effectively. Money must be available to allow experimentation also.
- He/she should support the budget and interpret the subordinates, any changes that may affect instruction services for the adopted budget. He/she secures for the adopted budge and responsibility of the administrator to see that expenditure should not exceed the appropriation made.
- The nurse administrator also is responsible for budget and covers the routine budget control.

General Rules and Functions of Administrator/ Manager in Budgeting

Rules: He/she

- Is visionary in identifying or forecasting short and long term unit needs, thus inspiring proactive rather than reactive fiscal planning.
- Is knowledgeable about political, social and economic factors that shape fiscal planning in health care today.
- Demonstrates flexibility in fiscal goals set in a rapidly changing system.
- Anticipates, recognizes and creatively solves problem under budgetary constraints.
- Influences and inspires group members to become active in short and long-range fiscal planning.
- Recognizes when fiscal constraints have resulted in an inability to meet organizational or unit goals and communicate this insight effectively, following the chain of command.
- Ensures that the client safety is not jeopardized by cost contents.

Functions

- Identifies the importance of, and develops short and long-range fiscal plans that reflect unit need.
- Articulates and documents unit needs effectively to higher administrative levels.
- Assess the internal and external environment of the organizations to identify driving forces and barriers of fiscal planning.
- Demonstrates knowledge of budgeting and uses appropriate techniques.
- It provides opportunities for subordinates to participate in relevant fiscal planning.
- Coordinates unit level fiscal planning to be congruent with organizational goals and objectives.
- Accusatively assesses personal needs using predetermined standards or an established patient classification system.
- Coordinates the monitoring aspects of budget control.
- Ensures that documentation of clients' needs for services are clear and complete to facilitate organizational reimbursement.

Advantages of Clinical Budgeting

- Head of the clinical units is involved in planning, allocation of resources and achievement of objectives.
- The Head of the clinical units seeks specific resources, personnel, and equipment to perform optimally the services.
- Each clinical unit is responsible for expenditure including referrals, investigations, drugs and materials and services from other departments.
- Clinical budgeting leads to cost containment and control over wastage.

Conclusion: The budget is very important in the management of patients in the health care setting. Proper planning of the budget will improve the quality of services provided in the organization. So the nurse should know about types, steps, and cost containment.

 REVIEW QUESTIONS

1. Define financial management. What are the objectives and elements of financial management?
2. Define finance. Explain the approaches and scope of financial management.
3. Explain approaches to budgeting.
4. Define Nursing Budget, Steps in Nursing Budget and Role of Nurse in budgetary processes.
5. Explain budget planning and its stages.
6. Explain the steps in making a hospital budget and mechanics of budgeting.
7. Explain budgeting for disaster. What are the principles and problems faced during budgeting?

Further Readings

1. Banerjee, Shyamal. Principles and Practice of Management. Oxford and IBM Publishing, New Delhi; 2000.
2. Basavanthappa BT. Nursing Administration. 2nd Edition: Jaypee Brothers Medical Publishers (P) Ltd., New Delhi; 2009.
3. Barrett, Jean. Ward Management and Teaching. Konark Publishers, Delhi; 1992.
4. Warren, Stevens, F. Management and Leadership in Nursing. McGraw – Hill Inc, New York; 1978.
5. Alexander et al. Nursing Service Administration. Mosby Publishers, US; 1962.
6. Park K. Preventive and Social Medicine, 19th Edition: M/s. Banarasidas Bhanot Publishers, Jabalpur; 2007.
7. Basavanthappa BT. Nursing Administration, 1st Edition: Jaypee Brothers Medical Publishers (P) Ltd., New Delhi; 2002.
8. Goel SL, Kumar R. Management of Hospitals – Hospital Administration in the 21st century, Vol. 4, Deep and Deep Publication, New Delhi; 2002.
9. Ranga Rao SP. Administration of Primary Health Centers in India, 1st Edition: Mittal Publications, New Delhi; 1993.
10. Lucita M. Nursing: Practice and Public Health Administration. Current Concepts and Trends. B. I. Churchill Living Stone Pvt. Ltd., New Delhi; 2002.
11. Sakharkar BM. Principles of Hospital Administration and Planning, 2nd Edition: Jaypee Brothers Medical Publishers (P) Ltd., New Delhi; 2009.
12. Patricia S Yoder-Wise. Leading and Managing in Nursing. 2nd Edition: Mosby Publication, US; 1999.
13. Bessie L Marquis, Carol J Huston. Leadership Roles and Management Functions in Nursing: Theory and Application. 5th Edition: Lippincott Williams and Wilkins, New York; 2006.
14. Linda Roussel. Management and Leadership for Nurse Administrators. 4th Edition: Jones and Bartlett Publication, USA; 2006.
15. Wehrich H, Koontz H. Management A Global Perspective. 11th Edition: Tata McGraw-Hill Publishing Company, Ltd., New Delhi; 2005.
16. Marquis BL, Huston CJ. Leadership and Management Functions in Nursing- Theory, and Application. 5th Edition: Lippincott Williams and Wilkins, Philadelphia; 2006.
17. Douglass LM. The Effective Nurse: Leader and Manager. 5th Edition: Mosby Publication, US; 1996.
18. Trained Nurses Association of India, Nursing Administration, and Management.
19. Samson Rebecca. Leadership and Management in Nursing Practice and Education 1st Edition: Jaypee Brothers Medical Publishers (P) Ltd., New Delhi; 2009.
20. Kunders GD. Designing for Total Quality in Health Care, Prism Book Pvt. Ltd., Bangalore; 2002.
21. Chandorkar AG. Hospital Administration and Planning. 2nd Edition: Paras Medical Publisher, New Delhi; 2009.
22. Joshi DC, Joshi Mamta. Hospital Administration. 1st Edition: Jaypee Brothers Medical Publishers (P) Ltd., New Delhi; 2009.
23. Eleanor J Sullivan, Philip J Decker. Effective Leadership and Management in Nursing. 4th Edition: Published by Addison Wesely; 2011.
24. Kulkarni GR. Financial Management for Hospital Administration, Jaypee Brothers Medical Publishers (P) Ltd., New Delhi; 2009.

Unit

11

Nursing Informatics/ Information Management: Review

Unit Outline

- Nursing Informatics and Information Management
- Patient Records (Computerized Patient Records)
- Electronic Nursing Records
- Role of Computers in Nursing
- Telemedicine
- Telenursing
- Electronic Medical/Health Records

NURSING INFORMATICS AND INFORMATION MANAGEMENT

Health care is delivered in a dynamic, complex, and ever-changing environment. Changes in medical treatments, regulations for federal and state reimbursement and public knowledge create growing demands for information. The computer has moved from "nice to know" luxury item to "need to know". On average, medical/surgical nurses spend 34% of their time handling information.

Informatics comes from the French word "Informatique", which means "computer science". Informatics is defined as computer science + information science. Nursing informatics is a field of nursing that incorporates nursing, computer, and information sciences to maintain and develop medical data and systems to support the practice of nursing, and to improve patient care outcomes. Technologies that have evolved due to health care/nursing informatics include:

- Computerized provider order entry (CPOE)
- Electronic medical records (EMRs) (Test results, progress notes, nursing notes, and medication records)

There are three "building blocks" of nursing communications—data, information, and knowledge. Data includes direct observations that do not need interpretation, such as the patient's name, age, vital signs and disease history. Information is data that has been interpreted. Examples include the prevalence of hospital-acquired infections, by care unit, percentage of patient care delays in outpatient clinics, by specialty. Knowledge is the amalgam of information to identify relationships that provide further observation on an issue. For example, the effect of nurse-patient ratios and patient outcomes. Developing care protocols (i.e., anaphylactic reaction protocols, pressure ulcer protocols, etc.)

While nurses incorporate all three communication "building blocks" in their daily routines, the three concepts are also stored in computer programs and software to assist health care providers across the continuum to provide high-quality, safe patient care.

Nurse informaticists work to develop communication and information technologies in health care. They also serve as educators, researchers, software engineers, and chief nursing officers. Using the "building blocks" listed above, they help develop evidence-based policies and procedures for organizations.

Definitions

Nursing informatics is a combination of computer science, information science and nursing science designed to assist in the management and processing of nursing data, information, and knowledge. **—Graves and Corcoran, 1989**

Nursing informatics is defined as the use of computer technology to support nursing, including clinical practice, administration, education, and research. **—Hebda, 1998**

Nursing informatics is defined as the development and evaluation of applications, tools, processes, and structures that assist nurses with the management of data in taking care of patients or supporting the practice of nursing.

—American Nurses Association (ANA) 1994

Nursing informatics is the integration of nursing, information and information management with information processing and communication technologies to support health efforts.

—ICN, 2006

Nursing informatics is a specialty that integrates nursing sciences, computer science, and information science to manage and communicate data; information, knowledge, and wisdom in nursing practice. **—ANA, 2008**

Nursing informatics is the application of computer technology in all fields of nursing, nursing services, nurse education, and nursing research. **—Scholes and Barber, 1980**

Dimensions of Nursing Informatics

Nursing informatics is using technology, research, and professional experience to manage nursing data, information, and knowledge to improve practice and deliver better health care (Fig. 1).

Data: Data are discrete observations that are not interpreted, organized or structured.

Information: Information is the data that can be interpreted, organized or structured to give meaning to the data. Information is an essential phenomenon of study for an information-based discipline such as nursing.

Knowledge: Knowledge is the synthesis of the information to identify the relationship that provides further insight into the subject area.

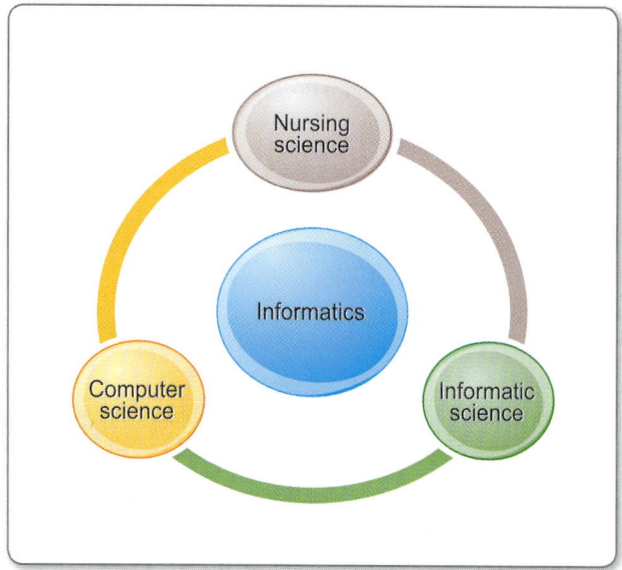

Fig. 1: Dimensions of nursing informatics

Historical Development of Nursing Informatics

- Healthcare began to use computers in the 1950s.
- Computers, in this era, were typically used in the business office.
- In the 1970s, nursing began to realize the importance of computers to the nursing profession and became involved in the design, purchase, and implementation of information systems.
- 1977—the first Nursing Information System Conference was held in the United States.
- In the 1980s, medical and nursing informatics specialties emerged.
- October 1995—the first ANA certification examination in Nursing Informatics was given.
- The post-2000 era saw an unprecedented explosion in the number and sophistication of both computer hardware and software.
- Telemedicine became possible and was recognized as a specialty in the late 1990s.
- 1999—a study was performed to identify International Standards for health information and their adaptability in the Philippines referred to as "Standards of Health Information in the Philippines, 1999 ver. (SHIP99).
- 2003—Master of Science in Health Informatics was proposed to be offered by UP-Manila College of Medicine (major in medical informatics) and the College of Arts and Science (major in bioinformatics) and was later approved to be offered to start the academic year 2005-2006.
- The Technology Informatics Guiding Education Reform (TIGER) Initiative was established in 2006 in the United States to develop key areas of informatics in nursing.
- 2008—Nursing Informatics course in the undergraduate curriculum was defined by the Commission on Higher Education (CHED).
- 2009—Mr. Kristian R. Sumabat and Ms Mia Alcantara-Santiago, both nurses and graduate students of Master of Science in Health Informatics at the University of the Philippines, Manila began drafting plans to create a nursing informatics organization.
- 2010—they began recruiting other nursing informatics specialists and practitioners to organize a group that later became the Philippine Nursing Informatics, a sub-specialty organization of PNA for nursing informatics.
- NI has experienced rapid growth in the last 40 years which does not appear to be slowing.

Purposes of Nursing Informatics

- To enhance all aspects of patient care and health management.
- To study the process and structure of nursing information to support clinical decision making and the delivery of nursing care at the micro-level.
- To help in retrieving evidence-based standards of practice, legislation acts, statistical analysis, of the profession of nursing and practitioners of nursing at any given time or interval of time at the macro level.
- To streamline the handling of data. The traditional method of documentation of a nurse was confined to paper and it was difficult to file the massive number of documents.
- Efficient information management to access relevant information.
- To have easy access to sharing vital data within co-workers and other health care disciplines.
- To safeguard personal records of patients while at the same time allowing the easiest possible access to the information for those who need it.
- To develop an information-sharing network and data handling standards to work nationally and worldwide.

Application of Nursing Informatics

- **Nursing clinical practice:**
  - Worklists to remind staff of planned nursing interventions.
  - Computer-generated client documentation.
  - Electronic medical record (EMR) and Computer-based Patient Record (CPR).
  - Monitoring devices that record vital signs and other measurements directly into the client record (EMR).
  - Computer-generated nursing care plans and critical pathways.
  - Automatic billing for supplies or procedures with nursing documentation.
  - Reminders and prompts that appear during documentation to ensure comprehensive charting.
- **Nursing administration (health care information system)**
  - Automated staff scheduling.
  - E-mail for improved communication.
  - Cost analysis and finding trends for budget purposes.
  - Quality assurance and outcomes analysis.
- **Nursing education:**
  - Computerized record keeping.
  - Computerized assisted instruction.
  - Interactive video technology.
  - Distance learning—web-based courses and degree programs.
  - Internet resources- formal nursing courses and degree programs.
  - Presentation software for preparing slides and
  - Handouts- power points and MS words.
- **Nursing research:**
  - Computerized literature searching—CINHAL, Medline and web sources.
  - The adoption of standardized language related to nursing terms—NANDA, etc.
  - The ability to find trends in aggregate data, that is data derived from large population groups—SPSS.

- **Patient education:** Nursing informatics can be used for symptom management and patient education. The nurses can access the information for the patient or teach the patient where to find appropriate and helpful information. For example, in an oncology unit, nursing informatics can be used to teach patients effective symptom management of the treatment modalities, which often cause pain, fatigue, and poor nutritional status. Nursing informatics can also aid in other nursing interventions of the oncology nurse, such as analgesic administration and stress-reduction techniques.

- **Clinical alert system:** The computerized clinical alert system can be used in conjunction with the hospital pharmacy. System design is created to alert both pharmacy and health staff when two or more drug prescriptions are incompatible.

- **Patient data:** Nursing informatics can also be useful in a physician's clinic. In a managed care environment, information systems make administrative management more efficient. The private practitioner, program or facility to manage every aspect of patient care can use one data management system. In each of these health care settings, data management systems can be applied to treatments, diagnostics, documentation, practice management, insurance claims and referrals, and protocols as well as treatment and diagnostic results.

- **Telehealth:** Telehealth includes the use of telephones and sophisticated image transmission systems like ECG, faxes and remote camera imaging. Telehealth places the ambulance personnel in touch with the Emergency Department and it also operates to put the generalist "nurses and doctors" at the ED in touch with specialists. Telehealth is used to evaluate the stroke victims while they are in transit so appropriate therapy can be initiated quickly upon arrival at the ED. Similarly, a nurse practitioner in a remote ED might be guided via telephone in the proper procedure for inserting chest tubes so a man with a collapsed lung could be stabilized for subsequent transport to a major hospital. Finally, nursing informatics can be useful for interdepartmental communication such as ordering supplies from a central supply, lab work, etc.

PATIENT RECORDS (COMPUTERIZED PATIENT RECORDS)

Nursing documentation is a vital component of safe, ethical and effective nursing practice, regardless of the context of practice or whether the documentation is paper-based or electronic. The documentation is intended to provide registered nurses (RNs) with professional accountability. Although different documentation systems and technology may be used throughout the province, quality nursing documentation is expected in every area of care or service delivery and every setting. Nurses must be familiar with and follow, agencies' documentation policies, standards, and protocols. Nurses are subject to increasing scrutiny regarding their record-keeping. Legislations such as the Human Rights Act 1998 and the Data have Protection Act 1998 have increased the profile of and access to, health records, while patients are increasingly willing to complain about their care. Whether complaints are resolved by health care providers or settled in court, comprehensive records are essential. It is important, therefore, that nurses keep abreast of legal requirements and best practice in record-keeping. The Code of Professional Conduct (NMC, 2002a) advises that good note-taking is a vital tool of communication between nurses.

Definitions

Documentation is anything written or electronically generated that describes the status of a client or the care or services given to that client. —**Perry, AG, Potter, PA, 2010**

Nursing documentation refers to written or electronically generated client information obtained through the nursing process. —**ARNNL, 2010**

A computer-based patient record system is a repository of electronically maintained information about an individual's lifetime health status and health care, stored so that it can serve multiple legitimate users. It may be linked with an information management tool to provide clinical reminders, link to knowledge sources for health care decision support and aggregate data for further analysis.

Functional Components of CPR

- **An integrated view of patient data:** Data usually needs to be acquired using interface engines and even mature standards (such as Health Level Seven or HL7 is a set of international standards to support clinical practice including its management, delivery and evaluation.). The data should comprise all details about the care and treatment of patients such as demographic features, laboratory features, radiology features, pharmacy features, bills and finance related aspects, diagnosis and treatment-related aspects including medication and surgical remarks. The data must be accessible to all health care professionals at multiple points.

- **Clinical decision support:** A clinical decision support system (CDSS) is a health information technology system that is designed to provide physicians and other health professionals with clinical decision support (CDS), that is, assistance with clinical decision-making tasks. CDSSs constitute a major topic in artificial intelligence in medicine. This implies that a CDSS is simply a decision support system that is focused on using knowledge management in such a way to achieve clinical advice for patient care based on multiple items of patient data. The main purpose of modern CDSS is to assist clinicians at the point of care.

This means that clinicians interact with a CDSS to help and analyze and reach a diagnosis based on patient data. The CDS may be of two types such as knowledge-based or non-knowledge-based systems. The knowledge-based system operates based on the information or decision-making inputs that are fed in the electronic system. E.g. If the drug X is administered to a patient then the drug Y should not be given. The non-knowledge-based system makes use of artificial intelligence to support decision making.

- **Clinician order entry:** Computerized physician order entry (CPOE), sometimes referred to as computerized provider order entry or computerized provider order management (CPOM), is a process of electronic entry of medical practitioner instructions for the treatment of patients (particularly hospitalized patients) under his or her care. The entered orders are communicated over a computer network to the medical staff or to the departments (pharmacy, laboratory, or radiology) responsible for fulfilling the order. CPOE reduces the time it takes to distribute and complete orders while increasing efficiency by reducing transcription errors including preventing duplicate order entry while simplifying inventory management and billing.
- **Access to knowledge resources:** This feature can help in the decision making process.
- **Integrated communication support:** This feature allows to confer messages to other members of the treatment team that may be localized elsewhere, or when the patient is transferred. Can be used as a tracking tool, e.g.: Are prescribed orders carried out?

Advantages of CPR

- CPR is flexible.
- The input process may be facilitated if linked to other data storage devices.
- Usable for both individualized patient care, and management needs, plus public health demands.
- Better accessibility than a paper record.
- Better legible, and better organized.
- Interactive control of completeness and accuracy.
- Reusability of data, e.g., in discharge letters.

Disadvantages of CPR

- CPR is more costly.
- The input process must be learned by staff.
- The use of CPR will change workflow, and interaction with patients.
- Conversion from paper to CPR takes time.

Fundamental Issues of CPR

- **Data entry:** It includes data capture, quality of input data, prevention of error in data entry and manual feeding of data.

- **Data display:** The issues related to data display include, flowsheets of patient data, summaries and abstracts. They are only available and dynamic displays.
- **Query and surveillance-related:** Issues in clinical care clinical research, retrospective studies, and administration related queries.

ELECTRONIC NURSING RECORDS

Health records have been the most accessible source of this information, and this accessibility has been facilitated and expanded with the advent of electronic health record (EHR) systems. Routine clinical practices are using EHR systems to create large, electronic databases, and this reduces the cost, effort, and time required for data collection. Traditional methods such as paper-based data inputs and data repositories, and traditional ways of managing this information, cannot meet the increasing demand for expedited data collection; their processing time is longer, and they have more potential to produce errors. Large electronic databases generated by routine care become more important as the focus shifts from efficacy research to effectiveness research.

Nursing documentation is a significant indicator of effective patient care delivery. Documentation can be either paper-based or electronic-based, as per the electronic health records (EHRs), which include all information related to patient care. Regardless of the method of documentation, nursing documentation has to be conducted at the highest standard, to ensure the delivery of safe and high-quality healthcare services. High quality of nursing documentation is expected in every area of care and every setting; it is considered an important responsibility of nursing, to ensure the continuity of effective patient care and to improve patients' outcomes.

Nurses, the largest group of healthcare providers in the healthcare system, play a crucial role in every area of performance improvement in healthcare organizations. The role demands to document and manage patient information through coordinating patient care and communicating with other interdisciplinary team members. It is believed that paper-based documentation does not meet the requirements of high-quality documentation and communication among healthcare providers, because it is time-consuming, repetitive and inaccurate. Problems arise when attempting to obtain information from paper-based records, as it is considered labor-intensive. Health care is built upon and revolves around information. The introduction of electronic health records (EHRs) as a method of documentation is more legible and more accessible.

The increasing amount of data makes managing information difficult to assemble and more importantly, more difficult to provide the best care to patients. Electronic health record documentation has been used by many nurses for documenting nursing care including the nursing process, such as entering orders and accessing laboratory results, as well as supporting healthcare professionals in processing, managing and communicating data in a variety of settings. It has the potential to improve patients' safety, enhance healthcare professionals' access to a patient's healthcare information, ensure the appropriate use of resources and finally, improve communication among healthcare professionals.

With the transition from paper-based nursing records to electronic nursing record (ENR) systems, nurses have focused on the development and use of nursing databases to accomplish nursing effectiveness research. Despite this, ENR systems that enable nurses to document on-screen virtually all the components of the nursing process (diagnosis, intervention, and outcome evaluation) and store them in databases are still rare.

Functional Components of Electronic Nursing Records

The nursing care of the patients is purely based on the concept of providing a nursing care plan. The electronic Nursing Records ensure accurate recording and recognizing the nursing diagnosis based on the pre-fed guidelines of the system. The elements of ENR are briefed below:

- **Standardized nursing languages:** For the nursing diagnosis component, the North American Nursing Diagnosis Association-International (NANDA-I), nursing diagnoses including defining characteristics (signs and symptoms) and related factors must be incorporated into the Electronic health management System. The Nursing Outcomes Classification (NOC), a comprehensive standardized classification of patient outcomes responsive to nursing interventions, also must be defined to measure patient outcomes.
- **Preparation of nursing care interface:** The Nursing care interface must allow for updating nursing documents by adding, revising, deleting, or saving. The nurses can see patients' personal information and medical diagnoses delivered from the clinical data server. The Nursing Care Interface lets nurses (1) search and select the nursing process elements from the existing database, (2) enter free texts of nursing care that do not exist in the depository, (3) save and print the information, and (4) review the documented nursing care by patient and date/period. It includes the provision for selecting appropriate nursing diagnoses and setting up the desired goals.
- **Developing the decision support system:** Although the use of Standardized Nursing Languages helps describe the nursing care delivered in a standardized way, developing the decision support system helps prevent errors and duplication. The decision support system includes assistance in the selection of appropriate nursing diagnoses, interventions, and outcomes.

- **Environment of the electronic nursing record system:** The ENR system must be incorporated with the Order Communication System within the hospital information system. The ENR system is organized as a client/server type, and its database lies within a server.
- **Evaluating the electronic nursing record system:** The system guides nurses to re-evaluate patients' status using the nursing outcomes evaluation screen. This evaluation is available after completing nursing interventions. Because this system allows nurses to assess more than once and shows all results, and thus nurses can document changes in the patient's condition.

ROLE OF COMPUTERS IN NURSING

Computers play a key role in almost every sphere of life. They facilitate the storage of huge amounts of data, they enable speedy processing of information and they possess an inbuilt intelligence. Owing to these unique capabilities, computers function on levels close to that of a human brain. Computers can hence be employed in a wide variety of fields like engineering, data processing, and storage, planning and scheduling, networking, education as well as health and medicine.

- Computers are an excellent means for the storage of patient-related data. Big hospitals employ computer systems to maintain patient records. It is often necessary to maintain detailed records of the medical history of patients. Doctors often require information about a patient's family history, physical ailments, already diagnosed diseases, and prescribed medicines. This information can be effectively stored in a computer database.
- Computers can keep track of prescriptions and billing information. They can be used to store the information about the medicines prescribed to a patient as well as those, which cannot be prescribed to him/her.
- Computers enable the efficient storage of huge amounts of medical data. Medicine comprises a vast base of knowledge. Computer storage can serve as the best means of housing this information.
- Medical journals, research and diagnosis papers, important medical documents and reference books can best be stored in an electronic format.
- Many of the modern-day medical equipment have small, programmed computers. Many of the medical appliances of today work on pre-programmed instructions. The circuitry and logic in most of the medical equipment is a computer.
- The functioning of hospital-bed beeping systems, emergency alarm systems, X-ray machines, and several such medical appliances is based on computer logic.
- Computer software is used for the diagnosis of diseases. It can be used for the examination of the internal organs

of the body. Advanced computer-based systems are used to examine the delicate organs of the body. Some of the complex surgeries can be performed with the aid of computers.

- The different types of monitoring equipment in hospitals are often based on computer programming. Medical imaging is a vast field that deals with the techniques to create images of the human body for medical purposes. Many of the modern methods of scanning and imaging are largely based on computer technology.
- Magnetic resonance imaging employs computer software. Computed tomography makes use of digital geometry processing techniques to obtain 3-D images. Sophisticated computers and infrared cameras are used for obtaining high-resolution images. Computers are widely used for the generation of 3-D images in medicine.
- Computer networking enables quicker communication. In the field of medicine, computers allow for faster communication between a patient and a doctor. Medical professionals sitting on opposite sides of the globe can communicate within minutes employing the Internet. Medical practitioners can discuss medical issues in medical forums.

The importance of computers cannot be stressed enough as computer technology has revolutionized the field of medicine.

TELEMEDICINE

Telemedicine has been defined as the use of telecommunications to provide medical information and services. It may be as simple as two health professionals discussing a case over the telephone, or as sophisticated as using satellite technology to broadcast a consultation between providers at facilities in two countries, using videoconferencing equipment or robotic technology. Telemedicine generally refers to the use of ICT for the delivery of clinical care.

Types of Telemedicine

- **Real-time (synchronous):** Real-time telemedicine could be as simple as a telephone call or as complex as robotic surgery. It requires the presence of both parties at the same time and a communications link between them that allows a real-time interaction to take place. Video-conferencing equipment is one of the most common forms of technologies used in synchronous telemedicine. There are also peripheral devices that can be attached to computers, which can aid in an interactive examination. For instance, a tele-otoscope allows a remote physician to 'see' inside a patient's ear; a tele stethoscope allows the consulting remote physician to hear the patient's heartbeat.
- **Store-and-forward (asynchronous):** It involves acquiring medical data (like medical images, biosignals, etc.) and then transmitting this data to a doctor or medical specialist at a convenient time for assessment offline. It does not require the presence of both parties at the same time. Dermatology, radiology, and pathology are common specialties that are conducive to asynchronous telemedicine. Teleradiology, the sending of X-rays, CT scans, or MRIs (store-and-forward images) is the most common application of telemedicine in use today.

Use of Telemedicine

- Telemedicine is the most beneficial for populations living in isolated communities and remote regions and is currently being applied in virtually all medical domains.
- Telemedicine is also useful as a communication tool between a general practitioner and a specialist available at a remote location.
- Telepathology is another common use of this technology. Images of pathology slides may be sent from one location to another for diagnostic consultation.
- The other widely used technology, two-way interactive television (IATV), is used when a 'face-to-face' consultation is necessary. The patient and sometimes their provider, or more commonly a nurse practitioner or telemedicine coordinator (or any combination of the three), are at the originating site. The specialist is at the referral site, most often at an urban medical center.

Scope of Telemedicine

- It can make specialty care more accessible to underserved rural and urban populations.
- Video consultations from a rural clinic to a specialist can alleviate prohibitive travel and associated costs for patients.
- Video conferencing also opens up new possibilities for continuing education or training for isolated or rural health practitioners, who may not be able to leave a rural practice to take part in professional meetings or educational opportunities.
- The use of telemedicine can also cut costs of medical care for those in rural areas.

Barriers to Telemedicine

- License related problems. Many states will not allow out-of-state physicians to practice unless licensed in their state.
- Many private insurers will not reimburse, the cost of medical service.
- Lack of appropriate telecommunications technology.
- Lack of funding for developing state-of-the-art telemedicine infrastructure.

Need for Telemedicine in India

The health of a nation is the product of many factors and forces that combine and interact. Economic growth, per capita income, literacy, education, age at marriage, birth rates, information on health care and nutrition, access to safe drinking water, public and private health care infrastructure, access to preventive health and medical care and health insurance are among the contributing factors. The advances in Medical science, biomedical engineering on one side and Telecommunication and Information Technology on the other side are offering wide opportunities for improved health care.

Despite making huge strides in overall development, the health coverage to the majority of our population is still a distant dream. India is a vast country gifted with rich and ancient historic background and geographically nature has provided India with all the varieties like the mountain regions like Ladakh, deserts, green planes and far-flung areas in the northeast and offshore islands of Andaman's and Lakshadweep.

India today has more than 1 billion population and there is a finite limit of elasticity in providing health care in terms of infrastructure, facility, the manpower, and the funds. Wide disparities persist between different income groups, between rural and urban communities, and between different states and even districts within States.

Further, this is compounded by the following factors like high cost of health care and lack of investment for health care in rural areas. Inadequate medical facilities in rural and inaccessible areas is due to the problem of retaining doctors in rural areas where they are required to serve and propagate widespread health awareness. Specialist doctors cannot be retained in rural areas as they will be professionally isolated and become obsolete and even monetary incentives also cannot prevent it.

A recent survey by the Indian Medical society has found 75% of a qualified consulting doctor practice in urban centers and 23% in semi-urban areas and only 2% from rural areas whereas the majority of the patients come from rural areas. Hospital beds/1000 people are 0.19 in rural and 2.2 in urban areas. This calls for innovative methods of utilization of science and technology for the benefit, of our society and telemedicine assumes a great significance to revolutionize the health care system in India.

TELENURSING

Telenursing is the use of telecommunications technology in nursing to enhance patient care. It involved the use of electromagnetic channels (e.g., wire, radio, and optical) to transmit voice, data, and video communications signals. It is defined as distance communication, using electrical or optical transmissions between humans and/or computers.

Telenursing refers to the use of information technology in the provision of nursing services whenever physical distance exists between patient and nurse, or between any number of nurses. As a field, it is part of telemedicine and has many points of contact with other medical and non-medical applications, such as telediagnosis, teleconsultation, and telemonitoring.

Telenursing is growing in many countries because of the preoccupation in driving down the costs of health care, an increase in the number of aging and chronically ill population, and the increase in coverage of health care to distant, rural, small or sparsely populated regions. Among its many benefits, telenursing may help solve increasing shortages of nurses; to reduce distances and save travel time, and to keep patients out of the hospital.

Nursing informatics, a branch of health informatics, has been defined by Judith Rae Graves and Sheila Corcoran as "a combination of computer science, information science, and nursing science designed to assist in the management and processing of nursing data, information, and knowledge to support the practice of nursing and the delivery of nursing care." Telenursing is a potential application of nursing informatics and as such, nursing informatics has served as a critical background concept of its development.

Need of Telenursing

- Demographic changes
- Nursing and health care workers shortage
- Chronic diseases and conditions
- Educated consumers
- Economic conditions

Applications/Scope of Telenursing

- **Home care:** One of the most distinctive telenursing applications is home care. For example, patients who are immobilized, or live in remote or difficult to reach places, citizens who have chronic ailments, such as chronic obstructive pulmonary disease, diabetes, congestive heart disease, or debilitating diseases, such as neural degenerative diseases (Parkinson's disease, Alzheimer's disease or ALS), may stay at home and be "visited" and assisted regularly by a nurse via video conferencing, internet or video phone.

- **Case management:** A common application of telenursing is also used by call centers operated by managed care organizations, which are staffed by registered nurses who act as case managers or perform patient triage, information, and counseling as a means of regulating patient access and flow and decrease the use of emergency rooms.

- **Telephone triage:** Telephone triage refers to the symptom or clinically-based calls. Clinicians perform symptom assessment by asking detailed questions about the patient's illness or injury. The clinician's task is to estimate and/or rule out urgent symptoms. They may use pattern recognition and other problem-solving processes as well. Clinicians may utilize guidelines, in paper or electronic format, to determine how urgent the symptoms are. Telephone triage requires clinicians to determine if the symptoms are life-threatening, emergency, urgent, acute or non-acute.

Advantages of Telenursing

- Increase public access to health care.
- Provide access to rural areas.
- Decrease wait times.
- Decrease unnecessary hospital visits.
- The decrease in healthcare costs.
- Increase continuity of care.
- Increase patient compliance with aftercare.

Disadvantages of Telenursing

- Decreased face-to-face interaction.
- Risk of decreasing quality of care.
- May increase liability.
- Concerns with security.
- Concerns with maintaining confidentiality.

Legal Issues and Ethical Issues related to Telenursing

- Maintaining patient privacy
- Verifying consent
- Nursing Licensure across state lines
- Maintaining compliance with the scope of practice
- Maintaining autonomy (identity, privacy)
- Maintaining the patient's integrity and preventing harm.

ELECTRONIC MEDICAL/HEALTH RECORDS

The significance of electronic health records (EHRs) to nursing cannot be underestimated. Although EHRs on the surface suggest simple automation of clinical documentation their implications are broad, ranging from how care is delivered, to the types of interactions nurses have with patients in conjunction with the use of technology to the research surrounding EHRs that will inform nursing practice for tomorrow. Basic knowledge of EHRs and nursing informatics is now considered by many to be an entry-level nursing competency.

Components of Electronic Health records

- **Health information and data:** Health Information and data comprises the patient data required to make sound clinical decisions, including demographics, medical and nursing diagnoses, medication lists, allergies, and test results.
- **Results management:** It is the ability to manage results of all types electronically, including laboratory and radiology procedure reports, both current and historical.
- **Order entry management:** A clinician can enter medication and other orders, including laboratory, microbiology, pathology, radiology, nursing, supply orders, ancillary services, and consultations directly into a computer.

- **Decision support:** It entails the use of computer reminders and alerts to improve the diagnosis and care of a patient, including screening for correct drug selection and dosing, screening for medication interactions with other medications, preventive health reminders in such areas as vaccinations, health risk screening and detection, and clinical guidelines for patient disease treatment.
- **Electronic communication and connectivity:** It includes online communication among healthcare team members, their care partners, and patients including email, web messaging, and an integrated health record within and across settings, institutions, and telemedicine.
- **Patient support:** It encompasses patient education and self-monitoring tools, including interactive computer-based patient education, home telemonitoring, and telehealth systems.
- **Administrative processes:** These are activities carried out by the electronic scheduling, billing, and claims management systems, including electronic scheduling for inpatient and outpatient visits and procedures, electronic insurance eligibility validation, claim authorization and so on.
- **Reporting and population health management:** These are data collection tools to support public and private reporting requirements, including data represented in a standardized terminology and machine-readable format.

Advantages of EMR/EHR

Electronic Medical Record systems are much more fitting, important, and efficient than manual medical records, says the Mayo Clinic. Several doctors can update the patient record at the same time. Furthermore, Electronic Medical Record does not need a huge capacity for space and manual work to record and accumulate data.

- **Organization:** The most important benefit of EMR is the way that a patient's records can be managed and arranged. Paper records or files can simply be misplaced in a file room at the clinic, but an electronic medical record is accumulated on a network that is available throughout the service.
- **Access:** Physicians can access quickly to patient files using the electronic medical record system. In each of the patients' rooms and practice rooms, there are computers that are provided with the facilities that are prepared with this technology. The patient's record can be logged on from any computer to update conditions, medications, and procedures that have been performed on the patient.
- **Decision support:** Improved health decisions can be prepared for the patient when his EMR is accessible by more than one physician. Repeatedly a patient is sent from one physician to another when health problem appears to be dangerous or need to be diagnosed. These physicians may not have the ability to communicate or transmit the

patient's medical records to every facility. In this case, the patient can be subjected to repetitive or unwarranted actions because of the lack of transmission.

- **Standardization:** Electronic medical record systems will also provide better standardization once it takes place to keep patient records throughout the health care system. Several medical services apply various terminologies for similar procedures. Other services apply structures that are dissimilar from other facilities. Electronic medical record systems will make it easier for physicians and nurses to get the information they want for every patient by providing a standard way of filling out data on a patient's file.

- **Patients:** A few Electronic medical record systems give the patients the ability to log on their test results and other vital information from their health record through a protected site on the internet. This help patients better understand their health-care choice.

Barriers to Using EMR

- **Technical barriers:** It is expensive to implement an Electronic Medical Record system in a physician's office, mainly for minor practices. Moreover, install such a system in minor hospital institutions require external industrial support.

- **Cultural barriers:** An Electronic Medical Record will extensively change a physician's flow and potentially decrease the quality of service the doctor provides by giving him more patients, however, before physicians expected a specific amount of workflow because they were spending time filling out paperwork.

 REVIEW QUESTIONS

1. Define nursing informatics. List down the purpose and explain the scope of nursing informatics.
2. What are computerized patient records? Explain its function to the health care sector.
3. Explain the role of computers in nursing.
4. What is Telemedicine? What are its types? Explain the uses and scope of telemedicine in India.
5. Briefly explain Telenursing and its scope.

Further Readings

1. Fendrick AM, Goodman CS, Trobe JD. The Effectiveness Initiative, II: The Spectrum of Effectiveness Research. Arch Ophthalmol. 1995;113:862–865.
2. Kupersmith J, Sung N, Genel M, et al. Creating a New Structure for Research on Health Care Effectiveness. J Investig Med. 2005; 53(2):67–72.
3. Ozbolt JG. Strategies for Building Nursing Databases for Effectiveness Research. http://www.ninr.nih.gov/NR/rdonlyres/B3322AAC-2C54–4309-BE83-E09AAD41D1AB/4747/
4. Ingersoll GL, Hoffart N, Schultz AW. Health Services Research in Nursing: Current Status and Future Directions. Nurs Econ. 1990; 8(4):229–238.
5. McCormick KA. Nursing Effectiveness Research Using Existing Databases. http://www.ninr.nih.gov/NR/rdonlyres/B3322AAC2C54-4309-BE83-E09AAD41D1AB/4746
6. Werley H, Lang N. Identification of the Nursing Minimum Data Set. Springer, New York; 1998.
7. Delaney C, Mehmert PA, Prophet C, Bellinger SLR, Huber DG, Ellerbe S. Standardized Nursing Language for Healthcare information systems. J Med Syst. 1992;9(4):145–159.
8. Delaney C, Moorhead S. The Nursing Minimum Data Set, Standardized Language, and Health Care Quality. J Nurs Care Qual. 1995;10(1):16–30.
9. Lee HY, Choi YH, Kim HS, Park HA, Park HK. Development of a Korean-translated version of the 17 Nursing Diagnoses. J Korean Acad Adult Nurs. 1998;10(3):395–402.

Unit

12

Personal Management Review

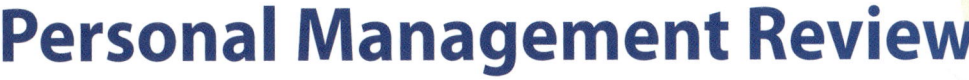

 Unit Outline

- ➤ Emotional Intelligence
- ➤ Resilience Building
- ➤ Stress Management
- ➤ Time Management
- ➤ Career Planning and Development

EMOTIONAL INTELLIGENCE

Emotions are involved in everything people do: every action, decision, and judgment. Emotionally intelligent people recognize this and use their thinking to manage their emotions rather than being managed by them. In the course of the last two decades, Emotional Intelligence (EI) concept has become a very important indicator of a person's knowledge, skills, and abilities in the workplace, school, and personal life. The overall result of researches suggests that EI plays a significant role in job performance, motivation, decision making, successful management, and leadership. Thus, applying EI methodology in higher education can have lots of benefits for students. It not only fulfills their desire but also makes them more efficient in their field. Everyone experiences and relates their feelings and emotions in day to day life. Emotions have valuable information about relationships, behavior and every aspect of human life around us. The most recent research shows that emotions are constructive and do contribute to enhance performance and better decision making both at the job and in private life.

Definitions

Emotional intelligence is: "The ability to monitor one's own and others' feelings and emotions, to discriminate among them and to use this information to guide one's thinking and actions."   —**Salovey and Mayer, 1990**

Emotional intelligence is: "An array of noncognitive (emotional and social) capabilities, competencies and skills that influence one's ability to succeed in coping with environmental demands and pressures."   —**Reuven Bar-On, 1996**

"Emotional intelligence is the set of abilities that we like to think of as being on the other side of the report card from academic skills."   —**Maurice Elias, 2001**

Emotional intelligence is "The ability to perceive emotions, to access and generate emotions to assist thought, to understand emotions and emotional meanings, and to reflectively regulate emotions in ways that promote emotional and intellectual growth."   —**Peter Salovey and John Mayer, 2002**

Emotional Intelligence in Leadership

Emotional intelligence or EI is the ability to understand and manage your own emotions, and those of the people around you. People with a high degree of emotional intelligence know what they're feeling, what their emotions mean, and how these emotions can affect other people. For leaders, having emotional intelligence is essential for success. According to Daniel Goleman, an American psychologist who helped to popularize emotional intelligence, there are five key elements to it:

- **Self-awareness:** If a leader is self-aware, he always knows how he feels, and he knows how his emotions and his actions can affect the people around him. Being self-aware when one is in a leadership position also means having a clear picture of one's strengths and weaknesses, and it means behaving with humility. A leader can improve self-awareness by spending some time writing down the thoughts, or slowing down in anger and strong emotions to reflect one's own emotions. Remember, no matter what the situation, one can always choose how one reacts to it.

- **Self-regulation**: Leaders who regulate themselves effectively rarely verbally attack others, make rushed or emotional decisions, stereotype people, or compromise their values. Self-regulation is all about staying in control. This element of emotional intelligence, according to Goleman, also covers a leader's flexibility and commitment to personal accountability. To improve one should know his values and absolutely will not be compromised. Spend some time examining one's "code of ethics." Secondly one should hold oneself accountable if something goes wrong. Thirdly a leader should practice being calm. Writing down something, deep breathing exercises are some techniques to calm down.

- **Motivation:** Self-motivated leaders work consistently toward their goals, and they have extremely high standards for the quality of their work. To improve one's motivation, re-examine the job that one does, set the goals properly, and make him hopeful and optimistic in nature. Every time we face a challenge, or even a failure, try to find at least one good thing about the situation. It might be something small, like a new contact, or something with long-term effects, like an important lesson learned. But there's almost always something positive if we look for it.

- **Empathy:** For leaders, having empathy is critical to managing a successful team or organization. Leaders with empathy can put themselves in someone else's situation. They help develop the people in their team, challenge others who are acting unfairly, give constructive feedback, and listen to those who need it. If you want to earn the respect and loyalty of your team, then show them you care by being empathic.

- **Social skills:** Leaders who do well in the social skills element of emotional intelligence are great communicators. They're just as open to hearing bad news as good news, and they're experts at getting their team to support them and be excited about a new mission or project. Leaders who have good social skills are also good at managing change and resolving conflicts diplomatically. They're rarely satisfied with leaving things as they are, but they don't sit back and make everyone else do the work: they set an example with their behavior. The leader must learn the method of conflict resolution and praising others and should have impressive communication skills and so on.

Influence of Emotional Intelligence

- **Motivation and creativity:** It is not a matter of surprise that moods and emotions affect our minds. When we feel good about ourselves, we find the world around us a great motivator. This motivation helps us to express our personality better, creative and optimistic. This stage can be achieved by social awareness and proper emotional responses in a given situation. Thus, an emotionally intelligent person can motivate his attitude for himself and for others, which produces better results at work and in personal life. Moreover, the sense of EI creates a positive work environment and brings healthy job attitudes also.

- **Decision making:** Many researchers agree that the key to good decision making is the combination of both thoughts and feelings in one's decisions. Positive moods and emotions help for better decision making. With positive emotions, people can develop problem-solving skills and make good decisions quickly.

- **Negotiation:** Everybody knows that negotiation is an emotional process. By proper use of emotions and understanding the moods of oneself and others, one can manage the conflict and stressful situations. A person can be successful in negotiations if he has an active listening technique and skill of reading non-verbal cues.

- **Leadership:** Effective leaders use their emotions to convey their messages. When leaders feel excited, enthusiastic and active, they may be more likely to energize their subordinates and convey a sense of efficacy, competence, optimism, and enjoyment. Therefore, successful leaders are emotionally intelligent.

- **Personal growth:** Research shows that emotionally intelligent people achieve better results at work, school, and personal life. They are flexible enough to accept positive changes in their life for personal growth, which can be achieved by developing EI competencies.

- **Education:** Emotional intelligence will affect educational approaches that are based on IQ that include logic, data, concrete thinking, and memory power. To be successful in school life, EI competencies can be introduced through educational programs. Thus, students in adolescent age acquire social, emotional and personal identity by emotional intelligence.

RESILIENCE BUILDING

Resilience is the process of adapting well in the face of adversity, trauma, tragedy, threats or even significant sources of stress such as family and relationship problems or workplace and financial stressors. It means bouncing back from difficult experiences. Resilience is typically defined as the capacity to recover from difficult life events.

"It's the ability to withstand adversity and bounce back and grow despite life's downturns,"
—**Amit Sood**

Resilience is not a trampoline, where we are down one moment and up the next. It's more like climbing a mountain without a trail map. It takes time, strength, and help from people around us, and we will likely experience setbacks along the way. Research has shown that resilience is ordinary, not extraordinary. People commonly demonstrate resilience. Being resilient doesn't mean that a person doesn't experience trouble or distress. Emotional pain and sadness are common in people who have suffered major adversity or trauma in their life. The road to resilience is likely to involve considerable emotional distress.

Resilience is not a trait that people either have or do not have. It involves behaviors, thoughts, and actions that can be learned and developed in anyone.

Developing resilience is both complex and personal. It involves a combination of inner strengths and outer resources, and there isn't a universal formula for becoming more resilient. All people are different: While one person might develop symptoms of depression or anxiety following a traumatic event, another person might not report any symptoms at all.

A combination of factors contributes to building resilience, and there isn't a simple to-do list to work through adversity. In one longitudinal study, protective factors for adolescents at risk for depression are family cohesion, positive self-appraisals, and good interpersonal relations, and are associated with resilient outcomes in young adulthood. While individuals process trauma and adversity in different ways, certain protective factors help build resilience by improving coping skills and adaptability.

Types of Resilience

The word resilience is often used on its own to represent overall adaptability and coping, but it can be broken down into categories or types:

- **Psychological resilience**: Psychological resilience refers to the ability to mentally withstand or adapt to uncertainty, challenges, and adversity. It is sometimes referred to as "mental fortitude." People who exhibit psychological resilience develop coping strategies and capabilities that enable them to remain calm and focused during a crisis and move on without long-term negative consequences.

- **Emotional resilience:** There are varying degrees of how well a person copes emotionally with stress and adversity. Some people are, by nature, more or less sensitive to change. How a person responds to a situation can trigger a flood of emotions. Emotionally resilient people understand what they're feeling and why. They tap into realistic optimism, even when dealing with a crisis, and are proactive in using both internal and external resources. As a result, they can manage stressors as well as their emotions in a healthy, positive way.

- **Physical resilience:** Physical resilience refers to the body's ability to adapt to challenges, maintain stamina and strength, and recover quickly and efficiently. A person can function and recover when faced with illness, accidents, or other physical demands. Healthy lifestyle choices, building connections, making time to rest and recover, deep breathing, and engaging in enjoyable activities all play a role in building physical resilience.
- **Community resilience:** Community resilience refers to the ability of groups of people to respond to and recover from adverse situations, such as natural disasters, acts of violence, economic hardship, and other challenges to their community.

Methods to Build Resilience

- **Make connections:** Good relationships with close family members, friends, or others are important. Accepting help and support from those who care about you and will listen to you strengthens resilience. Some people find that being active in civic groups, faith-based organizations, or other local groups provides social support and can help with reclaiming hope. Assisting others in their time of need also can benefit the helper.
- **Avoid seeing the crisis as insurmountable problems:** You can't change the fact that highly stressful events happen, but you can change how you interpret and respond to these events. Try looking beyond the present to how future circumstances may be a little better. Note any subtle ways in which you might already feel somewhat better as you deal with difficult situations.
- **Accept that change is a part of living:** Certain goals may no longer be attainable as a result of adverse situations. Accepting circumstances that cannot be changed can help you focus on circumstances that you can alter.
- **Move towards the goal:** Develop some realistic goals. Instead of focusing on tasks that seem unachievable, do something regularly, even if it seems like a small accomplishment and that enables you to move toward your goals.
- **Take decisive actions:** Act on adverse situations as much as you can. Take decisive actions, rather than detaching completely from problems and stresses and wishing they would just go away. The ability to make and carry out realistic plans helps individuals play to their strengths and focus on achievable goals.
- **Look for opportunities for self-discovery:** People often learn something about themselves and may find that they have grown in some respect as a result of their struggle with loss. Many people who have experienced tragedies and hardship have reported better relationships, a greater sense of strength even while feeling vulnerable, an increased sense of self-worth, a more developed spirituality, and heightened appreciation for life.

- **Nurture a positive view of self:** Developing confidence in your ability to solve problems and trusting your instincts helps build resilience. A positive sense of self-confidence in one's strengths can stave off feelings of helplessness when confronted with adversity.
- **Keep things in perspective:** Even when facing very painful events, try to consider the stressful situation in a broader context and keep a long-term perspective. Avoid blowing the event out of proportion.
- **Maintain a hopeful outlook:** An optimistic outlook enables you to expect that good thing will happen in your life. Try visualizing what you want, rather than worrying about what you fear.
- **Take care of oneself:** Pay attention to your own needs and feelings. Engage in activities that you enjoy and relax. Exercise regularly. Taking care of yourself helps to keep your mind and body primed to deal with situations that require resilience.

STRESS MANAGEMENT

Stress and anxiety are basic to life, no matter how wealthy, powerful; hard working and happy you might be, mild stress can be stimulating, motivating and sometimes even desirable. The word stress was originally used by Selye in 1956 to describe the pressure experienced by a person in response to life demands. These demands are referred to as stressors.

Definitions

Stress is a process of adjusting to or dealing with circumstances that disrupt or threaten to disrupt a person's physical or psychological functioning.   —**Hans Selye, 1976**

Stress is a state produced by a change in the environment that is perceived as challenging, threatening or damaging to the person's dynamic balance or equilibrium.

—**Brunner and Suddart**

Types of Stress

According to Hans Selye, it is of two types:
1. **Eustress:** Stress that helps us function better. A bit of stress can be energizing and motivating, that is why many of us work best under pressure.
2. **Distress:** Stress that causes mental agony. Stress can be mild-moderate or severe.

Sources of Stress

There are many sources of stress that are broadly classified as:
- **Internal stress:** They originate within a person e.g., cancer, feeling of depression.
- **External stress:** It originates outside the individual, e.g., moving to another city, a death in the family.

- **Developmental stress:** It occurs at predictable times throughout an individual's life, e.g., child—the beginning of school.
- **Situational stress:** They are unpredictable and occur at any time during life. It may be positive or negative. e.g., the death of the family member, marriage/ divorce.

Sources of Clinical Stress

For patients, the sources of stress may be uncertainty, fear, pain, cost, lack of knowledge, the risk of harm and unknown resources.

For nurses, the stress can arise from poor patient outcomes, risk of making an error, unfamiliar situations, excessive workload, and inadequate resources.

Indicators of Stress

- **Physiological indicators:** The physiological signs and symptoms of stress result from the activation of sympathetic and neuroendocrine systems of the body. Pupils dilate to increase visual perception, sweat production increases, heart rate and cardiac output increases, the skin becomes pale due to peripheral blood vessel constriction, the mouth may be dry, urine output decreases and blood sugar increases.
- **Psychologic indicators:** The manifestations of stress includes anxiety, fear, anger, depression and unconscious ego defense mechanism.
- **Cognitive indicators:** Problem-solving the person assesses the situation or analyzes problem, choose alternatives, carries out selected alternatives and evaluates. The person may use structuring: Arrangement/manipulation of a situation so that threatening events do not occur; self-control: The manner and facial expression convey a sense of being in control or change; suppression; wilfully putting a thought or feeling out of mind; daydreaming: unfulfilled wishes and desires are imagined as fulfilled or a threatening experience is reworked or replayed so that it ends differently from reality.

Techniques of Stress Management

Stress management encompasses techniques intended to equip a person with effective coping mechanisms for dealing with psychological stress, with stress defined as a person's physiological response to an internal or external stimulus that triggers the fight-or-flight response. Stress management is effective when a person uses strategies to cope with or alter the stressful situation. The stress management strategies include:

- **Take a breath:** When you feel uptight try taking a minute to slow down and breathe deeply. Breathe in through your nose and out through your mouth. Try to inhale enough so that your lower abdomen rises and falls. Count as you exhale slowly.

- **Practice specific relaxation techniques:** Techniques like meditation, self-hypnosis, and deep muscle relaxation work in a similar fashion. In this state, both body and mind are at rest and the outside world is screened out for a while. The practice of this for a regular basis provides a calming and relaxing feeling that seems to have a lasting effect on many people.
- **Manage time:** Give priority to important ones. And do those first. If a particularly unpleasant task comes, tackle it early in the day and get over with it; the rest of your day will include much less anxiety. Schedule time for both work and recreation.
- **Connect with others:** A good way to combat sadness, boredom, and loneliness is to see out activities involving others.
- **Talk it out:** Share your feelings. Bottled up emotions increase frustration and stress. Talking with someone else can help clear your confusion so that you can focus on problem-solving. Also, consider writing down thoughts and feelings. Putting problems on paper can assist you in clarifying the situation and allow you a new perspective.
- **Take a minute vacation:** Imaging a quiet country scene can take you out of a stressful situation. When you have the opportunity, take a moment to close your eyes and imagine a place where you feel relaxed. Notice all details of your chosen place, including pleasant sounds, smells and temperature or change your mental channel by reading a good book or playing relaxing music to create a sense of peace.
- **Monitor your physical comfort:** Wear comfortable clothing. If it's too hot, go somewhere where it's not. If the chair is uncomfortable, change it. If the computer causes eye strain change it. Don't wait until discomfort changes to the real problem.
- **Get physical:** When you feel nervous, angry or upset, release the pressure through exercise or physical activity. Running, walking or swimming are good options for some people, while others prefer to dance, etc. Working in the garden, washing your car or playing with children can relieve the uptight feeling. Aerobics can be done for 20 minutes daily to reduce stress.
- **Take off your body:** Healthy eating and adequate sleep fuel your mind as well as body. Avoid consuming too much caffeine and sugar. Take time to have breakfast in the morning. Well-nourished bodies will cope better with stress. Increase the number of fruits and vegetables in the diet. Take time for personal interests and hobbies. Listen to one's body.
- **Laugh:** Maintain your sense of humor, including the ability to laugh at yourself.
- **Know your limits:** There are many circumstances in life beyond your control, consider the fact that we live in an imperfect world. Know your limits. If a problem is beyond

your control and cannot be changed at the moment, don't fight the situation. Learn to accept what is, for now, until the time comes when you can change things.

- **Think positively:** Refocus the negative to be positive. Make an effort to stop negative thoughts.
- **Clarify your values and develop a sense of life:** Clarify your values and decide what you want out of your life. It can help you feel better about yourself and have that sense of satisfaction and centeredness that helps you deal with the stresses of life. Compromise: Consider cooperation or compromise rather than confrontation. A little give and take on both sides may reduce the strain and help you feel more comfortable.
- **Have a good cry:** A good crying during periods of stress can be a healthy way to bring relief to your anxiety, and it might prevent a headache or other physical consequences of bottling things up.
- **Avoid self-medication:** Alcohol and other drugs do not remove stress. Although they may seem to mask or disguise problems. In the long run, alcohol use increases rather than decreases stress, by changing the way you think and solve problems and by impairing your judgments and other cognitive capacities.
- **Look for the pieces of gold around you:** Pieces of gold are positive or enjoyable moments or reactions that may seem like small events but as these pieces of gold accumulate they can often provide a big lift to energy and spirits and help you begin new and balanced way.

Stress is mental or physical tension brought about by external pressures. Researchers have found significant biochemical changes that take place in the body during stress. Exaggerated, prolonged, or genetic tenderness to stress cause destructive changes, which lower the body's immune system response and can lead to a variety of disease and disorders. These include depression, cardiovascular disease, stroke, and cancer.

TIME MANAGEMENT

Time is an equally important resource. If managers are to direct employees effectively and maximize the resources, they must first able to find the time to do so. Time management is making optimal use of available time. Because time is a finite and valuable resource, learning to use it wisely requires both leadership skills and management functions. The effective use of time management tools becomes more important to enable managers to meet personal and professional goals and reduces stress. Good time management skills allow an individual to spend time on things that matter.

Definition

Time management is the use of tools, techniques, strategies and follow-up systems to control wasted time and to ensure that the time invested in activities leads towards achieving a desired, high priority goal.

Time management refers to a range of skills, tools, and techniques used to manage time when accomplishing specific tasks, projects and goals. These include planning, allocating, setting goals, delegation, analysis of time spent, monitoring, organizing, scheduling, and prioritizing.

Leadership Roles in Time Management

- Self-awareness regarding personal blocks and barriers to efficient time management as well as how one's value system influences one's use of time and the expectations of followers.
- Functions as a role model, supporter, and resource person to subordinates in setting priorities.
- Assists followers in working cooperatively to maximize time use.
- Prevents and/or filters interruptions that prevent effective time management.
- Role models flexibility in working cooperatively with other people whose primary time management style is different.
- Presents a calm and reassuring demeanor during periods of high unit activity.

Management Functions in Time Management

- Appropriately prioritize day-to-day planning to meet short-time and long-time unit goals.
- Builds time for planning into the work schedule.
- Analyzes how time is managed on the unit level using job analysis and time and motion studies.
- Eliminates environmental barriers to effective time management for unit staff.
- Handles paperwork promptly and efficiently and maintains a neat work area.
- Breaks down large tasks into smaller ones that can more easily be accomplished by unit members.
- Utilizes appropriate technology to facilitate timely communication and documentation.
- Discriminates between inadequate staffing and inefficient use of time when time resources are inadequate to complete the assigned task.

Time Wasters

Time is our most valuable resource and unless it is managed, nothing can be achieved. It is self-management and requires no qualification or training. It is an art that is very easy to understand but difficult to follow. Keeping track of how one spends time is not time management but is about making changes to the way to spend time.

- **Doing too much:** Doing too much at once, having three or four projects at the same time, a member of more than one organizational committee, etc.

- **Inability to say "no":** If you are suffering from overload, you probably have gotten thereby not being able to say no. Learning to not say yes to every request is difficult and, in the process, others may be displeased. If you do not say no, you may end up spending a great deal of time on projects in which you have no interest, projects that have no relationship to personal goals and priorities.
- **Procrastination:** Engaging in procrastination or doing one thing when you should be doing something else, you give up time to complete your task and therefore limit the quality of the work you produce. Procrastination is the avoidance of doing a task, which needs to be accomplished. This can lead to feelings of guilt, inadequacy, depression, and self-doubt. Procrastination has a high potential for painful consequences.
- **Complaining:** Often the time nurses spend complaining about a task or a particular situation is greater than the time needed to solve the problem. If you find yourself complaining, stop and ask yourself what would be the ideal solution to the problem and then take the risk to act on it.
- **Disorganization:** One of the most serious time-wasters of all is disorganization. How many times have you had to spend 5 minutes trying to find something you have misplaced or misfiled?
- **Too much information:** The newest time waster to evolve is data proliferation. The technology with the workplace forces to receive huge amounts of data and transform these data into useful information.

Rules to be Followed in Time Management: Butler and Hope (1996) 9 Rules

- Get started—This is one of the all-time classic time wasters. Often, as much time is wasted avoiding a project, as actually accomplishing the project. A survey showed that the main difference between good students and average students was the ability to start their homework quickly.
- Get into a routine—Mindless routines may curb your creativity, but when used properly, they can release time and energy. Choose a time to get a certain task accomplished, such as answering email, working on a project, completing paperwork; and then sticking to it every day. Use a daily planning calendar. There are a variety of formats on the market. Find one that fits your needs.
- Do not say yes to too many things—Saying yes can lead to unexpected treasures, but the mistake we often make is to say yes to too many things. This causes us to live to the priorities of others, rather than according to our own. Every time you agree to do something else, something else will not get done. Learn how to say no.
- Do not commit yourself to unimportant activities, no matter how far ahead they are—Even if a commitment is a year ahead, it is still a commitment. Often, we agree to do something that is far ahead, when we would not normally

do it if it was short. No matter how far ahead it is, it will still take the same amount of your time.
- Divide large tasks—Large tasks should be broken up into a series of small tasks. By creating small manageable tasks, the entire task will eventually be accomplished. Also, by using a piecemeal approach, you will be able to fit it into your hectic schedule.
- Do not put unneeded effort into a project—There is a place for perfectionism, but for most activities, there comes a stage when there is not much to be gained from putting extra effort into it. Save perfectionism for the tasks that need it.
- Deal with it for once and for all - We often start a task, think about it, and then lay it aside. This gets repeated over and over. Either deal with the task right away or decide when to deal with it.
- Set start and stop times—When arranging start times, also arrange stop times. This will call for some estimating, but your estimates will improve with practice. This will allow you and others to schedule activities better. Also, challenge the theory, "Work expands to fill the allotted time." See if you can shave some time off your deadlines to make it more efficient.
- Plan your activities—Schedule a regular time to plan your activities. If time management is important to you, then allow the time to plan it wisely.

Personal Time Management

Personal management refers in part to self-knowledge. Self-awareness is a leadership skill. For people who are not certain of their own short to long term goals, time management in general poses difficulties. Personal Time Management is about controlling the use of your most valuable (and undervalued) resource, which must be planned, monitored and regularly reviewed. Managing time is very difficult if a person is unsure of his or her priorities for time management, including personal short term, intermediate and long-term goals. These goals give structure to what should be accomplished today, tomorrow and in the future. However, goals alone are not enough; a concrete plan with timelines is needed. Plans outlined in manageable steps are clear, more realistic and attainable.

CAREER PLANNING AND DEVELOPMENT

Individuals' career planning is assumed to have greater significance with the unparalleled growth and speed of knowledge, phenomenal increase in educational and training facilities and widespread increase in job opportunities. Similarly, organizational career planning also gained importance with the change in technology, human needs, values, and aspirations, increase in organizational size, complexity and number of openings at different levels.

Career Planning essentially means helping the employees plan his/her career in terms of his/her capabilities within the context of organizational needs. Career planning implies the planning of specific career paths of the employees in the foreseeable future further in the organization. It may be useful to work out career path charts for incumbents of different job clusters. Career planning often means job rotation, successive planning, and promotion policy. Career planning is a process that optimizes the interdependence of the individuals and also their organizational relationship. Career planning is more akin to growth and development which is a must for every individual of the organization. It helps to facilitate dialogue between the individual and the organization to optimize their mutual needs.

Definitions

"Career plan is an individually perceived sequence of attitudes and behaviors associated with work-related experiences and activities over the span of the person's life". —**Douglas T Hall**

A career is defined as, "a sequence of separate but related work activities that provides continuity, order, and meaning in a person's life."
                                    —**Edwin B Flipo**

Need for Career Planning

Career planning is essential for:
- To attract competent persons and to retain them in the organization.
- To provide suitable promotional opportunities.
- To enable the employees to develop a mind and make them ready to meet future challenges.
- To increase the utilization of managerial reserves within an organization to correct employee placement.
- To reduce employee dissatisfaction and turnover.
- To improve motivation and morale.

Steps in Career Planning and Development

- Analysis of individual skills, knowledge, abilities, aptitude, etc.
- Analysis of career opportunities both within and outside the organization.
- Analysis of career demands on the incumbent in terms of skills, knowledge, abilities, aptitude, etc. and in terms of qualifications, experience and training received, etc.
- Relating specific jobs to different career opportunities.
- Establishing realistic goals both short-term and long-term.
- Formulating career strategy covering areas of change, and adjustment.

- Preparing and implementing an action plan including acquiring resources for achieving goals.

Importance of Career Planning

A career may be defined as 'a sequence of jobs that constitute what a person does for a living'. Career planning is a process by which one selects career goals and the path to those goals. It involves a clear selection of career goals and career paths. It encourages individuals to explore and gather information, which enables them to synthesize, gain competencies, make decisions, set goals, and take action. It is a crucial phase of human resource development that helps the employees in making the strategy for work-life balance. Career planning is needed for the following reasons:

- **Provides career goals and paths:** It is needed to provide career goals and career paths to an employee. It provides clear future directions in terms of career.
- **Develop competencies:** It motivates and encourages an employee to develop competencies for higher-level jobs. The competencies can be conceptual, interpersonal and technical.
- **Creativity:** It is needed to increase employee creativity. It is needed for innovation in an organization. It can lead to entrepreneurship within the organization.
- **Employee retention:** It is needed for the retention of qualified employees in the long-term. This is needed to decrease the costs of recruitment, selection, and training.
- **Motivation:** It motivates employees for higher performance. An upward movement in the organization is based on the quality and quantity of performance.

Benefits of Career Planning

- Career planning ensures a constant supply of promotable employees.
- It helps in improving the loyalty of employees.
- Career planning encourages an employee's growth and development.
- It discourages the negative attitude of superiors who are interested in suppressing the growth of the subordinates.
- It ensures that senior management knows about the caliber and capacity of the employees who can move upwards.
- It can always create a team of employees prepared enough to meet any contingency.
- Career planning reduces labor turnover.
- Every organization prepares succession planning towards which career planning is the first step.

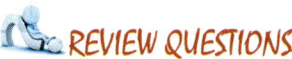 *REVIEW QUESTIONS*

1. Define emotional intelligence. What is the need for emotional intelligence in leadership? Explain the influence of emotional intelligence in management.
2. What is resilience? Explain their types and brief the methods of resilience building.
3. Explain the modes of stress management.
4. Define time management. What is the role of manager/leader in time management? What are the techniques of time management?

Further Readings

1. Mayer JD, Salovey P. The Intelligence of Emotional Intelligence. Intelligence, 1993 17(4), pp. 433-442.
2. Goleman D. Emotional Intelligence: why it can matter more than IQ. Bloomsbury. London; 1995.
3. Bar-On, R. The Emotional Quotient Inventory (EQ-i): a test of emotional intelligence. Toronto: Multi-Health Systems, from https://ecom.mhs.com/1996.
4. Dee Ann Gillies. Nursing Management and System Approach, 3rd Edition: W.B. Saunders Company, London; 1982, pp. 200-209.
5. Marquis Huston. Leadership Role and Management Functions in Nursing, 5th Edition: Lippincott Publication, New Delhi; pp. 191-206.
6. Tappen, Weiss, and Whitehead. Essentials of Nursing Leadership and Management, 3rd Edition: FA Davis Publication, Philadelphia, 2004, pp. 137-48.
7. Patronis Jones, Rebecca A. Nursing Leadership and Management Theories, Process and Practicel, 1st Edition: Jaypee Brothers Medical Publishers (P) Ltd., New Delhi; 2008, pp. 366-67.
8. Patricia S Yoder. Wise, Leading and Managing in Nursing, 2nd Edition: Mosby Publication, New York; 1999, pp. 195-200.
9. Rebecca Samson. Leadership and Management in Nursing Practice and Education, 1st Edition: Jaypee Brothers Medical Publishers (P) Ltd., New Delhi; 2009, pp. 37-42.
10. Mary C. Townsend. Psychiatric Mental Health Nursing, 1st Edition: Philadelphia Publisher, pp. 4-12.
11. Gail W, Stuart, Michelet, Laraia. Principles and Practice of Psychologic Nursing, 8th Edition: Published by Elsevier. pp. 60-73.
12. Suzanne C Smeltzer. Textbook of Medical and Surgical Nursing, 10th Edition: Published by Lippincott Williams & Wilkins, pp. 81-87.
13. Kozier & Erb's. Fundamentals of Nursing, 8th Edition: Published by Dorling Kindersley, pp. 1063–1071.
14. Sharma Jai Narain (2002). "Human Resource Management?', Mittal Publications, New Delhi, pp. 253.
15. Fred Luthans (1981). "Organizational Behavior", Mc Graw Hill International Book Co., New York, pp. 611.
16. Edwin B Flippo (1980). Principles of Personnel Management, Mc Graw Book Co., pp. 219.

Unit

13

Establishment of Nursing Educational Institutions

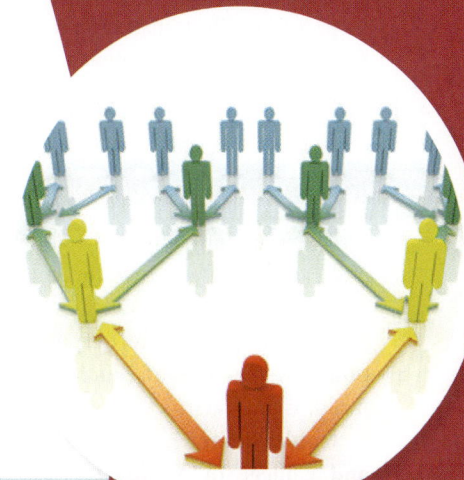

 Unit Outline

- ➡ Establishment of Nursing Educational Institution; INC Norms and Guidelines
- ➡ Physical and Academic Facilities Required for the Nursing Educational Institution Including Staffing Norms as per the Regulations of Indian Nursing Council
- ➡ Affiliation and Coordination with Regulatory Bodies
- ➡ National Regulatory Bodies
- ➡ International Regulatory Bodies
- ➡ Accreditation
- ➡ Inspections

ESTABLISHMENT OF NURSING EDUCATIONAL INSTITUTION; INC NORMS AND GUIDELINES

All the nursing education programs are established, keeping in view the health needs of the country. The success and goodwill of the organization are based on a strong base of advanced knowledge. The excellent output of an organization of nurses training helps in the quality nursing care of deserved. Educational organizations of the country are monitored by Indian Nursing Council (INC) through the process of affiliation. The Indian Nursing Council conducts periodic inspections of these institutions. Additionally, other regulatory bodies such as UGC, State University, State Nursing Council, Medical Education Department of the State also monitor the institutions through various measures.

Indian Nursing Council (INC)

It is the autonomous body under the Ministry of Health and Family Welfare, Government of India constituted under the Indian Nursing Council Act, 1947 and the consecutive amendments. The core purpose of this act is to maintain uniform standards of education for nurses, midwives, and health visitors across the country.

Guidelines for Establishment of new School of Nursing and College of Auxiliary Nurse and Midwives (ANM), General Nursing and Midwifery (GNM), Basic BSc Nursing, Post Basic BSc Nursing (PBBSc Nursing) and MSc Nursing.

(As per the information published in www.indiannursing-council.org)

- Any organization under Central/State Government, Local body or any other organization registered under Society Registration Act or Company incorporated under section 25 of the Company's Act is eligible to establish the School of Nursing or College of Nursing.
- A parent hospital of a minimum of 100 beds is required. However, the requirement of parent hospital is exempted for institutions located in a tribal and hilly area.
- Indian Nursing Council recognized BSc (N)/PBBSc (N) College of Nursing wherein one batch has passed out is eligible to establish PBBSc (N)/MSc. (N) Program. Any Super Specialty Hospital can also establish MSc (N) program.
- The above organizations shall obtain the Essentiality Certificate/No Objection Certificate for the respective courses from the respective State Government and permission from respective State Nursing Council.
- The Indian Nursing Council, after the receipt of the above documents/proposal, will conduct the statutory inspection for the suitability of the Institution.
- The institution will admit the students only after taking the approval of the Examination Board/University.

PHYSICAL AND ACADEMIC FACILITIES REQUIRED FOR THE NURSING EDUCATIONAL INSTITUTION INCLUDING STAFFING NORMS AS PER THE REGULATIONS OF INDIAN NURSING COUNCIL

The Nursing Training Institutions should be located near to the parent hospital but in a separate building. There should be a space for expansion if it is in the hospital building. The preferred built-up area for the college with an annual intake of 40–60 students is 23720 sq.ft. It may increase according to the number of programs and students. The specific construction area is according to the number of classrooms, laboratories, a residential area for students and staff, other amenities, and facilities.

A sample of area distribution and the built-up area of the teaching/academic block as recommended by the National Regulatory Body (Indian Nursing Council) for a Nursing Educational Institution (BSc Nursing) with an average intake of 60 students per year is given below for reference. As the number of intake of students increases or the addition of any program takes place the area has to be increased proportionally as per the guidelines.

Sr. no.	Teaching block area	Figures in sq. ft.
1.	Lecture hall	4@900 = 3600
2.	Nursing foundation lab	1500
3.	Community health nursing lab	900
4.	Nutrition lab	900
5.	OBG and pediatrics lab	900
6.	Pre-clinical science lab	900
7.	Computer lab	1500
8.	Multipurpose hall	3000
9.	Common room (male and female)	1000
10.	Staff room	800
11.	Principal room	300
12.	Vice principal room	200
13.	Library	2300
14.	AV Aids room	600
15.	One room for each head of departments	5@200 = 1000
16.	Faculty room	2400
17.	Provisions for toilets	1000
	Total	22800 sq. ft.

Note:
- Nursing Educational institutions should be in the Institutional area only and not in a residential area.
- If the institute has a non-nursing program in the same building, the Nursing program should have a separate teaching block.
- Shift-wise management with other educational institutions will not be accepted.
- Separate teaching block shall be available if it is on hospital premises.
- Proportionately the size of the built-up area will increase according to the number of students admitted.
- School and College of nursing can share laboratories if they are on the same campus under the same name and same trust, that is the institution is one but offering different nursing programs. However, they should have equipment and articles proportionate to the strength of admission. And the classrooms should be available as per the requirement stipulated by the Indian Nursing Council of each program.

Departments: College should have the following departments:

- **Medical-surgical nursing:** The department will have a Head of the Department who should be a professor (10 years of experience after MSc Nursing). It is also comprised of Associate professors, Assistant Professors, and Clinical Instructors/Tutors. The number of staff is determined by the number of students.
- **Community health nursing:** The department will have a Head of the Department who should be a professor (10 years of experience after MSc Nursing). It is also comprised of Associate Professor, Assistant Professors, and Clinical Instructors/Tutors. The number of staff is determined by the number of students.
- **Obstetric and gynecological nursing:** The department will have a Head of the Department who should be a professor (10 years of experience after MSc Nursing). It is also comprised of Associate Professor, Assistant Professors, and Clinical Instructors/Tutors. The number of staff is determined by the number of students.
- **Child health nursing:** The department will have a Head of the Department who should be a professor (10 years of experience after MSc Nursing). It is also comprised of Associate Professor, Assistant Professors, and Clinical Instructors/Tutors. The number of staff is determined by the number of students.
- **Psychiatry and mental health nursing:** The department will have a Head of the Department who should be a professor (10 years of experience after MSc Nursing). It is also comprised of Associate Professor, Assistant Professors, and Clinical Instructors/Tutors. The number of staff is determined by the number of students.

Responsibilities of the Head of the Department

- Divide and delegate syllabus according to specialties concerned.
- Conduct unit tests, give assignments and evaluate performances.
- Conduct practicals concerning specialties.
- Perform internal assessment.
- Prepare the students concerned with their specialties.

Equipment and Supplies for Nursing Educational Institutions

The well functioning equipment and adequate supplies are necessary for the smooth functioning of any educational institution. Insufficient and ill-functioning material results in increased work and waste of time. Like any other educational institution, a school/college of nursing also requires basic amenities such as building with a lecture hall, demonstration laboratories, library, office facilities for staff and faculty without which a proper education and training cannot go on.

Classrooms: There should be spacious classrooms according to the number of students and the number of programs. All the classrooms must have good lighting, ventilation, and associated requirements. It should be furnished with a sufficient amount of seating arrangements and should possess the necessary/advanced teaching-learning equipment such as LCD projectors, whiteboards, charts and models, racks, cupboards, etc. For each student, there should be a distinct chair and desk or chair cum desk, or alternately enough space for each student to sit and write so that group debates can be arranged. There should be a mobile blackboard for each room or at least one per two classrooms in addition to the fixed blackboards. Bulletin boards and other facilities such as LCD projectors for displaying material should also be available. It should be possible to shade the windows in hot weather and to have some convenient arrangement for darkening one room for the showing of films.

Laboratories: It is recommended to have a minimum of seven laboratories as listed below. These laboratories or workrooms are required for demonstrations and practical classes of different subjects.

- Nursing Foundations and Medical-Surgical
- Community Health Nursing
- OBG and Pediatrics
- Nutrition
- Computer lab with a minimum of 30 computers
- Pre Clinical Science Lab. (Biochemistry, Microbiology, Biophysics, Anatomy and Physiology)
- AV Aids Room.
- **Preclinical science lab:** The extent to which a science laboratory is necessary and its utilization depends on the arrangement made by school/college for the teaching of science subjects. The natural sciences such as anatomy and physiology, physics and chemistry and microbiology are all subjects that require laboratory facilities, and it is probably more convenient to have these available in the school/college. However, if the arrangement is adequate, appropriate and enduring, a university/college may arrange

to use the laboratories in the hospital, medical college or local science college, in which it will not be required to construct a science laboratory in nursing school/college. The science laboratory should be equipped with chairs and tables, cupboards, running water, and either piped gas or cylinder. It also should have all the models, charts, torso, microscope, biochemical solutions, and so on.

- **Nutrition laboratory:** The nutrition laboratory must be equipped to learn the basics of food and nutrition, and the preparation methods. The furnishings and equipment, therefore, should include workbenches with stainless steel, marble chip or heat-resistant tops, electric or gas or indigenous type of cooking stove, sinks and running water, dietetic scales, cooking utensils, shelves, and cupboards for storage.
- **Nursing arts lab:** It should have ample cupboard space, shelves, sinks, and running water, tables or workbenches and movable chairs. Adequate storage space should be available, with protection against heat, moisture, insects, and vermin for perishable products. Easy access to machinery and supplies should be available. Equipment should be chosen based not only on price, but also on its usefulness and durability, and should be consistent with what is frequently used in hospitals and society. In case more than one nursing program is offered by the same organization the laboratories can be shared, provided the number of articles, simulation models and equipment should be sufficient for the students of all programs. The area of the lab also can be expanded.
- **MCH lab:** It should be equipped with all models and equipment of the maternal and child health nursing, all the specimens and all the instruments in sufficient quantity.
- **Community health nursing lab:** Community lab should be equipped with sufficient models, community health care bags, and all the necessary articles for providing practical exposure to the students.
- **Computer lab:** It should be equipped with enough computers and other software for the use of students.
- **AV aids room:** It should be equipped with the latest audio-visual aids for the ease of study such as LCD Projectors, T.V, C.D Players, etc. There should be a seating facility for all the students.

Auditorium: The availability of a spacious auditorium or a multipurpose hall shall be ensured. This can be used to hold college functions such as annual day, graduation ceremony, conferences, workshops, examinations, etc. It should be appropriately equipped.

Library: A separate and spacious (minimum 2400 sq.ft) library should be made accessible for faculty and students. It should have required seating arrangements and necessary furniture and computers with internet/wifi facilities. A sufficient number of books, journals, magazines, other publications should be made available. There shall also be the facility for ebooks, e-journals, and e-magazines, etc. The INC recommends a minimum of 3000 books in the library.

A sound library makes an immeasurable contribution to an educational program. It not only opens the door to new knowledge but stimulates critical thinking and helps to develop independence in seeking and obtaining information. An up to date, varied section of books and other library materials also encourage and assist the staff in study and research both for self-improvement and for the benefits of the students. The furniture and equipment should include comfortable chairs, and tables of convenient height, metal bookshelves, catalog cabinets, magazine display racks and stationery items such as registers, borrowers cards, index cards, etc.

Other Requirements in the College/School of Nursing

- Separate office rooms for administrative sections, accounts section with all the necessary furniture and office equipment as per the need.
- There should be provision for record room, storeroom, canteen transportation, toilets, common rooms, residential facilities for students, faculty, and staff. Separate hostels for boys and girls are recommended.
- The college should have telephone, fax, internet facilities.

Office: It should have all the furniture and the equipment according to the number of staff and the nature of the job.

House keeping room: The school or college building should have a room for the use of housekeeping.

Store room: The college should have storage space for equipment and supplies. The store room should be easily accessible, should be protected from the weather and should have enough cupboard and shelf for the proper maintenance of articles.

Sanitary annex: There should be hygienic hand washing and restroom facilities for both staff and students with convenience to the classrooms and office.

Drinking water: The school or college should have facilities for the provision of drinking water.

Sr. no.	Hostel block area	Figures in sq. ft.
1.	Single room/double room	12000 (50 sq.ft for each students)
2.	Sanitary one latrine and one bathroom (for 5 students)	One latrine & one bathroom for 5 students -600 × 4 = 2400
3.	Visitor room	500
4.	Reading room	250
5.	Store	500
6.	Recreation room	500
7.	Dining hall	3000
8.	Kitchen and store	1500
9.	Warden's Room	450
	Total	21100 sq. ft.

Hostel: The hostel may or may not be located in the same building as the college; if it is separate, it should be within a convenient distance. It should have the student room, warden office, common room, pantry, dining facility, laundry facility, sanitary annexes, and recreation facility.

Clinical Facilities for an Educational Institution

The organization of clinical experience in the curriculum is done based on the syllabus laid down by the statutory bodies like INC and Universities. Organization of clinical skills as per the requirement of the program is the responsibility of the institution and faculty. Clinical experiences related to each course should be planned according to the objective so that students will get enough opportunities for developing the desired nursing skills and attitude.

Each Nursing College should have its parent hospital, preferably with a medical college attached. In the absence of its own hospital, a nursing college should be affiliated to a nearby hospital located within a distance of 10 – 15 km from the college. The minimum clinical facilities prescribed by the Indian Nursing Council for a college of the annual intake of 40 students is given below:

Parent hospital: Parent Hospital for a nursing institution having the same trust which has established nursing institutions and has also established the hospital. College of nursing should have a 150-bedded Parent Hospital. The size of the Hospital/Nursing Home for affiliation should not be less than 100 beds.

Sr. no.	Particulars
1.	Distribution of beds in different areas for a college with annual intake of 40 students is Medical beds: 30 Surgical beds: 30 Obstetrics and Gynecology: 30 Pediatrics: 20 Orthopedics: 10
2.	Bed occupancy of the hospital should be minimum 75%
3.	Other specialties/facilities for clinical experience required are as follows: Operation theater, eyes unit, ENT units, burns and plastic surgery unit, neonatology with nursery, units of communicable disease, super speciality services such as cardiology, oncology, neurology, neurosurgery, nephrology, gastro enterology, etc. Critical care units such as intensive care unit, intensive coronary care units, high dependency unit or step-down ICU, cardio thoracic care unit, pediatric ICU, neonatal ICU and so on.
4.	The nursing staffing norms in the affiliated hospital should be as per the INC/SIU/IPHS norms
5.	For the grant of 100 students minimum 300 bedded parent hospital is mandatory

Affiliated hospitals: The organization which has less facility in parent hospital can have affiliation with other hospitals and nursing homes. The affiliated hospital should give student status to the candidates of the nursing program.

Sr. No.	Particulars
1.	The size of the hospital/nursing home for affiliation should not be less than 100 beds.
2.	Bed occupancy of the hospital should be minimum 75%
3.	Affiliation of psychiatric hospital should be of minimum 100 beds if own psychiatric unit is not available
4.	The nursing staffing norms in the affiliated hospital should be as per the INC/SIU/IPHS norms
5.	Maximum distance between affiliated hospital and nursing educational institutions: Institutions generally can be in the radius of 15–30 kms. from the affiliated hospital Hilly and tribal area can be in the radius of 30–50 kms. From the affiliated hospital 1:3 student patient ratio is to be maintained

Community health care facilities: There should be permission obtained from the competent authority for the activities of urban and rural health centers in relation to the practical exposure of community health nursing. It is desirable to have affiliation with well-established community health centers to provide a consistent learning experience as per the curriculum. It is also suggested that the college/school also can adopt a village/subcenter to carry out the health services of the adopted area. Transport facilities should be available for both students and the staff.

AFFILIATION AND COORDINATION WITH REGULATORY BODIES

Regulatory agencies are usually a part of the executive branch of the government or they have statutory authority. Regulatory authorities are commonly set up to enforce standards and safety. The regulatory body is the formal organization designated by a statute or an authorized government agency to implement the regulatory form and process whereby order uniformity and control are brought to the profession and its practice.

A regulatory agency (also regulatory authority, regulatory body or regulator) is a public authority or government agency responsible for exercising autonomous authority over some area of human activity in a regulatory or supervisory capacity.

Vital Role of the Regulatory Body

- To support and assist professional members.
- Set and enforce standards of nursing practice
- Monitor and enforce standards of nursing practice
- To ensure the public rights to quality health care service
- Monitor and enforce standards for nursing education
- Set the requirement for registration of nursing professionals

The main roles of Regulatory Bodies in Nursing is to ensure the public's rights to quality health care services, to support and assist professional members, to set and enforce standards of nursing practices, to set the requirement for registration of nursing professionals and licensing of nurses. This regulation helps to achieve the uniformity of nursing education all across the country and hence every nursing institution must adhere to the regulations laid down by regulatory bodies.

NATIONAL REGULATORY BODIES

- Government of India and State Government
- Indian Nursing Council (INC)
- State Nursing Council (SNC/SNRC)
- UGC/University/Board of Examinations
- Trained Nurses Association of India (TNAI)

Government of India and State Government

India is a union of 28 states and 8 union territories. Under the constitution of India, the states are largely independent in matters relating to the delivery of health care to the people. Each state, therefore, has developed its system of healthcare delivery independent of the central government. The central responsibility consists mainly of policymaking, planning, guiding, assisting, evaluating, and coordinating the work of the state health ministries so that health services cover every part of the country and no state lags behind for want of these services. The Health regulation in India is the collective responsibility of the Central and the State Government (Fig. 1).

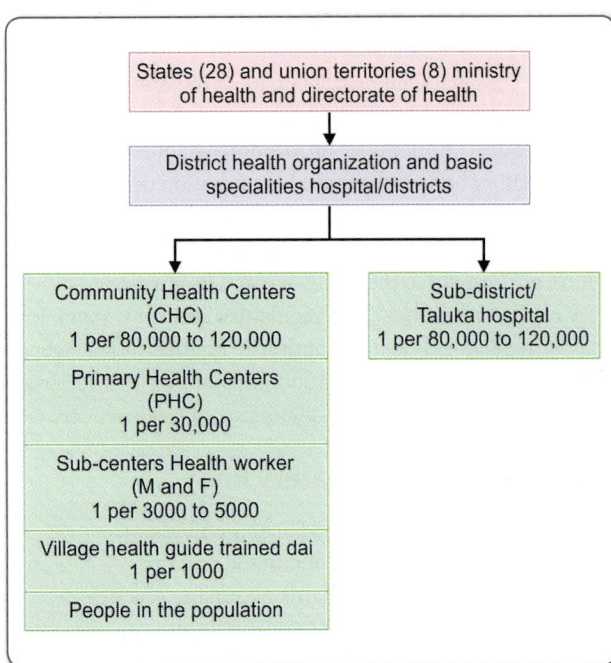

Fig. 1: Health regulation

Indian Nursing Council

It is the autonomous body under the Ministry of Health and Family Welfare, Government of India constituted under the Indian Nursing Council Act, 1947 and the consecutive amendments. The core purpose of this act is to maintain uniform standards of education for nurses, midwives, and health visitors across the country. It ensures the reciprocity of nurses' registration across the country.

Goals of the Indian Nursing Council

- To accomplish and evaluate a fixed standard of nursing education for the nurse-midwife, auxiliary nurse-midwives, and health visitors through regular appraisal of the nursing training institutions.
- To recognize registered nurses and midwives belonging to different nursing courses and their qualifications as per section 10(2)(4) of the Indian Nursing Council Act 1947 for registration and job purpose in India and Abroad.
- To provide approval for the registration of Indian and Foreign Nurses having foreign qualifications under section 11(2)(a) of the Indian Nursing Council Act 1947.
- To frame and update from time to time, the nursing syllabus, rules, and regulations for the nursing program.
- Provide guidelines to SNRCs, Examination Boards, University, Central, and State Governments regarding the up-gradation of nursing education and maintenance of standards.

State Nursing Council

The State Nursing Council or State Nurse's Registration Council is an autonomous body established in each state of India to establish uniform standards and provide registration to trained nurses and midwives under the law of State. Each State Nursing Council is governed by a Registrar and comes under INC, New Delhi. It is formed by a legislative act in the particular state similar to the Indian Nursing Council. E.g. JKSNC, PNRC, KNC, KSNC, etc.

Function of the State Nursing Council

- **Registration:** carries out student registration as a nurse and nurse-midwife/public health/psychiatric nurse upon the completion of the desired nursing course from a recognized institution.
- Control and monitor the conduct of different nursing programs in a particular state.
- Inspection of the training institutes and providing recognition.
- **Examinations:** are conducted for different courses throughout the year.
- Maintenance of different registers.
- Renewal of registration.

- Foreign verification and good standing certificate.
- Maintaining the record of additional qualifications.
- Monitor the code of conduct and adherence to professional ethics.
- Publication, in-service education, and research collaboration.

University Grant Commission

The first attempt to formulate a national system of education in India came in 1944, with the Report of the Central Advisory Board of Education on Post War Educational Development in India, also known as the Sargeant Report. It recommended the formation of a University Grants Committee, which was formed in 1945 to oversee the work of the three Central Universities of Aligarh, Banaras, and Delhi. In 1947, the Committee was entrusted with the responsibility of dealing with all the then existing Universities.

Soon after Independence, the University Education Commission was set up in 1948 under the Chairmanship of Dr. S Radhakrishnan "to report on Indian university education and suggest improvements and extensions that might be desirable to suit the present and future needs and aspirations of the country". It recommended that the University Grants Committee be reconstituted on the general model of the University Grants Commission of the United Kingdom with a full-time Chairman and other members to be appointed from amongst educationists of repute.

In 1952, the Union Government decided that all cases about the allocation of grants-in-aid from public funds to the Central Universities and other Universities and Institutions of higher learning might be referred to as the University Grants Commission. Consequently, the University Grants Commission (UGC) was formally inaugurated by late Shri Maulana Abul Kalam Azad, the then Minister of Education, Natural Resources and Scientific Research on 28 December 1953.

The UGC, however, was formally established only in November 1956 as a statutory body of the Government of India through an Act of Parliament for the coordination, determination, and maintenance of standards of university education in India. To ensure effective region-wise coverage throughout the country, the UGC has decentralized its operations by setting up six regional centers at Pune, Hyderabad, Kolkata, Bhopal, Guwahati, and Bangalore. The head office of the UGC is located at Bahadur Shah Zafar Marg in New Delhi, with two additional bureaus operating from 35, Feroze Shah Road and the South Campus of the University of Delhi as well.

University/Board of Examinations

A university is formally defined as an institution set up by public or private organizations to conduct formal stream of education and award degrees in the various academic discipline.

Generally, the universities are classified as undergraduate and postgraduate universities. In India, a university is understood to be valid in providing degrees; only when it is permitted to do so by the University Grant Commission.

Nursing Education in India has grown up to newer trends in the last few years. Many institutions are providing a different stream of education in the nursing profession starting with Diploma Programs to Doctorate programs. To bring the uniformity of nursing education across the country and to ensure the quality of nursing education all the nursing programs are offered through recognized Universities and Board of Examinations. Few of the names of Universities and Board of examinations are mentioned below.

Universities

- University of Delhi
- All India Institute of Medical Sciences, New Delhi
- Post Graduate Institute of Medical Education and Research, Chandigarh
- University of Jammu
- Shri Mata Vaishno Devi University
- Rajiv Gandhi University of Health Sciences
- Maharashtra University of Health Sciences
- Baba Farid University of Health Sciences
- Bombay University
- SNDT University
- Lovely Professional University
- Amity University
- Jawaharlal Nehru University
- Kerala University of Health Sciences
- Banaras Hindu University

Board of Examination

These are not recognized as fully fledge universities but formally permitted and are recognized to conduct the examination and award degrees in selected programs of Nursing Education.

- The Examination Board appointed by the Government of Tamil Nadu.
- The School of Nursing, Christian Medical College, Vellore.
- The Indian Psychiatric Society
- The Public Health Department, Madras
- Uttar Pradesh Nurses and Midwives Council State Faculty, Uttar Pradesh
- Maharashtra Nursing Council.
- The State Board of Examiners for Nurses
- The Director of Health and Medical Services (Health), Gujarat
- Kerala Nurses and Midwives Council Trivandrum
- The Punjab State Nursing Council
- Jammu and Kashmir State Nursing Council

Trained Nurses Association of India

It is the Autonomous National Association of the nursing profession in India. The present name and association were set up in 1922. In general, it points out the needs of the individual and issues in the nursing profession. It incorporates the development, upliftment, and streamlining of nursing training and education. It encourages you to be educated on recent developments in nursing and offers chances to distribute articles and opinions. The TNAI includes the following organization incorporated in it. (1) Health Visitors League (2) Auxiliary Nurse-Midwives Association, (3) Student Nurses Association. It is also affiliated to Commonwealth Nurses Federation. The membership in TNAI may be full, associate, or affiliate. The official organ of TNAI is The Nursing Journal of India.

Aims

- To develop, standardize, and upgrade nursing training and education.
- To enhance the employment conditions of the nurses in the country and foster their living.
- Provide membership in the organization for reciprocity of registration. A qualified nurse can get enrolled through the regular application process with the supporting evidence of the State Nursing Council registration certificate.

INTERNATIONAL REGULATORY BODIES

They help in framing policies, standards, and overall professional development.
- International Council of Nurses.
- American Nurses Association.
- The Commonwealth Nurses Federation.

International Council of Nurses

It was framed in 1899 by Mrs. Bedford Fenwick in collaboration with nurse leaders across the world. It is located in Geneva, Switzerland. Currently, around 128 countries are members of ICN. It is a federation of non-governmental and non-political nursing associations. It is a global relationship of all nurses on the planet. The ultimate destinations are to advance the improvement of national associations, help them to enhance the measures of nursing and the skill of nurses and fill in as the legitimate voice for nurses and nursing universally. All nurses who are registered with National associations are members of ICN by default. Individual membership in ICN is not permitted. Other International Professional Organizations such as the World Health Organization (WHO), UNESCO, UNICEF, Red Cross, etc. are also related to ICN.

American Nurses Association

It is a professional organization to improve quality, protect, and uplift Nursing. It was founded in 1911 and located in Maryland, United States. It encompasses the European regions.

Activities

- Establish and maintain the standards for nursing care.
- Develop and modify the educational standards governing nursing education and training.
- Promote nursing research.
- Establish a professional code of ethics.
- Monitor a credentialing system in nursing and regulate the legal aspects affecting professional practice.

The Commonwealth Nurses Federation

The Commonwealth Nurses Federation was formally sorted out in 1973 and works in six areas of the world which are East Africa, Atlantic, Australia, Pacific, South Asia, and Europe. The TNAI is additionally partnered with the Commonwealth Nurses Federation. It is comprised of nurses associations from federation member nations.

Cooperation in Professional Associations is of benefit to the nurses and nursing professions. It gives methods through which joined endeavors can be made to raise guidelines of nursing instruction and practice. It is also a platform for us to speak up our suggestions and getting updated with current trends and issues in nursing practice. Enrollment is essential for dynamic nursing practice either here or abroad. This is done through your State Nurses Registration Council. It gives legal protection to nurses and the recipients of nursing care.

ACCREDITATION

Accreditation is the demonstration of allowing credit or acknowledgment, particularly to an organization to provide education or training. It helps the organization to develop and maintain the concept standard or quality. It assures the quality, improvement, maintenance, and protection of institutions or a particular program against the socially harmful challenges and pressures.

Types of Accreditation Agencies

They are generally classified as under
- Regional accreditation agencies
- State accreditation agencies
- National accreditation agencies
- International accreditation agencies

India has the following accreditation agencies who provide accreditation to organizations/institutions in the preview of the quality of education, training, and services offered by the respective organizations. They are:

- All India Council of Elementary Education
- All India Council of Secondary Education
- All India Council of Technical Education (AICTE)
- University Grants Commission (UGC)
- Medical Council of India (MCI)
- Indian Nursing Council (INC)
- National Assessment and Accreditation Council (NAAC)
- National Accreditation Board for Hospital and Health Care (NABH)
- Joint Commission International (JCI) (International Agency)

Importance of accreditation: In the preview of the dimensions mentioned above, there are two major dimensions of accreditation, such as quality assurance and institutional and program improvement that addresses the need of the society. The importance of accreditation may be organized as under:

For the public	For the students	For the institutions
Confirms the general expectations in the field of education	Students' needs are met	It helps in improvement and self-evaluation
The availability of professional services as the accredited program is backed up by newer knowledge and practice	Universal acceptability and transferability of credits across the institutions/ platform	Strengthens the public regard
Minimum intervening by public agencies	Widely accepted by many industries	Protection of external encroachments that harm the quality of the program as well as the institution
		Eligible for special aids from the Government and assures the quality of the program.

Educational accreditation is a type of quality declaration process under which services and operations of an educational institution are evaluated by an external body to determine if the applicable standards are met. If standards are met, accredited status is granted by the agency.

University accreditation and quality assurance measures vary from country to country. Most commonly, universities are granted the right to issue 'degrees', with procedures put in place to measure the level of quality of instruction to ensure that it is maintained at a level acceptable to the body that issues the degree-granting right. In most countries in the world, the function of educational accreditation is conducted by a government organization, such as the Education Ministry.

Accreditation in India

Accreditation is compulsory for all universities in India except those created through an act of Parliament. Without accreditation, "It is emphasized that these fake institutions have no legal entity to call themselves as University and to award 'Degrees' which are not treated as valid for academic/ employment purposes." The University Grants Commission Act (1956) explains, "the right of conferring or granting degrees shall be exercised only by the following

- A university established or incorporated by or under a Central Act, or a State Act.
- An institution deemed to be university or an institution specially empowered by an Act of the Parliament to confer or grant degrees.

Thus, "any institution which has not been credited by an enactment of Parliament or a State Legislature or has not been granted the status of a Deemed-to-be-University is not entitled to award a degree." Accreditation for higher learning is overseen by autonomous institutions established by the University Grants Commission.

Accreditation Process

In general, there are six steps for accreditation of programs/ colleges/institutions. It includes:

1. Application for registration
2. Self-assessment
3. On the site survey
4. Report Preparation
5. Award of accreditation
6. Maintaining Accredited Status

National Assessment and Accreditation Council

India has one of the largest and diverse education systems in the world. Privatization, widespread expansion, increased autonomy and introduction of programs in new and emerging areas have improved access to higher education. At the same time, it has also led to widespread concern on the quality and relevance of higher education. To address these concerns, the National Policy on Education (NPE, 1986) and the Program of Action (PoA, 1992) spelled out strategic plans for the policies, advocated the establishment of an independent National accreditation agency. Consequently, the National Assessment and Accreditation Council (NAAC) was established in 1994 as an autonomous institution of the University Grants Commission (UGC) with its Head Quarter in Bengaluru. The mandate of NAAC as reflected in its vision statement is in making quality assurance an integral part of the functioning of Higher Education Institutions (HEIs).

The NAAC functions through its General Counsel (GC) and Executive Committee (EC) comprising educational administrators, policymakers and senior academicians from a cross-section of the Indian higher education system. The Chairperson of the UGC is the President of the GC of the NAAC, the Chairperson of the EC is an eminent academician nominated by the President of GC (NAAC). The Director is the academic and administrative head of the NAAC and is the member-secretary of both the GC and the EC. In addition to the statutory bodies that steer its policies and core staff to support its activities, the NAAC is advised by the advisory and consultative committees constituted from time to time. NAAC has formulated a three-stage process for assessment and accreditation as:

- **Institutional eligibility for quality assessment (IEQA):** It is obtained by an applicant institution at the beginning while it is still in the planning stage for assessment. The benefits of this step for an applicant institution are to get recognized as eligible to apply for the second step comprehensive assessment and accreditation process.
- **Preparation of the self study report:** Self-report is prepared by the institution as per the guidelines given by NAAC, its submission to NAAC and in house analysis of the report by NAAC.
- **Peer team visit:** Peer Team visit to the institution for validation of the Self Study Report is followed by the presentation of a comprehensive assessment report to the institution. Later grading, certification, and accreditation is done based on the evaluation by the executive committee of the NAAC.

Accreditation of Hospitals

Hospital accreditation has been defined as "A self-assessment and external peer assessment process used by health care organizations to accurately assess their level of performance concerning established standards and to implement ways to continuously improve. The common Hospital Accreditation Agencies are:

- **National Accreditation Board for Hospitals and Health Care Providers (NABH):** NABH is a constituent board of Quality Council of India, set up to establish and operate accreditation programs for healthcare organizations. The board is structured to cater to the much-desired needs of the consumers and to set benchmarks for the progress of the health industry. The board while being supported by all stakeholders including industry, consumers government has full functional autonomy in its operation.
- **Joint Commission International (JCI):** An independent not for profit organization accredits and certifies health care organizations and programs across the globe. It is recognized as the global leader's health care quality of is and patient safety. Joint Commission International identifies, measures, and shares best practices in quality and patient safety with the world.

INSPECTIONS

To maintain the uniformity and quality of the nursing education in the respective institutions, inspections are conducted by the regulatory bodies to ensure that standards are maintained and the quality of education and training is assured.

If qualitative education is a thing seriously desired in nursing schools and colleges so that standard of education in our schools can be highly improved, school supervision must, therefore, be accorded high priority. Through inspection and supervision, the inspectors and supervisors assist in improving classroom instructions and practical training because teachers are made more competent and efficient, the consumers of health care are satisfied with the performance of the professionals and they are motivated to work harder to achieve the required standard, hence, in the long run, the goal of professional education is achieved.

Types of Inspections

Inspections are broadly classified into the following categories:

- **First inspection:** This is usually done by the regulatory bodies before the commencement of any program in nursing to check the feasibility of the institution to offer the said program. During this inspection, the physical infrastructure, human resource planning, academic and clinical facilities, residential facilities and other associated factors are assessed. Based on the finding, provisional permission is granted to the organization to start the intended program. Usually, many regulatory bodies' certification is required to start a nursing program such as Central/State Government, Indian Nursing Council, State Nursing Council, the Examining Body or affiliated University and so on.
- **Re-inspection:** These are conducted for those institutions, which are found unsuitable by a particular regulatory body. The institutions and the government are informed about the deficiencies and advised to improve upon them. Once the institution takes necessary steps to rectify the deficiencies, the institution should submit the compliance report with documentary proof of the deficiencies pointed out and re-inspection fees. On receipt of the compliance report and fees from the institution, the application will be considered for re-inspection.
- **Routine visits:** This is a short visit made to the school on which no formal reports are written but brief comments are made. The aim depends on such an inspector on why such inspection is made. It may be a check on the punctuality of teachers or how the school is settling down. One of the aims of such supervisory visits is to look into what is happening, the work being done, the human relationships or the appropriate use of the building and school equipment.

- **Follow-up inspection/periodic inspection**: This is the follow up of previous visits. The inspector investigates whether the suggestions, corrections, and recommendations he or she made during the previous visit have been carried out by affected schools. He or she also ascertains how those corrections and suggestions are helping in achieving the school objectives.
- **Inspection with special purpose**: If the institution plans for the addition of new programs, the addition of the number of students or to make any other modification to the existing system of instruction, a special inspection is conducted upon the request of the institution.

Agencies Conducting Inspections in a Nursing Institution

- Higher Education or Medical Education Department of the Central or State Government
- Indian Nursing Council
- State Nursing Council
- University/The Board of Examination
- Any other agencies appointed by the Competent Authority

 REVIEW QUESTIONS

1. What are the norms in the establishment of nursing educational institutions? Which are the regulatory bodies of nursing education?
2. Define accreditation. Explain the concepts, purpose, and types of accreditation. Brief the process of NAAC accreditation.
3. Explain the physical facilities of a college of nursing.
4. What are the inspections? Explain types of inspections conducted in nursing educational institutions.

Further Readings

1. Banerjee, Shyamal. Principles and Practice of Management. Oxford and IBM Publishing, New Delhi; 2000.
2. Basavanthappa BT. Nursing Administration. 2nd Edition: Jaypee Brothers Medical Publishers (P) Ltd., New Delhi; 2009.
3. Barrett, Jean. Ward Management and Teaching. Konark Publishers, Delhi; 1992.
4. Warren, Stevens, F. Management and Leadership in Nursing. McGraw – Hill Inc, New York; 1978.
5. Alexander et al. Nursing Service Administration. Mosby Publishers, US; 1962.
6. Park K. Preventive, and Social Medicine, 19th Edition: M/s. Banarasidas Bhanot Publishers, Jabalpur; 2007.
7. Basavanthappa BT. Nursing Administration, 1st Edition: Jaypee Brothers Medical Publishers (P) Ltd., New Delhi; 2002.
8. Goel SL. Healthcare System, and Social Medicine, Health Organization and Structure, 1st Volume: Deep and Deep Publishers, New Delhi; 2001.
9. Ranga Rao SP. Administration of Primary Health Centers in India, 1st Edition: Mittal Publications, New Delhi; 1993.
10. Lucita M. Nursing: Practice and Public Health Administration. Current Concepts and Trends. B. I. Churchill Living Stone Pvt. Ltd., New Delhi; 2002.
11. Sakharkar BM. Principles of Hospital Administration and Planning, 2nd Edition: Jaypee Brothers Medical Publishers (P) Ltd., New Delhi; 2009.
12. Patricia S Yoder-Wise. Leading and Managing in Nursing. 2nd Edition: Mosby Publication, US; 1999.
13. Bessie L Marquis, Carol J Huston. Leadership Roles and Management Functions in Nursing: Theory and Application. 5th Edition: Lippincott Williams and Wilkins, New York; 2006.
14. Linda Roussel. Management and Leadership for Nurse Administrators. 4th Edition: Jones and Bartlett Publication, USA; 2006.
15. Wehrich H, Koontz H. Management A Global Perspective. 11th Edition: Tata McGraw-Hill Publishing Company, Ltd., New Delhi; 2005.
16. Marquis BL, Huston CJ. Leadership and Management Functions in Nursing—Theory, and Application. 5th Edition: Lippincott Williams and Wilkins, Philadelphia; 2006.
17. Douglass LM. The Effective Nurse: Leader and Manager. 5th Edition: Mosby Publication, US; 1996.
18. Trained Nurses Association of India, Nursing Administration, and Management.
19. Samson Rebecca. Leadership and Management in Nursing Practice and Education 1st Edition: Jaypee Brothers Medical Publishers (P) Ltd., New Delhi; 2009.
20. Kunders GD, Designing for Total Quality in Health Care, Prism Book Pvt. Ltd., Bangalore; 2002.

Unit

14

Planning and Organizing of Nursing Educational Institutions

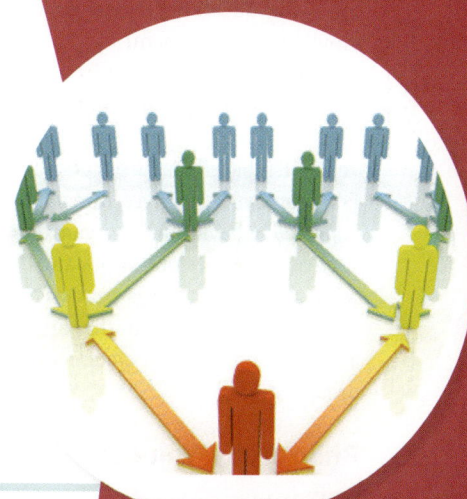

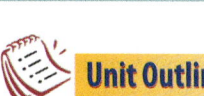 **Unit Outline**

- Mission, Vision, and Philosophy of the College
- Organization Structure of School/College
- Curriculum Planning, Implementation, and Evaluation
- Planning Teaching and Learning Experiences
- Master Plan, Clinical Rotation
- Budget for Educational Institution
- Physical and Academic Facilities Required for the Nursing Educational Institution Including Staffing Norms as per the Regulations of Indian Nursing Council
- Records and Reports in Nursing Educational Institutions
- Committees

MISSION, VISION, AND PHILOSOPHY OF THE COLLEGE

Mission Statements and Vision Statement

Mission Statement describes the primary objectives of the organization. It primarily tries to explain the reason for the existence of any organization. It is the beginning of an organization's strategic planning. It tries to explain to the stakeholders the purpose of existence and what is the current performance of the organization. Mission statements support the achievement of the vision statements. It normally asks the following questions. What do we do? Whom do we serve? How do we serve them?

Vision statements are future-oriented and try to explain the prospects of the organization. It usually is a projected plan of functioning for the forthcoming years. (Normally 10–15 years). It is based on the purpose and values of the organization. For employees, it gives direction and understanding of the expected behavior in the organization. It usually asks questions such as; What are our hopes and dreams for the future?

In a nutshell, an organization through its mission statement tries to describe what the organization wants to do now and through a vision statement, it outlines the plans of the organization.

Philosophy/Value Statements

Philosophy or value statements are understood as a method of achieving the mission and vision. It briefs the ideologies, concepts, and principles of an organization. They are considered as the core belief of an organization that decides the pathway to achieve the mission/vision of the organization.

Philosophy of Nursing Education

The nursing service philosophy could be a statement of beliefs that is in agreement with the institution's philosophy. It should reflect the ideologies of the members of the nursing service and should be mutually agreeable. These are the values, beliefs, attitudes, and ideas which the faculty and students have collectively agreed upon about nursing education programs. It is a combination of the philosophy of education and nursing. It focuses on the overall development of student life. It may also be influenced by many factors such as institutional policies, availability of resources, health needs of the society and the cultural and ethical background of the student and faculty.

Below given are few examples of the mission, vision and philosophy statements of some renowned organization of the country.

- **University of Delhi**
  - **Mission statement:** To provide the best quality education to students regardless of their socioeconomic background, nurture their talent, promote their intellectual growth and shape their personal development.
  - **Vision statement:** Be an internationally acclaimed University, recognized for excellence in teaching, research and outreach; provide the highest quality education to students, nurture their talent, promote intellectual growth and shape their personal development; remain dedicated and steadfast in the pursuit of truth aligned with the motto of the University of Delhi "Nishtha Dhriti Satyam" and serve humanity through the creation of well-rounded, multi-skilled and socially responsible global citizens.
  - **Philosophy/value:** Creativity, ethical conduct, social responsibility, diversity and inclusion, global citizenship, collaborative and experimental learning, excellence and innovation.
- **Manipal College of Nursing, Karnataka**
  - **Mission statement:** Be the most preferred choice of students, faculty, and industry. Be in the top 10 in every discipline of education, health sciences, engineering, and management.
  - **Vision statement:** Global leadership in human development, excellence in education and healthcare.
  - **Philosophy/Values:** Integrity, Transparency, Quality, Teamwork, Execution with passion, Human touch
- **Bharati Vidyapeeth College of Nursing, Maharashtra**
  - **Mission statement:** To provide inclusive borderless access to higher education and vocational education based on merit; To offer varied professional, technical, vocational and general education programs to meet the changing and diverse needs of society in a global context; To provide quality higher education for the liberation of mind and empowerment of hands; To promote quality research in diverse areas of development and engage in the application of knowledge for community development; To develop national and international networks with industry, service sector and other academic and research institutions to meet the expectations of various stakeholders; To promote extensive use of ICT for the enrichment of teaching-learning and effective governance.
  - **Vision statement:** The College of Nursing aspires to be a model of excellence through dynamic programs, innovative practices, and research.
  - **Philosophy/values:** Preparing a competent professional nurse by providing an innovative and academically challenging environment to meet the global health care needs.

ORGANIZATION STRUCTURE OF SCHOOL/ COLLEGE

An organizational structure is a system that outlines how certain activities are directed to achieve the goals of an organization. These activities can include rules, roles, and responsibilities. The organizational structure also determines how information flows between levels within the organization. For example, in a centralized structure, decisions flow from the top down, while in a decentralized structure, decision-making power is distributed among various levels of the organization. Having an organizational structure in place allows organizations to remain efficient and focused.

Types of Organizational Structure

- **Functional structure:** This is also referred to as a bureaucratic organizational structure and breaks up a company based on the specialization of its workforce. Most small-to-medium-sized businesses implement a functional structure. Dividing the firm into departments consisting of marketing, sales, and operations is the act of using a bureaucratic organizational structure.
- **Divisional or multidivisional structure:** The second type is common among large companies with many business units. Called the divisional or multidivisional structure, a company that uses this method structures its leadership team based on the products, projects, or subsidiaries they operate. A good example of this structure is Johnson and Johnson. With thousands of products and lines of businesses, the company structures itself so each business unit operates as its own company with its president.
- **Flatarchy structure:** Flatarchy, a newer structure, is the third type and is used among many startups. As the name alludes, it flattens the hierarchy and chain of command and gives its employees a lot of autonomy. Companies that use this type of structure have a high speed of implementation.
- **Matrix structure:** The fourth and final organizational structure is a matrix structure. It is also the most confusing and the least used. This structure matrixes employees across different superiors, divisions, or departments. An employee working for a matrixed company, for example, may have duties in both sales and customer service.
- Other structures in the organization include formal, informal, vertical and horizontal organizations.

The organizational charts and manuals explain the structure of the organization. An organization chart is a diagrammatic representation of the framework or structure of an organization. An organization chart is a diagrammatical form that shows the essential aspects of an organization including the significant functions and their relationship, the channels of supervision and the relative authority of each employee who is in charge of each function. Above given is an example of the organization structure of a nursing college (Fig. 1).

CURRICULUM PLANNING, IMPLEMENTATION, AND EVALUATION

Curriculum word is derived from the Latin language, which means a course of deeds and experiences through which children grow to become mature adults.

It is a course of study or a set of subjects or a set of performance objectives or a program of studies.

—**Oliva, 1997**

The curriculum is a tool in the hands of an artist to mold his material according to his ideals in his studio. In this definition, the artist is the teacher, the material is the student, ideals are the objectives, and the studio is the educational institution.

—**Cunningham**

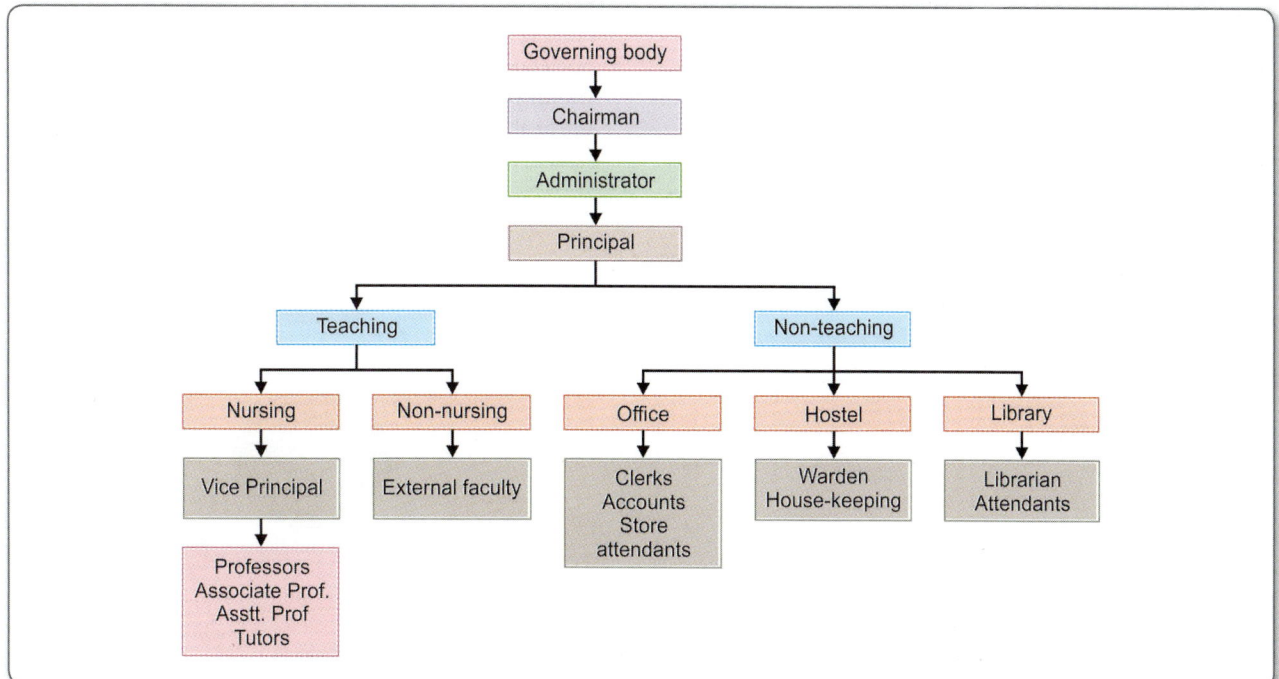

Fig. 1: Organizational chart of a nursing college

Curriculum Development

It is the process of planning, implementing, and evaluating learning opportunities intended to produce desired changes in learners. —**Print (1993)**

The curriculum development model is suggested to correlate and study the dimensions of curriculum and its association with its elements. It incorporates a symbolic representation that represents the association among the different phases, steps, and tasks involved in constructing a curriculum.

Constitution of a Curriculum Committee

- Investigation and analysis of the existing health needs of the region and nation (E.g., National Health Policy, 2005)
- Investigation of curriculum needs for nursing education
- Formulation of the philosophy of nursing education
- Establishment of educational objectives/outcomes/competencies
- Selection of learning experiences
- Selection of instructional strategies
- Organization of learning experiences
- Development of evaluation systems

Purposes of Curriculum

- It communicates to learners in advance what they are expected to know to achieve their instructional objectives over a defined period of time.
- Introduces examination or assessment criteria to allow learners to prepare for examinations accordingly.
- It defines the course, unit, and lesson goals, as well as the necessary teaching-learning techniques to help educators, plan their lessons accordingly.
- It communicates to the policymakers about the competencies and expertise of a particular group of students the positions and roles they can perform.
- It prepares the pupil for citizenship in a democratic society.
- It meets the needs of students with a wide range of abilities, aptitudes, and interests.
- It relates and systematically organizes the various learning experiences to produce the maximum cumulative effect in attaining the objectives of the school.

Levels of Curriculum Planning

According to Goodland, there are three levels of curriculum planning, namely, societal, institutional, instructional (Fig. 2).

Societal curriculum: This is the curriculum planned for a specific population of students by experts outside the educational institution and who are legally appointed. In nursing education, the societal curriculum is designed by different statutory bodies such as the Indian Nursing Council. A societal curriculum is synonymous with the official type of curriculum.

Institutional curriculum: This is the curriculum prepared by the faculty of the institute for a particular group of students for a definite period. An institutional curriculum is synonymous with the actual type of curriculum.

Instructional curriculum: This is the curriculum prepared by the individual teacher at the instructional level.

Factors Influencing Curriculum Development

Forces and problems affecting the curriculum of nursing science are complicated and continuously changing. There are fast changes in the health care system in the new millennium, which poses difficulties for nurse teachers to devise appropriate curricula for nursing education to maintain pace with these changes. The curriculum is never created in a vacuum but in the contextual depiction of worldwide trends, domestic health, and essential statistics, domestic health policy, domestic population policy, professional priorities and values of the teachers. The main factors are the philosophy of nursing education, educational psychology, society, students, social activities, knowledge, and skills required of training (Fig. 3). The following are the determinants of the curriculum in nursing sciences:

- Societal determinants such as demographic revolution, health problems, advanced medical technology, change in the healthcare delivery system, cultural diffusion, changing patients' expectations, etc.

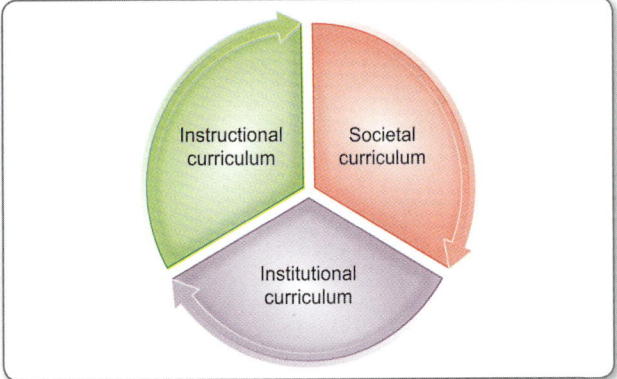

Fig. 2: Levels of curriculum planning

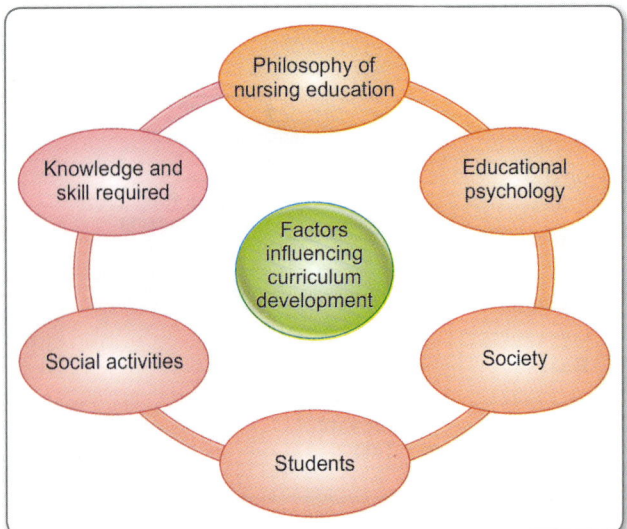

Fig. 3: Factors influencing curriculum development

- Educational determinants such as new instructional Strategies and new methods of assessment. It is the learning experience.
- Economic determinants involve cost-benefit analysis to determine the suitability of a nursing program.
- Philosophical determinants include the school of philosophy in which the profession or society or nations believe, influence the contents of the curriculum as well as the instructional strategies employed to achieve objectives of the education.
- Subject matter is too shallow without addressing the needs, interests, and abilities of the students, and does not encourage in-depth understanding.

Models of Curriculum

- **Behavioral objective model/product model:** It was proposed by Ralph Tyler in 1950. It reflects the need to organize the utility and purpose of a product of the quality and its practical application. Here the curriculum is viewed objectively for its function and recognizes teaching and learning as an integral part of it. According to him, the curriculum decides the order and scope of what is to be taught, and thus learning may be enhanced. He identified four fundamental questions to be answered in the process of developing a curriculum.
  - What educational purposes should the school seek to attain, i.e., the objectives?
  - How can learning experiences be selected?
  - How can the learning experiences be organized?
  - How can the effectiveness of learning be evaluated?
- **Stenhouse's process model/process model:** It is an input model suggested by Lawrence Stenhouse in 1975. Here the emphasis is on learning experiences or the process of education. It is possible to organize a curriculum without the planning of the expected behavioral change among students. The content of the curriculum should not be based on means of its achievement; instead, it should be based on learning experiences. The teacher assesses the student to develop self-assessment qualities among the students.
- **Lawton's cultural analysis model:** This model which came up in the year 1983 was a reaction against what he saw as the dangers of the behavioral objectives models. It is based on the concept of cultural analysis. Culture is defined as the holistic way of life of society, and the purpose of education is to make available to the next generation what we regard as the most critical aspects of culture. Cultural analysis is the process by which a selection is made from the cultural context and in terms of curriculum planning.
- **Beattie's Fourfold model:** Beattie suggests (1987) that there are four fundamental approaches in relation to the task of planning a curriculum for nursing:
  - Curriculum as a map of key subjects. This approach consists of mapping out the key subjects in the nursing curriculum.
  - Curriculum as a schedule of necessary skills. This approach emphasizes the specifics of the basic skills of nursing practice.
  - Curriculum as a portfolio of meaningful personal experiences. This approach places students at the center of learning by organizing the curriculum around their interests and skills.
  - Curriculum as an agenda of critical cultural issues. This approach avoids giving detailed subject matter, focusing instead on controversial issues and political dilemmas in nursing and health care.

Principles of Curriculum Development

A curriculum has been described as a tool in the hands of teachers for giving training to students in the art of living together in a community.

- **The conservative principle:** It has been stated that nations live in the present, on the past and for the future. This means that the present, past and future needs of the community should be taken into consideration.
- **The forward-looking principle:** Children of today are the citizens of tomorrow. Therefore, their education should be such that it enables them to become progressive-minded persons.
- **The creative principle:** In the curriculum, those activities should be included, which enable the child to exercise his/her creative and constructive powers.
- **Principle of totality:** The total learning experience and learning opportunity may have to be well planned as a whole curriculum, and the teaching-learning activity needed for the entire period has to be considered while developing a curriculum.
- **Child-centered curriculum:** While developing the curriculum, due consideration should be given to the students' age, educational level, need, and individual difference.
- **Principle of integration and correlation:** Each year's course should be built on what has been done in previous years and at the same time, should serve as a basis for subsequent learning.
- **Principle of variety and flexibility:** Variety should be provided in terms of learning and teaching activities. A curriculum should not be so rigid that appropriate modifications cannot be done as and when needed.
- **Training for leisure:** There should be some provision for co-curricular activities, relaxation, library utilization, and electives according to choice.

Evaluation of the Curriculum

Evaluation is a systematic and organized process of realizing the extent to which educational objectives laid down in a curriculum have been achieved.

Aims of Evaluation

- To find out to what extent the objectives of the program have been attained.
- For certification purposes.
- To provide guidelines for decisions about a curriculum, revision modification, and shift of emphasis.
- It is designed to protect society to prevent incompetent personnel from practicing nursing.

In Curriculum Evaluation, the Evaluation of Five M's is Done

- **Men:** whether the curriculum has been organized and implemented correctly by the faculty members and others involved in it.
- **Money:** whether money meant for curriculum development is utilized correctly.
- **Materials:** whether the evaluation of textbooks, literature, is used for the development of the curriculum.
- **Methods:** whether teaching-learning methods planned in the curriculum are appropriate.
- **Minutes:** appropriateness of allocation theory and practical hours in the curriculum.

Types of Assessments/Evaluation

- **Formative assessment:** It is an ongoing evaluation to measure the progress made by the students. The purpose is to provide feedback to students and teachers at regular intervals. Its results may form a part of the internal assessment.
- **Summative assessment:** It is the final evaluation of the student done at the end of the course. Part of the summative assessment may be based on the formative evaluation.

Curriculum implementation is an essential part of curriculum development because it is through the implementation that the intended changes as specified in the curriculum document are supplied in practice. The curriculum is the blueprint of an educational program. Even though a curriculum cannot be entirely preplanned and prescribed, to a great extent, it can be developed based on the needs of the students as well as society.

PLANNING TEACHING AND LEARNING EXPERIENCES

The teaching-learning process in nursing educational institutions are generally categorized into theoretical education and practical/clinical training.

Theoretical Learning in an Educational Institution

The theory classes are conducted in the nursing educational institutions as per the guidelines of university and syllabus/

curriculum recommended by the regulatory bodies. Lesson plans are prepared by the faculty for delivering classroom sessions in each course of a program. A lesson plan is a title given to the statements of achievements to be realized and specific meaning by which these are to be attained as a result of activities engaged during the period.

Purposes of Lesson Plan

- Ensures a definite objective for the days' work
- Keeps the teacher on track
- Ensures selection, presentation, and interpretation of the subject matter
- Helps to choose an effective method of teaching
- Enables to evaluate the teaching sessions
- Helps to review the subject and gives up to date knowledge
- Helps to clarify the ideas
- Gives the teacher greater confidence
- It stimulates the teacher to think of related material, illustrations, and audio-visual aids.
- Enables the teacher to organize classroom teaching activities
- Develops reasoning, imagination and decision-making ability of the teacher
- Facilitates micro-teaching.

Principles of Lesson Plan

- Used as a guide rather than as a rule of thumb
- The teacher must have mastery of and adequate training in the topic
- Needs to be fully conversant with new methods and techniques of teaching
- Needs to organize the material in an organized rather than a logical fashion
- Must ensure active student participation
- Should use different teaching-learning methods

MASTER PLAN, CLINICAL ROTATION

Planning is the function of a managing authority which decides in advance what have to do. It is an intellectual process in which creative thinking and imagination are essential. Planning is the first function of an executive. Planning plays an important role in everybody's life. Every moment every individual has to plan future action.

A master plan is the overall plan of all students in a particular educational institution, showing the placement of the students belonging to the total program, including both theory and practice denotes the study block, partial block, placement of student of the clinical block, team nursing, examinations, vacation, and co-curricular activities, etc.

The clinical rotation plan is the complete planning of clinical experience for a student. Clinical experience is an integral part of learning where the student will be actively participating to obtain skills in clinical practice by applying the principles of learning by doing. The time the student spends and learns in the clinical fields is an important and integral part of the total study program. In nursing education, rotation refers to the regular, successive and recurrent posting of various groups of nursing students belonging to different classes in specific nursing fields, i.e., OPDs, specialty wards, OT, delivery room, clinics, community health fields- clinics, outreach centers, sub-centers, health centers, schools, etc.

Note: The detailed explanation of the master plan, master rotation plan, clinical rotation plan is explained in Unit 6

BUDGET FOR EDUCATIONAL INSTITUTION

Every educational institution should have a separate budget. The budget committee of a school/college of nursing comprises of Chairman/Director, Members of the Governing Council, Principal, Vice Principal, Administrator, and Account Officer. The financial management of the institution, such as the amount of fee to be collected, salaries, and other expenses of the college/school depends on the annual budget policies.

Contents of the Budget

Revenue: It includes assets, fixed deposits, property, investments, loans, advances, and income/fees collected from the students.

Balance: It is the statement that explains the income and expenditure details of an organization. It also shows the monetary profit of the organization.

Expenditure: It includes recurring as well as nonrecurring expenses.

- Recurring annual mandatory spending includes:
  - Salary and allowances of the officers/staff
  - Printing and Stationery

- Transportation expenses
- Mess and accommodation expenses
- Books and Journals, magazines
- Annual affiliation fee
- Clinical training fee
- Hospitality
- Housekeeping and security
- Contingency charges
- Laboratory equipment
- Student welfare
- Staff welfare
- Miscellaneous
- Non-recurring expenditure includes:
  - Endowment fund with Government and university
  - Building and infrastructure
  - Security fixed deposits

To meet the educational objectives of the nursing program, there should have adequate supplies and equipment [physical facilities]. The number and type of physical facilities depends upon the size of the student's body and the needs of the educational program.

Sample Budget Proposal of College of Nursing

Every budget proposal begins with an introduction to the organization, its philosophy, mission, and objectives. The expenditure is classified broadly into two categories before preparing the budget such as

- **Recurring:** Salary of employees and other employee benefits, bus maintenance, electricity, water, telephone, lab consumables, stationery
- **Non-recurring:** Building/Infrastructure set up, furniture, lab equipments, vehicles, miscellaneous

Sr. no.	Particulars	Estimated cost in INR	% of the total anticipated allocation
1.	**Recurring Costs**		
	Salary		
	Professional activity (CNE, conferences)		
	Guest faculty expenses		
	Repair and maintenance of the building and equipment		
	Newspaper, magazines and other periodicals		
	Printing and stationery		
	Hospitality		
	Transportation/Vehicle maintenance		
	Internet, telephone, postage/courier		
	Electricity and water charges		
	Office and legal expenses		
	Affiliation and accreditation expenses		

Contd...

Sr. no.	Particulars	Estimated cost in INR	% of the total anticipated allocation
	Events/programs expenses		
	Student welfare, sports, etc.		
	Teaching aids		
	Examination expenses		
	Hostel (food, accommodation, security)		
	Scholarship expenses		
	Miscellaneous		
2.	**Non-recurring Costs**		
	Construction expenses		
	Books and Journals		
	Laboratory equipment		
	Furniture, office equipment, computers, etc.		
3.	**Anticipated Revenue/Income**		
	Prospectus/Application fee		
	Admission fee		
	University registration Fee		
	Tuition fee		
	Transportation fee		
	Hostel fee (food and accommodation)		
	Interest from income (deposits)		

Sample Annual Balance Sheet of a College of Nursing

Revenue/ income	Amount	Expenditure	Amount
Prospectus/Application fee		Salary	
Admission fee		Professional activity (CNE, conferences)	
University registration fee		Guest faculty expenses	
Tuition fee		Repair and maintenance of the building and equipment	
Transportation fee		Newspaper, magazines and other periodicals	
Hostel fee (food and accommodation)		Printing and stationery	
Interest from income (deposits)		Hospitality	
		Transportation/vehicle maintenance	
		Internet, telephone, postage/courier	
		Electricity and water charges	
		Office and legal expenses	
		Affiliation and accreditation expenses	
		Events/Programs expenses	
		Student welfare, sports, etc.	
		Teaching aids	
		Examination expenses	
		Hostel (food, accommodation, security)	
		Scholarships expenses	
		Miscellaneous	

Contd...

Revenue/ income	Amount	Expenditure	Amount
		Construction expenses	
		Books and Journals	
		Laboratory equipment	
		Furniture, office equipment, computers, etc.	
Total Gain		Total expenditure	

PHYSICAL AND ACADEMIC FACILITIES REQUIRED FOR THE NURSING EDUCATIONAL INSTITUTION INCLUDING STAFFING NORMS AS PER THE REGULATIONS OF INDIAN NURSING COUNCIL

The Nursing Training Institutions should be located near to the parent hospital but in a separate building. There should be a space for expansion if it is in the hospital building. The preferred built-up area for the college with an annual intake of 40–60 students is 23720 sq.ft. It may increase according to the number of programs and students. The specific construction area is according to the number of classrooms, laboratories, a residential area for students and staff, other amenities, and facilities.

Note: The infrastructure facilities required for a nursing educational institution as per the norms of Indian Nursing Council is explained in Unit 13.

RECORDS AND REPORTS IN NURSING EDUCATIONAL INSTITUTIONS

Every individual should be responsible for the execution of their obligations to general society, especially the professionals. Since nursing has been considered as a calling, nurses need to record their work on consummation. Records are the indispensable and unavoidable guide to the professional practitioner in giving the ideal support and service to their care recipients.

A record is defined as a permanent written communication that documents information relevant to a client's health care management.

A record is a scientific, clinical, administrative as well as legal document about the medical and nursing care given to the individual family or community.

Purposes of Records

- It provides vital information for planning and evaluation, and this data is also crucial in improving individual and family health.
- It is used as a correspondence material between health professionals and the family.

- A well-maintained record demonstrates the medical issue in the family and different variables that influence their wellbeing.
- It is vital in future planning and helpful in the research development of nursing services.

Principles of Writing the Record

- Nurses should build up their technique for articulation and frame in record composing.
- It is written plainly, properly and enough.
- Contain realities depending on perception, discussion, and activity.
- Since records are legally significant, it should be dealt with cautiously, and represented.
- Records should be composed on the same day about action/incident.
- Maintain confidentiality.
- Do not include any awkward phases, double meaning words, etc.
- The record has to be signed by the person who prepares it with proper date and time.

Advantages of Records

For the individual and family:
- It contains the complete history of the student and hence helps in continued services and follow up.
- Records fill in as proof to help or to oversee or confront the legal inquiries that emerge.
- As it contains all student-related information, it can be used as an educative and research tool.

For the teacher:
- It is the evidence of services provided to the students since it exhibits the overall performance of the students.
- It is the resource for further planning and advancements.
- Helps in self-growth/self-assessment and judgment of the services provided in terms of quality and quantity.
- Serves as a communicative tool among colleagues and helps in future planning.

For authorities:
- Provide the administration with measurable data essential for choice as to use of assets, making arrangements for authoritative control and future references.
- Help the manager assess the administrations rendered, teaching done, and an individual's activity and responses.

Types of Records

- **Cumulative records:** It is otherwise called as continuous records. It is economical and time-saving. It contains the complete information of the individual and helpful in the long-term evaluation.
- **Individual student record:** It contains all the information regarding each student from the day of admission to the course. It contains all the major communication, academic performance, leave details and other necessary information of the student. Every student will have a record/file maintained in the office in their name throughout the existence of the nursing educational institutions.
- **Anecdotal record:** An anecdotal record is a simple statement of an incident prepared by the observer, which seems to be significant with the pertaining incident. In elaboration, it is the recording of all incidents in an organization concerning a particular event or person.

Common Types of Records to be Kept in an Educational Institution

- **Admission register:** It is a record of all the candidates who are admitted to a college/school. According to departmental rules, the admission register is to be preserved permanently in the college/school. Therefore, it should be kept in safe custody. It should be free from mistakes because this register is at times required by superior authorities in a court of law as an evidence for the academic and other personal details of the candidate. At the time of admission, the candidate submits their relevant records like eligibility education certificates, provisional certificates of the previous qualification, migration certificate if any, etc. along with their application. All these papers are to be carefully preserved and entered in the admission register. It also contains the demographic details of the candidate,
- **Attendance register:** This is another important register which is maintained in each class and section, showing the names of the students on the roll of the class or section, during a month. Attendance is marked at the beginning of the classes and on a daily basis. Entries should be made in ink. Blanks should not be left. Holidays and Sundays are marked in red ink. Its main function as its name suggests is to show the presence and absence of every student enrolled in the class. Besides this, it also provides us with many other details like admission number details for quick reference, different categories of children present in a class and their background and thus guide us in planning a lesson in accordance with the differences. It involves calculations like average daily attendance. Nursing Institutions generally maintain a different type of attendance registers such as daily attendance register, clinical attendance register, subject attendance registers and so on. With the introduction of computer many organizations have started marking attendance online and digital base.

- **Attendance register of faculty/staff:** It contains the attendance of all the faculty and staff members. Nowadays the attendance registers of faculty and staff are monitored and maintained in the form of biometric attendance.
- **Leave register:** Separate leave register is maintained for staff and students. The leave register consists of information regarding the number of leaves, reason of leave, type of leave availed and so on.
- **Clinical experience records:** This book Clinical Experience Record Book for BSc Nursing Students is primarily designed to meet the practical needs of the nursing students working in the hospital setting, who are using the nursing process to identify the needs of patients, nursing goals, plans in nursing care implementation and evaluation of nursing care. The contents of the book are prepared according to the syllabus of the Indian Nursing Council (INC) to enable the nursing students to utilize it during all the practical procedures. Procedures are listed according to the year in which they are taught in the curriculum. All the nursing procedures should be completed by return demonstration in nursing school and nursing college laboratories, etc. under the supervision of the class teacher, clinical instructors and ward staff or nursing supervisors. This clinical experience record book should be approved by the class teacher and principal of the nursing training institution from time to time before the final/annual practical examination conducted by the board/council. It is also referred to as the Log Book of Nursing Course.
- **Common health record:** This contains the health-related information of the nursing student. It includes the weight, height, other vital information, serious illness if any, leave details related to any type of illness and so on. Periodical health check-up is done for all the students and the information is kept confidential.
- **Internal assessment register:** Every nursing program is evaluated through examination that is conducted annually or semester wise depending upon the practice of affiliated university of the board of examination. In addition to the final/major examination, periodical assessments are conducted at regular intervals for each course. The marks/grades of these periodical assessments are entered into an internal assessment register so that internal assessment marks can be calculated at the end of the session to be added to the final/major examination marks/grades.
- **External marks register:** It contains the final results of the student. The marks/grades obtained by the student at the end of each semester/academic year is entered in this register for future reference.
- **Reports of the various committee:** As mentioned before in this unit, the nursing college have various operational committees to carry out predefined roles and duties. All the committees conduct the meeting at regular intervals and minutes of each meeting is maintained in this record.

This need not to be necessarily maintained in the form of a book but can be maintained in the form of files with the proper index.

- **Other regulatory and affiliating bodies correspondence:** A Nursing College, for its smooth functioning, has to maintain correspondence and communication with many other agencies, departments, and organizations. The information regarding all the communication has to be formally maintained in the form of respective files of correspondence. The pattern of this filing and record maintenance varies from institution to institution.

Tips to Improve Record Keeping

- Get into the propensity for utilizing real, predictable, precise, objective, and unambiguous patient data.
- Ensure there is a contemplated method of reasoning (proof) for any information recorded.
- Ensure notes are precisely attested with time and date, along with the credentials of the person.
- Write the notes, where conceivable, with the inclusion and comprehension of the patient/bystanders.
- Errors should be remedied by putting a separate line through the inaccurate explanation and attest it with time and date. Do not use corrective fluids as it lacks transparency.
- Follow the SMART model (Specific, Measurable, Achievable, Realistic, and Time-based).
- Write up notes within 24 hours of the occasion. Subsequent modifications are not allowed.

Nursing Reports

Reports are oral or composed data traded between the health professionals in a hospital or similar place. A report is an outline of the activities of the individual or staff and the organization. Reports can be assembled every day, week after week, month to month, once in four months or annually.

Importance/Significance of Reports

- Useful reports spare duplication of exertion and take out the requirement for an examination to learn the certainties of a circumstance.
- Patients get better consideration when reports are intensive and give every single appropriate information.
- Complete reports help in getting all facts, and it provides a sense of security.
- It aides in proficient administration of the ward.

Criteria for Good/Decent Report

- Reports should be made instantly to serve its purpose.
- An excellent report is definite, total, and compact.
- It is to be composed of all appropriate, distinguishing information and incorporated the date and time, the general population concerned, the circumstance, with

proper credentials and attestations of the author of the report.

- Do not add self-perceptions and extra materials.
- Useful oral reports are communicated and shared intriguingly.

Types of Reports

- **Oral reports:** It is essential when the data is for quick use and not for the long term. E.g. The teacher reports another teacher regarding a particular student.
- **Written reports:** Reports are to be composed when the data is to be utilized by numerous faculties, which is pretty much of lasting worth, e.g., daily reports, interdepartmental reports, required by the circumstances, occasions, and conditions.
- **Incident reports:** The teacher who saw the episode or who found the student during the event should document the report. The teacher portrays in brief what happened explicitly. The teacher does not translate or endeavor to clarify the reason for the occurrence. The teacher portrays impartially the students and conditions when the event was found.

Attributes of a Good Report

- Before anything can be composed plainly, it must be clear as far as one could tell.
- Reports, lacking actualities, might be one-sided or useless.
- Conciseness, exactness, and fulfillment are fundamental to great reports.
- It is smarter to compose a few reports than single when there is more than one fundamental subject at which point to report.
- Terminology: Short, straightforward, commonly utilized words for nontechnical reports. Logical terms can be used when issuing statements to professionals.
- Observes mechanics of suitable composition. Use better language and sentences.
- If the report is composed of another person, check/proofread it before signing/marking it.

Roles of Nurse in Records and Reports

The obligations of the Nurse educator in records and reports can be summed as pursues:

- **Fact:** Information about patients and their treatment and care must be practical. A record should contain precise, targeted data about what a nurse has perceived about the patient with her senses.
- **Accuracy:** The record should be trustworthy. Precise data will make certainty among the colleagues.
- **Completeness:** Unfinished data in the record to be avoided. Make sure the entry of complete and thorough data of all the events related to the patient.
- **Currency:** Do not delay the recording/reporting as it creates suspicion of legal complications. A late entry in a register or any other record/report is negligence.

- **Organization:** The supervisor imparts data in a consistent and logical manner so that it is better to comprehend the data by the second person.
- **Confidentiality:** It is the legal, ethical, and moral responsibility of the health professionals to keep the privacy of the patient information.

COMMITTEES

Committees are found in every large organization since it is not always possible for the administrator to manage everything single-handed. A committee is a form of a formal group.

According to dictionary meaning, committee is "a group of people officially delegated to perform a function, such as investigating, considering, reporting, or acting on a matter." And also means a group of people appointed or elected to administer, discuss or make reports concerning a subject on which its members' have authorities to perform a specified service or function.

A committee can be defined as a body of persons appointed to meet an organized basis for the discussion and dealing of matters brought before it. **—LM Prasad**

The committee is defined as a group of persons to whom, as a group, some matter is committed. It involves group decision making. **—Koontz**

Characteristics of Committee

- A committee is a group of persons.
- It has definite jurisdictions, i.e., it deliberates only on matters that are brought before it.
- It can be constituted at any level of organization
- The authority delegated to the committee depends on the nature of the committee.

Purposes of Committees

- **Decision making:** The committee has the responsibility to decide to establish organizational objectives, setting policies, and designing a strategy to guide the nursing activities.
- **Informational:** The committee is constituted to obtain and disseminate the information to implement organizational programs in different departments.
- **Coordination:** The main purpose of the committee is to facilitate the coordination of activities of different departments of the institution.
- **Advisory:** The committee is constituted to have continuous advice from the specialists by the top-level executive.

Type of Committees

- According to authority:
  - **Line committee:** If the authority involves the decision making or carries out managerial function affecting subordinate, it is called as a line committee.

- **Staff committee:** Authority relationship to a superior is advisory in nature.
- According to the delegation of authority:
  - **Formal:** The committees with specifically delegated duties and authorities are called formal committees.
  - **Informal:** The committees without a specific delegation of authority are called an informal committee.
- According to existence:
  - **Permanent:** Usually formal committees are permanent. These committees last until the organization stands.
  - **Temporary:** These committees are constituted for a short duration depending on the purpose of the committee. Once the task is over, the committees are abolished.

Advantages of Committee

- The pooling of knowledge and experience
- Promotes coordination and cooperation
- It encourages a comprehensiveness and democratic approach
- It brings an effective face to face two-way communication
- It is a device or tool for management development
- Avoidance of a desired action or referral of a particular case from one person to other committees for decision making

Disadvantages of Committee

- Delay in execution as it requires collective effort and contribution
- Ineffective decision or wrong decision if the head is not competent
- Increased economical expenditure in the constitution and maintenance of the committee
- Divided responsibility of the group and less significance for the individual decision

Committee Organization

A nursing college will have several committees to coordinate the activities of the college. Committees are organized by the governing body and the principal. These committees are listed below:

- **Academic/curriculum committee:** Plans, organizes and evaluates the overall implementation of the programs. This may be also read with the Board of Studies in a University/Institute. It comprises of the Dean, Principal, Senior faculty members and external subject experts. They meet as and when required to plan and evaluate the academic programs including its implementation, revision, and modifications if any. The Board of Studies will report to the Academic Council of the University to which the institution is affiliated for the instruction and evaluation purpose.
- **Library committee:** The library committee consists of a group of persons who are empowered to do certain jobs relating to library and administration. The library committee includes a chairman, a secretary, members or

a convener or members. The library committee has an enormous power to select the personnel, to acquisition books and journals, responsible for fundraising, etc. The committee members though working closely with the librarian but it has some collective powers to run a library smoothly.

- **Staff welfare committee:** Identifies, communicates and co-ordinates matters concerned to welfare and development of staff.
- **Student welfare committee:** Identifies, communicates and co-ordinates matters concerned to the welfare and development of students.
- **Ethical committee:** Grants ethical clearance to the candidates conducting research in the field of nursing after scrutinizing the problem statement, feasibility, its benefits to the nursing profession and confirmation that the research will be conducted as per the guidelines of ICMR (Indian council of medical research).
- **Mess and hostel committee:** Looking after the affairs of the hostel and associated mess, ensuring the healthy and happy life of the inmates of the hostel, maintaining the discipline of the hostel and so on.
- **Discipline committee:** Plans, develops and displays the rules and regulations to be followed by the students at college, clinical /practice field and hostel. Maintains professional behavior/etiquette among students throughout the course.

- **Anti-ragging committee:** Maintains a ragging free atmosphere in the campus.
- **Sports committee:** Organizing sports events/sports meet for the students. Provision of equipment and facilities for excelling in sports competitions locally and nationally.
- **Grievance redressal cell:** Enhance the efficiency and effectiveness of the institution by prompt addressing to the needs of the staff and students.
- **Student's nurses association:** Encourages professional and recreational meetings and sports to uphold the dignity of the profession.
- **Placement cell:** To provide a better future and to place them in a better job.
- **Alumni association:** Promote and foster professional relationships among the Alumni, the present students, the staff and management.
- **Mentor-Mentee committee:** To provide support in career development for students by the establishment of a variety of mentoring/support arrangements with (an) experienced Fellow(s) whose professional knowledge and management skills will assist career development and provide the opportunity for students to meet their ongoing learning objectives.

The committees consist of faculty members and students. Few vital committees include only faculty members such as Academic Committee (Board of Studies).

 REVIEW QUESTIONS

1. Explain the organizational structure of a college of nursing. What are the types of organizations?
2. Define the curriculum and explain the modes of the curriculum.
3. Explain curriculum planning in detail.
4. Discuss the principles of curriculum development.
5. Explain the steps of curriculum development.
6. Enumerate the factors influencing curriculum development.
7. Explain the models of curriculum and evaluation of the curriculum.
8. Explain the teaching and learning methods in nursing educational institutions.
9. Prepare a sample budget for a nursing educational institution. (Program: BSc Nursing and Intake: 60 students per year)
10. What are the records and reports to be kept and maintained in a nursing educational institution? Explain in detail.
11. What are committees? Explain the purpose and types of committees in nursing college.
12. Enlist the committees constituted in a nursing college along with its function.

Further Readings

1. Banerjee, Shyamal. Principles and Practice of Management. Oxford and IBM Publishing, New Delhi; 2000.
2. Basavanthappa BT. Nursing Administration. 2nd Edition: Jaypee Brothers Medical Publishers (P) Ltd., New Delhi; 2009.
3. Barrett, Jean. Ward Management and Teaching. Konark Publishers, Delhi; 1992.
4. Warren, Stevens, F. Management and Leadership in Nursing. McGraw – Hill Inc, New York; 1978.
5. Alexander et al. Nursing Service Administration. Mosby Publishers, US; 1962.
6. Park K. Preventive, and Social Medicine, 19th Edition: M/s. Banarasidas Bhanot Publishers, Jabalpur; 2007.
7. Basavanthappa BT. Nursing Administration, 1st Edition: Jaypee Brothers Medical Publishers (P) Ltd., New Delhi; 2002.
8. Goel SL. Healthcare System, and Social Medicine, Health Organization and Structure, 1st Volume, Deep and Deep Publishers, New Delhi; 2001
9. Ranga Rao SP. Administration of Primary Health Centers in India, 1st Edition: Mittal Publications, New Delhi; 1993.
10. Lucita M. Nursing: Practice and Public Health Administration. Current Concepts and Trends. B. I. Churchill Living Stone Pvt. Ltd., New Delhi; 2002.
11. Sakharkar BM. Principles of Hospital Administration and Planning, 2nd Edition: Jaypee Brothers Medical Publishers (P) Ltd., New Delhi; 2009.
12. Patricia S Yoder-Wise. Leading and Managing in Nursing. 2nd Edition: Mosby Publication, US; 1999.
13. Bessie L Marquis, Carol J Huston. Leadership Roles and Management Functions in Nursing: Theory and Application. 5th Edition: Lippincott Williams and Wilkins, New York; 2006.
14. Linda Roussel. Management and Leadership for Nurse Administrators. 4th Edition: Jones and Bartlett Publication, USA; 2006.
15. Wehrich H, Koontz H. Management A Global Perspective. 11th Edition: Tata McGraw-Hill Publishing Company, Ltd., New Delhi; 2005.
16. Marquis BL, Huston CJ. Leadership and Management Functions in Nursing- Theory, and Application. 5th Edition: Lippincott Williams and Wilkins, Philadelphia; 2006.
17. Douglass LM. The Effective Nurse: Leader and Manager. 5th Edition: Mosby Publication, US; 1996.
18. Trained Nurses Association of India, Nursing Administration, and Management.
19. Samson Rebecca. Leadership and Management in Nursing Practice and Education 1st Edition: Jaypee Brothers Medical Publishers (P) Ltd., New Delhi; 2009.
20. Kunders GD. Designing for Total Quality in Health Care, Prism Book Pvt. Ltd., Bangalore; 2002.
21. Chandorkar AG. Hospital Administration and Planning. 2nd Edition: Paras Medical Publisher, New Delhi; 2009.
22. Joshi DC, Joshi Mamta. Hospital Administration. 1st Edition: Jaypee Brothers Medical Publishers (P) Ltd., New Delhi; 2009.
23. Eleanor J Sullivan, Philip J Decker. Effective Leadership and Management in Nursing. 4th Edition: Published by Addison Wesely; 2011.
24. Kulkarni GR. Financial Management for Hospital Administration, Jaypee Brothers Medical Publishers (P) Ltd., New Delhi; 2009.

Unit

15

Faculty and Student Selection in Nursing Educational Institutions

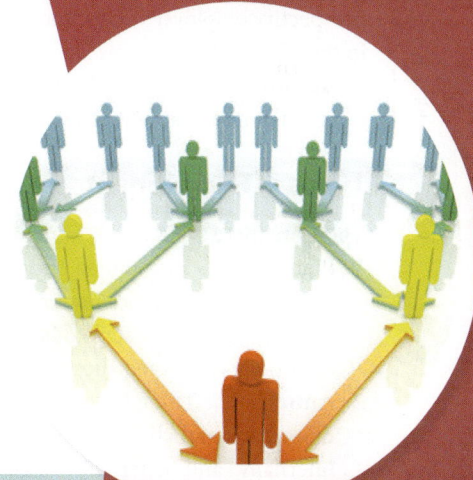

 Unit Outline

- Faculty/Staff Selection, Recruitment, and Placement in the Nursing Educational Institution
- Job Descriptions
- Performance Appraisal
- Faculty/Staff Development
- Continuing Nursing Education
- Faculty/Staff Welfare
- Selection and Admission Procedures
- Placement

FACULTY/STAFF SELECTION, RECRUITMENT, AND PLACEMENT IN THE NURSING EDUCATIONAL INSTITUTION

Recruitment is a vital capacity of organizations, which decides; regardless of whether the required will be accessible at the work spot when an occupation is really to be embraced. It incorporates the procedure and the techniques by which openings/vacancies are projected, published/advertised, applications are received and screened, interviews are directed, and offer of appointments are made.

"Recruitment is defined as the process of searching for prospective employees and stimulating them to apply for a job in the organization."

According to IGNOU Module: "It is a process in which the right person for the right post is procured."

Types of Recruitment

There are three types of recruitment:
1. **Planned:** It is preplanned and is based on the revision of the organizational recruitment policy. E.g., The number of nursing faculty and staff to be recruited for college/school of nursing is planned ahead.
2. **Anticipated:** Though not preplanned, these are expected due trends and challenges faced by the organization both internally and externally. E.g., Enhancement of seats, Addition of programs require additional manpower.
3. **Unexpected:** These are unexpected, and it may arise as a result of the transfer, severe illness of some staff, accidents, etc. E.g., Resignation of an existing employee.

Objectives of Recruitment

- To draw in individuals with multi-dimensional abilities and encounters that suit the present and future organizational strategies.
- To welcome newcomers and outsiders who are talented to lead the organization.
- To implant new blood at all levels of the association.
- To build up an organizational culture that pulls capable individuals into the organization.
- To devise approaches for surveying mental qualities.
- To search out the non-conventional advancement of ability.
- To scan for talents universally and not merely inside the organization.
- To foresee and discover individuals for new positions.

Principles of Recruitment

- Termination and production of any post should be finalized by capable officers.
- Only the empty positions should be filled and neither less nor more should be employed.

- A job profile/work examination should be made before recruitment.
- Procedure for recruitment has to be prepared by experts, it has to be from internal and external sources, and it should be based on set standards and required qualifications.
- Promotion policy has to be set.

Sources of recruitment: The origins of recruitment are:
- **Internal sources:** Internal sources include present employees, employee referrals, a former employee, and previous applicants.
  - **External sources:** It includes Professional or trade associations such as TNAI, Advertisements, Employment exchange, Campus recruitment, Walk-ins, Write-ins, and Talk-ins and Educational Consultants.

Recruitment process/steps: It is aimed at creating a pool of job applicants with the desired qualification by identifying and attracting them. This is carried out in five interconnected stages, i.e.,
- **Planning:** It includes identifying the need for recruitment and other aspects such as the number of posts to be filled.
- **Strategy development:** This involves developing the appropriate method of recruitment.
- **Searching:** This may vary according to the method of recruitment.
- **Screening:** According to the planned strategy, the candidates are screened and finalized.
- **Evaluation and control:** Final stage of offering the order of appointment.

Factors affecting recruitment: All association, regardless of whether vast or little, takes part in recruitment, however, not to a similar degree. This contrasts with:
- The size, area of the association, and the work conditions.
- The impacts of past recruitments which demonstrate the association's capacity to find and keep great performing individuals.
- Working conditions, for example, compensation/salary and advantage bundles offered by the association which may impact turnover and requires future selection.
- The rate of development of the association/organization.
- The level of the regularity of tasks and future development and generation programs.
- Culture, economical and legal factors, etc.

Selection begins when applications are screened in the workforce office. Choosing incorporates meeting, the business' offer, acknowledgment by the candidate, and marking of an agreement or composed offer are the further steps. Those candidates who appear to meet the job prerequisites are sent offer letters and are directed to top them off and send back to the employer for further proceedings. The job application form is a standout amongst the essential part of the job determination procedure. "It is the process of choosing from among applicants the best-qualified individuals, selecting includes interviewing, the employer's offer, acceptance by the applicant, and signing of a contract or written offer."

Steps in Selection of Faculty/Staff

The selection process of faculty and staff for a nursing education institution varies from organization to organization. The selection process carried out in Government, Autonomous and Private organizations are different. The recruitment including the job description and pay structure is also governed by the laws of the land, regulatory bodies, university. A sample process of the selection process of faculty and staff in a college of nursing is explained below.

- **Issue of advertisement:** The administration department issues advertisement in the national and regional newspapers regarding the vacant positions to be filled in the nursing college. The advertisement shall also contain the eligibility of the applicant, payment/salary structure and nature of employment.
- **Issue application forms:** The issue and receipt of application forms is the responsibility of the administration department, and a significant part of the primer work is taken care of by the administrative staff under the supervision of the managerial leader of the school/college. The application forms shall be offline or online based on the preference of the organization and supporting documents to prove the eligibility is also obtained along with the application.
- **Scrutiny of the application forms:** The data contained in the application form and reports got, regarding them, should be deliberately organized and documented. An expert committee review verifies the application and the attached supporting documents.
- **Constitution of selection committee:** A selection panel involving significant members from university, delegates of representations form statutory bodies, members from the governing body of the college, the administrator of the college and the head of the school should be constituted and the applications will be investigated, and after that, the suitable candidates will be chosen.
- **Plan and conduct written examinations if any:** Based on the number of applicants the organization may plan for a written examination to shortlist the number of applicants for interviews.
- **Interview session:** The selection committee conducts the interview as per the pre-planned session and the candidates for the interview are priorly notified regarding the date, time and place of the interview. The interview may also be conducted as a walk-in without the stage of the written examination. The results of the interview such as the selection list of the applicant along with the waiting list are published following the interview. The applicants are also informed about the selection list and the prerequisites of joining.

- **Joining of the organization:** The selected candidates join the organization and submit the joining report. After confirmation of the joining, an introduction, the program is to be directed to make the newly recruited employee mindful of the college structure, clinical training areas, labs, school/college rules, and inn/hostel. The introduction should be given by the senior staff of the school/college of nursing. The introduction program may take three to five days.

Qualification and Experience of Teachers of the College of Nursing

(As per the guidelines of Indian Nursing Council)

Sr. no.	Post, qualification and experience
1.	**Principal cum professor:** Essential Qualification: MSc(N). Experience: MSc(N), PhD(N) having total 15 years experience with MSc(N) out of which 10 years after MSc(N) in collegiate program. PhD(N) is desirable.
2.	**Vice-principal cum professor:** Essential Qualification: MSc(N). **Experience:** MSc(N), having total 12 years experience with MSc(N) out of which 10 years after MSc(N) in collegiate program. PhD(N) is desirable.
3.	**Professor:** Essential Qualification: MSc(N). Experience: MSc(N), having total 12 years experience with MSc(N) out of which 10 years after MSc(N) in collegiate program. PhD(N) is desirable.
4.	**Associate Professor:** MSc(N) with 8 years of experience including 5 years teaching experience PhD(N) is desirable.
5.	**Assistant Professor:** MSc(N) with 3 years teaching experience PhD(N) desirable.
6.	**Tutor:** MSc(N) or BSc(N)/PB BSc(N) with 1 year of experience.

Number of Teaching Faculty Required for Different Nursing Programs

The teaching faculty required for BSc Nursing College based on its intake capacity is as following:

Sr. no.	Designation	BSc Nursing 40–60	BSc Nursing 61–100
1.	Professor cum principal	1	1
2.	Professor cum vice principal	1	1
3.	Professor	0	1
4.	Associate professor	2	4
5.	Assistant professor	3	6
6.	Tutor/clinical instructor	10–18	19–28

The principal is excluded for 1:10 teacher-student ratio norms (Teacher) Tutor student ratio will be 1:10.

(For example, for 40 students intake a minimum number of teachers required is 17 including Principal. The strength of tutors will be 10, and 6 will be as per Sr. no. 02 to 05)

A college running both BSc Nursing (40–60 students) and Post Basic BSc Nursing (20–60 students intake) should have the following number of nursing faculty.

Sr. no.	Designation	BSc Nursing 40–60	PB BSc Nursing 20–60
1.	Professor cum principal	1	
2.	Professor cum vice principal	1	
3.	Professor	0	
4.	Associate professor	2	
5.	Assistant professor	3	2
6.	Tutor/clinical instructor	10–18	2–10

A college running BSc Nursing (40–60 students) and Post Basic BSc Nursing (20–60 students intake) and MSc Nursing (10–25 students including all specialties) should have the following number of nursing faculty.

Sr. no.	Designation	BSc Nursing 40–60	PB BSc Nursing 20–60	MSc(N) 10–25
1	Professor cum principal	1		
2	Professor cum Vice principal	1		
3	Professor	0		1
4	Associate professor	2		1
5	Assistant professor	3	2	3*
6	Tutor/clinical instructor	10–18	2–10	5

*1:10 teacher-student ratio for MSc(N) if BSc(N) is also offered by the institution.

A college running GNM (20–60 students), BSc Nursing (40–60 students) and Post Basic BSc Nursing (20–60 students intake) and MSc Nursing (10–25 students including all specialties) should have the following number nursing faculty.

Sr. no.	Designation	GNM 20–60	BSc Nursing 40–60	PB BSc Nursing 20–60	MSc(N) 10–25
1.	Professor cum principal		1		
2.	Professor cum Vice principal		1		
3.	Professor		0		1
4.	Associate professor		2		1
5.	Assistant professor		3	2	3*
6.	Tutor/clinical instructor	6–18	10–18	2–10	5

A college running ANM (20–60 students), GNM (20–60 students), BSc Nursing (40–60 students) and Post Basic BSc Nursing (20–60 students intake) and MSc Nursing (10–25 students including all specialties) should have the following number of nursing faculty.

Sr. no.	Designation	ANM 20–60	GNM 20–60	BSc Nursing 40–60	PB BSc Nursing 20–60	MSc(N) 10–25
1.	Professor cum principal			1		
2.	Professor cum Vice principal			1		
3.	Professor			0		1
4.	Associate professor			2		1
5.	Assistant professor			3	2	3*
6.	Tutor/clinical instructor	4–12	6–18	10–18	2–10	5

*1:10 teacher-student ratio for MSc(N) if BSc(N) is also offered by the institution.

Some courses/subjects included in the Nursing Program may be taught by externally hired faculty members. The external faculty members cannot be counted with the regular faculty members of the college. The external faculty members should have a postgraduate qualification in the respective discipline with teaching experience in the respective area. List of externally taught subjects are mentioned below:

Sr. no.	Courses/subjects
1.	Microbiology
2.	Biochemistry
3.	Sociology
4.	Biophysics
5.	Psychology
6.	Nutrition
7.	English
8.	Computer
9.	Hindi/Regional language
10.	Any other clinical discipline
11.	Physical education

Other Staff (Minimum Requirements)

In addition to the nursing teaching faculty members, the nursing educational institutions also require a number of non-teaching staff for its smooth functioning. The Indian Nursing Council has suggested the following non-teaching positions for a nursing college. However, the non-teaching posts may vary according to the organizational policy. Few of the services may be outsourced as per the organizational policy. The qualification and experience of the non-teaching staff may be considered in accordance with the norms of the University.

Ministerial	Library	Hostel
• Administrative officer—1 • Office superintendent—1 • PA to principal—1 • Accountant/cashier—1 • Upper division clerk—2 • Lower division clerk—2 • Store keeper—1 • Classroom attendants—2 • **Sanitary staff:** As per the physical space • Security staff as per the requirement • Peons/office attendants—4	• Librarian—2 • Library attendants as per the requirement	• Wardens—2 • Cooks, bearers, as per the requirement sanitary staff • Ayas/peons as per the requirement • Security staff as per the requirement • Gardeners and Dhobi depends on structural facilities (desirable)

JOB DESCRIPTIONS

There is a need for job descriptions because it is learned through some studies that most workers function in a mechanical fashion and are not conscious of the role assigned to them. It has been commented that a lack of knowledge of one's job and functions and that of other team members is one of the reasons for many problems in the functioning of the health team.

Principal (School of Nursing, College of Nursing)

The principal is the academic head of the nursing training institution. The principal will report to the Dean/Director. The principal should make sure that the education and training of nurses are carried out as per the curriculum and norms of the regulating bodies such as Government, INC, SNRC, UGC/University, etc.

Duties and Responsibilities

- Member of the governing council of the institution, Board of Studies, Academic Council, Budget Committee, etc.
- Correspondence with other organizations.
- **Administration:** Plans the aim of the educational programs and makes sure that they are as per the current needs of the society. Identify and meet the needs of the organization. Appraise and preserve the resources of the organization.
- **Organizing:** Discuss and determine the quantity and quality of the teaching faculty, staff, and other human resources. Decide the job description and line of authority/organizational chart for all employees in consideration with their interests and ability. The planning workload of the employees.
- **Directing:** Staff development and welfare activities such as selection, promotion, and retention of staff based on their performance, experience, qualification.
- **Coordinating:** Conduct regular meetings and coordinate academic activities. Maintain effective communication, cooperation, and networking relationship with all concerned departments regionally and nationally.
- **Controlling:** Maintain the quality of education and training. Ensure that all the programs meet the requirements of accreditation agencies.
- **Guiding:** Help and guide the colleagues in performing their tasks. Motivate students in their study, promote research, provide placements, etc.

Vice Principal

- Member of the governing council of the institution, Board of Studies, Academic Council, Budget Committee, etc.
- Performs the roles and responsibilities of the principal in her/his absence.

- **Financial:** Propose a budget and observe/monitor the financial expenditure of the organization in consultation with the principal.
- **Educational:** Collaborate with the principal in recognizing the learning needs of the students. Plan and suggest professional development activities for faculty and students, including in-service education, research, etc.
- **Supervisory:** Supervise the employees, plan academic activities, duty assignments to faculty and staff.
- **Establishment:** Maintain the code of conduct and etiquette of the institution.
- **Interpersonal:** Maintain effective communication, cooperation, and networking relationship with all concerned departments regionally and nationally. Recognize the conflicts among staff and solving the problems.

Professor and Associate Professor

The professor is the Head of the Department and associate professor is the senior faculty of the department. They are accountable for all the academic activities of the concerned department. They perform the following tasks:

- Overall administration of the department.
- Teaching/Instruction.
- Course Planning.
- Ensures the achievement of desirable knowledge, attitude, and skills by the students.
- Evaluate the students at regular intervals.
- Recording and Reporting of all the documents and events pertaining to the activities conducted in the department.
- Investigates methods to improve teaching.
- Provide guidance and counseling to the needy.

Assistant Professor

They perform their tasks under the direction of the HoD and assist the HoD in carrying out the daily functions of the department.

- Recognize the learning needs of the students.
- Help the students in understanding their educational goals and problem-solving skills.
- Assess and monitor the quality of performance and involve in the assessment of the educational curriculum.
- Prepare and maintain all the needed records and reports.
- Evaluate the effectiveness of instruction by appropriate methods.
- Improve one's knowledge and skills through in-service education and other faculty development services.
- Conduct research and utilize its findings.
- Counsel the problems of the students and guide according to their abilities and skills.

Tutor/Clinical Instructor

- Responsible for the planning and implementation of the teaching program.
- Teaching subjects as per the curriculum.
- Overall supervision of clinical teaching programs in hospital/community and another training area.
- Conducting examinations and tests as per the direction.
- Prepare lesson plans and unit plans and other teaching aids.
- Help the students in co-curricular activities.
- Assisting in administration.
- Assist in the maintenance of laboratories, library, and its records.
- Maintains various records.
- Conducting and participating in department meetings.
- Participate in in-service education/continuing education.
- Acts as a Counselor for students.
- Any other responsibility assigned by the Principal.

Librarian

- A librarian should be capable of locating books, cataloging, and classifying books in order.
- Maintain documents like issue register, stock register, complaint register, student register, and staff register.
- Update and display the books of the latest interest.
- Order and subscribe to publications and journals.
- Participate in all kinds of library meetings and conferences.
- Arrange books, journals, and publications according to date and year.

Thus duties and responsibilities are imperative that the role of each category of health workforce should be clarified through providing a written job description, training, and through the participative approach.

PERFORMANCE APPRAISAL

It implies the orderly assessment of the execution of an employee by his reporting authority. It helps in the evaluation of the quality and quantity of work in a given setting. Performance is understood as a measurement of one's activity in a particular field, and the appraisal reveals the demand satisfaction of the job. It acts as a record for apprentices and regular employees and is helpful in deciding promotions, transfer or demotions, increments, and bonuses.

Irancerich, Donnelly, and Gibson identified five possible parties who could evaluate or rate another person. They are:

- Supervisor
- Peers
- Raters inside the organizational environment
- Subordinates
- Raters outside the organizational environment

Definitions

Performance appraisal is the systematic, periodic and an impartial rating of an employee's excellence in the matters pertaining to his present job and his potential for a better job.

—**Flippo**

It is the method of evaluating the behavior of employees of the individual with regard to his or her performance on the job and his or her potential for development. —**Beach DS**

Performance appraisal is a systematic description of an employee's job-relevant strengths and weaknesses.

—**Cascio Wayne**

Characteristics of an Effective Appraisal System

A performance appraisal system should be effective as several crucial decisions are made on the basis of score or rating given by the appraiser, which in turn, is heavily based on the appraisal system. So an appraisal to be effective should possess the following essential characteristics:

- **Reliability and validity:** The appraisal system should provide consistent, reliable and valid information and data, which can be used to defend the organization-even in legal challenges.
- **Job relatedness:** The appraisal system should measure the performance and provide information in job-related activities/areas.
- **Standardization:** Appraisal forms, procedures, administration of techniques, ratings, should be standardized as appraisal decisions affect all employees of the group.
- **Practical viability:** The techniques should be practically viable to administer, possible to implement and economical to undertake continuously.
- **Legal sanction:** Appraisals must meet the laws of the land. They must comply with provisions of various statutes relating to labor.
- **Training to appraisers:** Because the appraisal is important and sometimes difficult, it would be useful to provide training appraisers. Some ideas on documenting, rating, conducting appraisal interviews should be provided.
- **Open communication:** A good appraisal system provides the needed feedback on a continuing basis. The appraisal interviews should permit both parties to learn about the gaps and prepare themselves for the future.
- **Employee access to results:** Employees should know the rules of the game. They should receive adequate feedback on their performance. If performance appraisals are meant for improving employee performance, then withholding appraisal result would not serve any purpose. Permitting employees to review the results of their appraisal allows them to detect any errors that may have been made.

Purposes/Importance

- It gives reinforcement information to administrative plans concerning pay norms, promotions, transfers, or selection/termination of service.
- It acts as an eligibility platform for recruitment and other HR services.
- It helps with employee motivation by providing the correct feedback.
- It helps in recognizing employee objectives and desires to acquaint them with organizational policies and objectives.
- To accept and reward the workers for their doings.
- To enhance correspondence among different levels of management which fosters the collective achievement of organizational objectives.
- To reserve/select persons for the supervisory and higher management designations to meet the organizational objectives.

Further, the purpose of performance appraisal may be categorized as follows:

- For employees
  - It is one of the criteria for promotion
  - It is a measurement of job performance
  - It helps in improving the job of the employees
  - It helps to identify training needs and planning for training programs.
  - It is helpful in the planning and administration of compensation for employees.
  - It facilitates feedback, self-examination, and maintains control in the organization.
- For organization
  - Measurement of organizational objectives.
  - Measurement of work standards.
  - It generates information regarding the employees and their personal planning.
  - It reduces the grievances of the employee.
  - It helps in manpower management.
- Specific uses
  - It facilitates promotion decisions.
  - It is helpful to plan and analyze the training and development programs.
  - Evaluation of supervisors and managers.
  - It helps in performance feedback and personal development.

Principles

- A single worker is evaluated by two persons, and both reports are analyzed for a precise result.
- It should be done by the immediate superiors.
- Useful performance appraisal is obtained by an ongoing and individual observation of a worker.
- The development of an independent department for performance appraisal is appreciable.

- The result of the appraisal should be shared with the concerned worker. The person can comprehend the position where he stands and where he should go.
- The benefits of a worker should be perceived, and less focus is given to the shortcomings but mentioned.
- The administration must be credible in terms of appraisal of its workers.

Approaches to Performance Appraisal

- **Traditional approach:** The traditional approach is based on past performance. The main purpose is to determine and justify the salary and perks of the employees and not considered for development purposes. This is to judge the organizational performance as a whole by the past performance of its employees.
- **Modern approach:** The purpose of performance appraisal has now been taken for development purposes, for taking the corrective actions timely so that the organizational goals can be achieved within the time frame and also help in re-planning. It is more formal and structured so that training needs can be identified and accordingly the training programs can be planned. Hence, the modern approach is future-oriented.

Process of Performance Appraisal

Performance appraisal is planned, developed and implemented through a series of steps. They are as:

- **Establish performance standards:** Appraisal systems require performance standards that serve as a benchmark against which performance is measured. To be useful, standards should be related to the desired results of each job. The performance standard should be clear to both appraiser and the appraise. Performance standards should be written down after a thorough analysis of the job. They must be measurable within a short period of time.
- **Communicating the standard:** Performance appraisal involves at least two parties, the appraiser and the appraisee. The appraiser should prepare job descriptions clearly, help appraise to set his goals and targets, analyze results objectively. Performance standards must be communicated to appraisee clearly.
- **Measure actual performance:** After the performance standard is set and accepted, the next step is to measure actual performance. This requires the use of dependable performance measures to be helpful and must be easy to use, reliable, and report on the critical behaviors that determine performance. Four common sources of information which are generally used by managers regarding how to measure actual performance are personal observation, statistical reports, an oral report, and written report.
- **Compare actual performance with standards and discuss the appraisal:** Actual performance may be better than expected and sometimes it may go off the track. Whatever

the consequences, there is a way to communicate and discuss the outcome. The assessment of another person's contribution and ability is not an easy task. It has serious emotional overtones as it may affect the self-esteem of the employee.

- **Taking corrective action, if necessary:** Corrective action is of two types: one puts out the fires immediately, while the other destroys the root of the problem permanently. Immediate action sets things right and gets things back on track whereas the basic corrective action gets to the source of deviation and seeks to adjust the difference permanently.

Methods of Performance Appraisal

There are numerous sorts of performance appraisal accessible, and they can use any method. Generally, there are two approaches to assessment; one is trait-oriented, and the other one is result-oriented. The traits approach evaluates the conduct and attitudes of the worker, while the other one focuses only on the results of the tasks assigned to the worker. The methods of performance appraisal are categorized as:

- **Individual evaluation methods:** This method is mostly used in government organizations. This is one of the old and traditional methods of evaluating the employees. The mechanisms are:
  - **Essay appraisal method:** Under this, the rater expresses in detail, the employee's strong and weak points. The suggestions for improvement are also mentioned.
  - **Critical incidence technique:** Under this method, the rater rates the employee based on the critical events that have taken place in the past and brief about positive and negative points of the employee. It is a rating method wherein rating is done for all the incidents about a particular employee that has happened during a specific period. The incidences might have occurred due to the ability/disability of the employee based on the nature of incidents.
  - **Checklists and weighted checklists:** A checklist is a set of descriptive statements about the employee and the rater has marked it accordingly. The assessment of the capacity of a worker through finding solutions to various inquiries is known as a checklist. These inquiries/questions are identified with the conduct of a worker.
  - **Graphic rating scales:** The appraisee marks the quantity and quality of the employee based on a particular trait. The trait may be predefined. The rater has the option to rate the employee on a scale-like Likert's scale.
  - **Behaviourally anchored rating scales:** BARS are systematically developed checklist using critical incidents in combination with graphic rating scales. It consists of predetermined statements of job performance and behavior based on critical incidents. They are time-consuming and costly to construct.

- **Management by objectives:** As already discussed in one fo the previous units, here the employee and employer sit together to set the objectives of the organization. The evaluation of the employee is based on the attainment of mutually set objectives.
- **Multiple person evaluation methods.**
  - **Ranking strategy:** It is the simplest and oldest type of performance appraisal. Here a worker is ranked/positioned against the other in the same group. In a group of 10 workers, the best performer is placed under the first rank, and the least performer is placed under the tenth rank.
  - **Paired comparison method:** This method is impractical in a large organization. Here the evaluator compares an employee against all his colleagues, and marking is done for favorable parameters upon which the appraisal is done. The evaluator repeats this exercise with each employee individually, and this is followed by the final tabulation and summary. At long last, a worker who gets the most extreme ticks is the best.
  - **Forced distribution strategy:** The evaluation is done in a group, and it is suitable for large organizations. Here the traits are not assessed; rather, the results are focused. A group of workers is selected by the supervisor/evaluator, and they are categorized into few subgroups based on outcomes such as very good, good, average, and below average. The number of subsets may be increased or decreased as per the requirement.
  - **Grading:** It also follows the moreover similar criteria of forced distribution method. Here the traits and results are assessed. A group of workers is selected by the supervisor/evaluator, and they are categorized into few subgroups based on attributes as well as consequences such as very good, good, average, and below average. The number of subsets may be increased or decreased as per the requirement.
- **Other methods:**
  - **Assessment centers:** This is a system or organization, where the assessment of many employees is done by various experts using the various techniques. The methods include simulation exercises, role play and so on.
  - **Group appraisal method:** Here the appraisal is done by many appraisers including the immediate superior. The group may use different techniques for appraisal. This method helps in the elimination of personal bias.
  - **Field review method:** Here the employee is evaluated by a different person than the superior. The appraiser interacts with the supervisor and employee and makes the report.
  - **360-degree appraisal:** This system is also known as multi-rater feedback. A 360-degree appraisal is a type of employee performance review in which subordinates, co-workers, and managers all anonymously rate the employee. This information is then incorporated into that person's performance review. The 360-degree performance appraisal system is an advanced kind of appraisal that is used by many organizations where the performance of the employee is judged using the review of around 7–12 people. These people are working with the employee and they share some of their work environment. The feedback is gathered in the form of reviews in terms of the competencies of the employee. The employee himself or herself also takes part in this appraisal with the help of self-assessment. The 360-degree performance appraisal system is a way to improve the understanding of the strength and weaknesses of the employee with the help of creative feedback forms.

Essentials of Good Appraisal System

- **Ease of understanding:** If an appraisal system is too complicated or too time-consuming, it may be grounded by its dead weight of complications, which nobody but only the experts understand.
- **Support of line workers:** If the line workers think that the system is too ambitious or unrealistic or that has been imposed on them by ivory-towered, staff or consultants who have no comprehension of the actual demands on the time of line workers, they will resent it.
- **Suitability to the operations and structure:** A system may function exceptionally well at an organization whose activities are compact.
- **Validity and reliability:** The efficacy of rating is the degree to which the system indeed indicates the intrinsic merit of the employees. Reliability refers to the consistency of the ratings.

Guidelines for Nurse Manager for Conducting Appraisal

The objective of a personal interview is to evaluate the past, present, and future potential of an individual. The following points are general guidelines for the nurse manager:

- Establish a friendly atmosphere by selecting the right time and place for the interview. Be sure the interview will be free of interruptions.
- Ensure freedom from a work assignment. Arrange for coverage during the time of the meeting. Begin and end the session on time.
- Establish rapport. A few brief chit-chats before the actual interview.
- Let the individual talk first. Include all the important issues in the discussion. Be alert and present criticism carefully. Never combine positive and negative comments and use the guidance approach. Use a concerned tone of voice. Discuss the work never the worker.

- Make a final overall judgment about the individual progress, as well as any recommendations on the evaluation form.
- Let the individual sign the report and explain that the signatures do not necessarily signify that she/he agrees with the content, but it indicates that the employee has seen the appraisal. If an employee refuse to sign the report, then it may also be recorded in the report with proper initial.

Limitations of Performance Appraisal

- The performance appraisal will be influenced by the familiarity of the employee with the employer.
- If the supervisor is not capable of the appraisal, then the employee cannot be evaluated.
- Some characteristics of a worker cannot be effortlessly evaluated through any assessment strategy.
- A manager may assess a worker to be great to make the employee happy.
- The individual difference among managers influences performance appraisal.

Potential Problems in Performance Appraisal

- **Leniency error:** The inclination of an administrator to overrate staff work.
- **Recency error:** The inclination of an administrator to rate a worker dependent on ongoing occasions as opposed to over the whole assessment time frame.
- **Halo error:** The inability to separate among different parameters of performance appraisal during its execution.
- **Horn Effect:** A tendency to rate another under a negative attitude or drive.
- **Ambiguous evaluation:** The propensity of evaluators to put vague remarks on the rating scale.

Performance Evaluation Report

Employee reviews and appraisals are some of the hardest meetings to have, and writing the report can create conflict or fear. Rather than being a manager who instills negative feelings in his employees, it can be written in such a way that the employee feels prepared to meet new challenges or fix current issues.

- **Step 1:** Decide on the criteria for review. Any manager that goes into a review completely subjective will be respected less, and all business notes that many employees already find written reviews to be "artificial and unfair." A good idea is to think about the role of the employee under review, create categories regarding that role (punctuality, work ethic, ability to meet deadlines, etc.) and use a numeric scale to rate the employee's effectiveness.
- **Step 2:** Prepare a report based on current conditions. In other words, how the employee is currently performing.

Rehashing the first few weeks of the employee's work history, often the most difficult and awkward will make the employee feel despondent and unmotivated. Compliment the ways the employee is contributing, note where she can perform better, and recommend ways that the employee can contribute further in the future.

- **Step 3:** Evaluate based on your own observations, not hearsay. Office gossip is not an accurate indicator of an employee's performance. For instance, saying, "I hear that many of the employees see you with personal email sites open," would cause the employee to feel upset and vulnerable. Only bring up a point if you have witnessed it yourself.
- **Step 4:** Use specific examples for your employee review. In any observation whether positive or negative be sure to have an example to back it up. For instance, if you want the employee to note his punctuality, say, "I appreciate the days you make it into the office by 8:30. Perhaps if you are going to be later, you could give a phone call." Employees will not grow unless they can understand what they did right or wrong in a specific scenario.
- **Step 5:** Encourage the employee under review to indicate the goals for the next year. This type of positive reinforcement makes the manager-worker relationship feel more reciprocal and motivates the employee to achieve more than she already has. Ask, "What do you feel you are capable of adding on to your duties?" or recommend a new task yourself, "I think that you are ready to move into increased client invoicing responsibility."

FACULTY/ STAFF DEVELOPMENT

Staff development alludes to all preparation and training given to selected and interested workers to enhance their abilities, attitude, and skills. It incorporates formal or casual education and training for an employee or a group of employees. It comprises different activities like in-service education, job orientation, continuing education, etc. Additionally, events such as attending nursing/medical rounds, observational visits to other health care organizations, professional workshops, conferences, etc., also help in professional development.

It is the procedure coordinated towards the individual and expert development of nurses and other workforce while they are working in any health care organization. Staff advancement and development program helps in refreshing the learning and routine of nurses and other employees. It applies to all the fields of professional practice.

Definition: Staff development refers to all training and education provided by an employee to improve the professional and personal knowledge, skills, and attitude of vested employees.

Philosophy of Staff Development

The department of continuing education is an essential part of the nursing division and adopts the philosophy of the division. It believes in the following:

- The primary goal of the health care agency is the achievement of high-quality health care for the people who use the agency's services.
- Focus on the development of all employees, including all nurses employed by the health care agency for the enhancement of nursing care.
- Educational activities should be designed and implemented to promote a high standard of safe, competent nursing practice.
- The educational environment should be non-threatening and should acknowledge the individuality of its learners.
- Teaching and learning is a dynamic, collaborative, shared process between teacher and learner.

Need for Staff Development

- Staff development helps to face social change through scientific advancement.
- It brings changes and helps in improving one's skills and knowledge.
- Professionals such as nurses get a direct opportunity to acquire and update knowledge and skill regarding patient care, new machinery, and other practice modules. The staff development program helps the nurse in overall updating skills, expertise and it contributes to modifying attitudes, values, and ideas that are essential to provide high-quality nursing care.
- It helps to meet the job-related learning needs of the nurse – (E.g., continuing education, in-service education, extramural education, and post-basic education).
- It also helps to bridge the gap between theory and practice. All graduate nurses possess sound knowledge regarding nursing science, but a staff development program will help in implementing this knowledge in regular patient care.
- It enables nurses to achieve personal or professional development, e.g., promotion.
- To prepare for future tasks or trends.

In-service education

Orientation

Skill training

Continuing education

Leadership training

Principles Involved in Staff Development

- Activities must be on the base of the needs and interests of employees and organizations.
- Learning is unique, based on motivation, and it is a blend of practice and theory.
- Learning is an internal, personal, and emotional process.
- Learning involves changes in behavior.

- The learner should be encouraged to contribute to the learning process.
- A problem-solving approach is well suited because; active learning takes place when there is a need/problem.
- The positive reward is sufficient.
- It is based on educational psychology, and it must fulfill the learning requirements of the individual.
- Learning is an active process, i.e., teacher and learner should be enthusiastic in learning.
- Teaching must satisfy the learning needs of an individual.
- Use a variety of sources for learning as adult learners have a wide range of previous experience.

Importance of Staff Development

- It is focused on developing nursing skills and knowledge.
- It introduces employees to new situations and gives them an orientation into the organization's philosophy.
- It provides job-related counseling, which improves the professional growth of employees.
- It provides learning experiences in work set up; it refines and develops new skills and knowledge related to job performance.
- It is planned and organized around learning experiences in a variety of settings.
- It reduces staff turnover and absenteeism.

Types of Staff Development Programs

Staff development programs may be categorized as formal and informal or individual and group. The following activities are usually conducted.

- **Induction training (3 days):** It is a traditional prologue to the philosophy, policies, terms of conditions given to every employee amid her or his initial few days of work to guarantee his or her understanding of institutional philosophy, objectives, and standards.
- **Job orientation (2–24 weeks):** The process of familiarizing the newly recruited individuals with occupation obligations, work environment, customers, and collaborators.
- **Skill training program:** Skill preparation might be a manual to improve the situation of individuals or their aptitude in managing and functioning with recipients of care. Through this, the nurses learn knowledge, attitude, and skill of changing strategies and new procedures. Frequently it is the continuation of the orientation program.
- **In-service education (2–8 hours):** It is an arranged and preplanned training and education method offered in the working environment and firmly related to benefit to assist the individual with performing all the more adequately as an individual and as a specialist.
- **Continuing education:** It is aimed to upgrade the professional qualification of the employees. It is formal full-time training for existing employees.

- **Extramural education:** It is university-based education with a combination of work at home. It is synonymical to distance learning. It is a society based instruction coordinated towards meeting the activity related to adapting the needs of the nurse and other workforce. In another term, it is an education program past the limit of the predetermined course.

Other Activities of Staff Development

- Attending the medical/clinical and nursing rounds.
- Observing other competing health care organizations for their mode of patient care.
- Attend proficient workshops, seminars, and conferences, present scientific papers.
- Make a habit of reading journals and other recent scientific articles related to professional practice and share the same with fellow workers.

Factors Influencing Staff Development Program in an Organization

- Philosophy and policies of the organization and that of the nursing experts in the organization.
- Human and material assets inside the organization.
- Environmental and physical infrastructure, including the financial ability of the organization.

Advantages of Staff Development

For the workers:

- This leads to enhanced proficient practice.
- Aids in refreshing information and abilities at all dimensions of association.
- Keep the nurse side by the side of the most recent patterns and advancements in the system of practice.
- Equips the nurses with the learning of flow research and advancements.

For the organizations/employer:

- Maintain the enthusiasm of the nurses and develop intrigue and employment fulfillment among the staff.
- Develops autonomy and accountability among nurses.
- Creates a proper situation and cool-headed choices as well as utilizing critical thinking approaches to acclimate to change.
- Aids in creating administration abilities, inspiration, and better dispositions.
- Aids in empowering and accomplishing self-improvement and fearlessness.

Roles and Functions of Administrator/Manager in Staff Development

Roles: He/she

- Applies adult learning principles when helping employees learn new skills or information.

- Uses teaching techniques that empower staff.
- Sensitive to the learning deficits of the staff and creatively minimize these difficulties.
- Prepare employees readily regarding knowledge and skill deficits.
- Actively seeks out teaching opportunities.
- Frequently assess the learning needs of the unit.

Functions

- Works with the reduction department to delineate shared individual responsibility.
- Ensures that all staff is competent for roles assigned.
- Ensure that there are adequate resources for staff development.
- Assumes responsibly for quality and fiscal control of staff development.
- Provides input in formulating staff development policies.

Evaluation of Staff Development

"Evaluation is the process of finding out how the development or training process has affected the individual, team, and the organization."

Types of Evaluation

Formative assessment: It is focused on the modification and improvement of the training program. It is usually performed at regular intervals. The feedback and comments are obtained from the participants, which is further analyzed for the fine-tuning of the plan, including the mid-course modifications if necessary. It helps in meeting the expectations of the participants. It may be used regularly.

Summative assessment: It is to decide the general adequacy of the training program. A summative assessment is done at the finish of the program. It is gathered at three dimensions: instructor practice, institutional changes, and the learning outcome of the participants.

Levels of Evaluation

Kirkpatrick suggested guidelines for the evaluation of educational training programs in 1994. Primarily it was developed for assessing the business/industry related training programs. Nowadays, its components make the broader base of all evaluation of adult training programs. It comprises of four stages of evaluation.

Reaction: It mainly focuses on the happiness index and the response by the participants towards the professional training activity. Usually, the participants express a positive reaction provided, their learning objectives are met, and the information gained has brought behavioral changes in them.

Learning: It is the measurement of knowledge, attitude, and practice (KAP) that the participants have gained through the training program. The behavioral changes in the participants are based on these learning objectives.

Behavior: It is the assessment of the extent to which the behavior is changed for the participants as well as the instructor.

Results: It takes into account the outcome of the entire training program. It answers questions such as What the participants have gained? and what the instructor has achieved? Learning is always a two-way process.

Employee Evaluation Report

Employee reviews and appraisals are the hardest tasks for a Manager. Often, an employee evaluation report becomes a reason for developing ill feelings among employees. It should be prepared in such a way to promote the employees to face challenges while rectifying the existing issues.

Characteristics of the Appraisal Report

- Is to be written jointly by the nurse manager and staff nurse.
- It should be reliable.
- It should be valid and accurate.
- Should show progress made by the staff nurse.
- Giving illustrations to substantiate value judgments.
- Any improvements are to be noted.

Instructions for Writing an Evaluation Report

Step 1: The Nurse Manager should decide on criteria for reviewing. Most of the time, the employee finds written reviews as artificial and unfair. It is good to create categories for evaluation, such as punctuality, work ethics, etc.

Step 2: The report should be grounded on the current working conditions. Preparing an employee evaluation report based on the beginning period of work where the employee had a hard time will make the employee demotivated. The employee also will develop an unhealthy attitude.

Step 3: The evaluation should be based on accurate observations, not on office gossips/hearsay and third party information. Those aspects that are witnessed and observed by the employer/evaluator should be considered, and if not, the employee will become vulnerable and upset.

Step 4: All observations, regardless it is positive or negative, should be backed up by compelling supporting examples. This promotes employee realization of their mistakes and supports healthy behavior. It also helps in avoiding biased observations.

Step 5: The employees should always be encouraged to express their future goals. This motivates the employee and also helps in maintaining the warmth of the manager-employee relationship.

CONTINUING NURSING EDUCATION

"Continuing education of health workers includes the experiences after initial training which help health care personnel to maintain and improve existing and acquire new competencies relevant to the performance of their responsibilities. Appropriate continuing nursing education (CNE) should reflect community needs in health and lead to planned improvements in the health of the community".

Features of CNE

- Unified approach
- Relationships with other systems
- Comprehensiveness
- Accessibility for woman health workers
- Integration with the management process
- Analysis of needs as a basis for learning continuity
- Internally coordinated
- Relevance in planning
- Credibility and economic
- Appropriateness in implementation

Need for CNE

- Safe and effective nursing care.
- Meet the need of the population.
- Update the knowledge.
- Career advancement.
- Acquire specialized skills of personnel and meet technologic adjuncts.
- Prepare in administrative and leadership positions.
- Shape their destiny.

Functions of CNE

- To meet the health needs and public expectations.
- To develop the practicing abilities of the nurse.
- Recruitment function.
- Recognize gaps in their knowledge.
- To improve the communication between the participants, faculty, community, and health sector.
- To test the participants' ability to do formal academic study.
- To shape or support university educational policies and practices.
- To ensure the quality of education.
- To grant budget for extension studies.
- To maintain academic standards.
- To meet educational requirements.

Role of Educator in CNE

- Guide and counselor to the learner.
- An arranger and organizer of learning experiences.
- Motivator and an encourager of students/learners.

- Evaluator of programs.
- Involving resources experts for teaching the students.
- Providing instructional materials.
- Select and evaluate materials prepared by others.
- Administrative role (planning, directing, budgeting and evaluation).
- Public relations role to change the image of nursing and in recognizing the contributions and potentials of nurses.

Principles of CNE

- Provision for school and nursing faculty involvement in planning and teaching the continuing nursing education courses tends to maintain high educational standards for the program.
- Adequate staff is essential to planning, implementing and evaluating a program that is based on learning needs and which has an impact on the quality of nursing care provided.
- An advisory committee has to be appointed, which includes: Faculty members from a variety of areas of nursing practice, Directors of hospital nursing services, Representatives from the state licensing authority, health department and voluntary agencies.
- The community may serve as a liaison between the school of nursing and the health community and fulfill a communication and public relations function for the university.
- Continuing nursing education program may be decentralized or centralized.

FACULTY/STAFF WELFARE

Employee welfare is a comprehensive term including various services, facilities, and amenities provided to employees for their betterment. It generally includes those items of welfare that is provided by statutory provisions or required by the customs of the industry or the expectations of employees from the contract of service from the employers. The basic purpose is to improve the lives of the working class. The purpose of providing welfare amenities is to bring about the development of the whole personality of the worker-his social, psychological, economic, moral, cultural and intellectual development to make him a good worker, a good citizen and a good member of the family. Employee welfare is a dynamic concept. These facilities may be provided voluntarily by progressive and enlightened entrepreneurs from their side out of their realization of social responsibility towards labor, or statutory provisions may compel them to make these facilities available, or these may be undertaken by the government or trade unions if they have the necessary funds for the purpose. Employee welfare measures are also known as fringe benefits and services. 'Labor Welfare' is a very broad term, covering social security and such other activities as medical aid, crèches, canteens, recreation, housing, adult education, arrangements for the transport of labor to and from the workplace.

Meaning and Definition

Employee welfare means, "the efforts to make life worth living for workmen." According to Todd, "employee welfare means anything done for the comfort and improvement, intellectual or social, of the employees over and above the wages paid which is not a necessity of the industry."

The objectives of employee welfare are: Employee welfare is in the interest of the employee, the employer and the society as a whole. The objectives are:

- It improves the loyalty and morale of the employees.
- It reduces labor turnover and absenteeism.
- Welfare measures help to improve the goodwill and public image of the enterprise.
- It helps to improve industrial relations and industrial peace.
- It helps to improve employee productivity.

Agencies of Employee Welfare

- **Central government:** The central government has made elaborate provisions for the health, safety and welfare under Factories Act 1948, and Mines Act 1952. These acts provide for canteens, crèches, restrooms, shelters, etc.
- **State government:** Government in different states and Union Territories provide welfare facilities to workers. The state government prescribes rules for the welfare of the workers and ensures compliance with the provisions under various labor laws.
- **Employers:** Employers in India, in general, looked upon welfare work as fruitless and barren though some of them indeed had done pioneering work.
- **Trade unions:** In India, trade unions have done little for the welfare of workers. But few sound and strong unions have been pioneering in this respect. E.g., the Ahmedabad textiles labor association and the Mazdoor Sabha, Kanpur.
- **Other agencies:** Some philanthropic, charitable and social service organizations like - Seva Sadan Society, YMCA, etc.

Types of Employee Welfare

- **Intramural:** These are provided within the organization like:
  - Canteen
  - Restrooms
  - Crèches
  - Uniform
  - Drinking water
  - Washing and bathing facilities
  - Provision of safety measures like fencing, and covering machines
  - Fire extinguishers
  - Provision of Pension, Provident Fund, Fringe benefits

- **Extramural:** These are provided outside the organization like:
  - Housing
  - Education
  - Child welfare
  - Leave travel facilities
  - Interest-free loans
  - Workers cooperative stores
  - Vocational guidance
- **Statutory welfare work:** Comprising the legal provisions in various pieces of labor legislation.
- **Voluntary welfare work:** Includes those activities which are undertaken by employers for their voluntary work. Different ways of Social Security Provision in India:
  - **Social insurance:** The common fund is established with periodical contributions from workers out of which all benefits in terms of cash or kind are paid. The employers and state prove a major portion of finances. Benefits such as PF, Group Insurance, etc are offered.
  - **Social assistance:** Benefits are offered to persons of small means by government out of its general revenues. E.g., Old age pension, Social Security Employee Welfare, Medical care benefit, Maternity benefit, Accident benefit, Survivor's benefit and so on.

Role of Management in Employee Welfare

- Organizations provide welfare facilities to their employees to keep their motivation levels high. The employee welfare schemes can be classified into two categories, viz. statutory and non-statutory welfare schemes.
- The statutory schemes are those schemes that are compulsory to provide by an organization as compliance with the laws governing employee health and safety. These include provisions provided in industrial acts. The statutory welfare schemes include drinking water, facilities for sitting, first aid appliances, canteen facilities, spittoons, lighting.
- The non-statutory schemes differ from organization to organization and from industry to industry. It includes personal health care, flexi-time, employee assistance programs. Various assistant programs are arranged like external counseling service so that employees or members of their immediate family can get counseling on various matters.

Impact of Welfare on Productivity

- The welfare measures aimed at integrating the socio-psychological needs of employees, the unique requirements of a particular technology, the structure and processes of the organization and the existing sociocultural environment.

- It creates a culture of work commitment in organizations and society which ensures higher productivity and greater job satisfaction to the employees.
- Due to the welfare measures, the employees feel that the management is interested in taking care of the employees that result in the sincerity, commitment, and loyalty of the employees towards the organization.
- The employees work with full enthusiasm and energetic behavior which results in the increase in production and ultimately the increased profit.

SELECTION AND ADMISSION PROCEDURES

(As per the norms of INC)

- Eligibility criteria for ANM program:
  - The minimum age for admission shall be 17 years on or before 31st December of the year in which admission is sought.
  - The maximum age for admission shall be 35 years.
  - The minimum educational requirements shall be 10 + 2 in Arts and English Core/English Elective or Science or Healthcare Science - Vocational stream ONLY passing out from recognized Board.
  - The student shall be medically fit.
  - Students qualified in 10+2 Arts or Science examinations conducted by the National Institute of Open School.
- Eligibility criteria for the GNM program:
  - Minimum and Maximum age for admission will be 17 and 35 years. There is no age bar for ANM/LHV.
  - Minimum education: 10+2 class passed preferably Science (PCB) and English with an aggregate of 40% marks. 10+2 in Arts and English Core/English Elective or Healthcare Science - Vocational stream ONLY, passing out from recognized Board under AISSCE/CBSE/ICSE/SSCE/HSCE or other equivalent Board with 40% marks.
  - Registered as ANM with State Nursing Registration Council.
  - The student shall be medically fit.
- Eligibility criteria for BSc(N) program:
  - The minimum age for admission shall be 17 years on 31st December of the year in which admission is sought.
  - Minimum education: 10+2 class passed with Science (PCB) and English Core/English Elective with an aggregate of 45% marks from the recognized Board under AISSCE/CBSE/ICSE/SSCE/HSCE or other equivalent Board.
  - The student shall be medically fit.
  - Students appearing in 10+2 examination in Science conducted by National Institute of Open School with 45% marks.

- Eligibility criteria for PB BSc(N) program
  - GNM passed from a recognized institution.
  - Candidate should be a registered nurse in the state nursing council.
  - The student shall be medically fit.
- Eligibility criteria for MSc(N) program
  - BSc Nursing (Basic or Post Basic) passed from a recognized institution. One year of experience is required for Basic BSc Nursing students.
  - Candidate should be a registered nurse in the state nursing council.
  - The student shall be medically fit.

PLACEMENT

It is a credit-bearing element of a degree course, and all placements are discretionary. On the off chance that a student quits a placement or there is no placement facility accessible, it implies placement is not ensured. Placement is characterized as the condition of being set or orchestrated.

Placement is a process of assigning a specific job to each of the selected candidates. It involves assigning a specific rank and responsibility to an individual. It implies matching the requirements of a job with the qualifications of the candidate. Placement is understood as assigning jobs to the selected candidates. Assigning jobs to employees may involve a new job or a different job. Thus, placement may include the initial assignment of a job to a new employee, on transfer, promotion or demotion of the present employees. Placement involves assigning a specific job to each one of the selected candidates. However, placement is not so simple as it looks. Instead, it involves striking a fit between the requirements of a job and the qualifications of a candidate.

Definitions

Placement may be defined as "the determination of the job to which an accepted candidate is to be assigned, and his assignment to that job. It is a matching of what the supervisor has reason to think he can do with the job demands (job requirements): it is a matching of what he imposes (in strain, working conditions)," and what he offers in the form of payroll, companionship with others, promotional possibilities, etc.

Proper placement of a worker reduces employee turnover, absenteeism and accident rates, and improves morale.

"Placement refers to the allocations of people to the job. It includes the initial assignment of new employees and promotion transfer or demotion of present employees."

Placement can also be defined as the internal filling of vacancies as distinguished from external recruitment. Placement is a process of assigning a specific job to each of the selected candidates. It involves assigning a specific rank and responsibility to an individual. It implies matching the requirements of a job with the qualifications of the candidate.

Significance of Placement

- It improves employee morale.
- It helps in reducing employee turnover.
- It helps in reducing absenteeism.
- It helps in reducing accident rates.
- It avoids the misfit between the candidate and the job.
- It helps the candidate to work as per the predetermined objectives of the organization.

Placement Team/Cell

The team of Placement Cell comprises a Chairperson, Coordinator, four faculty/trainers each with desirable knowledge and qualification of the placement area and few student representatives. The Placement Cell is constituted in all educational organizations to foster the placement of passing out students. This team will bolster the young aspirants all through the preparation of the placement process.

Problems of Placement

The difficulty with placement is that we tend to look at the individual but not at the job. Often, the individual does not work independently of others. Whether the employee works independently of others or is dependent depends on the type of jobs. Jobs in this context may be classified into three categories:

- **Independent jobs:** In certain cases, jobs are independent, for example, postal service or field sales. Here, nonoverlapping routes or territories are allotted to each worker.
- **Sequential jobs:** In sequential jobs, activities of one worker are dependent on the activities of a fellow worker.
- **Pooled jobs:** Where jobs are pooled in nature, there is high interdependence among activities. The final output is the result of the contribution of all the workers. Project teams, temporary task forces, and assembly teams represent pooled jobs.

Independent jobs do not pose great problems in placement, for each employee needs only to be evaluated relative to the match between his or her capabilities and interests, and those required on the job. But independent jobs are becoming rarer and rarer, as most jobs are dependent (sequential or pooled).

Process of Placement

- Collect details about the employee
- Construct his or her profile
- Which subgroup profile does the individual's profile best fit?
- Compare subgroup profile to job family profiles
- Which job family profile does the subgroup profile best fit?
- Assign the individual to job family
- Assign the individual to a specific job after further counseling and assessment.

Importance of Placement

The importance of placement lies in the fact that proper placement of employees reduces employee turnover, absenteeism, accidents, and dissatisfaction, on one hand, and improves their morale, on the other. Placements are also important for employment agencies, especially executive search firms, a type of employment agency that specializes in recruiting executive personnel for companies in various industries.

Benefits of Placement

- Employing a placement or work experience student can be viewed as part of the interview process for future company employees.

- Gain an intelligent, motivated, cost-effective labor resource with valuable skills, knowledge and fresh ideas.
- Projects which otherwise would not be done due to a shortage of resources can be moved forward.
- Offer a solution to short term staff shortages.

Placement is understood as the allocation of people to jobs. If the number of individuals is large in relation to the available jobs, only the best-qualified persons can be selected and placed. Once we establish this unique profile for each individual, people and jobs can be matched optimally within the constraints set by available jobs and available people.

 REVIEW QUESTIONS

1. Explain the recruitment of faculty for a nursing college. Elaborate the job description of various faculty positions.
2. Define performance appraisal. Explain its principles and types. Enlist the problems in performance appraisal.
3. What is performance appraisal? What are the methods of Performance Appraisal?
4. Define staff development. Explain the need and principles of staff development.
5. Explain the role of the administrator in staff development.
6. Define CNE. What is the need and function of CNE? Explain the principles and role of an Educator in organizing a CNE.
7. Explain the selection and admission procedures in different Nursing Programs.

Further Readings

1. Banerjee, Shyamal. Principles and Practice of Management. Oxford and IBM Publishing, New Delhi; 2000.
2. Basavanthappa BT. Nursing Administration. 2nd Edition: Jaypee Brothers Medical Publishers (P) Ltd., New Delhi; 2009.
3. Barrett, Jean. Ward Management and Teaching. Konark Publishers, Delhi; 1992.
4. Warren, Stevens, F. Management and Leadership in Nursing. McGraw – Hill Inc, New York; 1978.
5. Alexander et al. Nursing Service Administration. Mosby Publishers, US; 1962.
6. Park K. Preventive and Social Medicine, 19th Edition: M/s. Banarasidas Bhanot Publishers, Jabalpur; 2007.
7. Basavanthappa BT. Nursing Administration, 1st Edition: Jaypee Brothers Medical Publishers (P) Ltd., New Delhi; 2002.
8. Goel SL. Healthcare System, and Social Medicine, Health Organization and Structure, 1st Volume, Deep and Deep Publishers, New Delhi; 2001
9. Ranga Rao SP. Administration of Primary Health Centers in India, 1st Edition: Mittal Publications, New Delhi; 1993.
10. Lucita M. Nursing: Practice and Public Health Administration. Current Concepts and Trends. B. I. Churchill Living Stone Pvt. Ltd., New Delhi; 2002.
11. Sakharkar BM. Principles of Hospital Administration and Planning, 2nd Edition: Jaypee Brothers Medical Publishers (P) Ltd., New Delhi; 2009.
12. Patricia S Yoder-Wise. Leading and Managing in Nursing. 2nd Edition: Mosby Publication, US; 1999.
13. Bessie L. Marquis, Carol J. Huston. Leadership Roles and Management Functions in Nursing: Theory and Application. 5th Edition: Lippincott Williams and Wilkins, New York; 2006.
14. Linda Roussel. Management and Leadership for Nurse Administrators. 4th Edition: Jones and Bartlett Publication, USA; 2006.
15. Wehrich H, Koontz H. Management A Global Perspective. 11th Edition: Tata McGraw-Hill Publishing Company, Ltd., New Delhi; 2005.
16. Marquis BL, Huston CJ. Leadership and Management Functions in Nursing- Theory, and Application. 5th Edition: Lippincott Williams and Wilkins, Philadelphia; 2006.
17. Douglass LM. The Effective Nurse: Leader and Manager. 5th Edition: Mosby Publication, US; 1996.
18. Trained Nurses Association of India, Nursing Administration, and Management.
19. Samson Rebecca. Leadership and Management in Nursing Practice and Education 1st Edition: Jaypee Brothers Medical Publishers (P) Ltd., New Delhi; 2009.

Unit

16

Directing and Controlling Educational Institution

Unit Outline

➡ Curriculum Planning, Implementation, and Evaluation
➡ Guidance
➡ Counseling
➡ Quality Management: Educational/Academic Audit
➡ Program Evaluation: Evaluation of Performance
➡ Maintaining Discipline in Nursing Educational Institutions

CURRICULUM PLANNING, IMPLEMENTATION, AND EVALUATION

Curriculum word is derived from the Latin language, which means a course of deeds and experiences through which children grow to become mature adults.

It is a course of study or a set of subjects or a set of performance objectives or a program of studies. **—Oliva (1997)**

The curriculum is a tool in the hands of an artist to mold his material according to his ideals in his studio. In this definition, the artist is the teacher, the material is the student, ideals are the objectives, and the studio is the educational institution.

—Cunningham

Curriculum Development

It is the process of planning, implementing, and evaluating learning opportunities intended to produce desired changes in learners. **—Print (1993)**

The curriculum development model is suggested to correlate and study the dimensions of curriculum and its association with its elements. It incorporates a symbolic representation that represents the association among the different phases, steps, and tasks involved in constructing a curriculum. The stages in curriculum development are:

- Constitution of a curriculum committee
- Investigation and analysis of the existing health needs of the region and nation (E.g., National Health Policy, 2005)
- Investigation of curriculum needs for nursing education
- Formulation of the philosophy of nursing education
- Establishment of educational objectives/outcomes/ competencies
- Selection of learning experiences
- Selection of instructional strategies
- Organization of learning experiences
- Development of evaluation systems

Purposes of Curriculum

- It communicates to learners in advance what they are expected to know to achieve their instructional objectives over a defined period of time.
- Introduces examination or assessment criteria to allow learners to prepare for examinations accordingly.
- It defines the course, unit, and lesson goals, as well as the necessary teaching-learning techniques to help educators, plan their lessons accordingly.
- It communicates to the policymakers about the competencies and expertise of a particular group of students' the positions and roles they can perform.
- It prepares the pupil for citizenship in a democratic society.
- It meets the needs of students with a wide range of abilities, aptitudes, and interests.

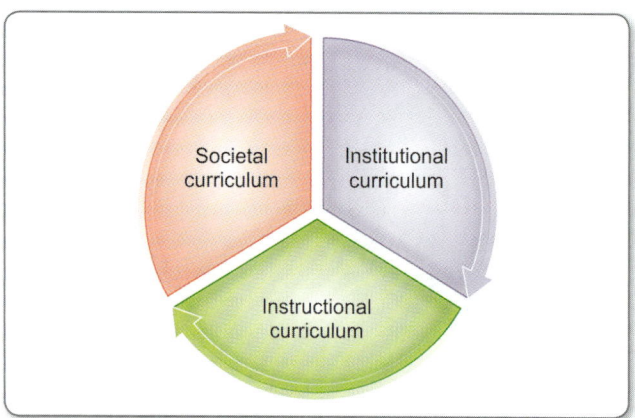

Fig. 1: Levels of curriculum planning

- It relates and systematically organizes the various learning experiences to produce the maximum cumulative effect in attaining the objectives of the school.

Levels of Curriculum Planning

According to Goodland, there are three levels of curriculum planning, namely, societal, institutional and instructional (Fig. 1).

Societal curriculum: This is the curriculum planned for a specific population of students by experts outside the educational institution and who are legally appointed. In nursing education, the societal curriculum is designed by different statutory bodies such as the Indian Nursing Council. A societal curriculum is synonymous with the official type of curriculum.

Institutional curriculum: This is the curriculum prepared by the faculty of the institute for a particular group of students for a definite period. An institutional curriculum is synonymous with the actual type of curriculum.

Instructional curriculum: This is the curriculum prepared by the individual teacher at the instructional level.

Factors Influencing Curriculum Development

Forces and problems affecting the curriculum of nursing science are complicated and continuously changing. There are fast changes in the health care system in the new millennium, which poses difficulties for nurse teachers to devise appropriate curricula for nursing education to maintain pace with these changes. The curriculum is never created in a vacuum but in the contextual depiction of worldwide trends, domestic health, and essential statistics, domestic health policy, domestic population policy, professional priorities and values of the teachers. The main factors are the philosophy of nursing education, educational psychology, society, students, social activities, knowledge, and skills required of training (Fig. 2). The following are the determinants of the curriculum in nursing sciences:

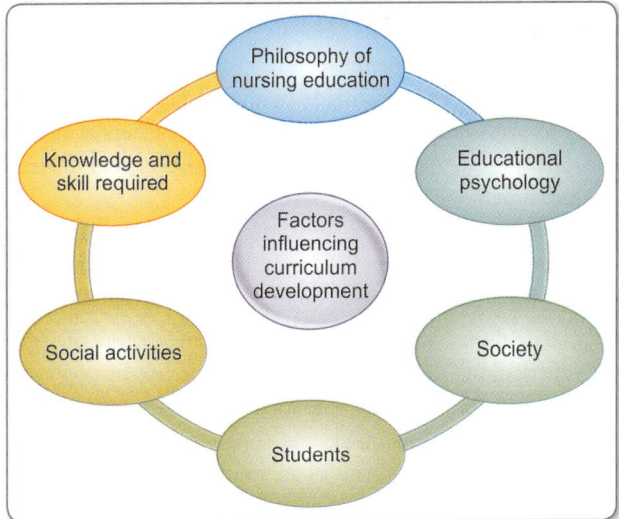

Fig. 2: Factors influencing curriculum development

- Societal determinants such as demographic revolution, health problems, advanced medical technology, change in the healthcare delivery system, cultural diffusion, changing patients' expectations, etc.
- Educational determinants such as new instructional Strategies and new methods of assessment. It is the learning experience.
- Economic determinants involves cost-benefit analysis to determine the suitability of a nursing program.
- Philosophical determinants Include the school of philosophy in which the profession or society or nations believe, influence the contents of the curriculum as well as the instructional strategies employed to achieve objectives of the education.
- Subject matter subject matter is too shallow without addressing the needs, interests, and abilities of the students, and does not encourage in-depth understanding.

Models of Curriculum

Behavioral Objective Model/Product Model

It was proposed by Ralph Tyler in 1950. It reflects the need to organize the utility and purpose of a product of the quality and its practical application. Here the curriculum is viewed objectively for its function and recognizes teaching and learning as an integral part of it. According to him, the curriculum decides the order and scope of what is to be taught, and thus learning may be enhanced. He identified four fundamental questions to be answered in the process of developing a curriculum.

1. What educational purposes should the school seek to attain, i.e., the objectives?
2. How can learning experiences be selected?
3. How can the learning experiences be organized?
4. How can the effectiveness of learning be evaluated?

Stenhouse's Process Model/Process Model

It is an input model suggested by Lawrence Stenhouse in 1975. Here the emphasis is on learning experiences or the process of education. It is possible to organize a curriculum without the planning of the expected behavioral change among students. The content of the curriculum should not be based on means of its achievement; instead, it should be based on learning experiences. The teacher assesses the student to develop self-assessment qualities among the students.

Lawton's Cultural Analysis Model

This model which came up in the year 1983 was a reaction against what he saw as the dangers of the behavioral objectives models. It is based on the concept of cultural analysis. Culture is defined as the holistic way of life of society, and the purpose of education is to make available to the next generation what we regard as the most critical aspects of culture. Cultural analysis is the process by which a selection is made from the cultural context and in terms of curriculum planning.

Beattie's Fourfold Model

Beattie suggests (1987) that there are four fundamental approaches in relation to the task of planning a curriculum for nursing:

1. Curriculum as a map of key subjects. This approach consists of mapping out the key subjects in the nursing curriculum.
2. Curriculum as a schedule of necessary skills. This approach emphasizes the specifics of the basic skills of nursing practice.
3. Curriculum as a portfolio of meaningful personal experiences. This approach places students at the center of learning by organizing the curriculum around their interests and skills.
4. Curriculum as an agenda of critical cultural issues. This approach avoids giving detailed subject matter, focusing instead on controversial issues and political dilemmas in nursing and health care.

Principles of Curriculum Development

A curriculum has been described as a tool in the hands of teachers for giving training to students in the art of living together in a community.

- **The conservative principle:** It has been stated that nations live in the present, on the past and for the future. This means that the present, past, and future needs of the community should be taken into consideration.
- **The forward-looking principle:** Children of today are the citizens of tomorrow. Therefore, their education should be such that it enables them to become progressive-minded persons.

- **The creative principle:** In the curriculum, those activities should be included, which enable the child to exercise his/her creative and constructive powers.
- **Principle of totality:** The total learning experience and learning opportunity may have to be well planned as a whole curriculum, and the teaching-learning activity needed for the entire period has to be considered while developing a curriculum.
- **Child-centered curriculum:** While developing the curriculum, due consideration should be given to the students' age, educational level, need, and individual difference.
- **Principle of integration and correlation:** Each year's course should be built on what has been done in previous years and at the same time, should serve as a basis for subsequent learning.
- **Principle of variety and flexibility:** Variety should be provided in terms of learning and teaching activities. A curriculum should not be so rigid that appropriate modifications cannot be done as and when needed.
- **Training for leisure:** There should be some provision for co-curricular activities, relaxation, library utilization, and electives according to choice.

Evaluation of the Curriculum

Evaluation is a systematic and organized process of realizing the extent to which educational objectives laid down in a curriculum have been achieved.

Aims of Evaluation

- To find out to what extent the objectives of the program have been attained.
- For certification purposes.
- To provide guidelines for decisions about a curriculum, revision modification, and shift of emphasis.
- It is designed to protect society to prevent incompetent personnel from practicing nursing.

In Curriculum Evaluation, the Evaluation of Five M's is Done

- **Men:** whether the curriculum has been organized and implemented correctly by the faculty members and others involved in it.
- **Money:** whether money meant for curriculum development is utilized correctly.
- **Materials:** whether the evaluation of textbooks, literature, is used for the development of the curriculum.
- **Methods:** whether teaching-learning methods planned in the curriculum are appropriate.
- **Minutes:** appropriateness of allocation theory and practical hours in the curriculum.

Types of Assessments/Evaluation

- *Formative Assessment:* It is an ongoing evaluation to measure the progress made by the students. The purpose is to provide feedback to students and teachers at regular intervals. Its results may form a part of the internal assessment.
- *Summative Assessment:* It is the final evaluation of the student done at the end of the course. Part of the summative assessment may be based on the formative evaluation.

Curriculum implementation is an essential part of curriculum development because it is through the implementation that the intended changes as specified in the curriculum document are supplied in practice. The curriculum is the blueprint of an educational program. Even though a curriculum cannot be entirely preplanned and prescribed, to a great extent, it can be developed based on the needs of the students as well as society.

GUIDANCE

Guidance is the assistance made available by qualified and trained persons to an individual of any age to help him to manage his own life activities, develop his own points of view, make his own decisions and carry on his own burdens.

—BG Barki, B Mukhopadhyay

Types of Guidance

- **Educational guidance:** It is aimed at providing support to the students during their education. Students are different in terms of achievement and cognitive abilities. This may lead to decreased motivation. Educational guidance can help them overcome these difficulties.
- **Social guidance:** Social problems such as over dependency, inferiority complex, deviant sexual behavior, and antisocial behavior are common among adolescents. It usually arises from the clash of adolescents and adulthood in terms of development. It is also linked to social adjustments and relationships. It also may be influenced by parents, society, and friends. Social guidance will help resolve this.
- **Personal guidance:** It is a client-centered approach to the personal problems of adolescents that are emotional in nature.
- **Vocational guidance:** It is the process of helping the individual to choose an occupation that fits him/her best.

Principles of Guidance

According to Crow and Crow, there are 14 significant principles for guidance, they are:
- Human beings have a complex personality pattern and attitudes; hence, the guidance should consider the overall adjustment and development of the individual.

- Recognize individual differences in providing guidance.
- Guidance is aimed to help an individual to formulate, accept, and attain the goals of desirable behavior.
- There is a crucial need for trained and experienced professionals to guide an individual's maladaptive behavior arising from social, political, and economic unrest.
- It is a continuing process throughout the life span.
- There should be equitable distribution of guidance services to all the needy irrespective of age, caste, creed, etc.
- The curriculum and its implementation should be evidenced by guidance.
- Guidance is the responsibility of parents and teachers.
- Individual evaluation and consultative record of each individual facilitates the intelligent administration of guidance.
- Flexible according to the needs.
- Guidance should be done by qualified, trained, and experienced persons. They should have cooperation with other agencies of guidance and community welfare.
- There should be periodical assessments/appraisal of the guidance program.
- The guidance affects all the dimensions of life.
- Special reference for specific guidance is promoted as per the availability of specially trained guides.

COUNSELING

"Counseling is a learning-oriented process carried out in a social environment in which the professionally competent counselor attempts to assist the counselee using appropriate procedures to become a happy and productive member of the society by formulating realistic and purposeful goals for total personal growth.   —**Gustad, 1953**

Aims of Counseling

- Achieve self-realization of individuals through desired changes.
- Provision of support in problem-solving and maintain intimacy in a personal relationship.
- Obtain and maintain positive mental health.
- Facilitate adjustments for academic improvement and productive life.

Principles of Counseling

- **Acceptance:** Accept the students irrespective of his/her physical, psychological, social, economic, and cultural conditions.
- **Communication:** Verbal and nonverbal communication should be used skillfully.
- **Non-judgmental:** Negative comments and criticizing approach is not helpful for a good counseling process.
- **Confidentiality:** It is essential to keep all the information coming to the knowledge of the counselor confidential.

- **Individuality:** Every human being is unique. The guidance should be organized well to meet the individual needs of the students at different levels. The interests, abilities, and aptitudes are different for every individual.
- **Learning:** Learning is an ongoing process. All the principles of learning should be applied in the process of counseling. The counselor learns the problems of the counselee through the counseling process.

Counseling Techniques: There are mainly three approaches:

- **Directive counseling** (prescriptive counseling) It is counselor-centered approach. The process of counseling is based on the accumulated information about the problems faced by the counselee. In this type, the counselor actively tries to get the specified reports about the difficulties of the counselee and suggest adaptable solutions.
- **Non-directive counseling:** On the other hand, the non-directive approach in counseling is based on making solutions for the personal problems of the counselee. It is a client-centered approach. It involves many phases such as establishing relationships/communication, identifying the issues, exploring alternate solutions, and end with terminating the session. It also should have a provision for follow up.
- **Eclectic counseling:** It is the use of both directive and non-directive approaches. Initially, the counselor may begin with directive counseling and may modify it to the non-directive method as per the need of the situation and type of problem assessed.
- **Individual and group counseling:** It is a classification based on the number of counselees undergoing the session simultaneously. In a group approach, the common problems of a group are addressed through group interaction method. The individual opportunity to discuss is ensured for all the group members. The latter one is concerned with the interview of the individual to identify his/her problems with a view to developing an action plan that is acceptable to the individual in solving the issues identified.

QUALITY MANAGEMENT: EDUCATIONAL/ACADEMIC AUDIT

The Academic Audit, like more traditional program reviews, is a peer-review process including a self-study and a site visit by peers from outside the institution. However, the similarities end there. Unlike the traditional approach to program evaluation, this process emphasizes self-reflection and self-improvement rather than compliance with predetermined standards. The purpose of an academic audit is to encourage departments or programs to evaluate their "education quality processes" which are the key faculty activities required to produce, assure, and regularly improve the quality of teaching and learning. Academic audit is a self assessment mechanism where one (faculty) understand his/her role in academic decision making. It includes the assessment of essence of team work and organization of work with the available resources with a sole purpose of enhancing quality of education in the best interests of the discipline and student learning.

Definitions

An academic audit can be understood as a scientific and systematic method of reviewing the quality of the academic process in the institution. It is related to quality assurance and enhancing the quality of academic activities in Higher Education Institutions.
—**National Assessment and Accreditation Council (NAAC)**

Administrative Audit can be defined as a process of evaluating the efficiency and effectiveness of the administrative procedure. It includes the assessment of policies, strategies and functions of the various administrative departments, control of the overall administrative system, etc.
—**National Assessment and Accreditation Council (NAAC)**

Objectives of Academic Audit

- To understand the existing system and assess the strengths and weaknesses of the Departments and Administrative Units and to suggest the methods for improvement and for overcoming the weaknesses.
- To identify the bottlenecks in the existing administrative mechanisms and to identify the opportunities for academic reforms, administrative reforms, and examination reforms, etc.
- To evaluate the optimum utilization of financial and other resources.
- To suggest the methods for continuous improvement of quality keeping in mind criteria and reports by NAAC and other bodies.

Elements of the Academic Audit

Based upon the approach laid by Dr William Massy (William Massy is a professor emeritus of education and business administration at Stanford University and president of the Jackson Hole Higher Education Group) the elements of Academic Audit are categorized into two such as **the self-study** and the **peer review**.

Self Study

Departments examine the following five focal areas of the educational process by asking common sense questions:
- Determining learning objectives:
  - Have we consciously considered what students who complete our courses/programs should know and be able to do? For employment? For their abilities/responsibilities as citizens?

- Do we use and document information gathered from employers, former students, senior institutions?
- Do we identify and learn from best practice, evaluate student outcome goals of comparable departments in other institutions?
- Designing curriculum and co-curriculum:
  - How do we determine what is taught, in what order, from what perspective?
  - Do we work collaboratively on curriculum design? How do we decide what resources and resource materials will be used as content vehicles?
  - Do we consciously consider how the course design relates to other courses and students will take as part of this program?
  - Do we consider out-of-classroom activities that could complement or be integrated into the curriculum?
  - Do we identify and learn from best practice, evaluate curricula of comparable departments in other institutions?
- Designing teaching and learning methods:
  - How are teaching and learning organized for students?
  - What methods will be used to expose students to the material for the first time?
  - To answer questions and provide interpretation?
  - To stimulate student involvement with the material?
  - To provide feedback on student work?
  - Do we analyze teaching and learning processes regularly?
  - Do we strive for coherence in the department's curriculum and educational processes?
  - Do we work collaboratively on process design?
  - Do we identify and learn from best practice, evaluate teaching and learning methods of comparable departments in ours and other institutions?
- Developing student learning assessment:
  - What measures and indicators do we use to assess student learning?
  - Have we defined indicators or measures of achievement based upon our stated learning objectives?
  - Do we assess performance only at the end of the course/program or do we compare the beginning and ending performance to ascertain value-added? Who is responsible for the assessment?
  - Do we work collaboratively on assessment design, implementation, and analysis?
  - Do we base decisions on facts?
  - Do we identify and learn from best practice, evaluate assessment practices of comparable departments in ours and other institutions?
- Assuring implementation of quality education:
  - Are we organized to ensure that our mutual departmental objectives and priorities are implemented consistently?

- How do we assure ourselves that content is delivered as intended, that teaching and learning processes are being implemented appropriately and consistently, that assessments are conducted as planned and the results used effectively?
- Do we work collaboratively to implement improvement initiatives?
- Do we identify and learn from best practice, evaluate quality assurance practices of comparable departments in ours and other institutions?

Departments write a self-study report (20 pages) describing the current state of their efforts to improve student learning and the academic quality of their programs, their strengths, and weaknesses in the five focal areas, citing and briefly describing documentation supporting exemplary practices and describing initiatives to address practices that need improvement.

Peer Review

- Auditors are volunteers (primarily faculty) who receive training on education quality processes and audit methodology.
- Audit teams (3–5 members) will most likely come from other TBR institutions.
- Because the auditors will be focusing on quality processes, they do not need to come from the academic discipline of the department being audited.
- Audit visits are typically one day per department.
- Auditors meet with departmental leadership, faculty, and students.
- Auditors ask questions similar to the self-study questions cited above.
- Auditors write a report: Highlighting examples of exemplary practice, noting areas for improvement, evaluating a department's approach to educational quality practices, and evaluating a department's level of quality process "maturity."

Principles of the Academic Audit

- Define quality in terms of outcomes. Learning outcomes should pertain to what is or will become important for the department's students. Learning, not teaching per se, is what ultimately matters.
- Focus on the process. Departments should analyze how teachers teach, how students learn, and how to best approach learning assessment. Departments should study their discipline's literature and collect data on what works well and what doesn't. Experimentation with active learning should be encouraged. Faculty should be encouraged to share and adapt to their colleague's successful teaching innovations.

- Work collaboratively. Teamwork and consensus lead to total faculty ownership of and responsibility for all aspects of the curriculum and make everyone accountable for the success of students. Dialogue and collaboration should be encouraged over territoriality and the "lone wolf" approach.
- Base decisions on evidence departments should collect data to find out what students need. Data should be analyzed and findings incorporated in the design of curricula, learning processes, and assessment methods.
- Strive for coherence. Courses should build upon one another to provide necessary breadth and depth. Assessment should be aligned with learning objectives.
- Learn from best practice. Faculty should seek out good practices in comparable departments and institutions and adapt the best to their own circumstances. Faculty should share best practices and help "raise the bar" for their department.
- Make continuous improvement a priority. Departments should continually and consciously strive to improve teaching and learning.

The National Assessment and Accreditation Council (NAAC) has evolved tools and guidelines for improving quality for different levels of Higher Education Institutions (HEIs) and for its sustenance. By establishing an Internal Quality Assurance Cell (IQAC) and undergoing an External Quality Assurance process it's possible to continuously strive for excellence. The monitoring and evaluation of the institutional processes require a carefully structured system of internal and external review.

National Assessment and Accreditation Council (NAAC)

India has one of the largest and diverse education systems in the world. Privatization, widespread expansion, increased autonomy and introduction of Programs in new and emerging areas have improved access to higher education. At the same time, it has also led to widespread concern on the quality and relevance of higher education. To address these concerns, the National Policy on Education (NPE, 1986) and the Program of Action (PoA, 1992) spelled out strategic plans for the policies, advocated the establishment of an independent National accreditation agency. Consequently, the National Assessment and Accreditation Council (NAAC) was established in 1994 as an autonomous institution of the University Grants Commission (UGC) with its head quarter in Bengaluru. The mandate of NAAC as reflected in its vision statement is in making quality assurance an integral part of the functioning of Higher Education Institutions (HEIs).

The NAAC functions through its General Counsel (GC) and Executive Committee (EC) comprising educational administrators, policymakers and senior academicians from a cross-section of the Indian higher education system. The Chairperson of the UGC is the President of the GC of the NAAC, the Chairperson of the EC is an eminent academician nominated by the President of GC (NAAC). The Director is the academic and administrative head of the NAAC and is the member-secretary of both the GC and the EC. In addition to the statutory bodies that steer its policies and core staff to support its activities, the NAAC is advised by the advisory and consultative committees constituted from time to time. NAAC has formulated a three-stage process for assessment and accreditation as:

- **Institutional eligibility for quality assessment (IEQA):** It is obtained by an applicant institution at the beginning while it is still in the planning stage for assessment. The benefits of this step for an applicant institution are to get recognized as eligible to apply for the second step comprehensive assessment and accreditation process.
- **Preparation of the self-study report:** Self-report is prepared by the institution as per the guidelines given by the NAAC, its submission to NAAC and in-house analysis of the report by NAAC.
- **Peer team visit:** Peer Team visit to is the institution for validation of the Self Study Report followed by the presentation of a comprehensive assessment report to the institution. Later grading, certification, and accreditation is done based on the evaluation by the executive committee of the NAAC.

PROGRAM EVALUATION: EVALUATION OF PERFORMANCE

Program evaluation involves a complex process of data collection and analysis in order to assign values to various program components leading to decisions about the program. In general, the purposes of program evaluation is to diagnose problems, weaknesses and strengths, test new and different approaches for accomplishing and advancing the school's philosophy, objectives, and conceptual framework, and improve the operation of all aspects of the school. More specifically, program evaluation in nursing education can help faculty and administrators account for scarce fiscal resources, make administrative and curricular decisions, appraise faculty and staff development needs, examine both intended and unintended effects of their nursing program within the community, and provide a mechanism to assure fulfillment of accreditation requirements.

Dimensions of Program Evaluation

- **Evaluation of administration and operations:** An important component of any program evaluation in nursing education is the evaluation of the administration and operations of the program. The questions asked in regard to this phase of evaluation include:

  - Do faculty, administrators and students participate in the governance of the institution in accordance with the bylaws of the regulatory bodies?
  - Does the organizational structure of the nursing program promote effective functioning and foster the attainment of program goals?
  - Is the program administered by a nurse educator who holds a minimum of a master's degree and/or earned doctorate has the minimum experience required to do the job?
  - Does the administrator of the nursing programs, with institutional consultation and nursing faculty input, have the responsibility and authority for planning and allocating program resources?

- **Curriculum evaluation:** The curriculum is defined as the totality of learning activities that are designed to achieve specific educational goals. Evaluation of the nursing curriculum has become a major concern of nurse educators in recent years. The curriculum should reflect the philosophy, conceptual framework, and program goals of the school and institution. Curriculum evaluation also involves an assessment of nursing content taught in each course, course objectives, teaching strategies, course evaluation methods, and the relationship of non-nursing courses to the overall plan of study. Course objectives should describe expected behaviors and reflect the level and nature of the content, whether cognitive, affective or psychomotor. They should also be assessed for clarity, appropriateness to the content, and the ease by which their achievement by students can be measured. Teaching strategies should relate to course content and objectives, and allow for the achievement of the objectives.

- **Faculty evaluation:** Faculty evaluation is based on measuring performance in the areas of teaching, research, and service. The necessity of faculty evaluation is seldom questioned. However, the format and evidence used for the evaluation are subjects of frequent discussion and debate. Self-evaluation has traditionally provided how the faculty can update their portfolio in terms of significant accomplishments in the areas of research, teaching, and services. Administrative evaluation of faculty generally involves synthesizing data from various sources and then reviewing results with faculty members. Peer evaluation is a somewhat controversial and biased measure of faculty evaluation, and often it is omitted from a comprehensive evaluation. It results in mutual backscratching, friendship, and popularity concerns. Student evaluations of faculty can provide important evaluative information regarding course assignments, textbooks, the fairness of evaluation methods, interest in the students, and interest in the subject matter.

- **Evaluation of outcomes**: Evaluation of outcomes in nursing education programs includes the evaluation of students. Students traditionally are evaluated throughout their academic careers so that their learning for each course of study can be assessed. Using such methods as written and oral assignments, paper and pencil examinations, and clinical performance appraisals, values are assigned that reflect the student's achievement in a given area and so on. In addition to reflecting a particular student's achievement, such evaluative measures also reflect program effectiveness in particular areas. If collective deficiencies exist, for example in students' knowledge of pharmacology this may pinpoint a weakness in the foundation courses.

Models for Evaluating Nursing Education Programs

Several programs and curriculum evaluation models have been advanced in recent years. Such strategies enhance both organization of the process and the comprehensiveness of the evaluation. Some of these models are briefly described below.

- **Comparative course evaluation**: Comparative course evaluation is a process designed to identify articulation, duplication, and omission of learning opportunities between courses in a curriculum. It involves a systematic examination of course syllabi in order to identify omissions and duplications of content and behavioral objectives between courses.
- **Discrepancy evaluation model:** Discrepancy evaluation refers to the search for differences between two or more elements or variables of an education/ training program that, according to logical, rational or statistical criteria, should be in agreement or correspondence. Most commonly the focus of program evaluation using the discrepancy model is upon one or more of the following (1) differences between program design and actual program operations, such as planned curriculum content, and actual content taught, (2) discrepancies between predicted and obtained program outcomes, such as predicted and actual NCLEX scores and so on.
- **Goal free evaluation:** The focus of goal free evaluation is to determine the importance and value of final outcomes, not intentions and design of the program. It is an approach to ensuring that evaluators take into account the actual effects and not just the intended effects of education and training programs.
- **Staropoli and Waltz model:** The Staropoli and Waltz Model is a comprehensive approach to educational program evaluation that has been widely used in schools of nursing. The Waltz evaluation plan considers the educational program as an open system consisting of inputs, operations, and outputs. Included in the plan are four distinct yet interrelated levels of analysis, school, program, subprogram, and course level.
- **Stufflebeam's CIPP model:** Context, input, process, and product (CIPP) comprise the four types of evaluation in Stufflebeam's model. Context evaluation serves decision-making for the planning of an ongoing program and therefore is formative or diagnostic in nature. Input evaluation involves questions regarding the feasibility, availability, costs, and potential advantages and disadvantages of the various strategies proposed. Process evaluation provides feedback to administrators and participants of the program which detects or predicts problems with the day-to-day functioning of the program. The final component, product evaluation, serves to measure the extent to which goals have been achieved, and is therefore summative in nature.

Although program evaluation can be time-consuming and expensive, it is necessary for the development and maintenance of quality nursing education programs. Escalating costs, shrinking appropriations, and the knowledge explosion have contributed to the need for examining educational programs for efficiency and efficacy.

MAINTAINING DISCIPLINE IN NURSING EDUCATIONAL INSTITUTIONS

Discipline can act as a natural control by which a student brings his or her conduct into a concurrence with the institution's legitimate conduct code, or it tends to be an administrative action to implement students' consistency with office principles and directions.

Discipline is defined as training or molding of the mind and character to bring about desired behaviors.

Discipline is the practice of making people to obey rules or standards of behavior, and punishing them when they do not.

—**Collins Dictionary**

Types of Discipline

- **Self-controlled discipline:** For the situation of self-controlled discipline, the student brings her or his conduct into a concurrence with the associations' authentic conduct code, i.e. the student controls their very own exercises for the benefit of all of the association. Therefore, individuals are acquainting with studies for a pinnacle execution under self-controlled discipline.
- **Enforced discipline/control:** Here, an administrative activity authorizes student consistency with the association's tenets and directions, i.e., it is a typical control forced from the higher level. Here, the supervisor practices his power to urge the students to carry on with a specific goal in mind.

Approaches to Discipline

- **Traditional methodology:** It accentuates correction/ punishment for unfortunate conduct. The reasons for conventional order are punishment for wrongdoing, implement an adjustment to custom, and fortify the power of the old over the youth.

- **Developmental methodology:** It accentuates discipline as a shaper of attractive conduct. The reason for formative discipline is to shape behavior by giving excellent results to the correct functioning and severe modifications for the wrong conduct; and shirking of physical punishments, defend the privileges of the blamed and swap for individual discretionary decisions of the blame.
- **Positive approach:** It depends on the presumption that a good student with a sense of pride, regard for power, and enthusiasm for the activity will stick to brilliant work benchmarks; and when an intrigued, conscious and self-regarding student briefly strays from his/her typically exclusive expectations, an amicable reminder/update is sufficient to divert their endeavors in the ideal bearing.

Indiscipline in Classroom

- Not attending
- Sleeping
- Lying
- Cheating
- Not studying
- Not completing homeworks and assignments
- Not punctual

Indiscipline in Clinical Areas

- Gross negligence, disobedience
- No attitude and improper behavior
- Not punctual
- Not considerate
- Not studying, laziness
- Not completing the assignments
- Absenteeism
- Leaving the clinical area without permission

Causes of Indiscipline

- Delay in administering discipline
- Ignoring rule violation in the hope that it is an isolated event
- Accumulations of rule violations, causing irritated supervisors to become outrageous
- Failure to administer progressively severe sanctions
- Failure to document disciplinary actions accurately
- Imposing discipline disproportionate to the seriousness of the offense
- Disciplining inconsistently

Classroom Disciplinary Measures

Desirable measures	Undesirable measures
Personal conference	Use of threat, forced apology

Contd...

Desirable measures	Undesirable measures
Suggestions regarding maintaining and adherence to guidelines	Punishing the group for the offense of one student
Deprivation of privileges	Use of students misdeed as an example for others.
Use of probation and honor	Nagging
Seating arrangements of the students	Scolding

Punishments/Penalties

- **Oral reprimands:** It is recommended in case of minor faults due to any reason. An oral warning will be given by the Faculty but add the same in the anecdotal record with nature of the event, time, and place.
- **Written reprimands:** It is advised in times of serious faults. A notice may be issued by the teacher to prevent the same in the future. It should include the name of the student and the teacher, the idea of the issue, the punishment, and the outcomes of future redundancy. The student needs to sign it, to demonstrate that the student has perused it. A duplicate should be given to the person who is getting punished and one held for the student record. On the off chance that again, the terms are not met, different punishments will most likely be vital.
- **Other punishments:**
  - Financial punishments may be initiated, such as imposing fines, etc.
  - Loss of benefits may incorporate exchange to deny a privilege or participation.
  - Suspension from the institution.
  - Termination (rejection) from the organization.

Measures to Maintain Class Discipline

- Ensure that classroom conditions are favorable to the lesson planned.
- Make sure that the teaching process doesn't depress class morale.
- Appropriate reinforcement on time.
- Neither too friendly nor too remote with the students.
- Watch for the signs of trouble very carefully.
- Plan the class with a desirable pace with appropriate learning measures.
- Be fair-mind and impartial- favoritism in any sense will lead to a withdrawal of co-operation and indiscipline among students.
- A teacher must know when and how to punish (i.e. to implement disciplinary measures).
- Ensure the necessity for a reprimand.
- Follow up all-important disciplinary matters.

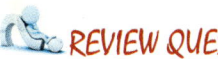 REVIEW QUESTIONS

1. Define the curriculum and explain the modes of the curriculum.
2. Explain curriculum planning in detail.
3. Discuss the principles of curriculum development.
4. Explain the steps of curriculum development.
5. Enumerate the factors influencing curriculum development.
6. Explain the models of curriculum and evaluation of the curriculum.
7. Define guidance. Explain the types and principles of guidance.
8. Define counseling. Explain the types and techniques of counseling.
9. Define academic audit. Explain the elements and principles of an academic audit.
10. Explain the concept and significance of program evaluation in nursing educational institutions.
11. Define discipline. Explain the types and approaches to discipline.
12. What are the principles of disciplinary action and enlist the type of punishments in a nursing educational institution?

Further Readings

1. Watson JE, Herbener, D. Program Evaluation in Nursing Education: The State of The Art. Journal of Advanced Nursing; (1990) 15(3), 316–323. DOI:10.1111/j.1365-2648.1990.tb01819.x
2. Anderson J. Why nursing education needs curriculum specialists Nursing Outlook 33; (1985) 96-97.
3. Anderson SB, Ball S, Murphy RT (1975). Encyclopedia of Educational Evaluation Jossey-Bass, San Francisco.
4. Bevis E Curriculum Building in Nursing, 3rd Edition: CV Mosby, St Louis; (1982) pp 26, 34, 35.
5. Clark T, Goodwin M, Manani M, Marshall M, Moore S (1983). Curriculum Evaluation, an Application of Stufflebeam's Model in a Baccalaureate School of Nursing Journal of Nursing Education 22; 54-58.
6. Fawcett J Analysis and Evaluation of Conceptual Models in Nursing FA Davis, Philadelphia; (1984) pp 37-47.
7. Fields M (1984). A model for comparable course evaluation Journal of Nursing Education 23, 76-78
8. Basavanthappa BT. Nursing Administration. 2nd Edition: Jaypee Brothers Medical Publishers (P) Ltd., New Delhi; 2009.
9. Alexander et al. Nursing Service Administration. Mosby Publishers, US; 1962.
10. Basavanthappa BT. Nursing Administration, 1st Edition: Jaypee Brothers Medical Publishers (P) Ltd., New Delhi; 2002.
11. Patricia S Yoder-Wise. Leading and Managing in Nursing. 2nd Edition: Mosby Publication, US; 1999.
12. Bessie L. Marquis, Carol J. Huston. Leadership Roles and Management Functions in Nursing: Theory and Application. 5th Edition: Lippincott Williams and Wilkins, New York; 2006.
13. Douglass LM. The Effective Nurse: Leader and Manager. 5th Edition: Mosby Publication, US; 1996.
14. Trained Nurses Association of India, Nursing Administration, and Management.

Unit

17

Professional Considerations

 Unit Outline

➥ Nursing as a Profession
➥ Philosophy of Nursing Practice
➥ Regulatory Bodies of Nursing; Indian Nursing Council
➥ State Nursing Council
➥ Current Trends and Issues in Nursing
➥ Trends in Nursing Education and Service
➥ Trends in Nursing Research
➥ Ethics and Code of Ethics
➥ Consumer Protection Act
➥ Legal Aspects of Nursing

NURSING AS A PROFESSION

The nursing services are aimed at both those who are sick and well. The health of a man is considered holistic in nature with four dimensions, specifically physical, mental, social, and spiritual aspects. The nursing profession adopts a humanistic approach with empathy and compassion and aims at promotive, preventive, and rehabilitative care of people who are sick and well. It is indeed a planned, deliberate action, the function of which is to bring about desirable changes in the person and his environment professionally.

The term 'Nurse' evolves from the Latin word nutrix, which means to nourish or to cherish. Today nursing emerged as a learned profession, which is both a science and an art. It is a body of knowledge. Knowledge is an awareness or perception of reality, which is acquired through learning or investigation. Science is defined as both a unified body of knowledge concerned with the specific subject matter, the skills and methodology necessary to provide such knowledge. The concept of profession was described as early as 1915. It is a vocation using a body of specialized knowledge on the level of practice. The prolonged training and the height of knowledge and skills obtained to differentiate the profession from other occupations. Nursing has been called the oldest of the arts and the youngest of the professions.

Profession: It is a type of occupation that meets certain criteria that raise it to a level above that of occupation.

Profession: It is a calling that requires special knowledge, skill, and preparation. An occupation that requires advanced knowledge and skills and that it grows out of society's needs for special services.

Professional: It is a person who belongs to and practices a profession.

Professionalism: It is the demonstration of a high level of a personal, ethical, and high level of skill characteristics for a member of a profession.

Professional nursing is defined as blending intellectual attainment, attitude and mental skills based upon the scientific medicine, acquired by means of prescribed course in a school of nursing, affiliated with a hospital, recognized for such purposes by the state and practiced in conjunction with curative and preventive medicine by an individual licensed to do so by the State.   **—American Nursing Association**

Difference Between Occupation and Profession

Occupation: is defined as what occupies or engages, one's time, business, and employment.   **—Webster**

Profession: is defined as a vocation requiring advanced training and usually involving mental rather than manual work as teaching, engineering, especially medicine, law, etc.

—Webster

Criteria of a Profession

- **High intellectual level of functioning**: Modern nurses use assessment skills and knowledge, have the ability to reason and make routine judgment depending on the patient's condition. Professional nurses function at a high intellectual level. Florence Nightingale raised the bar for education, and graduates of her school were considered to be highly educated.

- **High level of individual responsibility and accountability:** Nurses must be accountable and demonstrate a high level of individual responsibility for the care and services they provide. The concept of accountability has legal, ethical, and professional implications that include accepting responsibility for action taken to ensure client care as well as accepting responsibility for the consequences of an action that is not performed.

- **Specialized body of knowledge:** Nursing has developed into an identifiable separate discipline, a specialized body of knowledge called as nursing science. It was compiled through the research effort of nurses with advanced educational degrees. Although this body of specialized knowledge is relatively small, it forms a theoretical basis for the practice of nursing today. As more nurses obtain advanced degrees, conduct research and develop philosophies, and theories about nursing, this body of knowledge will increase in scope.

- **Evidence-based practice:** Almost all the currently used nursing theories address this issue in some way. Evidenced-based practice is the practice of nursing in which interventions are based on data obtained from research that demonstrate that the findings are appropriate and successful. It involves a systematic process of uncovering, evaluating, and using information from research as the basis for making decisions about providing client care.

- **Public service and altruistic activities:** Individual is the focal point of all nursing models and nursing practice. Nursing has been viewed universally as being an altruistic profession composed of selfless individuals who place the lives and well being of their clients above their personal safety. Dedicated nurses provide care for victims of deadly diseases with little regard for their welfare.

- **Well organized and strong representation:** Professional organizations represent the members of the profession and control the quality of professional practice. In India, TNAI and SNA are the two organizations that represent nursing in today's health care system. Many do belong to specialty organizations that represent a specific area of practice.

- **Code of ethics:** A Code of Ethics document may outline the mission and values of the business or organization, how professionals are supposed to approach problems, the ethical principles based on the organizations core values and the standards to which the professional is held. Some of the ethical principles are autonomy, justice, non-maleficence, and so on.

- **Competencies and professional license:** Nurses must pass a national licensure examination to demonstrate that they are qualified to practice nursing. Only after passing the exam, the nurses are allowed to practice. The granting of a nursing license is a legal activity conducted by the individual state under regulations contained in the state's nursing practice act.
- **Autonomy and independence of practice:** In reality, nursing is both an independent and interdependent discipline. Nurses in all health care settings must work with physicians, hospital administrators, pharmacists, and other groups in the provision of care. In some cases, nurses has an advanced practice role, e.g. Nurse practitioners can do establish their independent practices. To be considered a true profession, nursing will need to be recognized by other disciplines as having practitioners who practice nursing independently.
- **Professional identity and development:** Until nurses are fully committed to the profession of nursing, identify with it as a profession and are dedicated to its future development, nursing will probably not achieve professional status.

Characteristics of a Profession

- Mastery and thorough knowledge of the nursing theory.
- Ability to solve problems and application of theoretical knowledge.
- Continued development of knowledge and practice through self-enrichment and ongoing research.
- Existence of legal augmentation of professional standards.
- Authorization system to certify competence.
- Penalties against the incompetent or unethical practice.
- Public acceptance.

PHILOSOPHY OF NURSING PRACTICE

Nursing is a form of art and science devoted to developing the physiological and psychological wellbeing of patients in the community. Nursing services are committed to excellence in practice, education, informatics, research, and administration.

Nursing is the unique function of nurses in caring for individuals, sick or well, is to assess their responses to their health status and to assist them in the performance of those activities contributing to health or recovery that they would perform unaided if they had the necessary strength, will, or knowledge and to do this in such a way as to help them gain full or partial independence as rapidly as possible.

—**Virginia Henderson, 1977**

A nursing philosophy is a written declaration that states the views, values, and ethics of a nurse concerning their patient care and therapy while in the nursing industry. Although the philosophy may seem solely academic and too cerebral to be of any use, it is vital to approach your profession appropriately. It gives advantages to your profession and the lives of the individuals you care for and their relatives when you create a separate nursing philosophy.

Leddy and Pepper in 2003 defined the philosophy of nursing as:

- The cognitive and efficient outcomes of the efforts of professional nurses to understand the relationship between person, environment, and health.
- A scientific discipline.
- Incorporating a sense of value into nursing practice.
- Including artistic elements that facilitate health and well being.

Nursing is a profession that can make a significant impact on the lives of many. Being so, there are certain qualities that are necessary to be a fantastic nurse: compassion, honesty, and respect. During these present times, it is so easy to be task-oriented and continuously on the go. As nurses, there will be multiple patients at a time, so there is potential to treat the diagnosis and not the individual. These three qualities ensure that nurses will provide patients with the best care possible.

Compassion is a must-have quality when it comes to nursing. A nurse without compassion treats only the diagnosis, and a person's health is made up of more than one component: physical, social and mental wellbeing (Centers for Disease Control And Prevention, 2014). Being able to empathize with patients, a nurse builds rapport and creates an environment that is inclusive of the physical, social, and mental aspects of health.

Honesty is something that should be valued. A patient would want to know exactly what was happening to him and what are the plans for his/her treatment. Being honest builds trust and credibility with the patient. Patients are more cooperative with health professionals they deem trustworthy.

Respect is another quality that builds rapport with the patient. Patients want to be treated with dignity and involved with their treatment. Being respectful to patients encompasses getting to know them, their culture, and beliefs; it helps to distinguish a treatment plan that the patient will be cooperative with.

These qualities are crucial in nursing because each person should be treated as an individual and not a diagnosis. Health includes a person's social and mental wellbeing as well as their physical wellbeing, so developing relationships with patients is critical in delivering the best quality of care. With compassion, honesty, and respect, nurses will be able to create an environment that optimizes the health of their patients.

Therefore the philosophy of nursing considers the concept of humans. We understand man exists as a holistic individual with cultural and environmental diversity. In modern times, man is expected to be accountable for one's health and illness. This self-service and responsibility are manifested by the individual's ability to maintain self-care or to promote the self-care of others.

Roles of the Professional Nurse

NURSE – originated from a Latin word NUTRIX, means to nourish. Dictionary definition says that a person trained, licensed, or skilled in nursing is called a nurse. Florence Nightingale, in her Notes on Nursing, described the Nurse's role as "one that would put the patient in the best condition for nature to act upon him." A professional nurse is a person who has completed a basic nursing education program and is licensed in his country to practice professional nursing (Fig. 1).

- **Care provider:** Traditionally, the function of the caregiver has included those operations that physically and psychologically help the client while maintaining the privacy of the client. Care is physical, psychosocial, social, ethnic, and religious.
- **Communicator:** Communication is an essential part of all positions of nursing. In the group, nurses interact with the patient, relatives, other health care practitioners, and other people. Nurses recognize patient issues in the position of communicator and then communicate them verbally or in print to other health team members. The communication performance of a nurse is a significant variable in nursing care.
- **Teacher:** The nurse, as an educator, enables patients to know about their wellness and the practices they need to undertake to recover or retain their wellness. The nurse evaluates the learning requirements and willingness of the client to learn, establishes particular learning objectives in combination with the client, and develops policies for teaching and promotes learning.
- **Advocate:** The nurse talk for the patient. The needs, problems, desires, and other aspects are communicated through nurses to other health care team members. The nurse assists the patient in recognizing their issues and provides recommendations and referrals accordingly. The nurse helps the patient to exercise their rights and speak up for themselves.

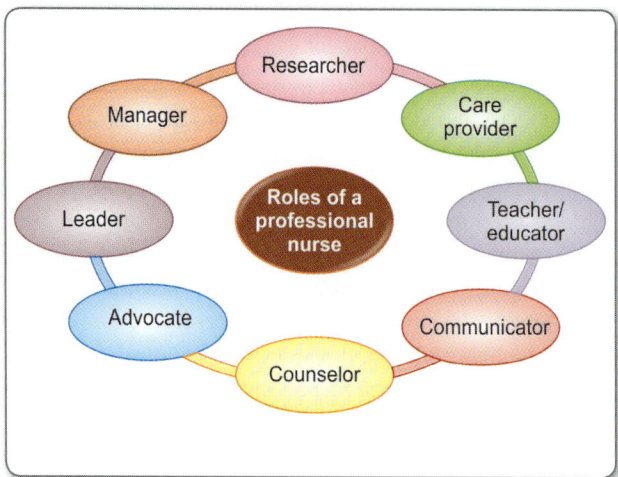

Fig. 1: Roles of a professional nurse

- **Counselor:** Counseling helps the patient to identify and deal with painful psychological or social issues. It is a suitable mechanism for stress management. It also helps in enhancing interpersonal relationships, thus fostering personal growth. It includes offering psychological, mental, and social assistance.
- **Leader:** It is a skill of influencing fellow workers to achieve common objectives. The role of a leader is exercised among individual patients, family or relatives of the patient, and community members in addition to fellow workers. Effective management is learned. This requires recognizing the needs and aims of the people that motivate them. It is based on scientific knowledge of leadership in addition to the communication and interpersonal skills needed to influence people.
- **Manager:** As a manager, the nurse looks after the affairs of individuals, families, and communities. The division of labor, coordinating patient care with other relevant departments, is the responsibility of the nurse manager. The nurse manager distributes the work and responsibilities to the staff and new supporting workforce in the unit.
- **Researcher:** The improvement of patient care and service is based on scientific research. As a discipline of health services, the nursing curriculum focus on the importance of nursing research. The nurse must have a sound understanding of the concept of nursing research and must apply the same in practice. The future of nursing is nursing research. The nurse should try to recognize the issues and problems of nursing care in the working area and seek scientific solutions through sound research.

Expanded Roles of the Nurse

- **Clinical specialists:** A nurse with a master's degree in a particular specialty and substantial clinical knowledge in that specialty is referred to as Clinical Specialists. She offers people with specialist care and is involved in teaching health care professionals. She is involved in research and function as a clinical advisor.
- **Nurse practitioner:** A nurse who possesses a master's degree or certificate in any specialty and with relevant license is referred to as Nurse Practioner. She can make nursing assessments and perform a physical examination. She also advises, teaches, and treats minor illnesses. She uses standing orders to function the role of a practitioner.
- **Nurse – Midwife:** The nurse must have completed the education and training in the midwifery program. She offers all the care services to a woman in pregnancy, and the care is extended to the prenatal, intra-natal, and postnatal periods. The services are aimed at safe pregnancy, labor, and childcare.

- **Nurse anesthetist:** Certified registered nurse anesthetists (CRNAs) play a key role in the practice of many medical procedures. Currently, it is practiced in developed countries. They collaborate with other health care professionals, such as surgeons, anesthetists, and so on. Their role is to ensure the safe administration of anesthesia and assessing anesthesia-related complications. Their services are utilized throughout the process of surgery and even after the surgery. Nurse anesthetists are usually well-compensated professionals because of their sophisticated training and the weight of their duties.

- **Nurse educator:** Nurse educators teach and train the registered nurse for entering into the field of practice. She also provides education and training to practicing nurses as part of in-service education. The in-service education is based on the current practice aspects and new methods of caring for the patients. Nurse educators should possess sound communication skills, robust clinical expertise, and critical thinking ability.

- **Nurse entrepreneur:** A nurse who is interested in growing their organization and health care strategies. She invests her knowledge and expertise and uses her creativity and business knowledge to develop new modes of using the knowledge of nursing for the betterment of human beings. The Nurse Entrepreneur makes use of her professional knowledge to start or grow in business.

- **Nurse administrator:** Nursing administration includes a broad range of nursing duties at the executive level. Nurse administrators are capable of handling all categories of professionals in the health care organization. They also perform administrative tasks such as preparation of performance reports, taking part in review meetings. They are also involved in the training and development of nursing personnel. Typically, a nurse administrator directly reports to a hospital CEO and supervise the nurse managers. This function is typical of an office and managerial nature, with little to no immediate communication between patients.

Characteristics of Professional Nurse

- **Honesty:** Nurses should have reliability and integrity. Avoiding exaggeration and accepting the shortcoming facilitates rectification. It is the quality on which other qualities depend.

- **Discipline and obedience:** Self-discipline is an integral part of the nursing profession that promotes obedience in carrying out vital orders. A calm well-poised nurse who has emotional intelligence inspires confidence and respect.

- **Dignity:** It is the maintenance of professional attitude towards each other and towards patients. Peals of laughter, loud and immature conversation, anger, and argumentation lower the nurse's dignity.

- **Optimism:** A nurse must maintain a positive and warm attitude towards the profession and the patients. A quick warm smile may be more therapeutic than a dose of medicine.

- **Observation and adaptability:** A nurse should develop consciously the qualities of observation and flexibility. A nurse must keep into account small things that improve patients' comfort. A keen observational skill is required to recognize any out of order/out of place equipment, lack of cleanliness, etc. in the ward.

- **Economy:** The nurse must be economical in terms of time, types of equipment, supplies, water, electricity, etc. It is an ideal characteristic of a nurse.

- **Responsibility:** The nursing profession in India today is in high demand for nurse leaders. It is the rarest type of quality/attribute to be acquired. The sense of responsibility produces leaders those who are reliable and efficient.

- **Personal appearance:** A nurse who appears healthy, neat, well-groomed, and meticulous about her hygiene, creates a favorable impression on patients as well as colleagues. Excessive jewelry, cosmetics, improper shoes, poorly fitting or inappropriate uniform ruin the professional appearance.

- **Sympathy:** It is an attribute that the nurse needs to develop along with tolerance and breadth of outlook.

- **Sense of humor:** It helps the nurse in dealing with the patients and her fellow nurses.

Qualities of a Nurse

- **Communication skills:** The fundamental basis for any profession is strong communication abilities. It is one of the most significant elements of the work of nurses with patients. An excellent nurse has good communication skills, particularly to speak and listen. They can fix the issues and interact efficiently with clients and their relatives. It is the responsibility of the nurse to make sure that all understand their patients, and thus, the skill of communication becomes significant. A genuinely outstanding nurse can support and anticipate their requirements for their clients.

- **Emotional stability**: Traumatic situations are faced everyday in nursing profession, and hence, it is considered a stressful job. When it comes to death and suffering, most of nurses feel it personally, and the other way is difficult. All days are not the same, and definitely, the personal life and situational factors place a great emphasis on nurses' emotional stability. Some of the added advantages of nurses' jobs are **to maintain emotional** balance in recovering a patient, interpersonal bonding, and relationship with colleagues. An excellent nurse is capable of managing the stress of unfortunate circumstances and gain positive motivation from better outcomes of the care.

- **Empathy**: The pain and suffering of patients make empathy among good nurses. This feeling of empathy and compassion comforts the patients. But the nurses must be prepared for the occasional bout and it happens often. Learn how to acknowledge and cope effectively with the diseases. Most of the time, the patients consider the nurses as their advocates, and it is the softer side of hospital administration. Being compassionate with the patients makes their living in the hospital a better one, and it accelerates the patient's progress. Most often, all patients enter the hospital looking for a compassionate nurse.

- **Flexibility**: Flexibility is an essential feature of any career, especially nurses. The nurse must be able to adapt to working conditions and responsibilities. Not only nurses but also all the health care professionals are expected to be flexible in terms of working hours as per the demand of the situation. It cannot be understood as exploitation as the compensatory mechanisms for overtime work has been developed in all the organization for these long working hours, shifts and weekend duty, and so on.

- **Interpersonal skills**: The connecting link between patients and doctors are nurses. The nurse connects the patient to all other health care professionals. The interpersonal skills help the nurse to work efficiently in a variety of situations and with a variety of people. They collaborate efficiently with other nurses, physicians, and other professionals and non-professionals. A nurse has the great function of holding the hospital together. Patients see nurses as a sympathetic side, and physicians rely on nurses for relevant information of the patient. It is the responsibility of the nurse to maintain a balance between the patient and the doctor in the preview of health care delivery.

- **Physical endurance**: Regular physical activities, long-term standing, carrying big items (or individuals), and performing many regular challenging exercises are the highlights of nursing lives. It certainly isn't a desk job. A good nurse always maintains the same level of energy throughout duty irrespective of place of work. To keep the level of energy at all times, a nurse must have a healthy life with sufficient intake, plenty of water, and healthy lifestyle practices.

- **Problem solving skills**: Quick thinking ability and facing the issues as and before they occur the critical skill of a nurse. Nurses always need to be on the side to fix a problematic scenario with ill clients, injury instances, and emergencies. The problem-solving approach helps the nurse to deal with the patient and his family irrespective of the place of duty. The nurse always has an alternative method to meet the goal.

- **Quick response**: Nurses must be prepared to react to crises and other emerging circumstances rapidly. Healthcare job is quite often merely the answer to unexpected occurrences, and nurses must always expect the unexpected and be ready for it. Standing by the crisis with a relaxed mind is an excellent quality of the nurse.

- **Respect**: Respect is an essential element in any job. The nurses' respect and obedience to the norms of the organization are necessary for a healthy practice. Nurses also must respect the patients and their relatives/community. The nurse must not be partial and adhere to

the quality of confidentiality. Patients belong to different cultures and traditions, but the nurse must be equal in service to all. The respect shall also be extended to fellow workers and other officers related to the service. The nurse who respects others gains self-respect.

REGULATORY BODIES OF NURSING; INDIAN NURSING COUNCIL

It is the autonomous body under the Ministry of Health and Family Welfare, Government of India constituted under the Indian Nursing Council (INC) Act, 1947 and the consecutive amendments. The core purpose of this act is to maintain uniform standards of education for nurses, midwives, and health visitors across the country. It ensures the reciprocity of nurses' registration across the country (Fig. 2).

Goals of the Indian Nursing Council

- To accomplish and evaluate a fixed standard of nursing education for the nurse-midwife, auxiliary nurse-midwives, and health visitors through regular appraisal of the nursing training institutions.
- To recognize registered nurses and midwives belonging to different nursing courses and their qualifications as per section 10(2)(4) of the Indian Nursing Council Act 1947 for registration and job purpose in India and Abroad.
- To provide approval for the registration of Indian and Foreign Nurses having foreign qualifications under section 11(2)(a) of the Indian Nursing Council Act 1947.
- To frame and update from time to time, the nursing syllabus, rules, and regulations for the nursing program.
- Provide guidelines to SNRCs, Examination Boards, University, Central, and State Governments regarding the up-gradation of nursing education and maintenance of standards.

Organizational Structure of INC

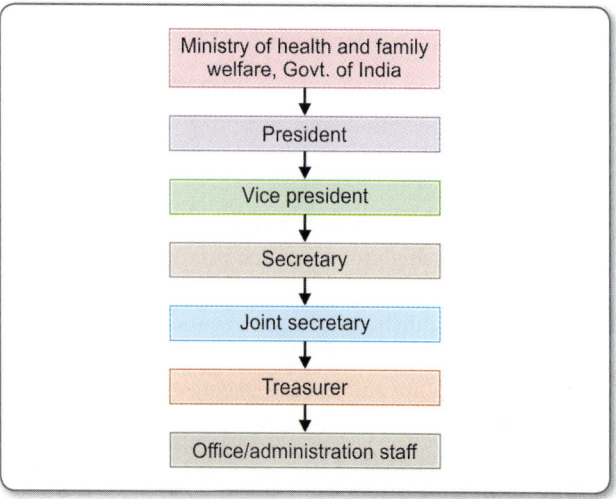

Fig. 2: Indian Nursing Council administration

Functions of INC

- Recognize nurses as a separate branch in health services.
- Regulates nursing training, sets a uniform standard or types of training for nurses throughout the country.
- Recognize nursing qualifications.
- Inspection of nursing colleges and schools for their suitability.
- Providing equivalency to qualified foreign nurses.
- Publications
- Nurses registration and tracking system (NRTS)

STATE NURSING COUNCIL

The State Nursing Council (SNC) or State Nurse's Registration Council (SNRC) is an autonomous body established in each state of India to establish the uniform standards and provide registration to trained nurses and midwives under the law of State. Each State Nursing Council is governed by a Registrar and comes under INC, New Delhi. It is formed by a legislative act in the particular state similar to the Indian Nursing Council. E.g. JKSNC, PNRC, KNC, KSNC, etc

Functions of the State Nursing Council

- **Registration:** Carries out student registration as a nurse and nurse-midwife/public health/psychiatric nurse upon the completion of the desired nursing course from a recognized institution.
- Control and monitor the conduct of different nursing programs in a particular state.
- Inspection of the training institutes and providing recognition.
- Examinations are conducted for different courses throughout the year.
- Maintenance of different registers.
- Renewal of registration.
- Foreign verification and good standing certificate.
- Maintaining the record of additional qualifications.
- Monitor the code of conduct and adherence to professional ethics.
- Publication, in-service education, and research collaboration.

CURRENT TRENDS AND ISSUES IN NURSING

Nursing is one of the oldest forms of art but has developed into a profession recently. From the beginning, it has undergone many drastic modifications and updations, and currently, it is an unavoidable part of society. The recent trend analysis shows that future nursing will see significant advantages in multidimensional patient care, including promotive and preventive health. Nurses will be the most preferred healthcare

providers in the coming time though there are challenges such as ethical considerations, rising health care costs, and quality of care. Healthier lifestyles, promotive environments, and continuity of quality care based on EBP are highlighted in nursing.

Nursing has the gigantic ability to change individuals. These requests require a broad learning base and essential reasoning capacities alongside able aptitudes. The focal point of nursing is moving towards perceiving patients as cooperative recipients as opposed to uninvolved beneficiaries of health care. Professional nursing is comprehensive as she/he will be effectively engaged with direct supervision, educating health care aspects, home care management, and OPD consultation.

The nursing profession continues to be challenged and rewarded by both new and changing opportunities and constraints, for all nurses, individually and collectively. Several forces have affected the development of professional nursing and continue to affect significant issues. These include:

- Societal images and expectations of nurses.
- Degree of the nursing profession's control over the quantity and quality of practitioners.
- Impact of technology and theory on nursing practices, its roles, and settings.
- The professional self-image of nurses.
- Sources of financing for health care services.

Current Trends in Nursing in India

- **Reduction in the distance:** The introduction of modern communication techniques such as mobile phone, email, video conferencing have reduced the gap between patients and health care professionals/care providers. The introduction of different mobile applications has made the health care consultation available at the fingertip.
- **Computerization of patient care:** Gone are the days of manual data maintenance. The introduction of computer-based applications in the health care organizations has made the patient data digital from OPD consultation/Admission to discharge and follow up. It includes computerized record-keeping, sharing of intra, and interdepartmental information pertaining to a patient (lab results, diagnostic reports, medical and surgical requirements). It also includes management and organizational aspects of an organization such as employee attendance, inventory management, inter-department communication, and so on.
- **Quality assurance in nursing:** In the changing health care environment, concerns over the quality of care are receiving more considerable attention than ever before. As consumers become more knowledgeable as a result of increased information available to them, much of the mystique surrounding health care is being dissipated.
- **Decentralized approach:** This approach makes the nurse accountable for the care of the allotted patient. It is appreciable and effective as it focuses on the satisfaction

of the patient, quality of the health care, and smooth functioning of the department.

- **Continuing nursing education (CNE):** It is aimed at the motivation of the workers and to build up their skills and capacities according to their respective current/future designations. The health care system is highly dynamic, and it is imperative for a nurse to keep abreast of the changes. It can be achieved through attending conferences, seminars, workshops, presenting scientific papers, and so on. Generally, CNE should be regularly organized by educational and health care organizations.
- **Evidence-based practice (EBP):** Nurses today should have a scientific bent of mind and a dynamic approach to patient care. Intensified researches and the application of the research findings in the clinical setting are yet another challenge.

TRENDS IN NURSING EDUCATION AND SERVICE

(Detailed information is provided in Unit 8)

Currently, nursing is focused on PBL and EBP grounded with nursing research. Earlier the entry-level of profession was certificate level and diploma level. The specialization programs in nursing education are symbolical to this trend growth. Currently, in India, several educational programs such as GNM, BSc (N), PBBSc (N), PG Diploma Programs, MSc (N) and PhD (N) are offered at different organizations to uplift the standard of the profession. The MSc Nursing program enables the nurses to specialize in their field of practice such as Medical-Surgical Nursing (MSN), Community Health Nursing (CHN), Psychiatric Nursing/Mental Health Nursing, Pediatric Nursing/Child Health Nursing, Obstetrics and Gynecological Nursing (OBG) and Forensic Nursing. The recent launch of Nurse Practitioner in Critical Care program by the Indian Nursing Council allows the graduate nurses to assume responsibility and accountability to provide competent care to critically ill patients and appropriate family care in tertiary care centers.

On the contrary, the increasing demands of healthcare need cause specific issues in Nursing. Few of the problems faced by the nursing education are compromised students, the gap of theory and practice, underutilization of clinical facilities, inadequate facilities in educational institutions, lack of qualified teachers, and overall compromised education system.

The nursing service industry faces challenges such as compromised working conditions, biased staffing patterns, fewer wages, lack of practice guidelines, lack of proper research, and deficient in-service education programs. Most of the time, nurses need to focus on routine administrative/paperwork rather than bedside care.

Challenges in Nursing Education

- Independent Infrastructure for Nursing college
- Independence for Principal
- Acute Shortage of Qualified Teaching Professionals
- Lack of UGC status
- Underutilization of Clinical facilities
- Academic dishonesty
- Lack of discipline
- Workplace violence
- Student voices

TRENDS IN NURSING RESEARCH

According to American Association of Colleges of Nursing, rigorous nursing research enables the sound development of body of knowledge and it is an essential element of scholarship in nursing. Nursing research improves the nursing practice and nursing practice gives rise to new research problems. Young professional nurses with research aptitude is of high demand in nursing profession across the globe. Research opportunities and needs await interested professionals in nursing. To fulfill their professional obligations in the health care delivery system, nurses have to keep the following objective in mind (a) Nursing research will be a core part of nursing education and nursing care service. (b) Nursing practice will accomplish an environment equal to the evaluation of professional practice.

Challenges in Nursing Research

- Funding
- Acceptance from Superiors
- Scarcity of resources
- Availability of nurse (nursing) expertise
- Appropriate Research setting
- Non-availability of Nursing research Program

Issues Affecting Nursing Practice

- **Demographical changes:** It includes an increased occurrence of illness at a younger age, increased poverty, lack of outreach of immunization and nutritional programs, compromised sanitation, cultural diversity, urbanization, etc.
  - Many older persons are healthy, but the likelihood of illness becomes more significant as people age. It indicates the nurse of the future should be equipped to work with the aged.
  - Several people in our country and abroad are still living under the poverty line. For them, the priority always focuses on food, clothing, and shelter. Health care is always a luxury for them.

- Immunization of children and pregnant women, provision of nutritious meals and other health maintaining aspects are still neglected though we have made some progress on it.
- Preventive health care is not often focused. This is due to lack of education, increased population density, lack of sanitation and waste management techniques, etc.
- The nursing profession is committed to providing care for people irrespective of socio-cultural and economic factors. The cultural beliefs and practices of citizens are quite different. The nurse needs to understand these differences while planning the care.
- Urbanization is a common phenomenon in society. People prefer to move from rural areas to the city. It causes many social issues such as homelessness, drugs, mental illness, violence, and crime. Nurses of the future should be equipped to confront health problems related to it.
- **Environmental changes:** It includes issues such as natural as well as human-made calamities, pollution, overpopulation, etc. Major ecological tragedies such as nuclear power plant accidents, burning oil wells, tsunamis, gradual decline in the purity of water, diminishing animal, and plant life lead to health problems. These are issues that the future nurse has to face.
- **Change in healthy practices:** Factors such as obesity, food habits, lack of exercise, stress, etc. Obesity is a significant reason causing risk for many illnesses among people. It contributes to hypertension, diabetes mellitus, PCOD, coronary artery diseases, cardiac abnormalities, and so on. The lifestyle and health habits such as sexual life, smoking/alcoholism contribute to HIV/AIDS, lung cancer, and liver diseases. In these conditions, nurses will have to play predominantly essential functions in educating the public regarding the health hazards of these lifestyles.
- **Emerging bioethical issues:** The ethical considerations are prevention of conception, termination of pregnancy, fetal surgery, organ transplantation, genetic research, fetal research, selection between life and death, etc.
  - Issues such as prevention of conception, termination of pregnancy, test-tube conception, other artificial fertilization (artificial insemination, IVF) and contraception methods contribute to emotional changes in people.
  - The ethical considerations in this regard must be weighed against its outcome.
  - Issues related to life or death, which include that the invention of life-saving apparatuses such as dialysis, ventilator, heart and the lung machine, new surgical procedures (organ transplant, fetal surgery) and new technologies (genetic research, fetal research) have all become necessary to redefine the terms of life and death.

- **Degree versus diploma for practice:** One of the major concerns in India is the lack of policies pertaining to nursing practice and the required professional training for intended designation. The distinction between the level of qualification and level of entry in-service should be clearly defined. Recently, an attempt is made by the Govt. of India and Indian Nursing Council, adopting a policy to discontinue GNM (General Nursing and Midwifery) and the level of entry to a health care organization as the nursing officer will be based on the graduation. (BSc Nursing/PB BSc Nursing).
- **Specialization in clinical area:** Currently, there are five clinical specializations in nursing education in India. The expanded role of the nurse based on these specializations is not in practice. The necessary policy and legal formulations have not yet been framed in this regard. Though few innovations in this regard have taken place in recent years such as the introduction of Nurse Practitioners in Critical Care, it is still in the infancy stage.
- **Nursing care standards:** Standards are written formal statements to describe how an organization or professional should deliver health service and are guidelines against which services can be assessed. Standards are directed at the structure, process, and outcome issues and guide the review of systems function, staff performance, and client care. The nurse has to be scientifically equipped for meeting the caring standards of patient's expectations.
- **Nurse patient ratio:** Staffing is an issue of both professional and personal concerns for nurses today. Inadequate staffing threatens patients' health and safety resulting in complexity of care by increasing fatigue and rate of injury in patients.
- **Long working hours:** Nurses are often required to work long shifts. But in several cases, nurses must work back-to-back or extended shifts, risking fatigue that could result in medical mistakes.
- **Workplace hazards:** Nurses face several workplace hazards each day while just doing their jobs. These hazards include exposure to bloodborne pathogens, injuries, and hand washing-related dermatitis and cold and flu germs.

The transition is a universal phenomenon, and nurses involved in the caring profession have to undergo it. Some techniques such as positive thinking, flexibility, organized and healthy personal life, and ideal mentor can help in the process of transition.

ETHICS AND CODE OF ETHICS

Ethics or Code of Ethics is understood as a line of practice or as the norm that is set to control the practice of nursing in alliance with service obligation that respects the life of a human. These are explained as a group of principles made and accepted by the members of the nursing profession. It frames the guidelines of nursing practice that enables the evaluation of performance and standards. It ensures the professional and personal accountability of the services.

Definitions

Ethics refers to the moral code for nursing and is based on the obligation to service and respect for human life.

—Melanie and Evelyn

A Code of Ethics is a set of ethical principles that are accepted by all members of a profession. —Potter and Perry

A Code of Ethics is a set of the ethical principle that is shared by members of a group, reflects their moral judgments over time and serves as a standard for their professional actions.

—Barbara Kozier

Nursing Ethics

It is a branch of applied ethics that concerns itself with activities in the field of nursing. It refers to ethical standards that govern and guide nurses in everyday practice such as being truthful with clients, respecting client confidentiality, and advocating on behalf of the client.

Need for Nursing Ethics

- Helps the students/RN to practice ethically.
- Helps the nurse to identify the ethical issues in her workplace.
- Protecting patients' rights and dignity.
- Providing care with possible risk to the nurses' health.
- Ethical reasoning.
- Guide for professional behavior.
- Staffing patterns that limit the patients' access to nursing care.
- Helps the nurse to respond to ethical conflicts.
- Helps to differentiate right/wrong behavior.
- Help teachers plan education.
- Prevent below standard practice.
- Protect a nurse if falsely accused and guide the direction for legal action.

Principles of Ethics

- **Respect for persons:** All nursing services are aimed for the wellbeing of the recipients of care. Hence the recipients should be respected.
- **Autonomy:** Every individual/professional should be responsible for their actions. Every registered nurse has the right to practice their profession individually according to their capacity. The principle of autonomy controls the functioning of nurses.
- **Beneficence:** All the actions are aimed at the promotion of wellbeing. The nurse needs to understand the possible harms while aiming at the benefits and maintain equilibrium.
- **Non-maleficence:** It says that no nursing actions should be aimed at causing harm for the patient, family, and society.
- **Veracity:** The health care professional should always speak the truth and provide evidence-based information about patients and their health status.
- **Justice:** It ensures the equal right of patients for treatment and other related services. All persons should be given equal importance in a health care organization.
- **Fidelity:** It is the principle of the fulfillment of duties faithfully and keeping one's commitment/promise.
- **Confidentiality:** The nurse should respect the patients and maintain the confidentiality of the information obtained from the patients. The information about the patients should be discussed or shared only for the therapeutic purpose and that too with their consent.

ICN Code of Ethics

- Every individual is unique. Hence the nursing care should not be based on the caste, culture, religion, etc. All individuals are given specialized care and service equally.
- The patients and nurses are partners in health care, and hence, informed consent is required to make choices.
- Provide and maintain confidentiality and privacy. The information should be shared judiciously.
- Improve and maintain professional competence that results in quality nursing care.
- Nursing should be practiced within the legal and ethical boundaries of the profession.
- Work as a team.
- Maintain a trustworthy relationship with the profession and society.

ICN Code of Ethics for Nurses

The first Code of Ethics for nurses at the international level was established in 1953 by ICN (International Council of Nurses). It was subsequently revised in 1965 and 2000. These Code of Ethics were adopted by ICN in 1973. The ICN suggests the nursing service as a four-dimensional care concern that aims at preventing illness, promoting health, restoring the wellbeing, and alleviating the suffering. It also ensures that every recipient of care has the right to receive dignified care and treatment. The care should be given to all without any discrimination. The ICN explains the nurses' responsibility under the following.

- **Nurses and people:** Every nurse is primarily responsible for those people who are in need of nursing care. Every individual should be respected as they are, and the nurse should adapt to a non-judgemental approach to the patients.
- **Nurses and practice:** The nurse conveys moral obligation regarding nursing practice and for keeping up capability

by continuous learning. The nurse keeps up the most astounding standard of nursing care conceivable within the fact of a particular circumstance. The nurse utilizes judgment ability in connection to singular ability when designating obligations. In a professional capacity, the nurse should consistently keep up benchmarks of individual leaders, which credits the profession.

- **Nurses and co-workers:** The nurse keeps up an agreeable association with colleagues in nursing and different fields. She also makes a proper move to protect the person when his care is jeopardized by a work associate or any individual.
- **Nurses and the profession:** The nurse assumes an exceptional job in deciding and actualizing attractive principles of nursing practice. The nursing is dynamic in building up a center of professional information. She takes an interest in building up and keeping up evenhanded social and financial working conditions in nursing.

ICN Code of Professional Conduct

Code of professional conduct for nurses in India

- **Professional responsibility and accountability:** To maintain professional responsibility and accountability, the nurse:
  - Appreciates a sense of self-worth and nurtures it.
  - Maintains standards of professional conduct, reflecting credit upon the profession.
  - Carries out responsibilities within the framework of professional boundaries.
  - Is accountable for maintaining practice standards set by the ICN.
  - Is accountable for his or her actions.
  - Is compassionate.
  - Practices healthful behavior.
  - Is responsible for the continuous improvement of current practices.
- **Nursing practice:** In the course of the practice of nursing, the nurse:
  - Provides care in accordance with set standards of practice.
  - Offer the physical, psychological, emotional, social, and spiritual elements of care, treat all individuals and families with human dignity.
  - Respect people and families in traditional and cultural activities and encourages good practices and discourages damaging practices.
  - Presents realistic pictures truthful in all situations for facilitating autonomous decision making by individuals and families.
  - Promotes the participation of individuals and significant others in the care.
  - Ensures safe practice.
- **Communication and interpersonal relationships:** This plays a crucial role in the interaction of the nurse with his or her clients. To effect optimal interaction, the nurse:
  - Establishes and maintains effective IPRs with all individuals and families.
  - Protects and upholds the dignity of team members and maintains valid IPR with them.
  - Appreciates the professional behavior of the team members.
  - Collaborates with other health care professionals in meeting the needs of the clients and their families.
- **Valuing human beings:** The nurse values human life.
  - Takes appropriate action to protect individuals from harmful, unethical practices.
  - Considers relevant facts while taking conscientious decisions in the best interest of individuals.
  - Encourages and supports the individual in their right to speak for themselves on issues affecting health and welfare.
  - Respect and support choices made by individuals.
- **Management:** Proper management of resources and infrastructure is essential for improving the overall efficiency of the nurse. Hence a nurse
  - Makes sure that the resources are adequately distributed and utilized.
  - Participates in supervision and education of students and other formal providers.
  - Uses judgment in relation to individual competence while accepting and delegating responsibility.
  - Communicates effectively following appropriate channels of communication.
  - Participates in performance appraisal.
  - Participates in the evaluation of nursing services.
  - Participates in a policy decision, following the principles of equity and accessibility of service.
- **Professional advancement:** To ensure that he or she is at par with contemporaries in the nursing field, the nurse must
  - Provide the protection of human rights while pursuing the advancement of knowledge.
  - Participate in determining and implementing quality care.
  - Take responsibility for updating one's own knowledge and competencies.
  - Contribute to the core of professional knowledge and conducting and participating in research.
  - The responsibility of nurses concerning patients is no more limited to care alone. It has a broader concern related to different environmental factors concerning patient such as the respect of culture, customs, religious beliefs and so on. The confidentiality and privacy aspects of patient care has more significance today. The nurse must be accountable for all professional and personal behavior.

American Nurses Association: Code of Ethics for Nurses

- Nursing should be practiced with empathy, respect, and dignity. Every patient/person is treated irrespective of their economic status, type of illness, and other personal attributes.
- The nurses' essential duty is to the patient; regardless, it is an individual, family, etc.
- The nurse should maintain professional responsibility/accountability through standardized practice and conduct within the line and framework.
- The nurses are actively involved in the establishment, improvement, and maintenance of health care as well as employment conditions required for quality health care provision in a professional and collective approach.
- The nurses also participate in professional advancements with numerous contributions such as contribution to practice, education, and knowledge development.
- Collaborate with other health care professionals locally, nationally, and internationally to promote health.
- Nurses/Professional association help in framing a social policy that articulate nursing values.

Canadian Nurses Association Code of Ethics for Nursing

- **Health and wellbeing:** Nurses provide care to the health and well being of the persons, family and community. Nurses use the least restrictive measures possible while giving care considering the community perception of care. Nurses also collaborate with other health care providers to maximize the health benefits.
- **Choice:** Nurses regard and advance the autonomy of patients/clients/customers and also promote to express their wellbeing needs and values and to get the proper services.
- **Dignity:** Nurses esteem and support the self-respect and dignity of people.
- **Confidentiality:** Provide and maintain confidentiality and privacy. The information should be shared judiciously.
- **Fairness:** Follow the principle of equity and justice. Every patient/person treated irrespective of their economic status, type of illness, and other personal attributes.
- **Accountability:** The nurse should maintain professional responsibility/accountability through standardized practice and conduct within the line and framework.
- **Practice environment:** Conducive to safe, competent, and ethical care. Nurses advocate the practice environments that have the organizational and human support systems and the resource allocation necessary for reliable, competent, and ethical nursing care.

Ethical Theories

- **Duty-oriented ethical theories/deontology class of theory:** It is an ethical reasoning scheme based on the notion of responsibility or duty. The obligation or duty is the foundation of this theory. According to the concept of deontology people while engaged in decision making must adhere to one's duties, responsibilities, and obligations. This implies that a person will fulfill his or her responsibilities towards another individual or community as it is deemed ethically right to preserve one's obligation. A deontologist, for example, will always keep his promises to a friend and obey the law. An individual who adheres to the principle of deontology will make very coherent choices as they are dependent on his/her duties.

  These types of theories are beneficial in homogeneous communities since the people in the group value the significance of duty. In a tribal society, a duty-oriented concept would operate well because it is simpler for a less number of individuals to communicate value and principles and therefore, beliefs. Classification of responsibilities is a disadvantage of a duty-oriented hypothesis. A nurse may have the dual duty of caring for the suffering person as well as supporting the life of another person. There are many beneficial characteristics in deontology, but it also includes faults. Most of the time, the determination of duties is done without a proper rational or logical basis. Sometimes there is a dispute between the responsibilities of a person.

- **Rights-oriented ethical theories:** In this context, right overlays the significance of duty. These concepts signify the glory of rights so that the duties become secondary to the right. In these theories, the established rights of the community are regarded as significant, and it is given higher priority to be protected. As a large population considers it valid, the rights are deemed to be ethically considerable. For example, A nurse commits a patient to give him the medication in the afternoon. Now the patient has the right to have the drug in the afternoon as the nurse has committed it.

  A significant potential problem of this hypothesis is that before the implementation of this right-oriented ethical theory, the community has to decide the right and wrong in the community, which has to be followed by all. Society needs to identify what privileges it intends its people to maintain and offer. The rights of society will be based on its goals and objectives.

- **Goal-oriented ethical theories:** It is otherwise referred to as a utilitarian ethical theory. This theory is based on the maximization of the overall goal of the person or decision. To a utilitarian, the consequences are more important in every decision and action. If any action would benefit a large group of people, then it is ethically considered right.

It firmly believes that good choices are meant for the excellent health of the patients irrespective of the fact of any other immediate consequences. A nurse might choose a plan of action without considering the immediate demerit but considering the long term merit on the health of the patient. It could be regarded as optimizing the welfare of the community to provide health care services.

- **Intuitionist ethical theory**: An ethical concept is an ethical reasoning scheme that balances objectives, rights, obligations, and responsibilities by the circumstance of the decision. Philosophers in favor of this assertion claim that human beings recognize the concept of good and evil through intuition, and thus, the rights and duties can be balanced accordingly.
- **Virtue ethical theory**: Here, the judging of a person's action or decision is based on the level of deviation from the concept of normal behavior. The morality, reputation, and fame is considered before judging the action of a person. For instance, if a person is noted for doing plagiarism, he may be dealt harshly in case the person is of academic misconduct. Instead, if the same happens with a bright and academically brilliant student, he may be dealt leniently considering it as a light error of negligence. The weakness of this theory is that it does take into account the concept of change in one's morality over some time.

Ethical Dilemmas

An ethical dilemma is described as a scenario that requires a decision between two options that are similarly acceptable or unacceptable. Every appropriate mode of action can be explained in an ethical dilemma by the way the person views it. The view of the person is based on the value system that he or she possesses. Nursing officers and their managers regularly face many difficulties in decision making among several factors such as technology, budget, and quality concerns. They need to make effective, ethical decisions despite these considerations. The following dilemmas are faced by nurses in all clinical and functional specialties.

- Need to limit the quality of patient care due to limited resources.
- The decision making of terminally ill patients for treatment and care.
- Obtaining consent for ethically significant decisions such as withdrawing nutrition, removing life support, and so on.
- Consent for mercy killing and assisted suicide.
- Concept of confidentiality and right of information (disclosing patient details to the near and dear ones)
- Rights of patients and vulnerable populations in the context of nursing research. Rights of the research participants in the controlled trials.

Decision making: The systematic approach to solving the problems of the patient is possible through the effective nursing process. The nursing process is aimed at improving the health and wellbeing of the patients. The ethical decision making is aimed at deciding the right and wrong according to the circumstances.

CONSUMER PROTECTION ACT

These are laws encircled to guarantee reasonable challenge and the free stream of right data in a particular field of service, including health care organizations. This aid in keeping any misrepresentation or any predefined unreasonable practices from picking up leverage. It gives extra security to the powerless and helpless to deal with themselves. Consumer Protection Act (CPA) is aimed to safeguard the opinions of consumers.

The CPA was implemented by Government of India in 1986 and came into existence since 1987. It is aimed at the provision of speedy, cheap, and straightforward redressal for consumer grievances relating to deficient services, defective goods, and unfair trade practices.

Objectives of CPA

- To prevent the manufacturing, sales, and spread of those services and products that are harmful to the life and land.
- To ensure that the customers are informed about the standard, quantity, quality, potency, purity, and price of services and products.
- Ensures the availability of a variety of services and products to choose from at competitive prices.
- The right to use the grievance redressal management system against unfair trade/service practices. The consumer is assured that their voice is heard.

Rights of the Consumer/Patient

- Right to be intimated
- Right to safety
- Right to selection
- Right to have listened
- Right to get relief

The CPA provides a forum for the customer and helps in resolving the disputes.

The District Consumer Redressal Forum consists of a District Judge (President) and two members out of which one will be a woman. The District Redressal Forum can award compensation up to Rs. 500,000/-.

The State Consumer Redressal Forum is comprised of a High Court Judge (President) and two members out of which one will be a woman. The State Redressal Forum can award compensation up to Rs. 20,00,000/-.

The National Redressal Forum comprises of a Supreme Court Judge (President) and four members. One of them will be a woman. The National Commission usually deals with appeals made against the judgments of the state commissions and can award any amount of compensation.

LEGAL ASPECTS OF NURSING

Understanding of legal aspects in nursing is vital for every nursing professional to protect the patients and self from different legal implications. All the laws of the land are of three sources such as Constitutional law/structured by the constitution, the common law from the court decisions and administrative law which is established by administrative agencies of the government.

The term law is derived from its Teutonic word "Lag," which means something definite or lies fixed or events. It means "uniform" in the English language. Law implies a body of rules to guide human action.

Definitions

The law is a system of rights and obligations which the state enforces.
—By Green
The law constitutes the body of principles recognized or enforced by public and regular tribunals have the administration of justice.
—By Pound

Sources of Law

- **Constitutional law:** It is a judgemental law. Law that governs the state/country. It determines the structure of the country or state, power, and duties.
- **Common law:** It is a body of legal principles that evolved from court decisions.
- **Administrative law:** Rules and regulations established by administrative agencies made by executives of government.

Purposes of Law in Nursing

- To help the nurse understand that in nursing practice, they have legal responsibilities.
- To provide them with an understanding of which power can enforce these legal obligations.
- Making them know what fields of nursing practice can generate mostly legal issues.
- Describe and defend rights of customers and nurses.
- There is a law to protect the nursing practice.
- The legislation is in place to identify the risk of liability.
- Law is in place to help in the nursing decision-making process.
- Protecting the public.
- Protection of the nurse.

Safeguarding the Nurse/Determinants of Legal Framework in India

- **Registration/licensure:** It is mandatory for all nurses to practice nursing. The registration is usually issued by the respective SNRCs. The person who holds a foreign qualification in nursing should obtain an equivalency certificate from INC before registration. The employers must recruit only those nurses who hold a valid registration of the respective State Nursing Council.
- **Good Samaritan laws:** Many States in India have adopted the Good Samaritan Law to protect health professionals. They justify the emergency health care services.
- **Legal liability:** It falls under section 304 of the IPC. (administration of wrong medications). Hence, the nurse must follow the rights of medication administration. Additionally, it also includes negligence. (E.g. not providing side rails to the unconscious patient causing a fall.)
- **Medication errors:** It mainly happens due to drugs with similar names, the same type of containers and an inadequate system of communication between professionals. According to JCA, the medication errors can be prevented by following the rights of medication administration and keeping the medicine at the patients' bedside in locked cupboards.
- **Medico-legal case (MLC):** An MLC is for a patient who is admitted to the hospital with an unnatural pathology. These kinds of cases have to be intimated to the nearby police station. The common MLC cases include RTA (Road Traffic Accidents), injuries related to fights/shooting/bomb blasts, homicide, burns, poisoning, rape, and suicide.
- **Good rapport:** Development and maintenance of interpersonal communication is an inevitable part of nursing practice. A genuine IPR with the patient and his/her family is crucial in preventing malpractice. The IPR strongly relies on the communication skills of health professionals.
- **Standards of care:** As like any other profession nursing care also requires specific standards, ethics, and policies. It is usually explained as organizational protocols for providing care. While giving care to clients, nurses must follow the protocols to avoid malpractice. Do not perform anything beyond the protocol and one's competence.
- **Standing orders:** Legally, the nurse does not diagnose and prescribe treatment for any illness. Still, the nurses are allowed to diagnose and provide treatment in case of emergencies as per the protocol of standing orders. The standing orders are usually established by the physician, and the nurse must follow the guidelines of standing orders.
- **Consent for surgical and other procedures:** Nurses must know their legal responsibilities concerning a letter which is duly signed by the patient regarding the routine treatment, surgery, or special treatment such as chemotherapy. The consent must be obtained from those above 18 years of

age, the parent in case of a child, guardian, blood relative, grandparents, etc. The nurse also must keep into account the concept of informed consent. The consentee must be explained in his/her level of understanding regarding the treatment/procedures and its outcome/side effects in detail. Consent should be obtained only from those persons who are mentally sound.

- **Correct identity:** The nurse/midwife is responsible for labeling/identification tags/bands for all newborn babies. The unconscious patients also should be labeled. Patients should be labeled in case of surgery, and the site of surgery also should be marked carefully.
- The OT scrub nurse must make sure that all swabs and instruments are returned before the closing of the surgical procedure.
- **Left against medical advice (LAMA):** These cases should be reported to the Medical Officer. Appropriate documents must be signed by the patient and witness.
- **Medical records:** It is very important to document all the details of treatments, surgeries, medications, and any other details pertaining to the patient. The case file of each patient must be stored at Medical Records Department (MRD).

Laws in Nursing

- **Common law:** These are framed in concordance with individual decisions made by the honorable Courts/Legal System with respect to individual cases.
- **Felony:** A crime that is serious in nature and is expected to have a penalty of imprisonment for more than one year.
- **Civil law:** These include legislations related to the rights of the person, including fair and equal distribution of services among the people.
- **Contract law:** Usually includes the terms and conditions pertaining to service. It is an MoU between two individuals or two organizations. E.g. Employment contract.
- **Criminal law:** It is related to crime. It regulates the conduct of the people to ensure their safety and welfare.

Legal Issues in Nursing

- **Personal liability:** Nurses are professionally qualified and educated. Hence they must be responsible for what they do. A nurse cannot do something unethical even if the employer forces to do it. Therefore, if a physician directs you to perform something opposite to your personal judgment and states, "I will assume accountability," then the concerned person is doing an unwise act. If the outcomes are harmful, the doctor and manager who gives the instructions may be responsible, but this would not be erase your liability. An organization or a person may be held accountable for someone else's actions even though everyone is accountable for their action.

- **Employer liability:** In particular, the organization or the contractor is liable for the behavior of its staff, especially the torts. The employer-employee relationship is the most prevalent condition in which a person or organization is held accountable for another's deeds. Most of the time, an employer becomes accountable for torts done by an employee. It is referred to as the doctrine of respondent superior. The employer is responsible for employing skilled staff, creating a suitable atmosphere for proper functioning, and offering supervision or guidance as necessary to prevent mistakes or damage.

  Consequently, if a nurse is accused of malpractice as a hospital worker, the hospital may be listed in the complaint. Employers' responsibility may occur even if it suggests that the employee has adopted measures to avoid mistakes. It is essential to realize that this doctrine does not take accountability from the nursing officer, but, it expands accountability to the organization.

- **Charitable immunity:** The health care organizations which are nonprofit in operation cannot be held legally liable for the harm. They get the immunity of charity. The employees of these organizations have personal liability. In some states, non-profit hospitals have charitable immunity. The employees of that nonprofit hospital are still legally responsible for their actions. The trend in legislation is toward the repeal of laws providing for charitable immunity. Those active in the consumer movement have argued that no institution should be relieved of responsibility in such a blanket fashion. If you are employed by a nonprofit institution, it is essential that you know whether the law in your state provides charitable immunity for the institution.

- **Supervisory liability:** The Nurse Supervisor/Incharge Nurse is responsible for the potential problems made by their subordinates. When a nurse is in the role of charge nurse, head nurse, supervisor, or any other role which involves supervision or direction of other people, the nurse is potentially liable for the actions of others. The supervising nurse is responsible for good exercising sound judgment in a supervisory role. This includes making appropriate decisions about assignments and delegation of tasks. If an error occurs and the supervising nurse is shown to have exercised sound judgments in all decisions made in that capacity, the supervising nurse may not be held liable for the error of the subordinate. If a poor judgment was used in assigning an inadequately prepared person to an important task, the supervisory nurse might be liable for resulting harm.

Informed Consent

Each individual has the power to agree to standard treatment or to deny it and hence the consent. According to the law, the patient must give informed consent voluntarily, and it may be either verbal or written. In health care, written consent is usually preferred to ensure that a consent record exists. The consent form must have the intended list of procedures and its details. The patient may sign the consent form in front of the nurse, and the nurse may countersign it as a witness. If the person does not appear to be well educated, the nurse should notify the doctor to provide the client with information. The nurse has ethical duties to help the client in practicing their rights and to help the doctor in giving adequate treatment.

- **Consent for nursing measures:** Patient approval and permission must be obtained before nursing interventions are undertaken. This does not imply that in each scenario, it is necessary to give exhaustive reasons because the law says that the patient must have a minimum understanding of the routine care. Consent can be obtained either in oral or written form. The nurse must acknowledge that the patients have the right to deny any part of the care. Like the doctor, however, the nurse is accountable for ensuring that the client is notified before a choice is made.

- **Competence to give consent:** The judgment making capacity of an individual based on his level of understanding is termed as competence. The common causes for this incompetence are some illnesses such as dementia, head injury, developmental disabilities, loss of consciousness, stroke, and so on that make judging impossible. Competence determination is a complicated problem. Competency is not determined by illness, gender, or situation alone. Court decides legal competence. If an individual is found to be legally incompetent, the approval of the legal guardian is acquired. A person's physical illness may alter competence.

- **Withdrawing consent**: Once provided, consent may be removed too. People are entitled to modify their minds. Therefore, if a person chooses not to have a second IV infusion after the first one, he is right. As a nurse, if the person declines medical procedure or therapy, you have a duty to notify the doctor.

- **Consent and minors**: Minor's consent is generally granted by a parent or legal guardian. Also, if he or she can offer it, then we should get the minor permission too. Increasingly, the judiciary emphasizes that when it comes to issues that they are worthy of understanding, minors are permitted to have a voice. This is particularly valid for adolescents, but any person who is seven years of age or older should be provided this option. You should not continue until legal clarification is provided when the minor rejects treatment and the legal guardian has permitted that care. The nursing manager may be consulted in case of any confusion.

- **Consent in an emergency**: If there is a real crisis, it is regarded that approval to care is meant. The law entitles a reasonable person to give consent on behalf of the patient in an emergency if he or she is aware of the situation. An exception is provided if the individual has dismissed such care before and this can found from the records.

Fraud

Fraud may be defined as an intentional deception for personal benefit. The legally significant cases of fraud are uncommon in the nursing profession. One instance would be an employee furnishes fake credentials and information to obtain a better designation and position in the organization. E.g., A nurse informs the higher authority that he has completed the training and education of Nurse Practitioner and produces a fake document to support the same; the nurse is defrauding the organization. It can also be considered as a criminal act as a person with fake qualification cause danger to the life of the people by providing care unscientifically and without sufficient knowledge or expertise. Trying to cover up a nursing error to escape from legal liability is also a fraud. The law of the land tends to be more vigilant and strict on people who perform fraud as it is an attempt to harm others.

Medication Errors

Some mistakes result from drugs with comparable titles, similar containers of medication, inadequate communication mechanisms in which handwriting issues are present. They can contribute to the occurrence of medication errors. When medication errors occur, it may be prosecuted for fraud or deliberate concealment and may add to punitive damages as well as normal damages.

Torts

They are civil violations committed by an individual against another individual. It may be physical, psychological, and livelihood issues.

Classification of Torts

- **Intentional Torts:** It is a willful action intended to cause injury to a person or property.
  - **Assault:** It is the deliberate cause of an offense. E.g. Giving an unwanted injection to the patient who is not cooperative. The law protects clients who are afraid of harmful contact. It is an assault for a nurse to threaten to give a client an X-ray procedure when the client has refused consent. The critical issue is client consent. In an assault lawsuit, if the clients give consent, the nurse is not responsible.
  - **Battery:** Touching the individual without permission. E.g. It includes touching of the private parts of the client without permission. The battery is a person's unconsented or illegitimate touch. The touch or contact that take place without permission is considered as the battery. Rather than a specific statement, even the implication of a particular gesture may also be regarded as consent. For example, if a client shows his arm to get an IM injection, he cannot claim battery stating that he was not asked for permission because extending arm

is a gesture of consent. In case the injection was given forcibly, then the patient has the right to claim battery.

- **False imprisonment:** Retaining the client in a particular place against his/her desire and will. It uses restraints. This happens, for instance, when staff restricts a patient in a confined zone to prevent the individual from being free. But when it happens in health service, it is most often the cause of a civil or statutory suit and not a criminal case. Whenever a person is needed to be restricted for his or her safety or well-being, it is better to make the person understand and agree for the same. The authorization may be obtained from the guardian or legally responsible persons. Another alternative for carrying out restraining is forwarding a written request to the physician and getting the physician's order for the same. As everyone has the right to make their own decisions, there is a need to teach and make the patient understand the need for a particular service. Keep in mind to report all the events to the Nurse manager.
- **Trespass:** An unauthorized entry into another person's property, using others' property without consent.

- **Quasi-intentional torts/Specific torts**
  - **Defamation:** It may be oral or written. It occurs when a person speaks or writes about another person to disturb the reputation of the affected person. E.g. The doctor tells the patient that the nurse is incompetent.
  - **Invasion of privacy:** It is the violation of patients' privacy. It is further classified as:

    Invasion of privacy—intrusion of solitude: Privacy seclusion is a subset of privacy intrusion committed by some health professionals or others where that individual is expected to have privacy. Usually, the location where the individual expects privacy is in a house or office environment. It can be in a health care setting too. It is also regarded that opening someone's mail is an intrusion of privacy. To perform an infringement of privacy complaints, the data collected by this type of intrusion need not be disclosed. Trespass is strongly linked to the privacy intrusion and can be reported at the same time.

    Invasion of privacy—appropriation of name, likeness, or identity: Every person has the right to maintain his privacy. The privacy in terms of the name of the person, his preferences, attitude, and other identity features should not be commercialized for an organizational gain. E.g. When making a video of the hospital or making a news coverage attention should be given not to disclose the identity of any patient. The patients may be included in the coverage after obtaining the necessary consent. Celebrities have decreased privacy rules applicable.

    Invasion of privacy—public disclosure of embarrassing private facts: Public disclosure of unpleasant personal information is an act of privacy violation when the revelation is so absurd that it is outraged and not of public concern. Though the information may be truthful in this invasion of privacy violation, it is not right to publish it as the act has taken place in private and hence require consent to publish it. These kinds of privacy invasion are common during divorce and breakup of a relationship.

- **Unintentional torts:** These are accidents that cause injury to another person. They are mainly negligence and malpractice.
  - **Negligence:** It is the failure of a nurse or any health care professional to provide ordinary care to the patient that resulted in an injury. The standard type of negligence includes medication errors, burns caused by instruments, falls, infection due to lack of aseptic technique, a mistake in identification, failure to follow the orders of the physician, failure in monitoring, failure of documentation, etc.

    Breach of duty: Doing something that a typical professional would not do or not doing something that a professional is supposed to do.

    Injury: If the information on records says that the nurse failed to perform the assigned responsibility and duty in taking care of a patient and if it causes harm to the patient, then it is termed as the case of injury due to negligence. In these cases, the relation between the failure of duty of nurse and the harm caused to the patient must be established. For instance, if a nurse continues to forget to administer drugs as instructed, then the situation of the patient will worsen, or he will die, the nurse may be accused of negligence and injury.

    Performance failures: Insufficient nursing skills or devotion to duties can lead to a complaint of negligence against a nurse who hopelessly refuses to provide care as per the established standards of the organization. Such occurrences include, but are not restricted to, regular medication errors, non-compliance with protocol or instructions, and inappropriate use of machinery.

    Avoiding negligence: It is essential for nurses to document their actions very carefully and accurately at the time because sometimes negligence cases come about later when details are challenging to remember. Charting everything makes it easy to determine the details of each activity or nonactivity to suggest a logical reason for the particular action. This, in combination with a nurse who follows the proper scope of practice, will likely keep a nurse from being prosecuted for nursing negligence.
  - **Malpractice:** The Malpractice is a professional liability based on negligence such as professional misconduct, breach of duty, illegal or immoral conduct, etc. that cause harm to the client.

Medical malpractice is professional negligence by act or omission by a health care provider in which care provided deviates from accepted standards of practice in the medical community and causes injury or death to the patient. Standards and regulations for medical malpractice vary by country and jurisdiction within countries. Medical professionals are required to maintain professional liability insurance to offset the risk and costs of lawsuits based on medical malpractice.

Types of Nursing Malpractice

Nursing malpractice takes many forms, including:

- Medication errors; giving a patient the wrong medication or the wrong dose, or dispensing medication to the wrong patient.
- Failure to follow a physician's orders.
- Delaying patient care and failure to monitor a patient.
- Incorrectly performing a procedure, or trying to perform a procedure without training.
- Documentation error.
- Failure to get informed patient consent.

Measures to Reduce the Liability Among Nurses

- Committed and dedicated to the profession.
- Genuine behavior to the patients.
- Develop honest attitudes, trust, and open relationships.
- Never converse with the patient that cause misinterpretation.
- Do not make a medical diagnosis.
- Do not involve in physical and verbal abuse.
- Maintain confidentiality.

Legal Responsibilities of Nurse

- Responsibility of appointing and assigning

- Responsibility in quality control
- Responsibility for equipment
- Responsibility for observation and reporting
- Responsibility to protect public
- Responsibility for record-keeping and reporting
- Responsibility for death and dying

Roles and Functions of the Nurse Manager in Legal Issues

- Serves as a role model by providing nursing care that meets or exceeds accepted standards of care.
- Reports substandard nursing care to appropriate authorities.
- Fosters nurse-patient relationships that are respectful, caring, and honest, thus reducing the possibility of future lawsuits.
- Joint and actively supports professional organizations to strengthen the lobbying efforts of nurses in health care legislation.
- Practices nursing within the area of individual competence.
- Prioritizes patients' rights and welfare first in decision making.
- Delegates to subordinates wisely, looking at the managers' scope of practice and that of those they supervise.
- Provides educational and training opportunities for staff on legal issues affecting nursing practice.

CONCLUSION

Every nurse should act as per the legal guideline of practice. Every nurse must understand that one has to be always responsible for one's actions. Therefore the nurses must have the responsibility of seeing that no harm comes to their patients and also to themselves.

 REVIEW QUESTIONS

1. Define the profession. What are the criteria of a profession?
2. Explain the role and functions of a professional nurse.
3. Explain the characteristics and qualities of a Professional Nurse.
4. Briefly explain the current trends and issues in nursing.
5. Define ethics. What are the principles of ethics?
6. Briefly explain the code of ethics by different national and international bodies.
7. Explain the consumer protection act.
8. Define laws. Explain legal issues in nursing. What are the legal responsibilities of a nurse?
9. Explain fraud and torts.
10. Explain the role and functions of the nurse manager in legal issues.

Further Readings

1. Banerjee, Shyamal. Principles and Practice of Management. Oxford and IBM Publishing, New Delhi; 2000.
2. Basavanthappa BT. Nursing Administration. 2nd Edition: Jaypee Brothers Medical Publishers (P) Ltd., New Delhi; 2009.
3. Barrett, Jean. Ward Management and Teaching. Konark Publishers, Delhi; 1992.
4. Warren, Stevens, F. Management and Leadership in Nursing. McGraw – Hill Inc, New York; 1978.
5. Alexander et al. Nursing Service Administration. Mosby Publishers, US; 1962.
6. Goel SL. Healthcare System, and its Management, Health Organization and Structure, Vol. 1, Deep and Deep Publication, New Delhi; 2001.
7. Basavanthappa BT. Nursing Administration, 1st Edition: Jaypee Brothers Medical Publishers (P) Ltd., New Delhi; 2002.
8. Ranga Rao SP. Administration of Primary Health Centers in India, 1st Edition: Mittal Publications, New Delhi; 1993.
9. Lucita M. Nursing: Practice and Public Health Administration. Current Concepts and Trends. B. I. Churchill Living Stone Pvt. Ltd., New Delhi; 2002.
10. Sakharkar BM. Principles of Hospital Administration and Planning, 2nd Edition: Jaypee Brothers Medical Publishers (P) Ltd., New Delhi; 2009.
11. Patricia S Yoder-Wise. Leading and Managing in Nursing. 2nd Edition: Mosby Publication, US; 1999.
12. Bessie L Marquis, Carol J Huston. Leadership Roles and Management Functions in Nursing: Theory and Application. 5th Edition: Lippincott Williams and Wilkins, New York; 2006.
13. Linda Roussel. Management and Leadership for Nurse Administrators. 4th Edition: Jones and Bartlett Publication, USA; 2006.
14. Wehrich H, Koontz H. Management A Global Perspective. 11th Edition: Tata McGraw-Hill Publishing Company, Ltd., New Delhi; 2005.
15. Marquis BL, Huston CJ. Leadership and Management Functions in Nursing- Theory, and Application. 5th Edition: Lippincott Williams and Wilkins, Philadelphia; 2006.
16. Douglass LM. The Effective Nurse: Leader and Manager. 5th Edition: Mosby Publication, US; 1996.
17. Trained Nurses Association of India, Nursing Administration, and Management.
18. Samson Rebecca. Leadership and Management in Nursing Practice and Education 1st Edition: Jaypee Brothers Medical Publishers (P) Ltd., New Delhi; 2009.
19. Kunders GD. Designing for Total Quality in Health Care, Prism Book Pvt. Ltd., Bangalore; 2002.
20. Chandorkar AG. Hospital Administration and Planning. 2nd Edition: Paras Medical Publisher, New Delhi; 2009.
21. Joshi DC, Joshi Mamta. Hospital Administration. 1st Edition: Jaypee Brothers Medical Publishers (P) Ltd., New Delhi; 2009.
22. Kulkarni GR. Financial Management for Hospital Administration, Jaypee Brothers Medical Publishers (P) Ltd., New Delhi; 2009.

Unit

18

Professional Advancement

 Unit Outline

➡ Continuing Education
➡ Career Opportunities
➡ Trends in Nursing Education
➡ Nursing Research Participation in Research Activities
➡ Publications in Nursing: Journals and Newspapers

CONTINUING EDUCATION

Learning is a continuous process, and when it does not stop at any stage is known as continuing education. It is an opportunity given to a person after the formal completion of learning to extend the study/learning to a particular field.

Continuing education is an extension of opportunities for reading, studying, and training to any person adult following the completion of or withdrawal from full-time school and/or college programs. Continuing education is an educational activity, primarily designed to keep the registered nurses abreast of their particular field of interest and do not lead to any formal advanced standing in the profession.

These are continuous learning activities that have been inculcated to create nursing education and experience of the professional nurse for the improvement of practical nursing education, administration, and research or theory development in nursing education.

—**American Nurses Association (ANA)**

Need for Continuing Education

- The Kothari Commission on education suggested that all the educational institutions should arrange courses that will make people able to respond effectively to the challenge of current social changes.
- Continuing education in nursing will help to improve health care, economic, and educational opportunities.
- Continuing education is a vital part of education in the rural area as much of the people there have limited access to education due to geographical, technological, and financial constraints.
- It helps to improve the new healthy patterns of health care.
  - Due to the increasing trend towards specialization.
  - Due to legislation and its impact on the education of health personnel.

Objectives of Continuing Education

- To ensure that nurses remain up to date and competent in their professional practice.
- To sharpen professional competence.
- To make further career advancements in the nursing profession.
- It gives more credentials.
- Enables effective response to the challenges about the social changes.
- Improvization of opportunities in health care and education.
- Meet the trend of specialization and legislation regarding the education of health professionals.

Principles of Continuing Education

- It requires careful planning.

- It should be based on the needs of staff and service.
- It should seek into areas of interest of staff.
- It should be based on clear, achievable objectives.
- Evaluation criteria must be clear.

Adult Education (According to the Draft of National Education Policy 2019 Published on the Website of MHRD, Government of India)

Adult education in India is aimed to achieve 100% youth and adult literacy rates by 2030, and significantly expand adult and continuing education programs. The abilities to attain foundational literacy, obtain an education, and pursue a livelihood must be viewed as fundamental rights of every citizen. Quality access to adult education is, therefore, critical to ensure that all citizens can fulfill this right. Adult education provides mature learners with opportunities to increase their knowledge, develop new skills, gain essential qualifications and credentials, enhance career prospects, and thereby truly enrich their lives. At the level of the country, a fully literate and educated workforce will naturally lead to a massive increase in productivity and a more enlightened nation, with corresponding gains in health, justice and equality, and a much higher per capita income and GDP.

Over the past three decades, India has achieved substantial progress towards improving access to adult education and learning, through initiatives such as the National Literacy Mission (NLM) (1988–2009), Sakshar Bharat (2009–2017), Scheme of Support to Voluntary Agencies for Adult Education and Skill Development, and most recently the Padhna Likhna Abhiyaan (2018 onwards). These initiatives have aimed to provide opportunities for adults to obtain not only foundational literacy and numeracy, i.e., the ability to read, write, and perform basic arithmetic operations, but also other education such as financial, digital, electoral, environmental and legal literacy, and skill development. In particular, the overall literacy rate in India increased by 9% to 74% over the period 2001–2011.

However, according to data from the last census, India still had over 3.26 crore youth non-literates (15–24 years of age) and a total of 26.5 crore adult non-literates (15 years and above) - a number comparable to the entire population of students in the school and higher education sectors taken together – and representing one-third of the world's non-literate people.

Importance of Adult Education

Being a non-literate member of a community has innumerable disadvantages, including the inability to:

- Carry out basic financial transactions.
- Compare the quality/quantity of goods purchased against the price charged.
- Filling up of application forms for jobs, loans, and other services.

- Understanding public circulars and notifications.
- Comprehending the news and other information.
- Usage of Email for communication and establishing a business.
- Use of other technologies of the internet to improve one's own life and profession.
- Understand the signs, symbols, and safety measures displayed on the street, on medicines.
- Supporting the education of one's children.
- Recognize one's rights and responsibilities as a citizen of this country.
- Understand and enjoy the work of literature.
- Improve the stage of employment and maximize productivity.

Thus, literacy and fundamental education open up a whole fresh universe of individuals private, social, financial, and lifelong learning possibilities that allow individuals to make private and professional strides. Literacy and fundamental education are strong multipliers of strength at the stage of community and country, which significantly improve the achievement of all other developmental initiatives.

The global data of different aspects indicates that one nation's growth, which is expressed in terms of GDP, is directly related to the level of education of that particular country. Unfortunately, our previous attempts to universalize education over millennia have led in today's significant proportion of people who have never had the chance to join or finish school. Currently, it is understood that the only way to compensate for this absence of entry is through a solid and efficient adult education scheme.

Methods to Make Adult Education Effective and Widely Accessible

An excellent curriculum structure must be created for adult education, taking into account what would be most helpful for enriching mature learners. It should be based on their interest and level of learning. The curriculum framework must be sufficiently versatile to adapt to local requirements and must include the following aspects:

- The primary education such as language, numbers, necessary skills must be included.
- More concentration should be given to essential life skills such as computer and internet, health care concepts, competent parenthood, necessary financial skills, and so on.
- Focus can also be given to vocational skill development based on the aptitude of the learner.
- The education should be provided with the equivalency of learning compared to established norms.
- There should be a provision for continuing education according to the interest of the learner.

The education and teaching-learning methods in adults are different from children. Ideally, the framework of the

adult education curriculum would be developed by a new and well-supported component of the NCERT, dedicated to adult education. This will ensure the development of synergies based on the expertise of the field. It should include outstanding curricula for literacy, numeracy, primary education, vocational skills, and beyond.

Methods to Combine and Implement Adult and Continuing Education Programs

- Setting up continuing education centers in rural areas.
- Educating workers through their employers' trade unions and concerned agencies of government.
- Providing post-secondary education institutions.
- Providing books, libraries, and reading rooms.
- Using radio, television, and film as mass and group learning media.
- Creating learners' groups and organizations.
- Designing programs for distance learning.
- Organizing assistance in self-study.
- Organizing vocational training programs based on the needs and interests of learners.

Philosophy of Continuing Education

Effective nursing requires learning, that is life long. The scheduled curriculum of any graduate or postgraduate nursing program does not guarantee all the skills and knowledge required for everything. With the advancing of technology and expertise, the medicine and healthcare sector is changing constantly and improving. For evidence-based treatment and beneficial patient results, ways of sharing this data are essential, and it is possible only through continuing education. Continuing nursing education, although not a replacement for advanced higher education, can also impact the performance of treatment and the results of patients. This will also improve the knowledge and skills of the nurse. It is strongly believed that the members of the profession must provide opportunities, promote and motivate the nursing officers to pursue continuing education to update the knowledge and skill of their field.

Planning for Continuing Education

The keystone of continuing education is planning for it. The result of continuing education will not be effective, and it will be unfertile if the planning is not done properly. The outcome of thorough and comprehensive planning is a good Continuing Education Program.

The effectiveness of planning is required at all levels of planning from top to bottom, such as the central level to the peripheral level. The grass root planning enables the minimization of the gap and prevents duplication of efforts.

Planning Formula

- **What is to be done?** A clear comprehension of what is expected to be planned with regard to the concept of continuing education. The education scheme has to be planned according to the subdivisions. The subunits or parts of the job may be done based on the ideologies and resources, in terms of men, money, and material. Every planning requires implementation, and it requires the resources, and it should be at the disposal of the person who plans it.

- **Why is it necessary?** The division of subunits should be based on objectives. The comprehension of objectives helps to understand the outcome of the expected plan of action. It also helps in preventing untoward actions, unnecessary use of resources, and so on.

- **How is it to be done?** About the achievement of each objective, the planning has to be done to how effectively the set targets can be obtained with the utilization of minimum resources. The resources include all amenities and support required for the implementation of the desired action of plan.

- **Where is it to be done?** It is necessary to find the appropriate place and surrounding for implementing the plan of action. New technologies, advanced equipment, and scientific methods may be adopted for large scale implementation. It may be decided according to the demand for the service and availability of resources.

- **When is it to be done?** Finding a suitable time for the said purpose is crucial as it requires many adjustments and compromises. Every plan has to be fixed into a particular schedule, and it should be in such a way that maximum persons can attend it, minimum manpower is used for its implementation, and there is a possibility of economical use of other resources such as materials and money.

- **Who should do the job?** Selecting the appropriate person to do each task is very important. Primarily, we should find the requirement of skills and knowledge for giving continuing education. The selection and training of the desired person should be done. This will help in avoiding wastage of resources.

Steps in Planning Continuing Education

1. The aims and objectives of continuing education must be set up in concordance with the mission and purpose of the organization.
2. The specific objectives must be decided accordingly.
3. Plan and decide the course of action to achieve the set specific objectives.
4. Recognize the available resources.
5. Plan and prepare the budget for the program.
6. Perform periodic evaluation of the effectiveness.
7. Perform post evaluative planning and goal setting for updating the course of action.

Methods of Continuing Education

- The prime strategy for the conveyance of continuing education can incorporate conventional kinds of classrooms and laboratories.

- Secondly, most of the Continuing Education programs are offered through distance learning. The distance learning largely focuses on self-study, and use of learning materials such as CD-ROM, Computer-based learning, online lectures, etc. Additionally, the massive open online courses (MOOC) platforms such as www.swayam.gov.in provide an enormous opportunity for continuing education. Here the learners are exposed to numerous programs that they may undertake as per the choice and pace of time.

- The third approach to continuing education can be a combination of conventional methods and distance learning modules.

- A combination of conventional, distance, and mixed type methods may be adapted for the Continuing Education Program. Some of the other ways of continuing education include webinars, seminars, conferences, workshops, etc.

Duration: The duration of the Continuing Education Program purely depends on the type of programs offered and the approach of the learner. Many of the programs are an open type or self-paced while some are time-limited.

Advantages of Continuing Education in Nursing

- **Updated knowledge:** It is essential for a nurse or any other health care professional to keep their knowledge and skills updated. Many advancements happen in patient care, such as new technologies, medicines, machinery, procedures, and further illness. The health professional must be updated to meet the arising needs of patients.

- **Career opportunities:** The health care industry always looks for current and better professionals. The higher qualification gives better opportunities and many benefits, especially monetary benefits. The specialization in any particular stream provides a specific career opening.

- **Licensing:** The nurses must be licensed to practice. As time goes many entry-level programs in nursing may become obsolete. Hence it is essential for every nurse to update their qualification to remain in the health care industry. E.g. The General Nursing and Midwifery Course (GNM) has been stopped from 2019. Additionally, many State Nursing Council demand the points (CNE points) to renew their license, which indicates the overwhelming need for continuing education.

- **Employments benefits:** Continuing Nursing Education is mandatory for promotion and other advanced benefits (financial) in practice.

The staff development program is a planned activity in which the employee and employer get benefitted from the programs. In most of the organizations, staff development programs are encouraging phenomena because, in this technological era, everyone has to be competent in their profession to make sure their position in the field. Moreover, in the nursing profession, the trend in healthcare is advancing day by day, so the staff development programs become a compulsory one to make sure their job.

CAREER OPPORTUNITIES

Nursing is a form of art and science devoted to developing the physiological and psychological wellbeing of patients in the community. Nursing services are committed to excellence in practice, education, informatics, research, and administration. As like any other health care professional, a nurse is also responsible for the health promotion, illness prevention, diagnosis, and treatment of the ill, etc. in a health care organization. Traditionally the nurses have the career choices of nursing practice and nursing education while the career opportunities of the nurse are much wide and prosper, including many nonclinical functions. It also depends on his/her educational qualification.

Career development is the implementation of planned strategies for a nurse's care plan. This can be done through complete assessment, job analysis, education, training, job search, and acquisition and work experience. The essential qualities required to pursue a nursing career are:

- **Maturity:** Become a matured student with proficiency in health sciences.
- **Accountability:** Keep in mind always the legal, moral, and ethical accountability for your actions.
- **Decision making and loyalty:** Apply good decisions and be loyal to patients and the nursing profession.
- **Compassion:** Practice without errors compassionately by respecting all people regardless of age, race, social status, sexual orientation, or religious beliefs.
- **Continuing/In-service education:** Provide the highest degree of enthusiasm to keep up with current changes in nursing research in the profession, and value life long learning.
- **Creativity:** Acquire the expertise to handle disaster and crisis, as well as everyday challenges in a confident, efficient, and caring way.
- **Health:** Possess good health in all dimensions, a sense of humor, and a determination to succeed.

Career Options for Nursing Students

- **Case manager:** It is a nurse who takes care of a particular type of patient. It is a case centered or patient-centered approach. It improves the efficiency of care and is cost-effective. E.g. transplant nurses, geriatric nurses, etc.

- **Certified nurse midwife:** A nurse who is certified to care for pregnant women during all stages of labor, including family planning services/counseling.
- **Manager/administrator:** A nurse with administrative responsibility to manage the junior nurses. He/She coordinates, plans, and executes the duty of staff nurses and monitors their service and care delivery. Acts as overall in charge of nursing services in the unit.
- **Nurse anesthetist:** They have special qualifications such as a diploma in nurse anesthesia. They provide anesthetic care to clients before, during, and after surgery. He/she is responsible for patient recovery from anesthesia after the surgery.
- **Nurse educator:** The responsibilities include education, lesson planning, instructing, patient care, demonstration, evaluation, and helping to solve problems related to learning.
- **Staff nurse:** It is the basic entry-level for nurses in health care organizations. She/He can use her/his scientific knowledge and skills in meeting the care needs of the patient.
- **Flight nurse:** A nurse who provides care to the passengers of an airplane during their journey. He/She also aids in the transfer of ill from air to the surface.
- **Forensic nurse:** A nurse who takes care of patients who are under the law and related situation. It is a nursing service for legally bound patients such as victims of rape, abuse, sexual assault, and other criminal activities.
- **Military nursing:** The nurse who chooses to serve in military services such as Army, Navy, and Airforce. The services are extended to war zones too.
- **Nursing informatics:** It is an upcoming area of nursing practice where the digital activities related to patient care such as data analysis, system management, medical transcription, online medical and nursing services including provision of medical library services are included.
- **Research nurse:** It involves all aspects of working with pharmaceutical/medical/nursing research opportunity to be part of groundbreaking studies, projects.
- **Travel nurse:** These are temporary assignments of nursing services that are provided to critical patients for their transportation nationally and internationally. E.g. ambulance services.

Nursing Specialties

- **AIDS care nurse:** It is a dedicated area of the nursing profession to take care of AIDS patient who is sure to die. The holistic approach of nursing care along with assistance in meeting the daily needs is provided. A wide range of responsibilities, such as relationship building, decision making, self-care, and health education, is taken up.
- **Cardiac rehabilitation:** The nurse who provides rehabilitative care and services to patients affected

with cardiac disorders such as CAD, congenital heart diseases, cardiac arrest, valvular disorders, etc. The nurse provides health education regarding the prevention of the reoccurrence of many conditions and also educate the clients regarding lifestyle modifications and exercise methods to prevent aggravation of the condition.

- **Infection control nurse:** A specialized branch of nursing practice. An infection control nurse is a member of the Hospital Infection Control Committee. She/He is responsible for the screening, identification, controlling, and preventing the occurrence and spread of infection in a health care setting. The job profile includes routine nursing rounds, observing the violation of the HIC Protocol, preparing reports, updating guidelines of CDC in the health care setting, educating the professionals, patients, and family members, etc.

- **Occupational health nurse:** This role is also referred to as Industrial Nursing. It is the application of knowledge and practice of nursing sciences in an industry, especially for the workers/laborers. It is an amalgam of public health and nursing theory. The job profile includes monitoring and maintaining the health of workers, providing preventive and promotive services, provision of first aid, maintenance of health records of the workers, occupational safety, identifying the health hazards, etc.

- **School health nurse:** An area of professional practice in nursing that focuses on the health care services provided at schools. The School Health Nurse teaches the students/ children/adolescents the healthy lifestyle practices, treatment of minor ailments, and provide necessary first aid and health care services when needed. She also observes the students for the normal pattern of growth and development and helps the children for improving academic as well as non-academic performance. Provides necessary guidance and counseling services to the students. She is a team member for the overall development of children.

- According to the Nursing Education pattern in India, the MSc Nursing gives an opportunity to practice the nursing profession in five specialized fields such as Medical/ Surgical Nurse, Pediatric Nurse, OBG Nurse, Community Health Nurse, and Psychiatric Nurse.

TRENDS IN NURSING EDUCATION

- **ANM:** Auxiliary Nurse Midwife: It is a two-year diploma program.
- **GNM:** General Nursing and Midwifery is a 3-year diploma program in nursing.
- BSc Nursing is four years Bachelor's degree program.
- PB BSc Nursing is two years additional qualification program offered to candidates after passing GNM.
- MSc Nursing is a master's degree program offered to candidates after successful completion of BSc(N)/

PB BSc(N). Currently, MSc Nursing is offered in following specialties;

- Medical-Surgical Nursing
- Child Health Nursing
- Mental Health Nursing
- Obstetrical and Gynecological Nursing.
- Community Health Nursing
- Forensic Nursing

- MPhil: It is an additional qualification with a duration of 2 years.
- PhD.: It is an additional qualification with a duration of 3–5 years. Some of the famous Universities currently offering PhD programs in Nursing are given below:
  - National Consortium for PhD in Nursing: Collaboration of Indian Nursing Council, New Delhi with Rajiv Gandhi University of Health Sciences, Bangalore University of Delhi
  - All India Institute of Medical Sciences - [AIIMS]
  - Jawaharlal Institute Of Post Graduate Medical Education And Research [JIPMER], Pondicherry
  - Bharati Vidyapeeth Deemed University, Pune.
  - Dr D Y Patil University, Pune
  - Dr MGR Medical University, Chennai
  - SNDT University, Mumbai
  - Punjab University, Chandigarh
  - Baba Farid University of Health Sciences, Faridkot, Punjab
  - Manipal University
  - SRM University
  - Amity University
  - Mahatma Gandhi Mission Institute of Health Sciences, Mumbai.

- PG Diploma Course: Currently PG Diploma courses are offered in following specialties:
  - Post Basic Diploma in Neonatal Nursing
  - Post Basic Diploma in Neurology Nursing
  - Post Basic Diploma in Psychiatric Nursing
  - Post Basic Diploma in Cardio-Thoracic Nursing
  - Post Basic Diploma in Orthopedic and Rehabilitation Nursing
  - Post Basic Diploma in Operation Room Nursing
  - Post Basic Diploma in Critical Care Nursing
  - Post Basic Diploma in Emergency and Disaster Nursing
  - Post Basic Diploma in Forensic Nursing
  - Post Basic Diploma in Geriatric Nursing
  - Post Basic Diploma in Oncology Nursing
  - Post Basic Diploma in Pediatric Nursing

Since the Nightingale era of nursing practice, the nursing profession has undergone numerous changes, and many faces have been responsible for this noble cause. From time to time, nurses have tried to develop better methods to cater to the needs of the patient and his/her family. Certainly, the scientific knowledge and clinical expertise of nurses will result in better nursing care of patients. Being a dynamic profession, nursing accounts for several trends. Experimental and Evidence-based knowledge forms a strong base for the nursing profession as like any other profession, and this knowledge creates innovations in nursing. The simple meaning of the trend is development in a specific course. These trends are the cornerstones of the nursing profession for its dynamic nature.

Curriculum Innovations in Nursing Education

Nursing educational programs and its curricula are competencies put together, and it centers with respect to result and stresses student support and obligation regarding learning. Accrediting bodies reexamine the educational program of nursing education every once in a while. Here the Indian Nursing Council, the autonomous body under the Ministry of Health and Family Welfare, responsible for uniformity of nursing education across the country has made the following modifications in the curriculum of different nursing programs in recent years.

- Revised the syllabus of the Auxiliary Nursing and Midwifery (ANM) course in 2006–07.
- Revised the syllabus of General Nursing and Midwifery (GNM) in the year 2005–2006. The course duration was extended to 3.5 years (including six months of internship).
- Revised syllabus for BSc. Nursing and Post Basic BSc. Nursing was implemented from 2005–2006 in all Indian Universities. The syllabus revision was made in tune with the National Health Policy 2002.
- A national consortium for PhD in Nursing was constituted by Indian Nursing Council (INC) in collaboration with Rajiv Gandhi University of Health Sciences, Karnataka in the year 2005.

Technology and Nursing

- **Nursing informatics:** It empowers nurses to achieve good patient-centered health care. Nursing Informatics is defined as "science and practice (that) integrates nursing, its information, and knowledge, with the management of information and communication technologies to promote the health of people, families, and communities worldwide." (Amia.org, 2015).
- **Simulations in nursing education:** Simulation is the "process of designing a model of a real system and conducting experiments with this model for either understanding the behavior of the system and/or evaluating various strategies for the operation of the system" (Bradshaw and Lowenstein, 2009).
- **Technology and nursing education:** Technology influences nursing education to a greater extent, and it is an essential part of the teaching and learning process. The use of computers in patient management and student management has become common. The use of LCD projectors, smart classrooms, computer-based simulation models is now widely used by nursing teachers to educate nursing students. Students are familiar with the use of computers, smartphones, and different computer/mobile-based applications for learning and reading. The quality of nursing research increases with greater access to literature through the internet.
- **Animations and cinematic technology:** Animations are now widely used to enhance the learning experience. Video-assisted teachings with the help of animation for nursing procedures, physical examination, breath sounds, and stages of labor can be made clear and thorough with the help of this visual learning technologies.

Student Population

- **Male nurses:** Nursing was predominantly considered as a female profession, especially in India. In recent decades, the trend is changing, and the numbers of male nurses have increased significantly.
- **Changing the demography of nursing students:** In earlier days, nursing care was provided by nun sisters, and many of the major hospitals were established by missionaries. Present-day nursing students represent a diverse population in terms of gender, age, and socioeconomic status.

Clinical Teaching-learning Process

- **Evidence-based practice:** Evidence-Based Practice (EBP) is defined as "a problem-solving approach to clinical care that incorporates the conscientious use of current best evidence from well-designed studies, a clinician's expertise, and patient values and preferences" (Fineout-Overholt, Melnyk and Schultz, 2005). Incorporating research-based evidence in nursing education enhances evidence-based practice. The quality of nursing practices improves in a more significant form by using evidence-based practices (D'Souza et al., 2014).
- **Advanced clinical nursing education:** Apart from being care provider nurses perform independent roles like Nurse Specialist, Nurse-Midwifery Practitioner, and Nurse Anesthetist.
- **Supervised training by nurse educators:** According to INC standards, the teacher-student proportion is 1:10. This guarantees the robust supervision of each student. Nursing institutions endeavor toward improving the clinical learning process. Teacher-practitioner model and faculty-student practice clinic are two newer concepts in clinical training.
- **Clinical instruction–training the trainers:** Over some time, more emphasis is given on clinical nursing education. Nursing faculty are now taking up responsibility and accountability to patient care, and they acknowledge the fact that clinical exposure of the student does not mean

the clinical practice/learning. To overcome this dilemma faced by novice as well as experienced faculty, now clinical teaching is given more emphasis and training of all nursing faculty in the clinical area is getting mandatory in Indian settings.

Evaluation System

- In recent years, the nursing education and its evaluation is brought under regulatory bodies. All the diploma courses are evaluated by the respective state nursing council or examination boards constituted by the respective State Governments. All the programs that are at the graduate level and above are reviewed by the Universities that are recognized by the University Grant Commission (UGC). Additionally, innovative evaluation methods, such as Objective Structured Clinical Evaluation (OSCE), Rubrics, are now widely being used in nursing education.

Quality Assurance

- Quality assurance is an inevitable part of every education system, especially nursing education. The emerging trends and scope of nursing give a flourishing stage of growth, and thus, it also tempts for dilution of the quality. Quality is the process of monitoring and evaluating the efficiency of the system. Accrediting agencies like ISO has taken the initiative of accrediting colleges of nursing in India.

Knowledge Expansion

- The last decade had witnessed a significant expansion in nursing literature. The CINAHL, Cochrane, PubMed databases serve as an excellent treasure for nurses and nursing students. Research has become a substantial area in the curriculum. Action research and the use of qualitative methodologies in research are getting full acceptance now.

Modes of Education

- The recent trends in education such as distance education, E-learning/Online Education have brought about professional up-gradation in the form of continuing nursing education and different certification programs. Many universities in the world offer these courses. Few of them are IGNOU, Stanford, and so on. The programs that are offered through these modes are accelerated RN program, LPN to RN, and many other certifications and short term courses.

Trends are a kind of change that takes place and becomes vogue. The technological changes, changes in demographics, and health patterns have contributed to various trends in nursing education. The dynamic nature of nursing education strives to enhance the quality of care, the core of nursing.

NURSING RESEARCH PARTICIPATION IN RESEARCH ACTIVITIES

Research is a systematic investigation to discover facts or collect information. The research has brought about innumerable changes and avenues for humanity. It makes a new horizon of practice and understanding across the disciplines. It helps in improving the cognitive levels through clear understanding, clarifying the misconceptions, and sufficiently explains the daily problems of the people. It forms the base of knowledge development and contributes to the concept of learning.

As like any other field of science, the Medical/Nursing Science also evolved with a scientific base that is rooted in scientific research. But as a matter of fact, the field of research, especially nursing research, is less explored in India. The primary concern in this regard is the generation of interest in the participation of research activities that ultimately cause the growth of individual professionals and the profession they belong to.

In many cases, the primary concern in allowing the student's participation in research activities is lack of time and the extra burden of the curriculum. The allocation of additional time for research may mean the compromise of teaching hours. This can occur only through the restructuring of the curriculum that focuses or give more weight to the research-oriented activity. Alternatively, the summer/winter vacation of the institutions within the specified academic year may also be utilized for research activities. This method is already in practice in many western Universities.

Currently, in India, there are dedicated research guidelines for postgraduate programs, but it also needs to be equally emphasized in undergraduate programs.

Purposes of Research in Nursing

- **Identification and Description:** In this, the researcher observes and classifies the problem.
- **Exploration:** The researcher investigates the full nature of the phenomenon.
- **Explanation:** The goal of explanatory research is to understand the underpinnings of specific phenomena and to explain the systematic relationship among phenomena.
- **Prediction and Control:** The researcher makes predictions and control phenomena based on research findings even in the absence of complete understanding.

Importance of Nursing Research

- Nursing research is an essential component of the healthcare industry. It helps in the implementation of new advancements in the nursing care and treatment of clients that result in optimum health status.
- This focuses and ensures the creation, maintenance, and promotion of standardized care and treatment facilities for the patients.

- It focuses on the holistic care approach. The holistic approaches help in the enhancement of quality of care, and recipients are benefitted.
- The health field makes considerable advances every day. The nursing research helps in the implementation of the new changes in medical and nursing sciences in the form of new therapeutic modalities that speed up the healing process and thus improve better quality of life.

Activities for Participating in Research

- Identification of problem: All nurses irrespective of their hierarchical level should try to find out the current issues faced by the patients as well as the healthcare industry.
- Assist with ongoing research: Nurses can be part of different research bodies.
- Disseminating and implementing the research findings: All the nurse researchers should make it sure that their research is well published and communicated so that the appropriate meaning of research is met.

Preparation and Participation in Research Activities

Researchers are not born; they learn the development of skills.

Training: Any intellectual nurse can go into research because nurses have been trained to be sharp observers in designing studies, selecting appropriate techniques, analyzing data, reporting the findings, judging and making decisions and applying the conclusions of the work situation.

Other disciplines: Nurse educators must select the best that different disciplines have to offer and then apply these learning in practice. Doctoral studies by nurses provide varied information. Findings of the student doctorate can be published and shared with others who could benefit from them.

Student nurses: A beginner student in nursing is academically prepared to learn the basic methodology and technologies of research.

PUBLICATIONS IN NURSING: JOURNALS AND NEWSPAPERS

The word publication means the act of publishing, and it also means any writing of which copies are published either in print or on electronic media. It includes publications in journals, newspapers, television, books, and publishers, and so on. Although it is expected that those nurses who are undertaking research will write up their findings and submit them for publication, there are also many elements of clinical practice that are worthy of dissemination. Often, however, the nurses delivering these aspects of care do not realize that they too should be writing for publication. Many have, in the course

of their work, designed or implemented ideas for practice or undertaken innovations that benefit service users, staff, and communities or all of these. These are often not widely shared. If there is a substantial body of practice/knowledge which is not shared, it is subsequently lost to the nursing evidence base. It emphasizes the importance of having a valid and qualified publication in nursing.

Types of Journals/Publications

- **Open Access Journals:** They are also called as academic or scholarly journals. They are scholarly and are available to readers with or without financial or other barriers other than the availability of internet facilities. Some are free, and some are payment-based. It is aimed at improving the field of practice and educating fellow members of the profession. E.g. The Nursing Journal of India, American Journal of Nursing, Nursing and Care, and so on. They are peer-reviewed too.
- **Peer-Reviewed Journals:** It may be referred to scholarly. Here the articles are written by an author, and it is reviewed by many other experts in the field before proceeding to publication. It is done to ensure the quality of the publication. E.g. American Journal of Nursing, Journal of Nursing and Care, Journal of Professional Nursing, and so on. These journals are widely available in scientific databases such as PubMed and CINAHL.
- **Trade Journals:** It is the method of giving the practical issues and trends of a particular industry. E.g. Nursing Times
- **Current Affair magazines:** E.g. Readers Digest, The Week, Frontline, etc.
- **Newspapers: E.g.** The Times of India, The Hindu.
- **Books:** A written/printed work of any subject.

Guidelines for Writing in Journals and Newspapers

- The article should be original, should not have been published nor sent for publication anywhere else.
- The details of the article, such as the name of the author, the title of the writing, and the necessary affiliation of the author, are required.
- The article should be arranged logically, it should be concise, written in scientific language, and accuracy of spelling and grammar should be focused.
- The article should not be too long or too short. It is suggested that the article should contain approximately 3000 words. However, different journals and newspapers have their protocol.
- The submission by the student nurses must be forwarded through the guide of the study.

Uniform requirements for manuscripts submitted to biomedical journals and the method of writing and editing for biomedical publication are described by the International Committee of Medical Journal Editors.

Format of Research Abstract

- Introduction
- Statement of the problem with objectives
- Literature Review
- Methodology
- Results/Findings and Summary
- Discussion and Conclusion.

Barriers to Writing

- Time, or rather the lack of it, is one of the most frequently cited reasons for not writing but successful and productive writers are often busy people with no more time than anyone else
- Lack of confidence
- Inexperience
- Lack of support
- Not understanding the publishing process
- Fear of criticism or rejection

Overcoming Barriers to Writing

- Goal setting is an essential element. The workshops and the group discussions aim to support each individual to persevere with their writing.
- Participants can be helped to identify what has relevance for their area of practice and needs to be disseminated to others.
- They can be motivated to select a subject that has a unique angle. An area where there is a lack of information published already.
- An unforeseen advantage of the eclectic writing support groups is the conversations between workers of all bands and disciplines that foster creativity and an exceptional shared understanding.
- Ideas for co-writing articles are now starting to emerge from these discussions.

Common Publications in Nursing (National)

- The Nursing Journal of India, TNAI, New Delhi.
- Indian Journal of Nursing Studies, Choithram College of Nursing, Indore.
- Journal of Nursing Research Society of India, Bharti Vidyapeeth, Pune.
- Kerala Nursing Forum, KNF, Theophilus College of Nursing, Kottayam.
- The Indian Journal of Medical Research, IJMR, Indian Council of Medical Research, New Delhi.
- Nursing and Midwifery Research Journal, PGIMER, Chandigarh.
- International Journal of Nursing Education, Noida.
- Manipal Journal of Nursing and Health Sciences, Manipal College of Nursing, Manipal, Karnataka.
- Indian Journal of Psychiatric Nursing, ISPN, Bangalore.
- Nursing Trends.
- Indian Journal of Nursing studies.
- Asian Journal of Cardiovascular Nursing.
- Indian Journal of Holistic Nursing.
- Nightingale Times.
- Indian Journal of Public Health.
- Code of Ethics and professional conduct, INC, New Delhi.
- Teaching Material for quality assurance model, INC, New Delhi.

Common International Publications in Nursing

- OJIN: The Online Journal of Issues in Nursing, ANA.
- American Journal of Nursing; AJN: ANA.
- IJN: International Journal of Nursing, American Research Institute.
- International Nursing Review, ICN.
- IJNS: International Journal of Nursing Studies, Elsevier Publishers.
- BMC Nursing.
- American Journal of Critical Care.
- European Journal of Cancer Care.
- European Journal of Cardiovascular Nursing.
- European Journal of Oncology Nursing.

It might be helpful to motivate young nurses to write and publish more and more to develop the profession. Some issues are present in writing such as language, grammar, copyright, etc. which may be taken care of.

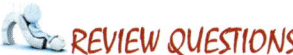
REVIEW QUESTIONS

1. Define continuing education. Explain its needs, objectives, and principles.
2. Explain the methods and advantages of continuing education.
3. Elaborate the career opportunities for nurses.
4. Explain the trends in nursing education.
5. Define nursing research. Explain the purpose and importance of nursing research.
6. Importance of publications in nursing. Explain the types of publications. What are the guidelines for writing in journals and publications?

Further Readings

1. Basavanthappa BT. Nursing Administration. 2nd Edition: Jaypee Brothers Medical Publishers (P) Ltd., New Delhi; 2009.
2. Goel SL. Healthcare System, and its Management, Health Organization and Structure, Vol. 1, Deep and Deep Publication, New Delhi; 2001.
3. Basavanthappa BT. Nursing Administration, 1st Edition: Jaypee Brothers Medical Publishers (P) Ltd., New Delhi; 2002.
4. Ranga Rao SP. Administration of Primary Health Centers in India, 1st Edition: Mittal Publications, New Delhi; 1993.
5. Lucita M. Nursing: Practice and Public Health Administration. Current Concepts and Trends. B. I. Churchill Living Stone Pvt. Ltd., New Delhi; 2002.
6. Sakharkar BM. Principles of Hospital Administration and Planning, 2nd Edition: Jaypee Brothers Medical Publishers (P) Ltd., New Delhi; 2009.
7. Patricia S Yoder-Wise. Leading and Managing in Nursing. 2nd Edition: Mosby Publication, US; 1999.
8. Bessie L. Marquis, Carol J. Huston. Leadership Roles and Management Functions in Nursing: Theory and Application. 5th Edition: Lippincott Williams and Wilkins, New York; 2006.
9. Linda Roussel. Management and Leadership for Nurse Administrators. 4th Edition: Jones and Bartlett Publication, USA; 2006.
10. Wehrich H, Koontz H. Management A Global Perspective. 11th Edition: Tata McGraw-Hill Publishing Company, Ltd., New Delhi; 2005.
11. Marquis BL, Huston CJ. Leadership and Management Functions in Nursing- Theory, and Application. 5th Edition: Lippincott Williams and Wilkins, Philadelphia; 2006.
12. Douglass LM. The Effective Nurse: Leader and Manager. 5th Edition: Mosby: Publication, US; 1996.
13. Trained Nurses Association of India, Nursing Administration, and Management.
14. Samson Rebecca. Leadership and Management in Nursing Practice and Education. 1st Edition: Jaypee Brothers Medical Publishers (P) Ltd., New Delhi; 2009.
15. Renjith, Vishnu, Renu G, George, Anice. Trends in Nursing Education. Indian Journal of Applied Research; (2015). pp. 496-498.

INDEX

Refer 'f' for figure and 't' for table, respectively.